Concepts of Fitness and Wellness

A COMPREHENSIVE LIFESTYLE APPROACH

Ninth Edition

Charles B. Corbin
Arizona State University

Gregory J. Welk
Iowa State University

William R. Corbin
Arizona State University

Karen A. Welk
Mary Greeley Medical Center, Ames, Iowa

Contributing author—Ancillary Resource Materials
Cara L. Sidman
University of North Carolina–Wilmington

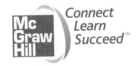
McGraw Hill

Connect
Learn
Succeed™

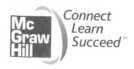

Published by McGraw-Hill, an imprint of The McGraw-Hill Companies, Inc., 1221 Avenue of the Americas, New York, NY 10020. Copyright © 2011, 2009, 2008, 2006, 2004, 2002, 2000, 1997, 1994 by The McGraw-Hill Companies, Inc. All rights reserved. No part of this publication may be reproduced or distributed in any form or by any means, or stored in a database or retrieval system, without the prior written consent of The McGraw-Hill Companies, Inc., including, but not limited to, in any network or other electronic storage or transmission, or broadcast for distance learning.

This book is printed on acid free paper.

1 2 3 4 5 6 7 8 9 0 DOW/DOW 9 8 7 6 5 4 3 2 1 0

ISBN: 978-0-07-352381-1
MHID: 0-07-352381-X

Vice President, Editorial: *Michael Ryan*
Publisher: *Beth Mejia*
Executive Editor: *Christopher Johnson*
Marketing Manager: *Caroline McGillen*
Market Development Manager: *Michael McKinney*
Developmental Editor: *Julia Akpan*
Director of Development: *Kathleen Engelberg*
Digital Project Manager: *Sora Kim*
Media Project Managers: *Thomas Brierly and David Blatty*
Production Editor: *Leslie Racanelli*
Manuscript Editor: *Judith Brown*
Cover Designer: *Allister Fein*
Interior Designer: *Lisa Buckley*
Photo Research: *Natalia Peschiera*
Cover Photo: *Martin Sundberg/Getty Images*
Production Supervisor: *Kara Kudronowicz*

This book was set in 10/12 Janson by Laserwords Private Limited, and printed on 45# New Era Matte by R.R. Donnelley & Sons.

The credits section for this book begins on page 525 and is considered an extension of the copyright page.

Library of Congress Cataloging-in-Publication Data

Concepts of fitness and wellness : a comprehensive lifestyle approach / Charles B. Corbin ... [et al.].— 9th ed.
    p. cm.
  ISBN 978-0-07-352381-1
  MHID 0-07-352381-X
  1. Physical fitness.   2. Exercise.   3. Health.   I. Corbin, Charles B.

                                                                    2010936011

Brief Contents

Section I

Lifestyles for Health, Wellness, and Fitness 1

1 Health, Wellness, Fitness, and Healthy Lifestyles: An Introduction 1
2 Self-Management and Self-Planning Skills for Health Behavior Change 21

Section II

An Introduction to Physical Activity 45

3 Preparing for Physical Activity 45
4 The Health Benefits of Physical Activity 65
5 How Much Physical Activity Is Enough? 85

Section III

The Physical Activity Pyramid 101

6 Moderate Physical Activity: A Lifestyle Approach 101
7 Cardiovascular Fitness 117
8 Vigorous Aerobics, Sports, and Recreational Activities 139
9 Muscle Fitness and Resistance Exercise 159
10 Flexibility 199

Section IV

Physical Activity: Special Considerations 223

11 Body Mechanics: Posture, Questionable Exercises, and Care of the Back and Neck 223
12 Performance Benefits of Physical Activity 263

Section V

Nutrition and Body Composition 287

13 Body Composition 287
14 Nutrition 321
15 Managing Diet and Activity for Healthy Body Fatness 345

Section VI

Stress Management 361

16 Stress and Health 361
17 Stress Management, Relaxation, and Time Management 375

Section VII

Avoiding Destructive Behaviors 397

18 The Use and Abuse of Tobacco 397
19 The Use and Abuse of Alcohol 409
20 The Use and Abuse of Other Drugs 425
21 Preventing Sexually Transmitted Infections 439

Section VIII

Making Informed Choices 453

22 Cancer, Diabetes, and Other Health Threats 453
23 Evaluating Fitness and Wellness Products: Becoming an Informed Consumer 473
24 Toward Optimal Health and Wellness: Planning for Healthy Lifestyle Change 491

Appendixes

A Metric Conversion Charts 513
B Canada's Food Guide to Healthy Eating 516
C Calorie, Fat, Saturated Fat, Cholesterol, and Sodium Content of Selected Fast-Food Items 518
D Calorie Guide to Common Foods 519
E Calories of Protein, Carbohydrates, and Fats in Foods 521

Selected References 523
Photo Credits 525
Index 527

Contents

Preface xi
Acknowledgments xvii

Section I

Lifestyles for Health, Wellness, and Fitness 1

1 Health, Wellness, Fitness, and Healthy Lifestyles: An Introduction 1
  National Health Goals 2
  Health and Wellness 2
  Physical Fitness 7
  Determinants of Lifelong Health, Wellness, and Fitness 9
  The HELP Philosophy 14
  Strategies for Action 15
  Web Resources 15
  Web Podcasts (Selected Websites) 16
  Suggested Readings 16
  Lab Resource Materials: The Healthy Lifestyle Questionnaire 17
  Lab 1A Wellness Self-Perceptions 19

2 Self-Management and Self-Planning Skills for Health Behavior Change 21
  Making Lifestyle Changes 22
  Factors That Promote Lifestyle Change 24
  Self-Management Skills 28
  Self-Planning for Healthy Lifestyles 29
  Strategies for Action 33
  Web Resources 35
  Suggested Readings 36
  Lab Resource Materials 37
  Lab 2A The Stage of Change Questionnaire 39
  Lab 2B The Self-Management Skills Questionnaire 41

Section II

An Introduction to Physical Activity 45

3 Preparing for Physical Activity 45
  Factors to Consider Prior to Physical Activity 46
  Factors to Consider during Daily Physical Activity 48
  Physical Activity in the Heat and Cold 50
  Physical Activity in Other Environments 53
  Soreness and Injury 54
  Attitudes about Physical Activity 54
  Strategies for Action 57
  Web Resources 57
  Suggested Readings 58
  Lab 3A Readiness for Physical Activity 59
  Lab 3B The Warm-Up and Cool-Down 61
  Lab 3C Physical Activity Attitude Questionnaire 63

4 The Health Benefits of Physical Activity 65
  Physical Activity and Hypokinetic Diseases 66
  Physical Activity and Cardiovascular Diseases 67
  Physical Activity and the Healthy Heart 68

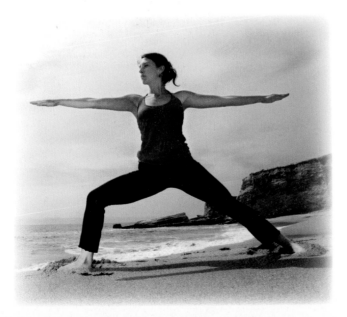

Physical Activity and Atherosclerosis 68

Physical Activity and Heart Attack 70

Physical Activity and Other Cardiovascular Diseases 71

Physical Activity and Other Hypokinetic Conditions 73

Physical Activity and Aging 77

Physical Activity, Health, and Wellness 78

Strategies for Action 81

Web Resources 82

Suggested Readings 82

Lab 4A Assessing Heart Disease Risk Factors 83

5 How Much Physical Activity Is Enough? 85

The Principles of Physical Activity 86

The FITT Formula 88

The Physical Activity Pyramid 89

Physical Activity Patterns 93

Physical Fitness Standards 94

Strategies for Action 95

Web Resources 95

Suggested Readings 96

Lab 5A Self-Assessment of Physical Activity 97

Lab 5B Estimating Your Fitness 99

Section III

The Physical Activity Pyramid 101

6 Moderate Physical Activity: A Lifestyle Approach 101

Adopting an Active Lifestyle 102

The Health Benefits of Moderate Physical Activity 105

How Much Moderate Physical Activity Is Enough? 106

Moderate Activity and the Environment 110

Strategies for Action 111

Web Resources 111

Suggested Readings 111

Lab 6A Setting Goals for Moderate Physical Activity and Self-Monitoring (Logging) Program 113

Lab 6B Evaluating Physical Activity Environments 115

7 Cardiovascular Fitness 117

Elements of Cardiovascular Fitness 118

Cardiovascular Fitness and Health Benefits 121

The FIT Formula for Cardiovascular Fitness 122

Threshold and Target Zones for Intensity of Activity to Build Cardiovascular Fitness 124

Guidelines for Heart Rate and Exercise Monitoring 127

Strategies for Action 129

Web Resources 130

Suggested Readings 130

Lab Resource Materials: Evaluating Cardiovascular Fitness 131

Lab 7A Counting Target Heart Rate and Ratings of Perceived Exertion 135

Lab 7B Evaluating Cardiovascular Fitness 137

8 Vigorous Aerobics, Sports, and Recreational Activities 139

Physical Activity Pyramid: Step 2 141

Vigorous Aerobic Activities 143

Vigorous Sport Activities 148

Vigorous Recreation Activities 151

Strategies for Action 151

Web Resources 152

Suggested Readings 152

Lab 8A The Physical Activity Adherence Questionnaire 153

Lab 8B Planning and Logging Participation in Vigorous Physical Activity 155

Lab 8C Combining Moderate and Vigorous Physical Activity 157

9 Muscle Fitness and Resistance Exercise 159

Factors Influencing Strength and Muscular Endurance 160

Health Benefits of Muscle Fitness and Resistance Exercise 162

Types of Progressive Resistance Exercise 163

Resistance Training Equipment 166

Progressive Resistance Exercise: How Much Is Enough? 167

Training Principles for PRE 169

Guidelines for Safe and Effective Resistance Training 173

Strategies for Action 175

Web Resources 175

Suggested Readings 177

Lab Resource Materials: Muscle Fitness Tests 187

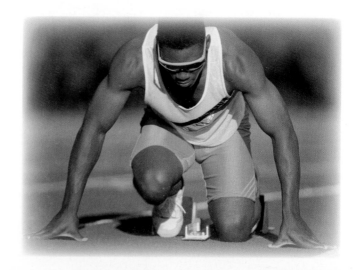

Lab 9A Evaluating Muscle Strength: 1RM and Grip Strength 191

Lab 9B Evaluating Muscular Endurance 193

Lab 9C Planning and Logging Muscle Fitness Exercises: Free Weights or Resistance Machines 195

Lab 9D Planning and Logging Muscle Fitness Exercises: Calisthenics or Core Exercises 197

10 Flexibility 199

Flexibility Fundamentals 200

Factors Influencing Flexibility 200

Health Benefits of Flexibility and Stretching 202

Performance Benefits of Flexibility and Stretching 203

Stretching Methods 204

How Much Stretch Is Enough? 206

Flexibility-Based Activities 209

Guidelines for Safe and Effective Stretching Exercise 210

Strategies for Action 211

Web Resources 211

Suggested Readings 211

Lab Resource Materials: Flexibility Tests 217

Lab 10A Evaluating Flexibility 219

Lab 10B Planning and Logging Stretching Exercises 221

Section IV

Physical Activity: Special Considerations 223

11 Body Mechanics: Posture, Questionable Exercises, and Care of the Back and Neck 223

Anatomy and Function of the Spine 224

Anatomy and Function of the Core Musculature 225

Causes and Consequences of Back and Neck Pain 226

Prevention of and Rehabilitation from Back and Neck Problems 229

Good Posture Is Important for Neck and Back Health 230

Good Body Mechanics Is Important for Neck and Back Health 233

Exercise Guidelines for Back Health 233

Strategies for Action 238

Web Resources 239

Suggested Readings 239

Lab Resource Materials: Healthy Back Tests 255

Lab 11A The Healthy Back Tests and Back/Neck Questionnaire 257

Lab 11B Evaluating Posture 259

Lab 11C Planning and Logging Exercises: Care of the Back and Neck 261

12 Performance Benefits of Physical Activity 263

High-Level Performance and Training Characteristics 264

Training for Endurance and Speed 266

Training for Strength and Muscular Endurance 268

Training for Power 269

Training for Balance and Flexibility 271

Training for High-Level Performance: Skill-Related Fitness and Skill 272

Guidelines for High-Performance Training 273

Performance Trends and Ergogenic Aids 275

Strategies for Action 277

Web Resources 277

Suggested Readings 277

Lab Resource Materials: Skill-Related Physical Fitness 279

Lab 12A Evaluating Skill-Related Physical Fitness 283

Lab 12B Identifying Symptoms of Overtraining 285

Section V

Nutrition and Body Composition 287

13 Body Composition 287

Understanding and Interpreting Body Composition Measures 288

Methods Used to Assess Body Composition 290

Health Risks Associated with Overfatness 292

Health Risks Associated with Excessively Low Body Fatness 294

The Origin of Fatness 295

The Relationship between Physical Activity and Body Composition 297

Strategies for Action 300

Web Resources 301

Suggested Readings 301

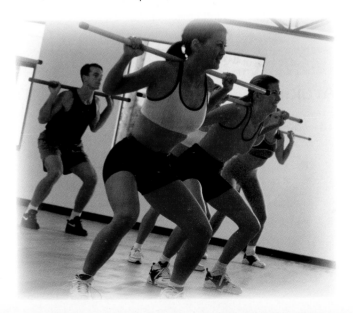

Lab Resource Materials: Evaluating Body Fat 303

Lab 13A Evaluating Body Composition: Skinfold Measures 311

Lab 13B Evaluating Body Composition: Height, Weight, and Circumference Measures 315

Lab 13C Determining Your Daily Energy Expenditure 317

14 Nutrition 321
Guidelines for Healthy Eating 322
Food Labels 325
Dietary Recommendations for Carbohydrates 327
Dietary Recommendations for Fat 329
Dietary Recommendations for Proteins 330
Dietary Recommendations for Vitamins 331
Dietary Recommendations for Minerals 333
Dietary Recommendations for Water and Other Fluids 334
Sound Eating Practices 335
Nutrition and Physical Performance 337
Strategies for Action 338
Web Resources 338
Suggested Readings 338
Lab 14A Nutrition Analysis 339
Lab 14B Selecting Nutritious Foods 343

15 Managing Diet and Activity for Healthy Body Fatness 345
Factors Influencing Weight and Fat Control 346
Guidelines for Losing Body Fat 349
Guidelines for Gaining Muscle Mass 354
Strategies for Action 355
Web Resources 355
Suggested Readings 356

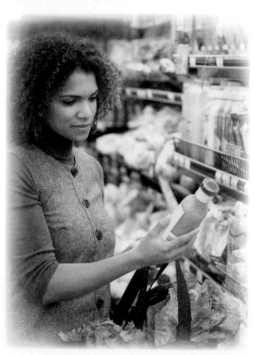

Lab 15A Selecting Strategies for Managing Eating 357

Lab 15B Evaluating Fast-Food Options 359

Section VI

Stress Management 361

16 Stress and Health 361
Sources of Stress 362
Reactions to Stress 365
Stress Responses and Health 366
Strategies for Action 370
Web Resources 370
Suggested Readings 370
Lab 16A Evaluating Your Stress Level 371
Lab 16B Evaluating Your Hardiness and Locus of Control 373

17 Stress Management, Relaxation, and Time Management 375
Physical Activity and Stress Management 376
Stress, Sleep, and Recreation 376
Time Management 378
Coping with Stress 380
Appraisal-Focused Coping Strategies (Cognitive Re-Appraisal) 382
Emotion-Focused Coping Strategies 382
Problem-Focused Coping Strategies 386
Social Support and Stress Management 386
Strategies for Action 387
Web Resources 388
Suggested Readings 388
Lab 17A Time Management 389
Lab 17B Evaluating Coping Strategies 391
Lab 17C Relaxation Exercises 393
Lab 17D Evaluating Levels of Social Support 395

Section VII

Avoiding Destructive Behaviors 397

18 The Use and Abuse of Tobacco 397
Tobacco and Nicotine 398
The Health and Economic Costs of Tobacco 398
The Facts about Tobacco Usage 401
Strategies for Action 405
Web Resources 406
Suggested Readings 406
Lab 18A Use and Abuse of Tobacco 407

19 The Use and Abuse of Alcohol 409
Alcohol and Alcoholic Beverages 410
Alcohol Consumption and Alcohol Abuse 411
Health and Behavioral Consequences of Alcohol Use 412
Risk Factors for Alcohol-Related Problems 415
Alcohol on Campus 416
Strategies for Action 418
Web Resources 419
Suggested Readings 420
Lab 19A Blood Alcohol Level 421
Lab 19B Perceptions about Alcohol Use 423

20 The Use and Abuse of Other Drugs 425
Classification of Illicit and Prescription Drugs 426
The Consequences of Drug Use 429
Use and Abuse of Drugs 430
Strategies for Action 435
Web Resources 436
Suggested Readings 436
Lab 20A Use and Abuse of Other Drugs 437

21 Preventing Sexually Transmitted Infections 439
General Facts 440
HIV/AIDS 441
Common Sexually Transmitted Infections 444
Strategies for Action 448
Web Resources 449
Suggested Readings 449
National AIDS and STI Hotlines 449
Lab 21A Sexually Transmitted Infection Risk Questionnaire 451

Section VIII

Making Informed Choices 453

22 Cancer, Diabetes, and Other Health Threats 453
Cancer 454

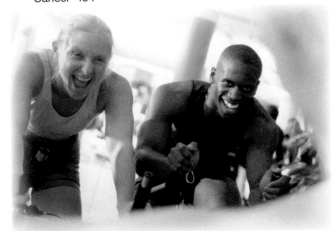

Diabetes 462
Other Health Threats 464
Strategies for Action 467
Web Resources 467
Suggested Readings 467
Lab 22A Determining Your Cancer Risk 469
Lab 22B Breast and Testicular Self-Exams 471

23 Evaluating Fitness and Wellness Products: Becoming an Informed Consumer 473
Quacks and Quackery 474
Physical Activity Quackery 475
Exercise Equipment 477
Health Clubs and Leaders 479
Body Composition 479
Nutrition 480
Other Consumer Information 483
Books, Magazines, and Articles 484
The Internet 484
Strategies for Action 486
Web Resources 486
Suggested Readings 486
Lab 23A Practicing Consumer Skills: Evaluating Products 487
Lab 23B Evaluating a Health/Wellness or Fitness Club 489

24 Toward Optimal Health and Wellness: Planning for Healthy Lifestyle Change 491
Strategies for Action 493
Web Resources 500
Suggested Readings 500
Lab 24A Assessing Factors That Influence Health, Wellness, and Fitness 501
Lab 24B Planning for Improved Health, Wellness, and Fitness 503
Lab 24C Planning Your Personal Physical Activity Program 505

Appendixes
A Metric Conversion Charts 513
B Canada's Food Guide to Healthy Eating 516
C Calorie, Fat, Saturated Fat, Cholesterol, and Sodium Content of Selected Fast-Food Items 518
D Calorie Guide to Common Foods 519
E Calories of Protein, Carbohydrates, and Fats in Foods 521

Selected References 523
Photo Credits 525
Index 527

Technology Updates

1:   Podcasts
2:   Health Apps for Smart Phones
3:   High-Tech Sneakers
4:   Blood Pressure Measurement
5:   Active Workstations
6:   Physical Activity Monitoring Devices
7:   Activity Monitoring
8:   Vigorously Active People
9:   High-Tech, Low-Tech Muscle Fitness
10: High-Tech, Low-Tech Stretching
11: New Training Aids
12: Performance Technology
13: WiFi Scale
14: Web Technology
15: Monitoring for Weight Control
16: Biochemical Markers of Stress
17: Gene-Based Therapies for Stress
18: Medical Advancements
19: Alcohol Consumption Detection
20: Epigenetic Effects of Cocaine
21: HIV-Resistant Gene
22: Genetic Testing
23: Health Websites
24: Online Second Opinions

In the News

1:   The Good News
2:   Public Opinion Polls
3:   National Physical Activity Plan
4:   The Surgeon General's Vision
5:   Participation in Physical Activity
6:   Public Health Promotions
7:   Heredity and CV Fitness
8:   Injuries—Issues and Solutions
9:   Worldwide Fitness Trends
10: Flexibility and Stretching Trends
11: New Gaming Technology
12: Risk of Injuries in Sports
13: Social Change to Reverse Obesity
14: New Dietary Guidelines
15: Social Media
16: PTSD
17: Stress Hormones
18: Family Smoking Prevention
19: Drinking Problems in the Military
20: Misuse of Prescription Drugs
21: Sexually Explicit Media
22: Mammograms
23: Vitamin Supplements
24: Healthiest Cities and States

Preface

A proven philosophy of health, wellness, and physical fitness

"Health is available to Everyone for a Lifetime, and it's Personal."

A proven approach to teaching fitness and wellness

Concise, accessible content modules highlighting key concepts and promoting active lifestyles.

Now with *Connect Fitness and Wellness*

A powerful online, interactive set of tools for learning and behavior change.

A winning combination!

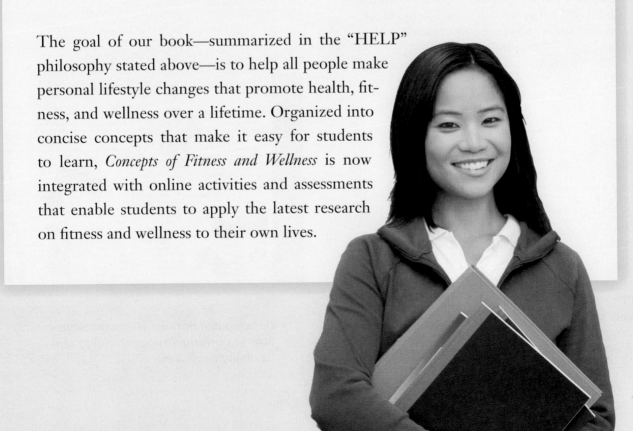

The goal of our book—summarized in the "HELP" philosophy stated above—is to help all people make personal lifestyle changes that promote health, fitness, and wellness over a lifetime. Organized into concise concepts that make it easy for students to learn, *Concepts of Fitness and Wellness* is now integrated with online activities and assessments that enable students to apply the latest research on fitness and wellness to their own lives.

A proven philosophy for teaching lifetime fitness and wellness . . . "Health is available to Everyone for a Lifetime, and it's Personal"

Strategies for Action

Screening for risks can help make activity safer. Athletes in competitive sports often undergo pre-participation physical examinations to screen for potential cardiac arrhythmias or conditions known to increase risks during exercise. Recreational athletes may not take the same precautions. The best advice is to get a physical prior to beginning serious training. This is especially critical if you have a family history of heart problems. Lab 3A will help you determine if you should consult a physician.

A proper warm-up and cool-down can make activity more effective and more enjoyable. A proper warm-up can prepare your body for activity and a gradual cool-down can improve recovery. Lab 3B provides a sample flexibility-based warm-up and cool-down routine that may be helpful. Determine what works best for your needs.

Assess your attitudes concerning physical activity. When preparing for physical activity, assessing your attitudes can be helpful. Active people generally have more positive attitudes than negative ones. This is referred to as a "positive balance of attitudes." The questionnaire in Lab 3C gives you the opportunity to assess your balance of attitudes. If you have a "negative balance" score, you can analyze your attitudes and

determine how you can change them to view activity more favorably.

(i) Be prepared for emergencies. To be prepared for physical activity, you also need to be prepared for emergencies. This concept has highlighted risks associated with different environmental conditions. Consider potential risks prior to exercise and be prepared (see position statements in Web Resources). Having a cell phone with you, when possible, during exercise is a good idea.

It is also important to know basic first aid and to be prepared to give CPR if needed. Guidelines from the American Heart Association have been revised to increase the likelihood that bystanders might give help. The most important change is a shift from mouth-to-mouth resuscitation to chest compressions. Proper certification is recommended, but the guidelines were revised to get more people to help, even when not certified (some CPR is better than no CPR). If a person is unresponsive, call for help and begin chest compressions immediately at a rate of 100–120 per minute. Continue compression until help arrives. Automatic defibrillators are now available in many public places, including fitness centers. Information on CPR guidelines and automatic defibrillators is available on the Web.

- **Strategies for Action boxes provide practical tips for applying that information to their own lives, and In the News boxes inform students about current topics, trends, reports, and research findings.**

Health is available to Everyone for a Lifetime, and it's **PERSONAL**

According to the National Institutes of Health, although genes don't necessarily cause diseases, they do influence our risk of developing diseases, such as cancer, heart disease, and addiction. The interaction between our genes and our environments and experiences is a complex one that is still being studied.

Would knowing you were genetically predisposed to a particular disease change the lifestyle decisions you make?

- **New HELP activities encourage students to reflect, think critically, and apply the HELP philosophy to their lives.**

- **New icons link text to additional online features and resources, interactive quizzes, video activities, and study aids.**

Table 9 Exercises for Core Strength

1. Crunch (Curl-Up)

This exercise develops the upper abdominal muscles. Lie on the floor with the knees bent and the arms extended or crossed with hands on shoulders or palms on ears. If desired, legs may rest on bench to increase difficulty. For less resistance, place hands at side of body (do not put hands behind neck). For more resistance, move hands higher. Curl up until shoulder blades leave floor; then roll down to the starting position. Repeat. Note: Twisting the trunk on the curl-up develops the oblique abdominals.

Rectus abdominis
Transversus abdominis
Internal oblique (cut)
External oblique (cut)

3. Crunch with Twist (on Bench)

This exercise strengthens the oblique abdominals and helps prevent or correct lumbar lordosis, abdominal ptosis, and backache. Lie on your back with your feet on a bench, knees bent at 90 degrees. Arms may be extended or on shoulders or hand on ears (the most difficult). Same as crunch except twist the upper trunk so the right shoulder is higher than the left. Reach toward the left knee with the right elbow. Hold. Return and repeat to the opposite side.

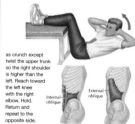

Internal oblique
External oblique

- **Detailed illustrations show students exactly how to perform strength training and flexibility exercises.**

A proven approach to fitness- and wellness-related behavior change

Connect Fitness and Wellness gives students the tools that will help them think critically about the lifestyle change process and develop behavior change strategies that are personal to them.

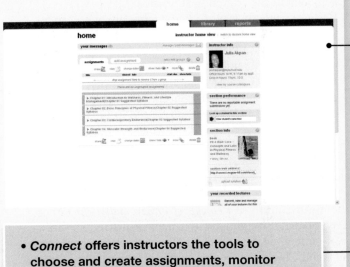

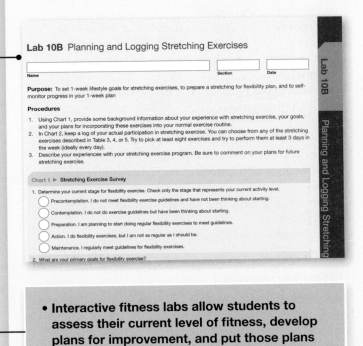

- *Connect* offers instructors the tools to choose and create assignments, monitor student progress, and manage their course more easily and efficiently.

- Interactive fitness labs allow students to assess their current level of fitness, develop plans for improvement, and put those plans into action.

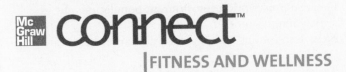

- New video clips and video activities engage students, make the concepts relevant, and motivate them to change.

McGraw Hill

connect™
| FITNESS AND WELLNESS

Other Key Features and Learning Aids

- Each concept contains a technology feature, which describes technological advances relating to health, wellness, and fitness lifestyles.
- It greatly pleased us that the Surgeon General's Report on Physical Activity and Health adopted our physical fitness definitions. Just as we have led the way in defining fitness, we include state-of-the-art definitions related to wellness and quality of life. These (and all other definitions) appear at the first point-of-use to make them easy to find.
- At the end of every concept, key websites are listed to provide students with additional online resources that supplement the content just learned.
- Because students want to know more about a particular topic, a list of readings is given at the end of each concept. Most suggested readings are readily available at bookstores or public libraries. Also included is the Web address (URL) for additional references related to topics covered in each concept. This expanded reference list will help those interested in further study of specific topics.

Highlights of the Ninth Edition

The ninth edition of *Concepts of Fitness and Wellness* has been updated throughout with current statistics, the latest developments in fitness and wellness, and timely topics and trends. Included are the new recommendations from the 2008 Physical Activity Guidelines for Americans, the new Physical Activity Pyramid, and new national health goals from Healthy People 2020. The features In the News, Technology Update, and Strategies for Action have been extensively revised and updated. A new feature based on the authors' HELP philosophy prompts students to develop their critical thinking and reflection skills and to apply concepts of fitness and wellness to their own lives. An updated design adds visual appeal, and new icons placed throughout the text guide students to additional online resources and features, videos and video activities, and study and review aids. A detailed summary of new and updated content follows:

1 Health, Wellness, Fitness, and Other Healthy Lifestyles—An Introduction

- Updated information about the Healthy People 2020 initiative
- Description of the Blueprint for America's Health recommendations
- Explanation of the Healthy Lifestyle Expectancy (HALE) index
- Changing public health emphasis on "determinants" of health
- Implications of aging population on public health

2 Self-Management and Self-Planning Skills for Health Behavior Change

- Review of public opinions on health
- Explanation of SMART goals
- Description of new technologies for fitness and health

3 Preparing for Physical Activity

- Explanation of new guidelines for exercise risk screening
- Updated facts about benefits of pre-exercise stretching and warm-up
- Information about the National Physical Activity Plan

4 Health Benefits of Physical Activity

- Updated health, obesity, and mortality statistics
- Updated references and documentation of links between activity and health
- Summaries of 2008 Physical Activity Guidelines for Americans
- Revised guidelines from the National Osteoporosis Foundation
- Description of the Exercise Is Medicine (EIM) initiative

5 How Much is Enough

- Review of various physical activity guidelines
- Description of new Physical Activity Pyramid
- Justification for new emphasis on vigorous physical activity
- Review of FITT principle and applications for exercise prescription
- Updated statistics on physical activity patterns

6 Lifestyle Physical Activity: Being Active in Diverse Environments

- Moderate activity in the Physical Activity Pyramid
- Benefits of moderate activity for health
- Tracking and monitoring moderate intensity activity
- Public health promotions for physical activity

7 Cardiovascular Fitness

- FIT guidelines for cardiovascular fitness
- Exercise prescription for different populations (fit vs unfit/young vs old)
- New descriptions and depictions of target heart rate calculations
- Review of impact of heredity and cardiovascular fitness

8 Active Aerobics, Sports, and Recreational Activities

- Vigorous activity in the Physical Activity Pyramid
- Distinctions between vigorous aerobic activities, sports and recreation
- Trends in participation in vigorous physical activity
- New statistics from the Sporting Goods Manufacturer Survey (SGMA)

9 Muscle Fitness and Resistance Exercises

- Resistance exercise in the Physical Activity Pyramid
- Review of resistance exercise recommendations in physical activity guidelines
- Review on core strength
- Comparison of high tech/low tech resistance exercises

10 Flexibility and Stretching Exercises

- Updated information on fundamentals and myths of flexibility
- Flexibility exercise in the Physical Activity Pyramid
- Updated recommendations for different stretching methods
- Descriptions and trends in pilates, yoga and tai-chi
- Comparison of high tech/low tech flexibility exercises

11 Body Mechanics: Posture, Questionable Exercises, and Care of the Back and Neck

- Updated back health and back pain statistics
- New descriptions and images of core musculature
- Examples of core exercise training equipment and routines
- Modified back health assessments

12 Performance Benefits of Physical Activity

- Importance of skills for performing physical activity
- New information on psychological ergogenics
- Updated statistics on injuries in sports
- Use of nanotechnology in sports

13 Body Composition

- Updated statistics on prevalence of overweight
- Health implications and burden of obesity
- Issues with eating disorders–binge eating
- Weight gain in college students

14 Nutrition

- MyPyramid and MyPyramid tracker
- New dietary guidelines
- Importance of food labels for dietary education
- Issues with "supplemental" food labels

15 Managing Diet and Activity for Healthy Body Fatness

- Public policies to curtail the obesity epidemic
- Emphasis on calorie control for weight loss and maintenance

- Changes in restaurant menus and labeling
- Updated information on commercial weight loss medications

16 Stress and Health

- New information linking stress with premature aging
- Individual variability in response and reaction to stress
- Links between stress and alcohol/drug abuse
- Role of locus of control in moderating stress

17 Stress Management, Relaxation, and Time Management

- Updated statistics on implications of stress method for stress management
- New information on fitness and mental health
- Importance of sleep on stress management
- Role of play and recreation for good mental health

18 The Use and Abuse of Tobacco

- Health implications and societal burden from smoking
- Trends in smoking and tobacco consumption (pipes/cigars/smokeless)
- New anti-smoking campaigns/advertisements
- New policies and effects on smoking

19 The Use and Abuse of Alcohol

- Definitions of alcohol consumption and abuse
- Binge drinking and alcohol on campuses
- Updates on DUI laws
- Treatment for alcoholism

20 The Use and Abuse of Drugs

- Updated statistics on patterns and trends in drug use in society
- New drugs and issues for prevention
- Biopsychosocial model of drug abuse
- Genetic and psychological determinants of drug use
- Issues with drugs on college campuses

21 Preventing Sexually Transmitted Infections

- New information on HIV screening, transmission, and treatment
- New strains of HIV and issues for prevention
- Explanations about vaccines for HPV–Pap screen
- Updated information on the health implications of lesser known STIs

22 Cancer, Diabetes, and Other Health Threats

- Updated health risks/causes of death
- New information on mammography and issues with screening
- New research on cancers (colo-rectal, prostate, cervical/uterine, skin)
- New cancer screening guidelines for prevention
- New updates on sunscreen ratings and safe exposure

23 Recognizing Quackery: Becoming an Informed Consumer

- New content on physical activity quackery
- New information on exercise equipment and selection
- Research, warnings and recalls on supplements
- Updates on vitamins and disease prevention

24 Toward Optimal Health and Wellness: Planning for Healthy Lifestyle Change

- Determinants of health and implications for prevention
- Issues with H1N1 and immunization policies
- Updates on healthy lifestyles
- New coverage on eye health and ear health
- New strategies for action for improving lifestyles

Teaching and Learning Tools

The *Concepts of Fitness and Wellness* **Online Learning Center** (www.mhhe.com/corbin9e) provides easy access to a variety of resources for instructors through a password protected website:

- PowerPoint presentations
- Course Integrator Guide
- Test Bank
- Concept outlines
- Videos and video activities
- Image Bank

Classroom Performance System (CPS) brings interactivity into the classroom or lecture hall with "clickers." Instructors can get immediate feedback on polling or quiz questions from the entire class using this system. Questions for each chapters are included on the *Fitness and Wellness* Online Learning Center.

Tegrity Campus is a service that captures audio and computer screen shots from your lectures, allowing students to review class material when studying or completing assignments. Lectures are captured in a searchable format so that students can replay any part of any class across an entire semester of class recordings. With classroom resources available all the time, students can study more efficiently and learn more successfully.

CourseSmart, the largest provider of eTextbooks, offers students the option of receiving *Concepts of Fitness and Wellness* as an eBook. At CourseSmart your students can take advantage of significant savings off the cost of a print textbook, reduce their impact on the environment, and gain access to powerful Web tools for learning. CourseSmart eTextbook can be viewed online or downloaded to a computer. The eTextbooks allow students to do full text searches, add highlighting and notes, and share notes with classmates. Visit www.CourseSmart.com to learn more and to try a sample chapter.

McGraw-Hill Create allows you to create a customized print book or eBook tailored to your course and syllabus. You can search through thousands of McGraw-Hill texts, rearrange chapters, combine material for other content sources, and include your own content or teaching notes. Create even allows you to personalized your book's appearance by selecting the cover and adding your name, school, and course information. To register and to get more information, go to http://create/mcgraw-hill.com.

Supplements for Students

Online Learning Center:

www.mhhe.com/corbin9e

The Online Learning Center provides students with access to course resources and study materials:

- **Features, resources, and study aids** linked to the text through icons
- **Video activities** highlight issues and trends in different areas of fitness and wellness with accompanying review questions
- **Application assignments** offer interactive Web-based activities for applying the information presented in each concept
- **Web resources** provide hyperlinks for the websites listed at the end of each concept
- **Interactive quizzes** offer practice questions to help in preparing for exams
- **Concept terms/flashcards** make learning key terms and definitions easy and fun
- **Concept outlines** include all the major "concepts" (heading topics) in the text to enhance the understanding and retention of content

Acknowledgments

Over the years we have been privileged to work with many different people who have helped the *Concepts* books to be successful. We listen to those who review our books and to our users, who provide comments by email, regular mail, phone, and personal conversations. Comments and critiques help us make our books better for students and instructors. The list of people who have helped us over the years is now nearly two pages long. But we feel that the pages that allow us to acknowledge those who have helped us are well worth it. At the risk of inadvertently failing to mention someone, we want to acknowledge the following people for their role in the development of this book.

First, we would like to acknowledge a few people who have made special contributions over the years. Linus Dowell, Carl Landiss, and Homer Tolson, all of Texas A & M University, were involved in the development of the first *Concepts* book in 1968.

Other pioneers were Jimmy Jones of Henderson State University, who started one of the first *Concepts* classes in 1970 and has led the way in teaching fitness in the years that have followed; Charles Erickson, who started a quality program at Missouri Western; and Al Lesiter, a leader in the East at Mercer Community College in New Jersey. David Laurie and Barbara Gench at Kansas State University, as well as others on that faculty, were instrumental in developing a prototype concepts program, which research has shown to be successful.

A special thanks is extended to Andy Herrick and Jim Whitehead, who have contributed to much of the development of various editions of the book, including excellent suggestions for change. Mark Ahn, Keri Chesney, Chris MacCrate, Guy Mullins, Stephen Hustedde, Greg Nigh, Doreen Mauro, Marc vanHorne, Ken Rudich, and Fred Huff, along with other current or former employees of the Applied Learning Technologies Institute and the University Technology Office, deserve special recognition.

We would like to thank the following reviewers (in alphabetical order), whose comments and suggestions were helpful in making this ninth edition as complete as possible: Dorothy Anthony, Keystone College; Michele Barton, Lakeland Community College; Julie Bisson, Plymouth State College; Amy Fletcher, University of Iowa-Iowa City; Joyce Grohman, Atlantic Cape Community College; Tom Jandovitz, Frederick Community College; Ronald Otterstetter, University of Akron; David Perron, Bryan College; Marc Postiglione, Union County College; Lorrie Radcliff, Moravian College; Erin Reilly, Auburn University–Montgomery; Debby Singleton, Western Carolina University; Jeffrey Walkuski, State University of NY–Cortland; Karen Wallace, Texas Wesleyan University

In addition, we want to acknowledge the following: Kelly Adam, Nena Amundson, James Angel, Vincent Angotti, Candi D. Ashley, Jeanne Ashley, Debra Atkinson, Kym Y. Atwood, Mark Bailey, Diane Bartholomew, Carl Beal, Debra A. Beal, Roger Bishop, Eugene B. Blackwell, Ann Bolton, Laura L. Borsdorf, Marika Botha, Amy Bowersock, David S. Brewster, Stanley Brown, Joseph W. Bubenas, Kenneth L. Cameron, Ronnie Carda, Bill Carr, Curt W. Cattau, Robert Clayton, Bridget Cobb, Ruth Cohoon, Sarah Collie, P. Greg Comfort, Cindy Ekstedt Connelly, Karen Cookson, Betsy Danner, J. Jesse DeMello, Linda Gazzillo Diaz, Terry Dibble, John Dippel, Caprice Dodson, Dennis Docheff, Joseph Donnelly, Paul Downing, J. Ellen Eason, Melvin Ezell Jr., Linda Farver, Bridget A. Finley, Pat Floyd, Diane Sanders Flickner, Judy Fox, James A. Gemar, Jeffrey T. Godin, Ragen Gwin, Janet Hamilton, Janelle Handlos, Earlene Hannah, Carole J. Hanson, James Harvey, John Hayes, Lisa Hibbard, Virginia L.Hicks, Robin Hoppenworth, David Horton, Amy Howton, Sister Janice Iverson, Wayne Jacobs, Tony Jadin, Martin W. Johnson, Arthur A. Jones, William B. Karper, Dawn Ketterman-Benner, Todd Kleinfelter, Larry E. Knuth, Jon Kolb, Craig Koppelman, Richard Krejci, William Kuehl, Mary Jeanne Kuhar, Garry Ladd, Ron Lawman, Jennifer L. H. Lechner, James E. Leone, Keri Lewis, Alexis Hayes Lowe, Paul Luebbers, James Marett, R. Cody McMurtry, Pat McSwegin, Betty McVaigh, John Merriman, Beverly F. Mitchell, Sandra

Morgan, Robert J. Mravetz, J. Dirk Nelson, Scott Owen, J. D. Parsley, Charles Pelitera, George Perkins, Judi Phillips, Wiley T. Piazza, Lindy S. Pickard, William Podoll, Karen (Pea) Poole, Robert Pugh, Kelly Quick, Harold L. Rainwater, Robert W. Rausch Jr., Larry Reagan, Matthew Rhea, Laura Richardson, Peter Rehor, Stan Rettew, Mary Rice, Amy P. Richardson, Sharon Rifkin, Rose Schmitz, Garth D. Schoffman, James J. Sheehan, Jan Sholes, Mary Slaughter, Robert L. Slevin, Laurel Smith, Dixie Stanforth, Robert Stokes, Jack Clayton Stovall, Dawn Strout, Frederick C. Surgent, Laura Switzer, Terry R. Tabor, Thomas E. Temples, McKinley Thomas, Paul H. Todd, Susan M. Todd, Don Torok, Maridy Troy, Kenneth R. Turley, Karen Watkins, Kenneth E. Weatherman, John R. Webster, James R. Whitehead, Louise Whitney, Marjorie Avery Willard, Patty Williams, Tillman (Chuck) Williams, Newton Wilkes, Bruce Wilson, Dennis Wilson, Ann Woodard, and Patricia A. Zezula.

We want to acknowledge others who have contributed, including Virginia Atkins, Charles Cicciarella, David Corbin, Ron Hager, Donna Landers, Susan Miller, Robert Pangrazi, Lynda Ransdell, Karen Ward, Darl Waterman, and Weimo Zhu. Among other important contributors are former graduate students who have contributed ideas, made corrections, and contributed in other untold ways to the success of these books. We wish to acknowledge Jeff Boone, Laura Borsdorf, Lisa Chase, Tom Cuddihy, Darren Dale, Bo Fernhall, Ken Fox, Connie Fye, Louie Garcia, Steve Feyrer-Melk, Sarah Keup, Guy LeMasurier, James McClain, Kirk Rose, Jack Rutherford, Cara Sidman, Scott Slava, Dave Thomas, Min Qui Wang, Jim Whitehead, Bridgette Wilde, and Ashley Woodcock. A very special thanks goes to Dave Corbin and Jodi Hickman LeMasurier. Dave and Jodi

spent many hours researching photos for this book. We especially appreciate the Spanish translation of vocabulary terms by Julio Morales from Lamar University, as well as the thorough and excellent proofreading by Bob Widen.

Over the years many people have helped with the development of ancillary materials. We wish to thank Jim Whitehead (also acknowledged earlier) for the suggestion to include the "Take a Stand" feature in the *Connect* materials that accompany the book. Thanks to Ron Hager and Lynda Ransdell for their early help with ancillary materials. We appreciate contributions by Michelle Immels and Marsha Todd for their assistance on the latest supplemental materials. A very special thanks goes to Contributing Author Cara L. Sidman for her continued help in creating presentations and other ancillary materials for the book.

The authors want to extend thanks to the video production crews at Arizona State University (especially Ken Rudich and Fred Huff), University of Missouri (special thanks to Steve Ball), and at East Carolina University, as well as Mark Ahn from Mark Ahn Creative Services, for the excellent work in producing video for the Online Learning Center and *Connect*.

Finally, we would like to thank all past editors (there have been many), including Michelle Turenne, Carlotta Seely, Gary O'Brien and Jill Eccher, and our current editors, Christopher Johnson, Julia D. Akpan, Kathleen Engelberg, and Leslie Racanelli—who used their expertise to make the *Concepts* books outstanding.

Charles B. Corbin
Gregory J. Welk
William R. Corbin
Karen A. Welk

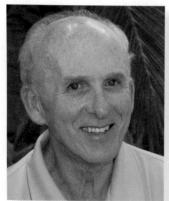
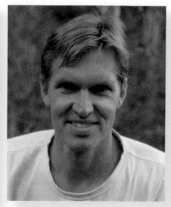
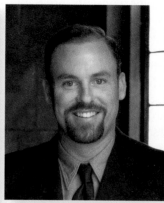
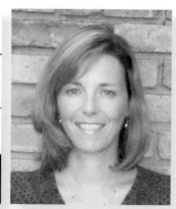

Dedication

The authors wish to dedicate this book in loving memory to Charles Samuel "Charlie" Corbin (April 22, 2004–July 18, 2004), son of Will and Suzi Corbin, grandson of Cathie and Chuck Corbin, and to Alyson Welk (April 30, 1995–June 2, 2003), daughter of Karen and Greg Welk. We also want to dedicate this new edition to our nonauthor wives, nonauthor children, and grandchildren, whose sacrifices have allowed us to spend the time necessary to create this book. Without their support, this book would not be possible. Thank you, Cathie Corbin, Suzi Corbin, Charles Corbin Jr., Dave Corbin, Katie Corbin, Julia Corbin, Molly Corbin, Colin Welk, Evan Welk, and Grant Welk.

Ruth Lindsey 1926–2005
In Memoriam:
A Tribute to Our Co-author and Friend

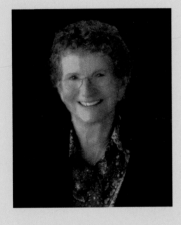

On May 29, 2005, we lost a great leader and an outstanding advocate for healthy lifestyles, physical activity, and physical education. Our long-time co-author and friend, Ruth Lindsey, will long be remembered for her contributions to the *Concepts* books and to our profession. Ruth was born in 1926 in Kingfisher, Oklahoma, and graduated from high school in Checotah. She earned her BS from Oklahoma State University in 1948, her MS from the University of Wisconsin in 1954, and her doctorate from Indiana University in 1965.

Ruth began her college teaching career at Oklahoma State University (OSU) in 1948, and after brief stints at Monticello College and DePauw University, she returned to OSU in 1956, where she advanced through the ranks to full professor. In 1976, she was a visiting professor at the University of Utah. Ruth then served as professor of physical education at California State University at Long Beach until her retirement in 1988. She continued to contribute as author of the *Concepts* books until 2003.

Ruth was a recognized scholar in physical education with special expertise in biomechanics, kinesiology, questionable exercises, nutrition, and physical activity for senior adults. She actively campaigned against consumer health fraud. She was the author of more than a dozen books, including *Body Mechanics, The Ultimate Fitness Book, Fitness for Life, Concepts of Physical Fitness,* and *Concepts of Fitness and Wellness.* Ruth published numerous papers and served as a leader in many professional organizations. She was an accomplished athlete who won the Oklahoma Women's Fencing Championship and was a low-handicap golfer.

Over the years, hundreds of thousands of students have read Ruth's writings. Her own students and her co-authors will remember her for her command of her subject matter, her attention to detail, the red ink on papers and manuscripts, her concern her profession, and her personal concern for each individual. Ruth was a woman of principle and character. She will long be remembered for her contributions to our field and for being the kind and caring person that she was. We will miss our co-author, our colleague, and our friend.

Navigating the Icons

Icons have been placed throughout the text to guide you in locating relevant information to the topic at hand. By accessing the Online Learning Center at www.mhhe.com/corbin9e, students and instructors can select the icon listed in the book from a clearly laid out concept-by-concept listing. These icons make it possible to quickly and easily access additional information, ranging from study aids to video activities.

The information icon guides you toward additional information, including expanded discussions of the In the News and Technology Updates boxes, specific feature information and Web resources.

The video icon indicates topics that have dynamic videos to supplement learning and classroom discussion.

The study aid icon guides you toward supplemental study and review materials, including concept outlines, key term definitions, Web resources, and suggested readings.

McGraw Hill connect™

With *Connect Fitness and Wellness*, you can gain access to a wealth of online content, including interactive fitness labs and self-assessments, a media-rich eBook, and additional video activities.

Health, Wellness, Fitness, and Healthy Lifestyles: An Introduction

Health Objectives for the Year 2020

- Attain high-quality, longer lives free of preventable disease, injury, and premature death.
- Achieve health equity, eliminate disparities, and improve the health of all groups.
- Create social and physical environments that promote good health for all.
- Promote quality of life, healthy development, and healthy behaviors across all stages of life.
- Increase public awareness and understanding of the determinants of health, disease, and disability.

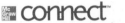

connect
|FITNESS AND WELLNESS   http://connect.mcgraw-hill.com

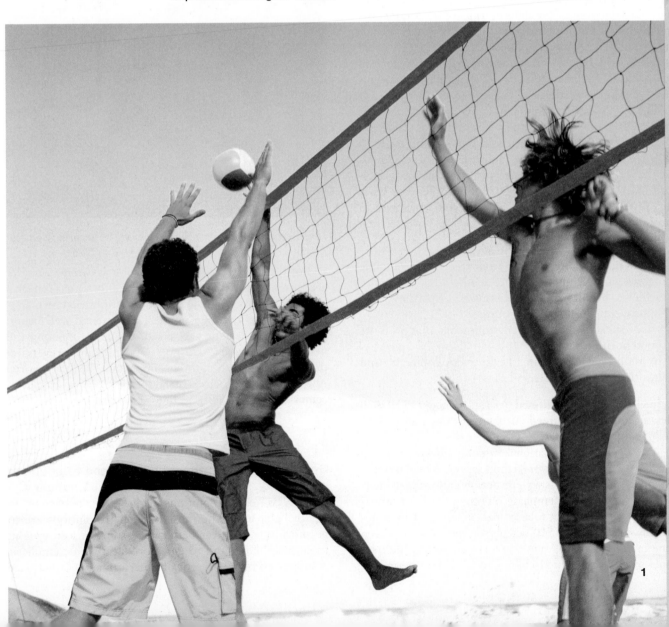

Good health, wellness, fitness, and healthy lifestyles are important for all people.

National Health Goals

(i) FEATURE 1 *Healthy People 2020* is a comprehensive set of health promotion and disease prevention objectives with the primary intent of improving the nation's **health.** The objectives, developed by experts from hundreds of national health organizations and published in 2010, provide benchmarks to determine progress over the period from 2010 to 2020. The objectives also serve as goals to motivate and guide people in making sound health decisions as well as to provide a focus for public health programs.

The broad vision of *Healthy People 2020* (abbreviated HP2020) is to create "a society in which all people live long, healthy lives." Two major missions are to identify health improvement priorities and to increase public awareness and understanding of the determinants of health, disease, and disability. The focus on determinants of health, including the social determinants of health, is consistent with that of the **World Health Organization**, which also focuses on health determinants. Concept 2 introduces the various health determinants featured throughout this book.

The HP2020 document highlights objectives related to 38 different health and wellness topics. Selected HP2020 objectives are featured on the opening pages of each concept in this book in abbreviated form. Details on the HP2020 objectives are provided at the associated Web link (visit the HP2020 site directly at www .healthypeople.gov/HP2020). The specific objectives in the HP2020 document contribute to four "overarching goals":

- attain high-quality, longer lives free of preventable disease, injury, and premature death;
- achieve health equity, eliminate disparities, and improve the health of all groups;
- create social and physical environments that promote good health for all; and
- promote quality of life, healthy development, and healthy behaviors across all stages of life.

As will be further outlined in this concept, HP2020 focuses not only on freedom from disease, but also on wellness (quality of life).

(i) FEATURE 2 A second national report (*Blueprint for a Healthier America*) emphasizes the need to focus future efforts on prevention and preparedness, including an increased emphasis on physical activity, nutrition, and prevention of tobacco use. The report indicates that an investment of $10 per person per year in proven community-based programs that focus on healthy lifestyles could save the country $16 billion over a 5-year period.

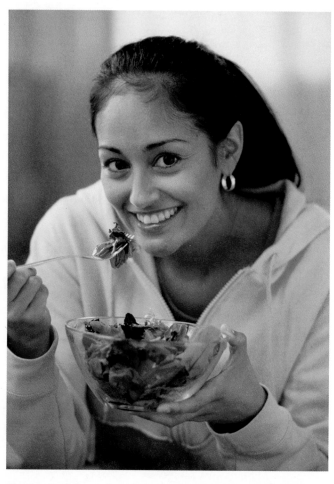

Healthy lifestyles are the principal contributor to health and wellness.

Both HP2020 and *Blueprint for a Healthier America* are consistent with the World Health Organization's focus on quality of life and its efforts to break down artificial divisions between physical and mental well-being. This book is designed to aid all people in meeting the new *Healthy People 2020* goals and meeting prevention priorities outlined in other important health reports. Accordingly, the focus is on adopting healthy lifestyles to achieve lifetime health, wellness, and fitness.

Health and Wellness

Good health is of primary importance to adults in our society. A Harris Poll indicates that most adults who make New Year's resolutions pledge to make changes in health behaviors. The most frequent resolutions are to be more active, to eat better, take steps to lose weight, to stop smoking, and to get more sleep. This emphasis is supported by 99 percent of American adults who place "being in good health" as a primary social value. Among those polled, none felt that good health was unimportant. Results of surveys in Canada and other Western nations show similar interests in good health.

Increasing the span of healthy life is a major health goal. Over the past century, the average life expectancy in the United States has increased by 60 percent. Although different reports yield slightly different results, it is clear that Americans now live longer than ever before. Results included in Figure 1 are from the most recent World Health Organization life expectancy report. These data were used because they provide statistics for other North American countries. In the most current *World Factbook*, Canada ranks 8th, the United States ranks 50th, and Mexico ranks 71st in life expectancy among countries of the world.

In addition to increasing total years of life, increasing years of "healthy life span" is a health goal. An index called HALE (Healthy Life Expectancy) is often used to determine the number of years of life for which a person has a good quality of life as opposed to having illness or impaired function. Figure 1 also shows healthy life expectancy and unhealthy years for the United States, Canada, and Mexico.

Eliminating health disparities is a major national health goal. Health varies greatly with ethnicity, income, gender, and age. For example, African Americans, Hispanics, and Native Americans have a shorter life expectancy than White non-Hispanics, and men have a shorter life expectancy than women. Health disparities also exist in quality of life. One method of assessing disparities in

quality of life is to compare the number of **healthy days** diverse groups experience each month. Minorities, including African Americans, Hispanics, and Native Americans, experience about 24 healthy days each month compared to 25 for White non-Hispanics. People with very low income typically have 22 healthy days per month, compared with 26 days for those with high income. Men have a higher number of healthy days than women. Healthy days decrease as we age, with young adults experiencing more healthy days each month than older adults. Over the past two decades, there has been a steady decline in healthy days for the average person, no doubt because of the increase in the number of older adults in our society.

The relatively higher number of unhealthy days for women is, at least in part, because they live longer and for this reason have more unhealthy years late in life. Number of healthy days takes its biggest drop after age 75. Disparities in healthy days by level of income may be due to environmental, social, or cultural factors as well as less access to preventive care. Both physical and mental health problems are the most frequent reasons for unhealthy days. Physical illness, pain, depression, anxiety, sleeplessness, and limitations in ability to function or perform enjoyable activities are the problems most frequently reported.

Health is more than freedom from illness and disease. Over 60 years ago, the World Health Organization defined health as more than freedom from illness, disease, and debilitating conditions. Prior to that time, you were considered to be "healthy" if you were not sick. HP2020 refers to quality of life in two of its four overarching goals, highlighting the importance of this wellness component of health.

Figure 2 illustrates the modern concept of health. This general state of being is characterized by freedom from disease and debilitating conditions (outer circle), as well as wellness (center circle).

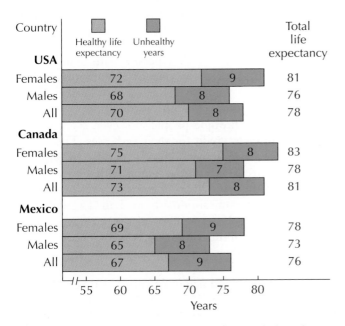

Figure 1 ▶ Healthy life expectancy for North America.
Sources: World Health Organization and National Center for Health Statistics.

Health Optimal well-being that contributes to one's quality of life. It is more than freedom from disease and illness, though freedom from disease is important to good health. Optimal health includes high-level mental, social, emotional, spiritual, and physical wellness within the limits of one's heredity and personal abilities.

World Health Organization (WHO) WHO is the United Nations' agency for health and has 193 member countries. Its principal goal is the attainment of the highest possible level of health for all people. WHO has been instrumental in making health policy and in implementing health programs worldwide since its inception in 1948.

Healthy Days A self-rating of the number of days (per week or month) a person considers himself or herself to be in good or better than good health.

HEALTH

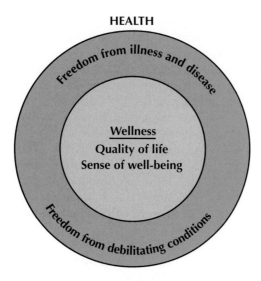

Figure 2 ▶ A model of optimal health, including wellness.

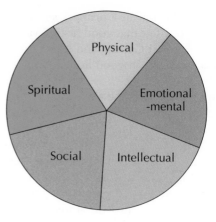

Figure 3 ▶ The dimensions of health and wellness.

Wellness is the positive component of optimal health. Death, disease, **illness,** and debilitating conditions are negative components that detract from optimal health. Death is the ultimate opposite of optimal health, and disease, illness, and debilitating conditions obviously detract from optimal health. **Wellness,** in contrast, is recognized as the positive component of optimal health. It is characterized by a sense of well-being reflected in optimal functioning, health-related **quality of life,** meaningful work, and a contribution to society. Wellness allows the expansion of a person's potential to live and work effectively and to make a significant contribution to society. HP2020 objectives use the term *health-related quality of life* to describe a general sense of happiness and satisfaction with life.

Health and wellness are personal. Every individual is unique—and health and wellness are influenced by each person's unique characteristics. Making comparisons to other people on specific characteristics may produce feelings of inadequacy that detract from one's profile of total health and wellness. Each of us has personal limitations and strengths. Focusing on strengths and learning to accommodate weaknesses are essential keys to optimal health and wellness.

Health and wellness are multidimensional. The dimensions of health and wellness include emotional-mental, intellectual, social, spiritual, and physical. Table 1 describes the various dimensions, and Figure 3 illustrates the importance of each one for optimal health and wellness. Some people include environmental and vocational dimensions in addition to the five shown in Figure 3. In this book, health and wellness are considered to be personal factors, so environmental and vocational wellness are not included in Tables 1 and 2. However, the environment (including the vocational environment)

is very important to overall personal wellness, and for this reason, environmental factors are prominent in the model of wellness described on page 10 and are featured throughout this book. The final concept in the book links environmental and vocational factors to the personal wellness dimensions described in Table 1.

Wellness reflects how one feels about life, as well as one's ability to function effectively. A positive total outlook on life is essential to each of the wellness dimensions. As illustrated in Table 2, a "well" person is satisfied in work, is spiritually fulfilled, enjoys leisure time, is physically fit, is socially involved, and has a positive emotional/mental outlook. He or she is happy and fulfilled.

The way one perceives each dimension of wellness affects one's total outlook. Researchers use the term *self–perceptions* to describe these feelings. Many researchers believe that self-perceptions about wellness are more important than actual circumstances or a person's actual state of being. For example, a person who has an important job may find less meaning and job satisfaction than another person with a much less important job. Apparently, one of the important factors for a person who has achieved high-level wellness and a positive outlook on life is the ability to reward himself or herself. Some people, however, seem unable to give themselves credit for their successes. The development of a system that allows a person to perceive the self positively is essential, along with the adoption of positive **lifestyles** that encourage improved self-perceptions. The questionnaire in Lab 1A will help you assess your self-perceptions of the various wellness dimensions. For optimal wellness, it is important to find positive feelings about each dimension.

Health and wellness are integrated states of being. The segmented pictures of health and wellness shown in Figure 3 and Tables 1 and 2 are used only to illustrate the multidimensional nature of health and wellness. In reality, health and wellness are integrated states of being

Table 1 ▶ Definitions of Health and Wellness Dimensions

Emotional/mental health—Freedom from emotional/mental illnesses, such as clinical depression, and possession of emotional wellness. The goals for the nation's health refer to mental rather than emotional health and wellness. In this book, mental health and wellness are considered to be the same as emotional health and wellness.

Emotional/mental wellness—The ability to cope with daily circumstances and to deal with personal feelings in a positive, optimistic, and constructive manner. A person with emotional wellness is generally characterized as happy instead of depressed.

Intellectual health—Freedom from illnesses that invade the brain and other systems that allow learning. A person with intellectual health also possesses intellectual wellness.

Intellectual wellness—The ability to learn and to use information to enhance the quality of daily living and optimal functioning. A person with intellectual wellness is generally characterized as informed instead of ignorant.

Physical health—Freedom from illnesses that affect the physiological systems of the body, such as the heart and the nervous system. A person with physical health possesses an adequate level of physical fitness and physical wellness.

Physical wellness—The ability to function effectively in meeting the demands of the day's work and to use free time effectively. Physical wellness includes good physical fitness and the possession of useful motor skills. A person with physical wellness is generally characterized as fit instead of unfit.

Social health—Freedom from illnesses or conditions that severely limit functioning in society, including antisocial pathologies.

Social wellness—The ability to interact with others successfully and to establish meaningful relationships that enhance the quality of life for all people involved in the interaction (including self). A person with social wellness is generally characterized as involved instead of lonely.

Spiritual health—The one component of health that is totally composed of the wellness dimension; it is synonymous with spiritual wellness.

Spiritual wellness—The ability to establish a values system and act on the system of beliefs, as well as to establish and carry out meaningful and constructive lifetime goals. Spiritual wellness is often based on a belief in a force greater than the individual that helps her or him contribute to an improved quality of life for all people. A person with spiritual wellness is generally characterized as fulfilled instead of unfulfilled.

that can best be depicted as threads woven together to produce a larger, integrated fabric. Each dimension relates to each of the others and overlaps all the others. The overlap is so frequent and so great that the specific contribution of each thread is almost indistinguishable when looking at the total (Figure 4). The total is clearly greater than the sum of the parts.

Table 2 ▶ The Dimensions of Wellness

Wellness Dimension	Negative — — — — — Positive
Emotional/mental	Depressed — — — — — — Happy
Intellectual	Ignorant — — — — — — — Informed
Physical	Unfit — — — — — — — — — Fit
Social	Lonely — — — — — — — Involved
Spiritual	Unfulfilled — — — — — — Fulfilled
Total outlook	Negative — — — — — — Positive

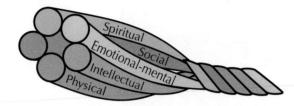

Figure 4 ▶ The integration of wellness dimensions.

It is possible to possess health and wellness while being ill or possessing a debilitating condition. Many illnesses are curable and may have only a temporary effect on health. Others, such as Type I diabetes, are not curable but can be managed with proper eating, physical activity, and sound medical treatment. Those with manageable conditions may, however, be at risk for other health problems. For example, unmanaged diabetes is associated with a high risk for heart disease and other health problems.

Illness The ill feeling and/or symptoms associated with a disease or circumstances that upset homeostasis.

Wellness The integration of many different components (social, emotional/mental, spiritual, and physical) that expand one's potential to live (quality of life) and work effectively and to make a significant contribution to society. Wellness reflects how one feels (a sense of well-being) about life, as well as one's ability to function effectively. Wellness, as opposed to illness (a negative), is sometimes described as the positive component of good health.

Quality of Life A term used to describe wellness. An individual with quality of life can enjoyably do the activities of life with little or no limitation and can function independently. Individual quality of life requires a pleasant and supportive community.

Lifestyles Patterns of behavior or ways an individual typically lives.

Muscular Endurance

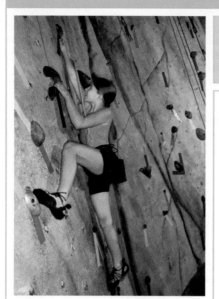

The ability of the muscles to exert themselves repeatedly. A fit person can repeat movements for a long period without undue fatigue.

Body Composition

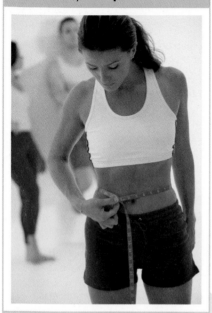

The relative percentage of muscle, fat, bone, and other tissues that make up the body. A fit person has a relatively low, but not too low, percentage of body fat (body fatness).

Cardiovascular Fitness

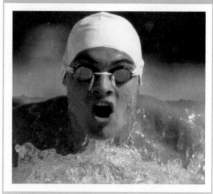

The ability of the heart, blood vessels, blood, and respiratory system to supply nutrients and oxygen to the muscles and the ability of the muscles to utilize fuel to allow sustained exercise. A fit person can persist in physical activity for relatively long periods without undue stress.

Dimensions of Health-Related Physical Fitness

Strength

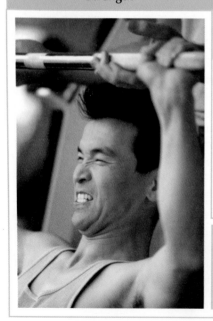

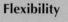

The ability of the muscles to exert an external force or to lift a heavy weight. A fit person can do work or play that involves exerting force, such as lifting or controlling one's own body weight.

Flexibility

The range of motion available in a joint. It is affected by muscle length, joint structure, and other factors. A fit person can move the body joints through a full range of motion in work and in play.

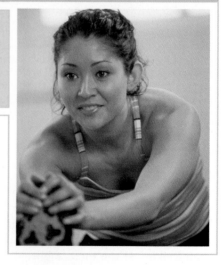

Figure 5 ▶ Components of health-related physical fitness.

Debilitating conditions, such as the loss of a limb or loss of function in a body part, can contribute to a lower level of functioning or an increased risk for illness and thus to poor health. On the other hand, such conditions need not limit wellness. A person with a debilitating condition who has a positive outlook on life may have better overall health than a person with a poor outlook on life but no debilitating condition.

Just as wellness is possible among those with illness and disability, evidence is accumulating that people with a positive outlook are better able to resist the progress of disease and illness than are those with a negative outlook. Thinking positive thoughts has been associated with enhanced results from various medical treatments and surgical procedures.

***Wellness* is a useful term that may be used by the uninformed as well as experts.** Unfortunately, some individuals and groups have tried to identify wellness with products and services that promise benefits that cannot be documented. Because well-being is a subjective feeling, unscrupulous people can easily make claims of improved wellness for their product or service without facts to back them up.

Holistic health is a term that is similarly abused. Consider that optimal health includes many areas; thus, the term *holistic* (total) is appropriate. In fact, the word *health* originates from a root word meaning "wholeness." Unfortunately, questionable health practices are sometimes promoted under the guise of holistic health. Care should be used when considering services and products that make claims of wellness and/or holistic health to be sure that they are legitimate.

Physical Fitness

Physical fitness is a multidimensional state of being. **Physical fitness** is the body's ability to function efficiently and effectively. It is a state of being that consists of at least five health-related and six skill-related physical fitness components, each of which contributes to total quality of life. Physical fitness is associated with a person's ability to work effectively, enjoy leisure time, be healthy, resist **hypokinetic diseases or conditions,** and meet emergency situations. It is related to, but different from, health and wellness. Although the development of physical fitness is the result of many things, optimal physical fitness is not possible without regular physical activity.

The health-related components of physical fitness are directly associated with good health. The five components of health-related physical fitness are body composition, cardiovascular fitness, flexibility, muscular endurance, and strength (see Figure 5). Each health–related fitness characteristic has a direct relationship to good health and reduced risk for hypokinetic disease. It is for this reason that the five health-related physical fitness components are emphasized in this book.

Possessing a moderate amount of each component of health-related fitness is essential to disease prevention and health promotion, but it is not essential to have exceptionally high levels of fitness to achieve health benefits. High levels of health-related fitness relate more to performance than to health benefits. For example, moderate amounts of strength are necessary to prevent back and posture problems, whereas high levels of strength contribute most to improved performance in activities such as football and jobs involving heavy lifting.

The skill-related components of physical fitness are associated more with performance than with good health. The components of skill-related physical fitness are agility, balance, coordination, power, reaction time, and speed (see Figure 6). They are called skill-related because people who possess them find it easy to achieve high levels of performance in motor skills, such as those required in sports and in specific types of jobs. Power is sometimes referred to as a combined component of fitness, since it requires both strength (a health-related component) and speed (a skill-related component). Because most experts consider power to be associated more with performance than with good health, it is classified as a skill-related component of fitness in this book. Skill-related fitness is sometimes called sports fitness or motor fitness.

Physical Fitness The body's ability to function efficiently and effectively. It consists of health-related physical fitness and skill-related physical fitness, which have at least 11 components, each of which contributes to total quality of life. Physical fitness also includes metabolic fitness and bone integrity. Physical fitness is associated with a person's ability to work effectively, enjoy leisure time, be healthy, resist hypokinetic diseases, and meet emergency situations. It is related to, but different from, health, wellness, and the psychological, sociological, emotional/mental, and spiritual components of fitness. Although the development of physical fitness is the result of many things, optimal physical fitness is not possible without regular exercise.

Hypokinetic Diseases or Conditions *Hypo-* means "under" or "too little," and *-kinetic* means "movement" or "activity." Thus, *hypokinetic* means "too little activity." A hypokinetic disease or condition is one associated with lack of physical activity or too little regular exercise. Examples include heart disease, low back pain, adult-onset diabetes, and obesity.

Power

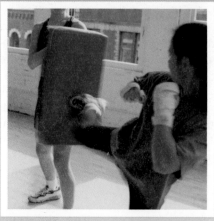

The ability to transfer energy into force at a fast rate. Throwing the discus and putting the shot are activities that require considerable power.

Agility

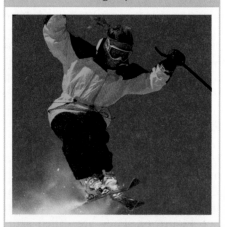

The ability to rapidly and accurately change the direction of the movement of the entire body in space. Skiing and wrestling are examples of activities that require exceptional agility.

Reaction Time

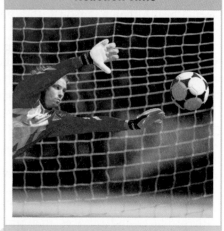

The time elapsed between stimulation and the beginning of reaction to that stimulation. Driving a racing car and starting a sprint race require good reaction time.

Dimensions of Skill-Related Physical Fitness

Coordination

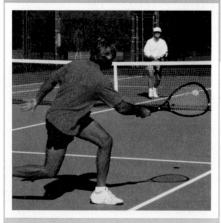

The ability to use the senses with the body parts to perform motor tasks smoothly and accurately. Juggling, hitting a tennis ball, and kicking a ball are examples of activities requiring good coordination.

Speed

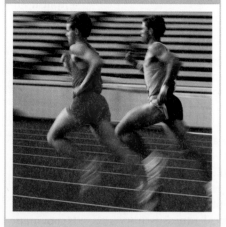

The ability to perform a movement in a short period of time. Sprinters and wide receivers in football need good foot and leg speed.

Balance

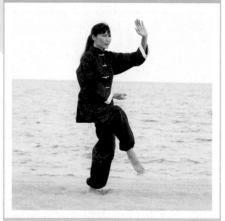

The maintenance of equilibrium while stationary or while moving. Water skiing, performing on the balance beam, and working as a riveter on a high-rise building are activities that require exceptional balance.

Figure 6 ▶ Components of skill-related physical fitness.

There is little doubt that other abilities could be classified as skill-related fitness components. Also, each part of skill-related fitness is multidimensional. For example, coordination could be hand-eye coordination, such as batting a ball; foot-eye coordination, such as kicking a ball; or any of many other possibilities. The six parts of skill-related fitness identified here are those commonly associated with successful sports and work performance. Each could be measured in ways other than those presented in this book. Measurements are provided to help you understand the nature of total physical fitness and to help you make important decisions about lifetime physical activity.

Metabolic fitness is a nonperformance component of total fitness. Physical activity can provide health benefits that are independent of changes in traditional health-related fitness measures. Physical activity promotes good **metabolic fitness,** a state associated with reduced risk for many chronic diseases. People with a cluster of low metabolic fitness characteristics are said to have metabolic syndrome (also known as Syndrome X). Metabolic syndrome is discussed in more detail in Concept 4.

Bone integrity is often considered a nonperformance measure of fitness. Traditional definitions do not include **bone integrity** as a part of physical fitness, but some experts feel they should. Like metabolic fitness, bone integrity cannot be assessed with performance measures the way most health-related fitness parts can. Regardless of whether bone integrity is considered a part of fitness or a component of health, strong, healthy bones are important to optimal health and are associated with regular physical activity and sound diet.

The many components of physical fitness are specific but are also interrelated. Physical fitness is a combination of several aspects, rather than a single characteristic. A fit person possesses at least adequate levels of each of the health-related, skill-related, and metabolic fitness components. Some relationships exist among various fitness characteristics, but each component of physical fitness is separate and different from the others. For example, people who possess exceptional strength may not have good cardiovascular fitness, and those who have good coordination do not necessarily possess good flexibility.

Good physical fitness is important, but it is not the same as physical health and wellness. Good physical fitness contributes directly to the physical component of good health and wellness and indirectly to the other four components. Good fitness has been shown to be associated with reduced risk for chronic diseases, such

as heart disease, and has been shown to reduce the consequences of many debilitating conditions. In addition, good fitness contributes to wellness by helping us look our best, feel good, and enjoy life. Other physical factors can also influence health and wellness. For example, having good physical skills enhances quality of life by allowing us to participate in enjoyable activities, such as tennis, golf, and bowling. Although fitness can assist us in performing these activities, regular practice is also necessary. Another example is the ability to fight off viral and bacterial infections. Although fitness can promote a strong immune system, other physical factors can influence our susceptibility to these and other conditions.

Determinants of Lifelong Health, Wellness, and Fitness

 Many factors are important in developing lifetime health, wellness, and fitness, and some are more in your control than others. Figure 7 provides a model for describing many of the factors that contribute to health, wellness, and fitness. Central to the model are health, wellness, and fitness because these are the states of being (shaded in green and yellow) that each of us wants to achieve. Around the periphery are the factors that influence these states of being. Those shaded in dark blue are the factors over which you have the least control (heredity, age, and disability). Those shaded in light blue (health care and environmental factors) are factors over which you have some control but less than the factors shaded in red. Those shaded in light red are the factors over which you have greater control (healthy lifestyles and personal actions/interactions, cognitions and emotions).

Heredity (human biology) is a factor over which we have little control. Experts estimate that human biology, or heredity, accounts for 16 percent of all health problems, including early death. Heredity influences each part of health-related physical fitness, including our tendencies to build muscle and to deposit body fat.

Metabolic Fitness A positive state of the physiological systems commonly associated with reduced risk for chronic diseases such as diabetes and heart disease. Metabolic fitness is evidenced by healthy blood fat (lipid) profiles, healthy blood pressure, healthy blood sugar and insulin levels, and other nonperformance measures.

Bone Integrity Soundness of the bones is associated with high density and absence of symptoms of deterioration.

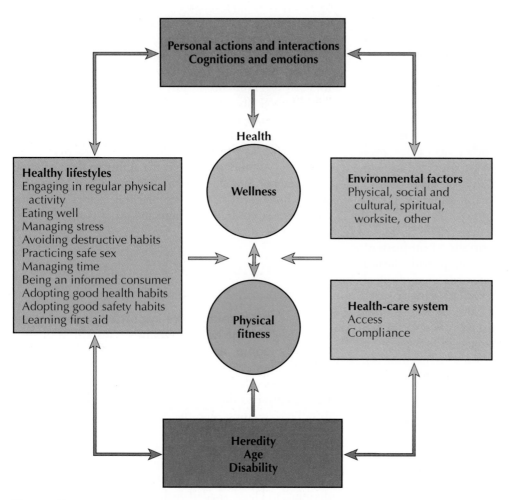

Figure 7 ▶ Determinants of health, fitness, and wellness.

Each of us reaps different benefits from the same healthy lifestyles, based on our hereditary tendencies. Even more important is that predispositions to diseases are inherited. For example, some early deaths are a result of untreatable hereditary conditions (e.g., congenital heart defects). Obviously, some inherited conditions are manageable (e.g., diabetes) with proper medical supervision and appropriate lifestyles. Heredity is a factor over which

HELP   Health is available to Everyone for a Lifetime, and it's **PERSONAL**

According to the National Institutes of Health, although genes don't necessarily cause diseases, they do influence our risk of developing diseases, such as cancer, heart disease, and addiction. The interaction between our genes and our environments and experiences is a complex one that is still being studied.

Would knowing you were genetically predisposed to a particular disease change the lifestyle decisions you make?

we have little control and is, therefore, illustrated in dark blue in Figure 7. Each of us can limit the effects of heredity by being aware of our personal family history and by making efforts to best manage those factors over which we do have control.

In the concepts that follow, you will learn more about heredity and how it affects health, wellness, and fitness.

Health, wellness, and fitness are influenced by the aging of our population. In 2030 when post–World War II baby boomers are over the age of 65, adults 65 or older will make up 20 percent of the population. The number of people over 85 will triple by 2050. More than 100,000 people are now 100 years of age or more. The definition of *old* is changing, with most people believing that a person is not old until age 71 or older. Nearly a quarter of the population believes that being old begins at 81.

Whatever the standard for being old, age is a factor over which we have no control. The major health and wellness concerns of older adults include losing health, losing the ability to care for oneself, losing mental abilities, running out of money, being a burden to family, and being alone. Chronic pain is also a major problem among older adults. Nearly 30 percent of adults over 65 experience chronic pain, as opposed to 3 percent of those under 30. Nearly 60 percent of older adults experience frequent pain, as opposed to 17 percent of those under 30. Older adults have 36 percent more unhealthy days than young adults.

Age is shaded in dark blue in Figure 7 because it is a factor that you cannot control. However, healthy lifestyles can reduce the effects of aging on health, wellness, and fitness. As detailed later in this book, healthy lifestyles can extend life and have a positive effect on quality of life.

Disabilities can affect, but they do not necessarily limit, health, wellness, and FEATURE **fitness.** Disabilities typically result from factors beyond control (shaded in dark blue in Figure 7).

Technology Update
Podcasts

TECH Podcasts are compressed digital files containing audio or video that can be downloaded from the Internet to a portable media player or personal computer. "Pod" refers to a personal media player, the receiver of the information delivered by a "podcaster." Originally used to transmit music and news, podcasts of health information are now common. For more information related to health, fitness, and wellness podcasts, visit the associated Web link.

Many types of disabilities affect health, fitness, and wellness. An objective disability (e.g., loss of a limb, impaired intellectual functioning) can make it difficult to function in certain circumstances but need not limit health, wellness, and fitness. All people have a limitation of one kind or another. Societal efforts to help all people function within their limitations can help everyone, including people with disabilities, have a positive outlook on life and experience a high quality of life. With assistance from an instructor, it is possible for all people to adapt the information in this book for use in promoting heath, wellness, and fitness.

The health-care system affects our ability to overcome illness and improve our quality of life. Approximately 10 percent of unnecessary deaths occur as a result of disparities in the health-care system. The quality of life for those who are sick and those who tend to be sick is influenced greatly by the type of medical care they receive. Health care is not equally available to all. A study by the Institute of Medicine, entitled "Insuring America's Health," indicates that 18,000 people die unnecessarily in the United States each year because they lack health insurance. Those without health insurance are more likely to go to but less likely to be admitted to emergency rooms and are less likely to get high-quality medical care than those with insurance. Many of those without insurance have chronic conditions that go undetected and as a result become untreatable. One of the great health inequities is that those with lower income are less likely to be insured.

Many people fail to seek medical help even though care is accessible. Others seek medical help but fail to comply with medical advice. For example, they do not take prescribed medicine or do not follow up with treatments. Men are less likely to seek medical advice than women. For this reason, treatable conditions sometimes become untreatable. Once men seek medical care, evidence reveals, they get better care than women. Also,

more of the medical research has been done on men. This is of concern because treatments for men and women often vary for similar conditions.

Wellness as evidenced by quality of life is also influenced by the health-care system. Traditional medicine, sometimes referred to as the **medical model,** has focused primarily on the treatment of illness with medicine, rather than illness prevention and wellness promotion. Efforts to educate health-care personnel about techniques for promoting wellness have been initiated in recent years. Still, it is often up to the patient to find information about health promotion. For example, a patient with risk factors for heart disease might be advised to eat better or to exercise more, but little specific information may be offered. In Figure 7, the health-care system is in light blue to illustrate the fact that it is a factor over which you may have limited control.

The environment is a major factor affecting our health, wellness, and fitness. Environmental factors account for nearly one-fourth of all early deaths and affect quality of life in many ways. We do have more control over environmental factors than heredity, but they are not totally under our control. For this reason, the environmental factors box is depicted in Figure 7 with a lighter shade of blue than the heredity, age, and disability box.

You can exert personal control by selecting healthy environments rather than by exposing yourself to unhealthy or unsafe environments. This includes your choice of living and work location, as well as the social, spiritual, and intellectual environments. On the other hand, circumstances may make it impossible for you to make the choices you would prefer. Important environmental factors are discussed throughout the text, particularly in Concept 6 and the final concept in the book. Some suggestions for how you can work to alter the environment in a positive way are also discussed in the last concept.

Personal actions, interactions, cognitions, and emotions all have an effect on health, wellness, and fitness. Some people think that good health, wellness, and fitness are totally out of personal control. Others think that they are totally in control. Neither statement is entirely true. While heredity, age, and disability are factors you cannot control, and health care and

Medical Model The focus of the health-care system on treating illness with medicine, with little emphasis on prevention or wellness promotion.

the environment are factors over which you have limited control, there are things that you can do relating to these factors. You can use your cognitive abilities to learn about your family history and use that information to limit the negative influences of heredity. You can learn how to adapt to disabilities and personal limitations, as well as to the aging process. You can research the health-care system and the environment to minimize the problems associated with them.

Your personal interactions also influence your health, wellness, and fitness. You are not alone in this world. Your various environments, and how you interact with them, influence you greatly. You have a choice about the environments in which you place yourself and the people with whom you interact in these environments.

Humans have the ability to think (cognitions) and to use critical thinking to make choices and to determine the actions they take and the interactions they engage in. Emotions also affect personal actions and interactions. A major goal of this book is to help you learn self-management skills designed to help you use your cognitive abilities to solve problems and make good decisions about good health, wellness, and fitness, as well as to help you to be in control of your emotions when taking action and making decisions that affect your health.

None of us makes perfect decisions all of the time. Sometimes we take actions and make choices based on inadequate information, faulty thinking, pressure from others, or negative influences from our emotions. While

the focus of this book is on healthy lifestyles, all of the factors that influence health, wellness, and fitness will be discussed in greater detail in the concepts that follow. The goal is to help you consider all factors and to make informed decisions that will lead to healthful behaviors. Some strategies for action for each of the factors are presented in the final concept of this book.

Lifestyle change, more than any other factor, is the best way to prevent illness and early death in our society. Statistics show that more than half of early deaths are the result of chronic diseases caused by unhealthy lifestyles. Many of these chronic diseases are targeted in the HP2020 report, and many of the new health objectives focus on them. As shown in Figure 7, these lifestyles affect health, wellness, and physical fitness. The double-headed arrow between heath/wellness and physical fitness illustrates the interaction between these factors. Physical fitness is important to health and wellness development and vice versa.

The major causes of early death have shifted from infectious diseases to chronic lifestyle-related conditions. Scientific advances and improvements in medicine and health care have dramatically reduced the incidence of infectious diseases over the past 100 years (see Table 3). Diphtheria and polio, both major causes of death in the 20th century, have been virtually eliminated in Western culture. Smallpox was globally eradicated in 1977.

In the News

Health, Wellness, and Fitness: The Good News

The "In the News" feature at the end of each concept is designed to provide the reader with the latest information about health, wellness, and fitness. Health news that we receive via newspapers, television, and the Web sometimes seems to overemphasize "bad news." Presentation of the bad news may lead some people to conclude that events are out of their control and there is nothing they can do. To be sure, this book will point out some of the bad news, because it is necessary to be aware of the facts (both positive and negative) if we are to make changes to improve our health, wellness, and fitness. It is important to note, however, that there is considerable good news to report. Some examples of the good news about health, wellness, and fitness are included here.

- Of the Healthy People goals established in 2000 for the year 2010, 18 percent were met and progress was made toward 70 percent. Among the key successes were the increase in life expectancy (all-time high) and decreases in deaths from stroke, cancer, and heart disease.
- Seventy percent of Americans favor increasing investments in prevention of health problems.
- Most adults, including young adults, say they are taking action to improve their health for the future.
- Most people in the United States (85 percent) and Canada (88 percent) report having good, very good, or excellent health.
- Adults who exercise regularly report greater happiness and less stress than those who do not exercise.

More good news information is available at the In the News Web link.

Table 3 ▶ Major Causes of Death in the United States

Current Rank	Cause	1900 Rank	Cause
1	Heart disease	1	Pneumonia
2	Cancer	2	Tuberculosis
3	Stroke	3	Diarrhea/enteritis
4	Lower respiratory disease	4	Heart disease
5	Injuries/accidents	5	Stroke
6	Diabetes	6	Liver disease
7	Alzheimer's disease	7	Injuries
8	Influenza/pneumonia	8	Cancer
9	Kidney disease	9	Senility
10	Septicemia	10	Diphtheria

The only diseases among the top ten that are primarily infectious in nature are influenza/pneumonia and septicemia (blood infections).

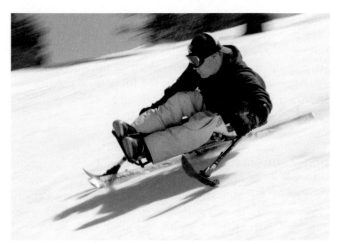

Physical activity is for everyone. Health and wellness are available to everyone for a lifetime.

Infectious diseases have been replaced with chronic lifestyle-related conditions as the major causes of death. Four of the top seven current causes of death (heart disease, cancer, stroke, and diabetes) fall into this category. Alzheimer's disease (also in the top seven) has been linked to physical inactivity and other lifestyle factors. While heart disease remains the leading killer among all adults, National Cancer Institute statistics indicate that cancer is the leading cause of death for adults under the age of 85. Decreases in death rates occurred for six of the top eight causes of death, with only lower respiratory disease death rates increasing, and Alzheimer's disease death rates remaining unchanged.

HIV/AIDS, formerly in the top 10, has dropped well down the list, primarily because of the development of treatments to increase the life expectancy of those infected. Many among the top 10 are referred to as chronic lifestyle-related conditions because alteration of lifestyles can result in reduced risk for these conditions.

Healthy lifestyles are critical to wellness. Just as unhealthy lifestyles are the principal causes of modern-day illnesses, such as heart disease, cancer, and diabetes, healthy lifestyles can result in the improved feeling of wellness that is critical to optimal health. In recognizing the importance of "years of healthy life," the Public Health Service also recognizes what it calls "measures of well-being." This well-being, or wellness, is associated with social, emotional/mental, spiritual, and physical functioning. Being physically active and eating well are two healthy lifestyles that can improve well-being and add years of quality living. Many of the healthy lifestyles associated with good physical fitness and optimal wellness will be discussed in detail later in this book. The Healthy Lifestyle Questionnaire at the end of this concept gives you the opportunity to assess your current lifestyles.

Regular physical activity, sound nutrition, and stress management are priority healthy lifestyles. Three of the lifestyles listed in Figure 7 are considered to be priority healthy lifestyles. These are engaging in regular **physical activity** or **exercise,** eating well, and managing stress. There are several reasons for placing priority on these lifestyles. First, they affect the lives of all people. Second, they are lifestyles in which large numbers of people can make improvement. Finally, modest changes in these behaviors can make dramatic improvements in individual and public health. For example, statistics suggest that modest changes in physical activity patterns and nutrition can prevent more than 400,000 deaths annually. Stress also has a major impact on drug, alcohol, and smoking behavior, so managing stress can help individuals minimize or avoid those behaviors.

Physical Activity Generally considered to be a broad term used to describe all forms of large muscle movements, including sports, dance, games, work, lifestyle activities, and exercise for fitness. In this book, *exercise* and *physical activity* will often be used interchangeably to make reading less repetitive and more interesting.

Exercise Physical activity done for the purpose of getting physically fit.

The other healthy lifestyles listed in Figure 7 are also very important for good health. The reason that they are not emphasized as priority lifestyles is that not all people have problems in these areas. Many healthy lifestyles will be discussed in this book, but the focus is on the priority healthy lifestyles because virtually all people can achieve positive wellness benefits if they adopt them.

The "actual causes" of most deaths are due to unhealthy lifestyles. As illustrated in Table 3, chronic diseases (e.g., heart diseases, cancer) are the direct causes of most deaths in our society. Public health experts have used epidemiological statistics to show that unhealthy lifestyles such as tobacco use, inactivity, and poor eating actually cause the chronic diseases and for this reason are referred to as the "actual causes of death." Tobacco is the leading actual cause of death, but inactivity and poor diet account for the next largest percentage of deaths (see Table 4). The percentage of deaths attributed to inactivity and poor diet has recently been questioned, but their overall influence on health is indisputable. The information presented throughout this book is designed to help you change behaviors to reduce your risk for early death from the actual causes listed in Table 4.

The HELP Philosophy

The HELP philosophy can provide a basis for making healthy lifestyle change possible. The four-letter acronym HELP summarizes the overall philosophy used in this book. Each letter in HELP characterizes an

important part of the philosophy: *Health* is available to *Everyone* for a *Lifetime*—and it's *Personal*. The concepts in the book provide principles and guidelines that help you adopt positive lifestyles. The labs provide experiences that help you build the behavioral skills needed to learn and maintain these lifestyles.

A personal philosophy that emphasizes health can lead to behaviors that promote it. The *H* in HELP stands for *health*. One theory that has been extensively tested indicates that people who believe in the benefits of healthy lifestyles are more likely to engage in healthy behaviors. The theory also suggests that people who state intentions to put their beliefs into action are likely to adopt behaviors that lead to health, wellness, and fitness.

Everyone can benefit from healthy lifestyles. The *E* in HELP stands for *everyone*. Accepting the fact that anyone can change a behavior or lifestyle means that *you* are included. Nevertheless, many adults feel ineffective in making lifestyle changes. Physical activity is

Table 4 ▶ Actual Causes of Death in the United States		
Rank	Actual Cause	Percentage of Deaths
1	Tobacco use	18.1
2	Inactivity/poor diet	16.6
3	Alcohol consumption	3.5
4	Microbial agents (flu, pneumonia)	3.1
5	Toxic agents	2.3
6	Motor vehicles	1.8
7	Firearms	1.2
8	Sexual behavior	0.8
9	Illicit drug use	0.7
10	Other	<.05

Source: Mokdad et al.

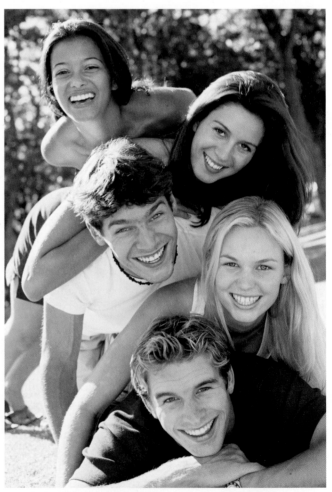

Health and wellness is available to everyone for a lifetime.

not just for athletes—it is for all people. Eating well is not just for other people—you can do it, too. All people can learn stress-management techniques. Everyone can practice healthy lifestyles. As noted earlier in this concept, important health goals include eliminating health disparities and promoting "health for all."

Healthy behaviors are most effective when practiced for a lifetime. The *L* in HELP stands for *lifetime*. Young people sometimes feel immortal because the harmful effects of unhealthy lifestyles are often not immediate. As we grow older, we begin to realize that we are not immortal and that unhealthy lifestyles have cumulative negative effects. Starting early in life to

emphasize healthy behaviors results in long-term health, wellness, and fitness benefits. One study showed that the longer healthy lifestyles are practiced, the greater the beneficial effects. This study also demonstrated that long-term healthy lifestyles can even overcome hereditary predisposition to illness and disease.

Healthy lifestyles should be based on personal needs. The *P* in HELP stands for *personal*. No two people are exactly alike. Just as no single pill cures all illnesses, no single lifestyle prescription exists for good health, wellness, and fitness. Each person must assess personal needs and make lifestyle changes based on those needs.

 ## Strategies for Action

Self-assessments of lifestyles will help you determine areas in which you may need changes to promote optimal health, wellness, and fitness. As you begin your study of health, wellness, fitness, and healthy lifestyles, it is wise to make a self-assessment of your current behaviors. The Healthy Lifestyle Questionnaire in the lab resource materials will allow you to assess your current lifestyle behaviors to determine if they are contributing positively to your health, wellness, and fitness. Because this questionnaire contains some very personal information, answering all the questions honestly will help you get an accurate assessment. As you continue your study, you may want to refer back to this questionnaire to see if your lifestyles have changed.

 Initial self-assessments of wellness and fitness will provide information for self-comparison. The Healthy Lifestyle

FEATURE 5

Questionnaire allows you to assess your lifestyles or behaviors. It is also important to assess your wellness and fitness at an early stage. These early assessments will only be estimates. As you continue your study, you will have the opportunity to do more comprehensive self-assessments that will allow you to see how accurate your early estimates were.

In Lab 1A, you will estimate your wellness using a Wellness Self-Perceptions questionnaire, which assesses five wellness dimensions. Remember, wellness is a state of being that is influenced by healthy lifestyles. Because other factors, such as heredity, environment, and health care, affect wellness, it is possible to have good wellness scores even if you do not do well on the lifestyle questionnaire. However, over a lifetime, unhealthy lifestyles will catch up with you and have an influence on your wellness and fitness.

Web Resources

 Additional websites with information related to Concept 1 are available at the associated Web link.

WEB

American Medical Association (AMA)
   www.ama-assn.org
Centers for Disease Control and Prevention (CDC)
   www.cdc.gov
Health Canada www.healthcanada.ca
Healthier United States www.healthierus.gov
Healthy People 2020 www.healthypeople.gov/HP2020

Institute of Medicine www.iom.edu
National Center for Chronic Disease Prevention and Health
   Promotion Publications www.cdc.gov/nccdphp/publicat.htm
President's Council on Physical Fitness and Sports
   www.fitness.gov
Robert Wood Johnson Foundation www.rwjf.org
Trust for America's Health http://healthyamericans.org
   report/55/blueprint-for-healthier-america
U. S. Government Healthcare www.HealthCare.gov
Well-Being Index—Gallup Poll www.gallup.com/poll
   /wellbeing.aspx
World Health Organization www.who.int

Web Podcasts (Selected Websites)

Arizona State University on iTunes U—Introduction to
   Exercise and Wellness **http://itunes.asu.edu**

CDC **www2a.cdc.gov/podcasts**

Johns Hopkins Medicine Podcasts
   **www.hopkinsmedicine.org/mediaII
   /Podcastsinstructions.html**

Journal of the American Medical Association Podcasts
   http://jama.ama-assn.org/misc/audiocommentary.dtl

University of Maryland—Medical Podcasts (Medically
   Speaking) **www.umm.edu/podcasts/?source=google&
   gclid=CNS2g7_8oo0CFRfOggodmDi_5g**

U.S. Food and Drug Administration
   www.fda.gov/oc/podcasts/podcasthelp.html

U.S. Government Podcasts—Health Podcasts from the U.S.
   Government **www.usa.gov/Topics/Reference_Shelf
   /Libraries/Podcasts/Health.shtml**

Suggested Readings

REFERENCES

Selected readings and references are listed below. A more comprehensive list is available at the associated Web link.

Centers for Disease Control and Prevention. 2009. *Healthy
   People 2020 Public Meetings: 2009 Draft Objectives.* Atlanta:
   CDC. Available at **www.healthypeople.gov/hp2020/
   objectives**

Central Intelligence Agency. 2009. *The World Factbook.*
   Washington, DC: CIA.

Owen, N., et al. 2010. Too much sitting: The population
   health science of sedentary behavior. *Exercise and Sport
   Sciences Reviews.* 38(3):105–1113.

Sebastiani, P., et al. 2010. Genetic signatures of exceptional
   longevity in humans. *Science.* Published online July 1, 2010,
   www.sciencemag.org

Trust for America's Health. 2008. *Blueprint for a Healthier
   America.* Washington, DC: Trust for America's Health.
   Available at **http://healthyamericans.org/report/55
   /blueprint-for-healthier-america**

World Health Organization. 2009. *Global Health Risks.*
   Geneva: WHO. Available at **www.who.int
   /publications/en**

Lab Resource Materials: The Healthy Lifestyle Questionnaire

The purpose of this questionnaire is to help you analyze your lifestyle behaviors and to help you make decisions concerning good health and wellness for the future. Information on this Healthy Lifestyle Questionnaire is of a personal nature. For this reason, this questionnaire is not designed to be submitted to your instructor. **It is for your information only.** Answer each question as honestly as possible, and use the scoring information to help assess your lifestyle.

Directions: Place an X over the "yes" circle to answer yes. If you answer "no," make no mark. Score the questionnaire using the procedures that follow.

(yes) 1. I accumulate 30 minutes of moderate physical activity most days of the week (brisk walking, stair climbing, yard work, or home chores).

(yes) 2. I do vigorous activity that elevates my heart rate for 20 minutes at least 3 days a week.

(yes) 3. I do exercises for flexibility at least 3 days a week.

(yes) 4. I do exercises for muscle fitness at least 2 days a week.

(yes) 5. I eat three regular meals each day.

(yes) 6. I select appropriate servings from the major food groups each day.

(yes) 7. I restrict the amount of fat in my diet.

(yes) 8. I consume only as many calories as I expend each day.

(yes) 9. I am able to identify situations in daily life that cause stress.

(yes) 10. I take time out during the day to relax and recover from daily stress.

(yes) 11. I find time for family, friends, and things I especially enjoy doing.

(yes) 12. I regularly perform exercises designed to relieve tension.

(yes) 13. I do not smoke or use other tobacco products.

(yes) 14. I do not abuse alcohol.

(yes) 15. I do not abuse drugs (prescription or illegal).

(yes) 16. I take over-the-counter drugs sparingly and use them only according to directions.

(yes) 17. I abstain from sex or limit sexual activity to a safe partner.

(yes) 18. I practice safe procedures for avoiding sexually transmitted infections (STIs).

(yes) 19. I use seat belts and adhere to the speed limit when I drive.

(yes) 20. I have a smoke detector in my house and check it regularly to see that it is working.

(yes) 21. I have had training to perform CPR if called on in an emergency.

(yes) 22. I can perform the Heimlich maneuver effectively if called on in an emergency.

(yes) 23. I brush my teeth at least twice a day and floss at least once a day.

(yes) 24. I get an adequate amount of sleep each night.

(yes) 25. I do regular self-exams, have regular medical checkups, and seek medical advice when symptoms are present.

(yes) 26. When I receive advice and/or medication from a physician, I follow the advice and take the medication as prescribed.

(yes) 27. I read product labels and investigate their effectiveness before I buy them.

(yes) 28. I avoid using products that have not been shown by research to be effective.

(yes) 29. I recycle paper, glass, and aluminum.

(yes) 30. I practice environmental protection, such as carpooling and energy conservation.

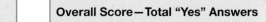

Overall Score—Total "Yes" Answers

Scoring: Give yourself 1 point for each "yes" answer. Add your scores for each of the lifestyle behaviors. To calculate your overall score, sum the totals for all lifestyles.

Physical Activity
1. ☐
2. ☐
3. ☐
4. ☐
☐ Total +

Nutrition
5. ☐
6. ☐
7. ☐
8. ☐
☐ Total +

Managing Stress
9. ☐
10. ☐
11. ☐
12. ☐
☐ Total +

Avoiding Destructive Habits
13. ☐
14. ☐
15. ☐
16. ☐
☐ Total +

Practicing Safe Sex
17. ☐
18. ☐
☐ Total +

Adopting Safety Habits
19. ☐
20. ☐
☐

Knowing First Aid
21. ☐
22. ☐
☐ Total +

Personal Health Habits
23. ☐
24. ☐
☐ Total +

Using Medical Advice
25. ☐
26. ☐
☐ Total +

Being an Informed Consumer
27. ☐
28. ☐
☐ Total +

Protecting the Environment
29. ☐
30. ☐
☐ Total =

Sum All Totals for Overall Score
☐

Interpreting Scores: Scores of 3 or 4 on the four-item scales indicate generally positive lifestyles. For the two-item scales, a score of 2 indicates the presence of positive lifestyles. An overall score of 26 or more is a good indicator of healthy lifestyle behaviors. It is important to consider the following special note when interpreting scores.

Special Note: Your scores on the Healthy Lifestyle Questionnaire should be interpreted with caution. There are several reasons for this. First, all lifestyle behaviors do not pose the same risks. For example, using tobacco or abusing drugs has immediate negative effects on health and wellness, whereas others, such as knowing first aid, may have only occasional use. Second, you may score well on one item in a scale but not on another. If one item indicates an unhealthy lifestyle in an area that poses a serious health risk, your lifestyle may appear to be healthier than it really is. For example, you could get a score of 3 on the destructive habits scale and be a regular smoker. For this reason, the overall score can be particularly deceiving.

Strategies for Change: In the space to the right, you may want to make some notes concerning the healthy lifestyle areas in which you could make some changes. You can refer to these notes later to see if you have made progress.

Healthy Lifestyle Ratings

Rating	Two-Item Scores	Four-Item Scores	Overall Scores
Positive lifestyles	2	3 or 4	26 to 30*
Consider changes	Less than 2	Less than 3	Less than 26

*See Special Note.

Lab 1A Wellness Self-Perceptions

Name	**Section**　**Date**

Purpose: To assess self-perceptions of wellness

Procedures

1. Place an X over the appropriate circle for each question (4 = strongly agree, 3 = agree, 2 = disagree, 1 = strongly disagree).
2. Write the number found in that circle in the box to the right.
3. Sum the three boxes for each wellness dimension to get your wellness dimension totals.
4. Sum all wellness dimension totals to get your comprehensive wellness total.
5. Use the rating chart to rate each wellness area.
6. Complete the Results section and the Conclusions and Implications section.

Question	Strongly Agree	Agree	Disagree	Strongly Disagree	Score
1. I am happy most of the time.	4	3	2	1	
2. I have good self-esteem.	4	3	2	1	
3. I do not generally feel stressed.	4	3	2	1	
			Emotional Wellness Total	**=**	
4. I am well informed about current events.	4	3	2	1	
5. I am comfortable expressing my views and opinions.	4	3	2	1	
6. I am interested in my career development.	4	3	2	1	
			Intellectual Wellness Total	**=**	
7. I am physically fit.	4	3	2	1	
8. I am able to perform the physical tasks of my work.	4	3	2	1	
9. I am physically able to perform leisure activities.	4	3	2	1	
			Physical Wellness Total	**=**	
10. I have many friends and am involved socially.	4	3	2	1	
11. I have close ties with my family.	4	3	2	1	
12. I am confident in social situations.	4	3	2	1	
			Social Wellness Total	**=**	
13. I am fulfilled spiritually.	4	3	2	1	
14. I feel connected to the world around me.	4	3	2	1	
15. I have a sense of purpose in my life.	4	3	2	1	
			Spiritual Wellness Total	**=**	
			Comprehensive Wellness (Sum of five wellness scores)		

In the results below, record your scores from the previous page; then determine your ratings for each score using the Wellness Rating Chart. Record your ratings in the Results section.

Results

Wellness Dimension	Score	Rating
Emotional/mental		
Intellectual		
Physical		
Social		
Spiritual		
Comprehensive		

Wellness Rating Chart

Rating	Wellness Dimension Scores	Comprehensive Wellness Scores
High-level wellness	10–12	50–60
Good wellness	8–9	40–49
Marginal wellness	6–7	30–39
Low-level wellness	Below 6	Below 30

Conclusions and Implications: In the space provided below, use several paragraphs to describe your current state of wellness. Do you think the ratings indicate your true state of wellness? Are there areas in which there is room for improvement?

Self-Management and Self-Planning Skills for Health Behavior Change

Health Objectives for the Year 2020

- Create a society in which all people live long, healthy lives.
- Attain high-quality, longer lives free of preventable disease, injury, and premature death.
- Increase public awareness and understanding of the determinants of health, disease, and disability.
- Achieve health equity, eliminate disparities, and improve the health of all groups.
- Create social and physical environments that promote good health for all.
- Promote quality of life, healthy development, and healthy behaviors (including being active, eating well, and avoiding destructive habits) across all stages of life.
- Increase health literacy of the population.

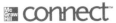

http://connect.mcgraw-hill.com

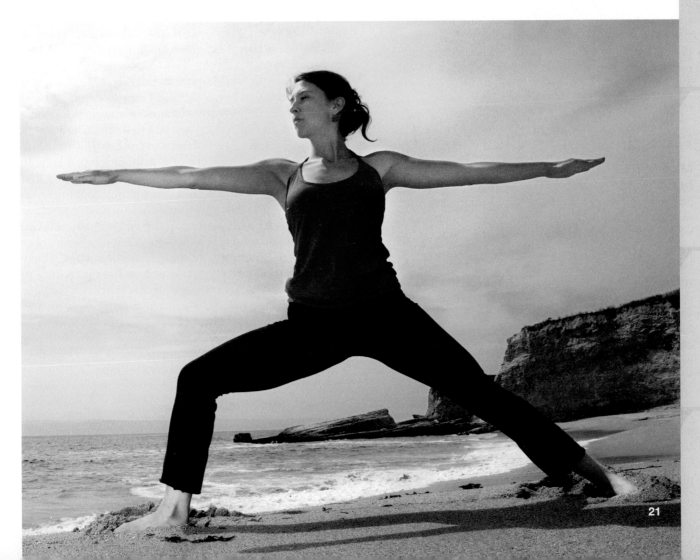

Learning and regularly using self-management skills can help you adopt and maintain healthy lifestyles throughout life.

Reducing illness and debilitating conditions and promoting wellness and fitness are important public health goals. As noted in Concept 1, adopting healthy lifestyles is a key factor in health, wellness, and fitness promotion, but evidence suggests that many people are not able to make changes, even when they want to do so. Experts have determined that people who practice healthy lifestyles possess certain characteristics. These characteristics, including personal responsibility, can be modified to improve the health behaviors of all people. Researchers have also identified several special skills, referred to as **self-management skills,** that can be useful in altering factors related to adherence and ultimately in making lifestyle changes. Like any skill, self-management skills must be practiced if they are to be useful. The factors relating to adherence and the self-management skills described in this concept can be applied to a wide variety of healthy lifestyles. The early sections of this book focus on using self-management skills to become and stay active throughout life. Later sections focus on using these skills to adopt other healthy lifestyles that promote good health and wellness. In the final section, you get an opportunity to use the skills to make informed choices and plan for healthy living.

Making Lifestyle Changes

Many adults want to make lifestyle changes but find changes hard to make. Results of several national public opinion polls show that adults often have difficulty making desired lifestyle changes. Examples include those who believe that physical activity is important but do not get enough exercise to promote good health, those who have tried numerous times to lose weight but have failed, those who know good nutrition is good for health but do not eat well, and those who feel stress on a regular basis but have not found a way to become less stressed. Changes in other lifestyles are frequently desired but often not accomplished. More information about public opinion polls related to health is presented in the "In the News" section at the end of this concept.

Practicing one healthy lifestyle does not mean you will practice another, though adopting one healthy behavior often leads to the adoption of another. College students are more likely to participate in regular physical activity than are older adults. However, they are also much more likely to eat poorly and abuse alcohol. Many young women adopt low-fat diets to avoid weight gain and smoke because they mistakenly believe that smoking will contribute to long-term weight maintenance. These examples illustrate the fact that practicing one healthy lifestyle does not ensure **adherence** to another. However, there is evidence that making one lifestyle change often makes it easier to make other changes. For example, smokers who have started regular physical activity programs often see improvements in fitness and general well-being and decide to stop smoking.

 People do not make lifestyle changes overnight. People progress forward and backward through several stages of change. When asked about a specific healthy lifestyle, people commonly respond with yes or no answers. If asked, "Do you exercise regularly?" the answer is yes or no. When asked, "Do you eat well?" the answer is yes or no. We know that there are many different stages of lifestyle behavior.

Prochaska (a well-known health psychology expert) and his colleagues developed the Transtheoretical Model to explain the importance of **stages of change** for understanding behavior. They suggest that lifestyle changes occur in at least five different stages, as illustrated in Figure 1. The stages were originally developed to help clarify negative lifestyles. Smokers were among the first studied. Smokers who are not considering stopping are at the stage of precontemplation. Those who are thinking about stopping are classified in the contemplation stage. Those who have bought a nicotine patch or a book about smoking cessation are in the preparation stage. They have moved beyond contemplation and are preparing to take action. The action stage occurs when the smoker makes a change in behavior, even a small one, such as cutting back on the number of cigarettes smoked. The fifth stage, maintenance, is reached when a person finally stops smoking for a relatively long time (e.g., 6 months).

The stages of change model (as illustrated in Figure 1) has been applied to positive lifestyles as well as negative ones. Those who are totally sedentary are considered to be in the precontemplation stage. Contemplators are thinking about becoming active. A person at the preparation stage may have bought a pair of walking shoes and appropriate clothing for activity. Those who have started activity, even if infrequent, are at the stage of action.

Public Opinion Polls about Health, Wellness, and Fitness

Results of a recent poll by *Parade* magazine indicate that most Americans are very concerned about health. Most (50 percent or more) indicate that they:

- are doing something now to stay healthy later in life (e.g., doing regular physical activity),
- are doing more than their parents did to stay healthy,
- believe that personal habits and choices are the most important factor in staying healthy, and
- have talked to a doctor about preventing health problems.

Another poll conducted by Research America, called "America Speaks," indicates that most Americans (50 percent or more):

- are willing to pay for research to improve health and
- believe that more money should be spent on medical and health research.

A recent Harris Interactive Poll shows that, compared to people with less education, those with a college education are:

- less likely to do unhealthy and risky behaviors,
- less likely to smoke, and
- more likely to use seat belts.

As you read the information in the previous paragraphs (and elsewhere in this book), you may have wondered about the source of the information. The information is obtained from a variety of sources, often public opinion polls. Many different organizations regularly conduct polls concerning politics, religion, and other subjects, such as health, wellness, fitness, and the behaviors that affect them. Many of these are private companies dedicated exclusively to polling, such as the Gallup Poll, the Harris Interactive, and Research America. Several foundations conduct regular polls. For example, the Kaiser and Pew Foundations regularly conduct polls related to health.

Various newspapers and television networks (e.g., CBS/New York Times, USA Today/CNN/Gallup, NBC/Washington Post) conduct polls that occasionally deal with health issues. The National Sporting Goods Association conducts polls related to sports and recreation. Government organizations, such as the Census Bureau, CDC, and National Center for Health Statistics, also gather data that relate to public opinion, often related to health. Links to various health polls are available at the associated Web link. Accessing these polls can help you better understand the nature of the information used by the authors in providing statistics such as those given in this book.

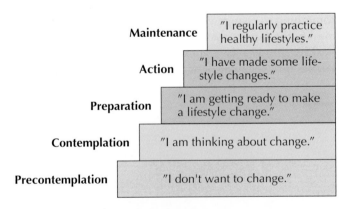

Figure 1 ▶ Stages of lifestyle change.

who succeed in quitting permanently report having stopped and started dozens of times before reaching lifetime maintenance. Similarly, those attempting to adopt positive lifestyles, such as eating well, often move back and forth from one stage to another, depending on their life circumstances.

Once maintenance is attained, relapse is less likely to occur. Although complete relapse is possible, it is generally less likely after the maintenance stage is reached.

Self-Management Skills Skills that you learn to help you adopt healthy lifestyles and adhere to them.

Adherence Adopting and sticking with healthy behaviors, such as regular physical activity or sound nutrition, as part of your lifestyle.

Stage of Change The level of motivational readiness to adopt a specific health behavior.

Those who have been exercising regularly for at least 6 months are at the stage of maintenance.

Whether the lifestyle is positive or negative, people move from one stage to another in an upward or a downward direction. Individuals in the action stage may move on to maintenance or revert to contemplation. Smokers

At the maintenance stage, the behavior has been integrated into a personal lifestyle, and it becomes easier to sustain. For example, a person who has been active for years does not have to undergo the same thought processes as a beginning exerciser—the behavior becomes automatic and habitual. Similarly, a nonsmoker is not tempted to smoke in the same way as a person who is trying to quit. Some people have termed the end of this behavior change process as termination.

Factors That Promote Lifestyle Change

Various factors have been found to influence adoption and maintenance of healthy lifestyles. A variety of theories have been proposed to understand health behavior (e.g., Social Cognitive Theory, Self-Determination Theory, Theory of Planned Behavior, Theory of Reasoned Action). Each theory offers some unique attributes or concepts, but a close examination shows that they share many of the same components. The previously mentioned Transtheoretical Model integrates elements from multiple theories and can be viewed as a "meta-theory." The distinction between a "theory" and a "model" is important in this case. The Transtheoretical Model does not provide a new explanation of behavior (a theory) but rather a guide or map that makes using and applying the theories easier (a model). The unique advantage of the Transtheoretical Model is that it demonstrates that behavior is influenced in different ways depending on the stage of change a person has reached.

Another meta-theory that has been used to explain the challenges of changing health behaviors is the Social-Ecological Model. This model also integrates multiple theories, but a key point in this model is that a person's behavior is strongly influenced by the nature of the environment in which she or he lives. If you are in a supportive social environment and have access to healthy foods and activity resources, adopting healthier lifestyles is easier.

You do not need a thorough understanding of the theories and models, but you should be aware of the basic principles. Concepts from both the Transtheoretical and Social-Ecological models have been combined to provide a simpler way to understand the various factors that influence behavior. For ease of understanding, the various factors are classified as **personal, predisposing, enabling,** and **reinforcing factors** (see Figure 2). Predisposing factors help precontemplators get going—moving them toward contemplation or even preparation. Enabling factors help those in contemplation or preparation take a step toward action. Reinforcing factors move

people from action to maintenance and help those in maintenance stay there.

Personal factors affect health behaviors but are often out of your personal control. Age, gender, heredity, social status, and current health and fitness levels are all personal factors that affect your health behaviors. For example, there are significant differences in health behaviors among people of various ages. According to one survey, young adults between the ages of 18 and 34 are more likely to smoke (30 percent) than those 65 and older (13 percent). On the other hand, young adults are much more likely than older adults to be physically active.

Gender differences are illustrated by the fact that women use health services more often than men. Women are more likely than men to have identified a primary care doctor and are more likely to participate in regular health screenings. As you will discover in more detail later in this book, heredity plays a role in health behaviors. For example, some people have a hereditary predisposition to gain weight, and this may affect their eating behaviors.

Age, gender, and heredity are factors you cannot control. Other personal factors that relate to health behaviors include social status and current health and fitness status. Evidence indicates that people of lower socioeconomic status and those with poor health and fitness are less likely to contemplate or participate in activity and other healthy behaviors. No matter what personal characteristics you have, you can change your health behaviors. If you have several personal factors that do not favor healthy lifestyles, it is important to do something to change your behaviors. Making an effort to modify the factors that predispose, enable, and reinforce healthy lifestyles is essential. As shown in Figure 2, the factors influence behavior at different stages of change.

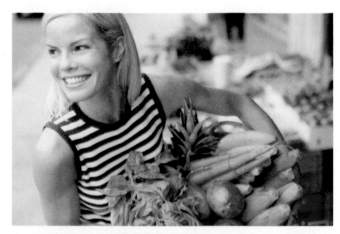

Access to healthy foods is an important predisposing factor for good nutrition.

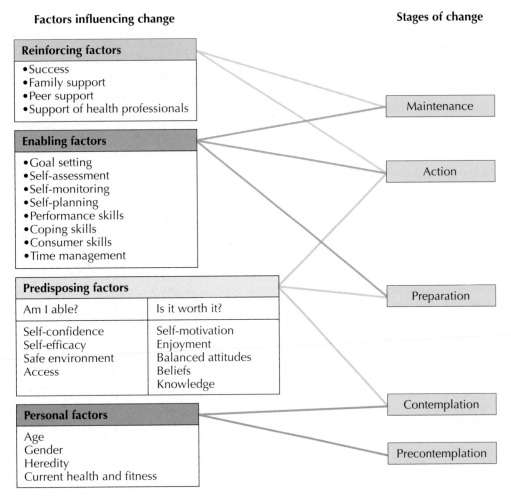

Factors influencing change

Stages of change

Reinforcing factors
- Success
- Family support
- Peer support
- Support of health professionals

Enabling factors
- Goal setting
- Self-assessment
- Self-monitoring
- Self-planning
- Performance skills
- Coping skills
- Consumer skills
- Time management

Predisposing factors

Am I able?	Is it worth it?
Self-confidence	Self-motivation
Self-efficacy	Enjoyment
Safe environment	Balanced attitudes
Access	Beliefs
	Knowledge

Personal factors
Age
Gender
Heredity
Current health and fitness

Maintenance

Action

Preparation

Contemplation

Precontemplation

Figure 2 ▶ Factors that influence health behaviors at various stages of change.

Predisposing factors are important in getting you started with the process of change. Several predisposing factors can help you move from contemplation to preparation and then to taking action with regard to healthy behavior. A person who possesses many of the predisposing factors is said to have self-motivation (also called intrinsic motivation). If you are self-motivated, you will answer positively to two basic questions: "Am I able?" and "Is it worth it?"

"Am I able to do regular activity?" "Am I able to change my diet or to stop smoking?" Figure 2 includes a list of four factors that help you say, "Yes, I am able." Two of these factors are **self-confidence** and **self-efficacy.** Both have to do with having positive perceptions about your own ability. People with positive self-perceptions are more self-motivated and feel they are capable of making behavior changes for health improvement. Other factors that help you feel you are able to do a healthy behavior include easy access and a safe environment. For example, people who have easy access to exercise equipment at home or the workplace or who have a place to exercise

within 10 minutes of home are more likely to be active than those who do not. Similarly, access to healthy food options is critical for adopting a healthy diet. A supportive physical and social environment can also make it easier to adopt healthy habits.

Personal Factors Factors, such as age or gender, related to healthy lifestyle adherence but not typically under personal control.

Predisposing Factors Factors that make you more likely to adopt a healthy lifestyle, such as participation in regular physical activity, as part of your normal routine.

Enabling Factors Factors that help you carry out your healthy lifestyle plan.

Reinforcing Factors Factors that provide encouragement to maintain healthy lifestyles, such as physical activity, for a lifetime.

Table 1 ▶ Self-Management Skills for Changing Predisposing Factors

Self-Management Skill	How Is It Useful?
Overcoming Barriers	**Lifestyle Example**
This involves developing skills that make it possible to overcome problems or challenges in adopting or maintaining healthy behaviors. By conquering challenges, you learn skills that help you overcome other barriers to healthy lifestyles.	A person is tempted by snack foods and candy provided by coworkers. Learning to resist these foods takes discipline, but overcoming barriers builds confidence that helps the person stay focused on long-term goals.
Building Self-Confidence and Motivation	**Lifestyle Example**
This involves taking small steps that allow success. With each small step, confidence and motivation increase and you develop the feeling "I can do that."	A person says, "I would like to be more active, but I have never been good at physical activities." Starting with a 10-minute walk, the person sees that "I can do it." Over time, the person becomes confident and motivated to do more physical activity.
Balancing Attitudes	**Lifestyle Example**
This involves learning to balance positive and negative attitudes. Developing positive attitudes and reducing negative attitudes helps you adhere to a healthy lifestyle.	A person does not do activity because he or she lacks support from friends, has no equipment, and does not like to get sweaty. These are negatives. Shifting the balance to positive things, such as fun, good health, and good appearance, can help promote activity.
Building Knowledge and Changing Beliefs	**Lifestyle Example**
An educated person knows the truth and builds his or her beliefs on sound information. Knowledge does not always change beliefs, but awareness of the facts can play a role in achieving good health.	A person says, "I don't think what I eat has much to do with my health and wellness." Acquiring knowledge is fundamental to being an educated person. Studying the facts about nutrition can provide the basis for changes in beliefs and lifestyles.

"Is it worth it?" People who say yes to this question are willing to make an effort to change their behaviors. Predisposing factors that make it worth it to change behaviors include enjoying the activity, balancing positive and negative attitudes, believing in the benefits of a behavior, and having knowledge of the health benefits of a behavior (see Figure 2). If you enjoy something and feel good about it (have positive attitudes and beliefs), you will be self-motivated to do it. It will be worth it. The lifestyle examples provided in Table 1 will help you understand how to apply these predisposing factors to your own lifestyle.

Enabling factors move you from the beginning stages of change to action and maintenance. A variety of skills help you follow through with decisions to make changes in behaviors. Figure 2 lists eight different self-management skills and each contributes to behavior change in different ways. The labs in each concept provide opportunities to learn and apply these self-management skills to your lifestyle. Table 2 explains the importance of each skill and how each one can contribute to behavior change.

Reinforcing factors help you adhere to lifestyle changes. Once you have reached the action or maintenance stage, it is important to stay at this high level.

Reinforcing factors help you stick with a behavior change (see Figure 2).

One of the most important reinforcing factors is success. If you change a behavior and experience success, this makes you want to keep doing the behavior. If attempts to change a behavior result in failure, you may conclude that the behavior does not work and give up on it. Planning for success is essential for adhering to healthy lifestyle changes. Using the self-management

HEALTH is available to Everyone for a Lifetime, and it's Personal

According to a thirty-two year study of social networks recently published in *The New England Journal of Medicine,* people are more likely to become obese if a friend becomes obese. Similar relationships were found for adult siblings and spouses, though not to as great a degree. The same relationship was not found for neighbors.

Do you think your friends hurt or help you maintain a healthy lifestyle?

Table 2 ▶ Self-Management Skills for Changing Enabling Factors

Self-Management Skill	How Is It Useful?
Goal-Setting Skills	**Lifestyle Example**
This involves learning how to establish what you want to achieve in the future. Goals should be realistic and achievable. Learning to set goals for behavior change is especially important for beginners.	A person wants to lose body fat. Setting a goal of losing 50 pounds makes success unlikely. Setting a process goal of restricting 200 calories a day or expending 200 more a day for several weeks makes success more likely.
Self-Assessment Skills	**Lifestyle Example**
This involves how to assess your own fitness, health, and wellness. In addition, it requires you to learn to interpret your own self-assessment results. It takes practice to become good at doing self-assessments.	A person wants to know his or her health strengths and weaknesses. The best procedure is to select good tests and self-administer them. Practicing the assessments in this book will help you become good at self-assessment.
Self-Monitoring Skills	**Lifestyle Example**
This involves monitoring behavior and recordkeeping. Many people think they adhere to healthy lifestyles, but they do not. They have a distorted view of what they actually do. Self-monitoring helps give you a true picture of your own behavior and progress.	In spite of restricting calories, a person can't understand why he or she is not losing weight. Keeping records may show that the person is not counting all the calories. Learning to keep records of progress contributes to adherence.
Self-Planning Skills	**Lifestyle Example**
This involves learning how to plan for yourself rather than having others do all the planning for you. Knowledge and practice in planning can help you develop these skills.	A person wants to be more active, to eat better, and to manage stress. Self-planning skills will help him or her plan a personal activity, nutrition, or stress-management program.
Performance Skills	**Lifestyle Example**
This involves learning the skills necessary for performing specific tasks, such as sports or relaxation. These skills can help you feel confident and enjoy activities.	A person avoids physical activity because he or she does not have the physical skills equal to those of peers. Learning sports or other motor skills allows this person to choose to be active, anyway.
Coping Skills	**Lifestyle Example**
This involves developing a new way of thinking about things. With this skill you can see situations in more than one way and learn to think more positively about life situations.	A person is stressed and frequently anxious. Learning stress–management skills, such as relaxation, can help a person cope. Like all skills, stress-management skills must be practiced to be effective.
Consumer Skills	**Lifestyle Example**
This involves gaining knowledge about products and services. It also may require rethinking untrue beliefs that can lead to poor consumer decisions.	A person avoids seeking medical help when sick. Instead, the person takes an unproven remedy. Learning consumer skills provides knowledge for making sound medical decisions.
Time-Management Skills	**Lifestyle Example**
This involves recordkeeping similar to self-monitoring. It relates to total time use rather than monitoring specific behaviors. Skillful monitoring of time can help you plan and adhere to healthy lifestyles.	A person wants more quality time with family and friends. Monitoring time can help him or her reallocate time to spend it in ways that are more consistent with personal priorities.

skills described in this concept and throughout this book can help you plan effectively and achieve success.

Social support from family, peers, and health professionals can also be reinforcing. There are, however, different kinds of support and some are more helpful than others. Support for well-informed personal choices is referred to as support of autonomy. One example is encouragement from family, friends, or a doctor for

Self-Confidence The belief that you can be successful at something (for example, the belief that you can be successful in sports and physical activities and can improve your physical fitness).

Self-Efficacy Confidence that you can perform a specific task (a type of specific self-confidence).

Table 3 ▶ Self-Management Skills for Changing Reinforcing Factors	
Self-Management Skill	**How Is It Useful?**
Social Support	**Lifestyle Example**
This involves learning how to get the support of others for healthy lifestyles. You learn how to get support from family and friends for your autonomous decisions. Support of a doctor can help.	A person has gradually developed a plan to be active. Friends and loved ones encourage activity and help the person develop a schedule that will allow and encourage regular activity.
Relapse Prevention	**Lifestyle Example**
This involves staying with a healthy behavior once you have adopted it. It is sometimes easy to relapse to an unhealthy lifestyle. Skills such as avoiding high-risk situations and learning how to say no can help you avoid relapse.	A person stops smoking. To stay at maintenance, the person can learn to avoid situations where there is pressure to smoke. He or she can learn methods of saying no to those who offer tobacco.

starting and sticking to a nutritious diet. The supporting person might ask, "How can I help you meet your goals?" One goal of this book is to help you take control of your own behaviors concerning your personal health, fitness, and wellness.

Not all feedback is perceived as reinforcing and supportive. Although the people providing the feedback may feel they are being helpful and supportive, some feedback may be perceived as applying pressure or as an attempt to control behavior. Scolding a person for not sticking to a diet, for example, or offering the suggestion that "you are not going to get anywhere if you don't stick to your diet," will often be perceived as applying pressure. If you want to help friends and family make behavior changes, avoid applying pressure and attempt to provide positive forms of support. Research also suggests it is desirable to promote autonomy and freedom of choice so that change is self-directed. Reinforcement can come from families, peers, and health professionals. Table 3 provides lifestyle examples of the key reinforcing factors of social support and relapse prevention.

Self-Management Skills

Learning self-management skills can help you alter factors that lead to healthy lifestyle change. Personal, predisposing, enabling, and reinforcing factors influence the way you live. These factors are of little practical significance, however, unless they can be altered to promote healthy lifestyles. Learning self-management skills (sometimes called self-regulation skills) can help you change the predisposing, enabling, and reinforcing factors described in Tables 1 (page 26), 2 (page 27), and 3. In fact, some of the enabling factors are self-management skills. Learning these skills takes practice, but with effort anyone can learn them. This book offers many opportunities to learn self-management skills. Many of the labs allow you to practice these skills.

It takes time to change unhealthy lifestyles. People in Western cultures are used to seeing things happen quickly. We flip a switch, and the lights come on. We want food quickly, and thousands of fast-food restaurants provide it. The expectation that we should have what we want when we want it has led us to expect instantaneous changes in health, wellness, and fitness. Unfortunately,

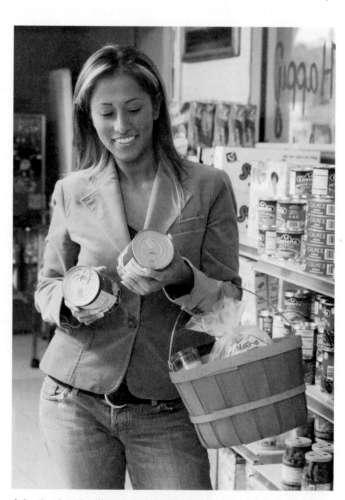

Adapting healthy lifestyle habits requires extra discipline and effort.

there is no quick way to health. There is no pill that can reverse the effects of a lifetime of sedentary living, poor eating, or tobacco use. Changing your lifestyle is the key. But lifestyles that have been practiced for years are not easy to change. As you progress through this book, you will have the opportunity to learn how to implement self-management skills. Learning these skills is the surest way to make permanent lifestyle changes.

Self-Planning for Healthy Lifestyles

Self-planning is a particularly important self-management skill. A goal of this book is to help you develop a personal plan for adopting and maintaining healthy lifestyles, beginning with a six-step self-planning process. In the final concept in this book, after you have studied a variety of concepts and self-management skills, you will have the opportunity to develop a personal plan for several healthy lifestyles. Several self-management skills, including self-assessment, self-monitoring, and goal-setting, are used in the self-planning process (see Table 4).

Step 1: Clarifying Reasons

Clarifying your reasons for behavior change is the first step in program planning. People at precontemplation stage are not considering change in behavior; they see no need. When they reach the contemplation stage, they are considering changes in behavior. One of the most common and most powerful reasons for contemplating a change in a lifestyle is the recommendation of a doctor, often after a visit associated with an illness. Other common reasons are to improve personal appearance, lose weight, increase energy levels, improve the ability to perform daily tasks, and improve quality of life (wellness). Identifying your reasons for wanting to change helps you determine which behaviors you want to change first and helps you establish specific goals. Reflect

Table 4 ▶ Self-Planning Skills

Self-Planning	Description	Self-Management Skill
1. Clarifying reasons	Knowing the general reasons for changing a behavior helps you determine the type of behavior change that is most important for you at a specific point in time. If losing weight is the reason for wanting to change behavior, altering eating and activity patterns will be emphasized.	Results of the Self-Management Skills Questionnaire (Lab 2B) will help you determine which self-management skills you use regularly and the ones you might need to develop.
2. Identifying needs	If you know your strengths and weaknesses, you can plan to build on your strengths and overcome weaknesses.	Self-assessment: In the concepts that follow, you will learn how to assess different health, wellness, and fitness characteristics. Learning these self-assessments will help you identify needs.
3. Setting personal goals	Goals are more specific than reasons (see step 1). Establishing specific things that you want to accomplish can provide a basis for feedback that your program is working.	Goal setting: Guidelines in this concept will help you set goals. In subsequent concepts, you will establish goals for different lifestyles.
4. Selecting program components	A personal plan should include the specific program components that will meet your needs and goals based on steps 1–3. Examples include meal plans for nutrition and specific activities for your physical activity plan.	Many self-management skills, including time management, consumer, and performance skills, are useful in developing plans for a variety of healthy behaviors.
5. Writing your plan	Once program components, such as meal plans for nutrition and specific activities for physical activity, have been determined, you should put your plan in writing. This establishes your intentions and increases your chances of adherence.	Self-planning: This includes writing down the time of day, day of the week, and other details you will include in your plan.
6. Evaluating progress	Once you have used your plan, you will know what works and what does not. Periodic self-assessments can help you modify the plan to make it better.	Self-monitoring: This skill is used in keeping records (logs) and determining if goals are met. Self-assessment: This skill is used to help you determine if goals are met.

on your reasons for wanting to make lifestyle changes before moving on to step 2.

Step 2: Identifying Needs

Self-assessments are useful in establishing personal needs, planning your program, and evaluating your progress. You have already done some self-assessments of wellness, current activity levels, and current lifestyles. In the labs for this concept and others that follow, you will make additional assessments. The results of these assessments help you build personal profiles for a variety of health behaviors that can be used as the basis for program planning. With practice, self-assessments become more accurate. For this reason, it is important to repeat self-assessments and to pay careful attention to the procedures for performing them. If questions arise, get a professional opinion rather than making an error.

Periodic self-assessments can help determine if you are meeting health, wellness, and fitness standards and making progress toward personal health goals. When performed properly, self-assessments help you determine if you have met your goals and if you are meeting health standards (e.g., meeting health fitness standards, eating appropriate amounts of nutrients). Self-assessments also provide a measure of independence and can help you avoid unnecessary and expensive tests. Because self-assessments may not be as accurate as tests by health and medical professionals, it is wise to have periodic tests by an expert to see if your self-assessments are accurate. In some cases, your self-assessments may be used as a type of screening procedure to determine if you need professional assistance. In the final concept in this book, you will have an opportunity to use the many self-assessments you have learned to build a health, wellness, and fitness profile.

Self-assessments have the advantage of consistent error rather than variable error. The best type of assessments are done by highly qualified experts using precise instruments. Eliminating error is always desirable. Following directions and practicing assessment techniques will reduce error significantly. Still, errors will occur. One advantage of a self-assessment is that the person doing the assessment is always the same—you. Even if you make an error in a self-assessment, it is likely to be consistent over time, especially if you use the same equipment each time you make the assessment. For example, scales have limitations for monitoring changes in weight (and fat). But if you measure your own weight using a home scale and your measurement always shows your

weight to be 2 pounds higher than it really is, you have made a consistent error. You can determine if you are improving because you know the error exists. Variable errors are likely when different instruments are used, when different people make the assessments, and when procedures vary from test to test. Differences in scores are harder to explain with variable forms of error because they are not consistent.

Step 3: Setting Personal Goals

Learning to set realistic goals is useful as a basis for self-planning. If any lifestyle change is to be of value, you need to determine—ahead of time—what you hope to accomplish. Goals are objectives that you hope to accomplish as a result of lifestyle changes. They have several important characteristics, which you can remember using the acronym SMART. They should be specific (S). Many individuals make the mistake of setting vague goals, such as "be more active" or "eat less." These are not goals, but the reasons you want to set goals. A specific goal provides details, such as limiting calories to a specific number each day. Goals should be measurable (M). You need to perform assessments before establishing goals and again after a lifestyle change is made to see if you met the goals. Goals should also be attainable (A), neither too hard nor too easy. If the goal is too hard, failure is likely. Failure is discouraging. If the goal is too easy, it is not challenging. Goals should be relevant (R) to you, since they are your personal goals. Personally relevant goals provide motivation. Finally, a goal should be timely (T). Timely goals are especially relevant to you at the present time. If you set too many goals, you may not reach any of them. Choosing goals that are timely helps you focus on the most salient lifestyles or behaviors.

Beginners are encouraged to focus on short-term goals. Realistic **short-term goals**—goals that you can accomplish in days or weeks—make you successful because one success leads to another. Once you meet short-term goals, establish new ones. **Long-term goals** take a long time to accomplish—months to years—and may be discouraging to beginners. After a series of short-term goals have been successfully accomplished, set long-term goals. In fact, setting and achieving a series of short-term goals is the best way to achieve long-term goals.

Short-term goals should be behavioral goals rather than outcome goals. A **behavioral goal** is associated with something you do. An example of a specific short-term behavioral goal is "to perform 30 minutes of brisk

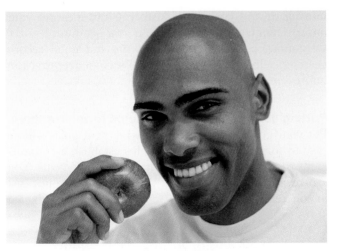

A goal to consume more fruits and vegetables is an example of a behavioral goal.

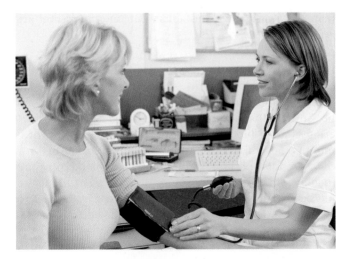

Reducing blood pressure is an example of an outcome goal.

walking 6 days a week for the next 2 weeks." It is a behavioral goal because it refers to a behavior (something you do). It is a SMART goal because it is specific, measurable, attainable, realistic, and timely. The principal factor associated with success is your willingness to give effort. No matter who you are, you can accomplish this behavioral goal if you give a daily effort. In addition, behavioral goals are easy to self-monitor. Keeping an activity log of your weekly participation in brisk walking will help you comply with the walking goal.

An **outcome goal** is associated with a physical characteristic (e.g., lowering your body weight or lowering your blood pressure) or something that you can do (e.g., perform 10 push-ups or perform CPR). Outcome goals are not recommended for beginners.

- *Typically, it takes weeks or months to reach outcome goals.* For this reason, short-term fitness goals are not recommended for beginners because they are often not achieved in the designated time, resulting in a perception of failure.
- *Outcome goals depend on many things other than your lifestyle behavior.* For example, your heredity affects your body fat and muscle development. Setting a goal of achieving a certain percentage of body fat or lifting a certain weight is influenced by heredity as well as your physical activity program. This makes it hard for beginners to set realistic goals. Too often the tendency is to set the goal based on a comparative standard rather than on a standard that is possible for the individual to achieve in a short time. As you become more experienced, you learn to set more realistic outcome goals and learn that these goals often take time to achieve.
- *Different people progress at different rates.* The same lifestyle change program may produce different results

for different people. For this reason, goals, especially outcome goals, must vary from person to person. For example, two people may establish an outcome goal of losing 5 pounds over a 6-week period. Because we inherit predispositions to body composition, one person may meet the goal, while another may not, even if both strictly adhere to the same diet.

A similar example can be used for fitness and physical activity. People not only inherit a predisposition to fitness but also inherit a predisposition to benefit from training. In other words, if 10 people do the same physical activities, there will be 10 different results. One person may improve performance by 60 percent, while another might improve only 10 percent. Experience will

Short-Term Goals Statements of intent to change a behavior or achieve an outcome in a period of days or weeks.

Long-Term Goals Statements of intent to change behavior or achieve a specific outcome in a period of months or years.

Behavioral Goal A statement of intent to perform a specific behavior (changing a lifestyle) for a specific period of time. An example is "I will walk for 15 minutes each morning before work."

Outcome Goal A statement of intent to achieve a specific test score (attainment of a specific standard) associated with good health, wellness, or fitness. An example is "I will lower my body fat by 3 percent."

help you learn how to establish outcome goals that are realistic for you.

Long-term goals can be either behavioral or outcome goals. Long-term goals can be either outcome or behavioral. For example, a person who has high blood pressure (160 systolic) may set an outcome goal of lowering systolic blood pressure to 120 over a period of 6 months. Several behavioral goals can be established for the 6-month period, including taking blood pressure medication (daily), performing 30 minutes of moderate physical activity each day, and limiting salt in the diet to less than 100 percent of the recommended dietary allowance. If the outcome goal is realistic, adhering to the behavioral goals will result in achieving the outcome goal.

Maintenance goals are also appropriate once goals have been achieved or when improvements aren't necessary. For example, the person who lowers systolic blood pressure from 160 to 120 need not continue to lower the new healthy blood pressure. Once a healthy outcome goal has been achieved, a new outcome goal of maintaining a systolic blood pressure of 120 is appropriate. Behavioral goals will also have to be modified. For the person who has reduced blood pressure to a healthy level, medication levels might be reduced for maintenance.

Maintenance goals are appropriate in other areas as well. For example, dietary restriction and extra exercise for weight maintenance will likely be different from those for losing weight. When a person reaches a healthy level of fitness, maintenance may be the goal rather than continued improvement. You cannot improve forever; at some point, attempting to do so may be counterproductive to health.

Making improvement can motivate you to reach long-term goals. As noted earlier, setting short-term goals that are both attainable and realistic will help you reach your long-term goals. Meeting short-term goals encourages and motivates you to continue with your healthy lifestyle plan. Don't expect to set perfect goals all the time. No matter how much self-assessing and self-monitoring you do, you may sometimes set goals too low or too high. If the goal is set too low, it is easily achieved, and a new, higher goal can be established. If the goal is set too high, you may fail to reach it, even though you have made considerable progress toward the goal.

Rather than becoming discouraged when a goal is not met, consider the improvement you have made. Improvement, no matter how small, means that you are

moving toward your goal. Also, you can measure your improvement and use it to help you set future goals. Of course, periodic self-assessments and good record keeping (self-monitoring) are necessary to keep track of improvements accurately.

Putting your goals in writing helps formalize them. Put your goals in writing. Otherwise, your goals will be easy to forget. Writing them helps establish a commitment to yourself and clearly establishes your goals. You can revise them if necessary. Written goals are not cast in concrete.

Step 4: Selecting Program Components

You can choose from many different program components to meet your goals. Many different components can be included in a lifestyle change program. Concept 1 described 10 types of lifestyle change (see Figure 7, page 10), ranging from priority lifestyles (physical activity, nutrition, and stress management) to avoiding destructive habits and adopting positive safety and personal health habits. The components depend on the goals of your program. For example, if the goal is to become more fit and physically active, the program components will be the activities you choose. You will want to identify activities that match your abilities and that you enjoy. You will want to select activities that build the type of fitness you want to improve.

Technology Update
Health Apps for Smart Phones

TECH   The rapid changes in cell phone technology have allowed phones to essentially take over the market for what used to be called "Personal Digital Assistants" (PDAs). The advances have opened up a huge new market for customized applications (apps) that are designed to run on these platforms. These tools have greatly expanded the capabilities and functionality of cell phones—allowing them to more fully realize the original vision of PDAs. Hundreds of software applications (apps) are now available to help people manage and organize their lifestyle, including many designed to promote good health. These tools can be useful for self-monitoring, an important self-management skill discussed in this concept. More information on a variety of health, fitness, and wellness apps is available at the associated Web link.

Other examples of program components are preparing menus for healthy eating, participating in stress-management activities, planning to attend meetings to help avoid destructive habits, and attending a series of classes to learn CPR and first aid. Preparing a list of program components that will help you meet your specific goals will prepare you for step 5, writing your plan.

Step 5: Writing Your Plan

Preparing a written plan can improve your adherence to the plan. A written plan is a pledge, or a promise, to be active. Research shows that intentions to be active are more likely to be acted on when put in writing. In the concepts that follow, you will be given the opportunity to prepare written plans for all of the activities in the physical activity pyramid, as well as for other healthy lifestyles. A good written plan includes daily plans with scheduled times and other program details. For example, the daily written plan for stress management could include the time of day when specific program activities are conducted (e.g., 15-minute quiet time at noon, yoga class from 5:30 to 6:30). An activity plan would include a schedule of the activities for each day of the week, including starting and finishing time and specific details concerning the activities to be performed. A dietary plan would include specific menus for each meal and between-meal snacks.

In the labs that accompany the final concept of this book, you will write plans for several different lifestyles. By then you will have learned a variety of self-management skills that will assist you.

Step 6: Evaluating Progress

 Self-assessment and self-monitoring can help you evaluate progress. Once FEATURE 4 you have written a plan, you will want to determine your effectiveness in sticking with your plan. Keeping written records is one type of self-monitoring.

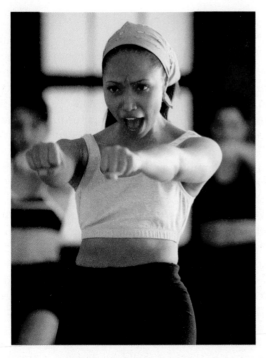

Self-planning can help you implement a variety of changes to enhance health, wellness, and fitness.

Self-monitoring is a good way to assess success in meeting behavioral goals. Keeping a dietary log or using a pedometer to keep track of steps are examples of self-monitoring. Self-assessments are a good way to see if you have met outcome goals.

Throughout this book, you will learn to self-assess a variety of outcomes (e.g., fitness, body fatness) and self-monitor behaviors (e.g., diet, physical activities, stress-management activities). In step 2 in program planning, you used self-assessments to determine your needs and to help you plan your goals (step 3). Once you have tried your program, you can use the same self-assessments and self-monitoring strategies to evaluate the effectiveness of your program. You can see if you have met the goals you established for yourself.

▶▶ Strategies for Action

To be effective, self-management and self-planning skills require a commitment to make changes in lifestyle. As indicated in Figure 1, change occurs stage by stage, and an individual is likely to be at different stages for different health behaviors. For example, a person may be at the maintenance stage for physical activity but at the contemplation stage for adopting sound nutrition practices. In this book, many self-management skills are described for use in progressing from one stage to another. Different skills are important, depending on your current stage and the lifestyle behavior you are attempting to change.

No matter how well you learn self-management skills, they will not be effective in moving you from one stage to another if you do not make a commitment to change. A commitment, a personal pledge or promise to change a behavior, is most effective if you write it down and make the commitment known to another person.

In this book, you will learn to use self-management and self-planning skills to change several physical activity behaviors (lifestyle physical activity, active aerobic, active sports and recreation, flexibility exercises, and muscle fitness exercises), nutrition behaviors, and stress-management behaviors. You can also use these skills to make other changes to improve health, wellness, and fitness, as outlined in Concept 1 (modify the environment, including the vocational environment; use the health-care system effectively; and effectively modify personal actions, interactions, and cognitions).

As you study each concept, you will have the opportunity to make plans for specific behavior change related to each topic of study. It is important that you learn to plan for each type of change, but it is unrealistic to expect that you can change all behaviors in the time you will spend in one class using this book. It is hoped that you will learn the planning process, so that by the time you reach the last concept of this text, you can begin the "process of change" for the specific healthful behaviors that you deem most important. Over time (most likely longer than you will spend in this class), you can make all of the behavior changes to which you are committed.

It takes time to make changes in lifestyle. Change does not occur overnight. It takes time. A commitment to use self-management skills to change "one behavior at a time" is more effective than trying to do "a total makeover" all at once.

The lab worksheets that accompany each concept will help you learn the self-assessment, self-management, and self-planning skills necessary for behavior change. Self-assessments of current health, wellness, and fitness status, as well as self-monitoring of your current lifestyle, can help you determine your reasons for making change and help you establish SMART goals for change. Like all skills, practice is necessary to improve self-management skills. Table 5 refers you to labs in the

Table 5 ▶ Opportunities for Learning Self-Management Skills	
Self-Management Skill	**Lab Number**
Overcoming barriers	6B, 15A, 17A, 24B
Building self-confidence and motivation	2A, 2B
Balancing attitudes	1A, 2A, 2B, 3C, 8A, 19B
Building knowledge and beliefs	1A, 4A, 7A, 12B, 14A, 15A, 15B, 18A, 18B, 19A, 19B, 20A, 21A, 22A, 22B, 23A, 23B
Goal setting	6A, 8B, 9B, 10C, 10D, 11C, 14B, 24B, 24C
Self-assessment	1A, 2A, 3A, 3C, 4A, 5A, 5B, 6B, 7B, 8A, 9A, 10A, 10B, 10D, 11A, 11B, 12A, 12B, 13A, 13B, 13C, 14A, 15B, 16A, 16B, 22A, 22B, 23B, 24A, 24B, 24C
Self-monitoring	2A, 5A, 6A, 7A, 8A, 8B, 9B, 10C, 11C, 17A, 17D, 19A, 22B, 24B, 24C
Self-planning	6A, 8B, 9B, 10C, 10D, 11C, 14B, 24B, 24C
Performance skills	3B, 12A, 17C
Adopting coping skills	16A, 16B, 17A, 17B, 17C, 17D
Learning consumer skills	14B, 15A, 18A, 20A, 23A, 23B, 24B, 24C
Managing time	17A
Finding social support	17D
Preventing relapse	15A, 19B, 24B, 24C

text designed to enhance specific self-management skills.

Many people can benefit from a new way of thinking about health, wellness, and fitness. Many people have unrealistic expectations about health and fitness. They compare their fitness with that of athletes and their appearance with that of models and movie stars, often setting standards for themselves that are impossible to achieve. Some say, "I could never do that," when considering becoming physically active, altering eating patterns, or learning to manage stress. Many lack information about what is really possible concerning healthy lifestyles. Those who feel a lack of control set unrealistic standards for themselves and lack confidence in their own abilities to change.

Adopting a new way of thinking can have dramatic implications. A major purpose of this text is to help you adopt a new way of thinking toward health behaviors. This new way of thinking acknowledges that you have some control over many of the factors that influence health, wellness, and fitness. Learning and practicing self-management skills can help you develop this new way of thinking.

Assessing self-management skills that influence healthy lifestyles provides a basis for changing your health, wellness, or fitness. Self-assessments of your current health, wellness, and fitness status, as well as self-monitoring of your current lifestyles, can help you determine your reasons and establish reasonable goals for healthy lifestyle change. The Healthy Lifestyle Questionnaire and the Wellness Self-Perceptions Questionnaire you took in Concept 1 got you started. In this concept you can use the Stage of Change Questionnaire (Lab 2A) to help you decide which lifestyles you might need to

modify. You can use the Self-Management Skills Questionnaire (Lab 2B) to determine which self-management skills you may need to improve to help you make effective changes in your lifestyles. In later concepts, you will have the opportunity to make self-assessments for a variety of lifestyles.

Public Opinions about Health, Wellness, and Fitness

Many organizations, both profit and nonprofit, regularly poll Americans concerning their health, wellness, and fitness, as well as their attitudes about these subjects. Among the most well known are polls by CBS/New York Times, USA Today/CNN/Gallup, NBC/Washington Post, and Trust for America's Health/Robert Woods Johnson Foundation. Some results of surveys by the various polls include the following:

- 76 percent of Americans favor increasing funding for prevention programs.
- 77 percent believe that prevention programs will save money over the long run.
- 72 percent want more investment in prevention, even if it does not save money, because it will prevent disease and save lives.
- 57 percent want to invest in prevention, even if money is not saved, if it improves quality of life (wellness).

More information from various polls is available at the associated Web link.

Web Resources

Additional websites with information related to Concept 2 are available at the associated Web link.

ACSM's Fit Society Page
www.acsm.org/health+fitness/ fit_society.htm

ACSM's *Health and Fitness Journal* www.acsm.org /publications/health_fitness_journal.htm

American Heart Association Health and Fitness Center www.justmove.org

American Red Cross www.redcross.org

Centers for Disease Control and Prevention (overcoming barriers) www.cdc.gov/nccdphp/dnpa/physical/life /overcome.htm

Healthy People 2020 www.healthypeople.gov/HP2020

National Heart Lung and Blood Institute—Health Behavior Change www.nhlbi.nih.gov/health/public/heart/obesity /lose_wt/behavior.htm

Robert Woods Johnson Foundation www.rwjf.org

SMART goals www.projectsmart.co.uk/smart-goals.html

Trust for America's Health—BluePrint for Healthier America http://healthyamericans.org/report/55/blueprint-for -healthier-america

Well-Being Index—Gallup Poll www.gallup.com/poll/wellbeing.aspx

Suggested Readings

Selected readings and references are listed below. A more comprehensive list is available at the associated Web link.

Glantz, K., B. K. Rimer, and K. Viswanath (eds.). 2008. *Health Behavior and Health Education.* 4th ed. San Francisco: John Wiley and Sons.

Marcus, B. E., and L. Forsyth. 2009. *Motivating People to Be Physically Active.* 2nd ed. Champaign, IL: Human Kinetics.

Pekmezi, D., et al. 2010. Using the transtheoretical model to promote physical activity. *ACSM's Health and Fitness Journal* 14(4):8–13.

Sullivan, G. S. and J. P. Strode. 2010. Motivation through goal setting: A self-determined perspective. *Strategies* 23(6):19–23.

Taylor, S. E. 2008. *Health Psychology.* 7th ed. New York: McGraw-Hill Higher Education.

White, S. M., E. L. Mailey, and E. McAuley. 2010. Leading a physically active lifestyle: Effective individual behavior change strategy. *ACSM's Health and Fitness Journal* 14(1):8–15.

Preparing for Physical Activity

Health Objectives for the Year 2020

- Increase percentage of adolescents and adults who meet national guidelines for aerobic and muscle fitness activities.
- Reduce percentage of population who do no leisure-time activity.
- Increase percentage of population who have access to exercise facilities and programs at work and in schools.
- Increase percentage of people who walk and bike.
- Increase percentage of physicians who counsel or educate patients about exercise.
- Promote quality of life, healthy development, and healthy behaviors (including being active) across all stages of life.
- Reduce sports and recreation injuries.
- Reduce injuries from overexertion.

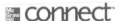 **connect**

|FITNESS AND WELLNESS http://connect.mcgraw-hill.com

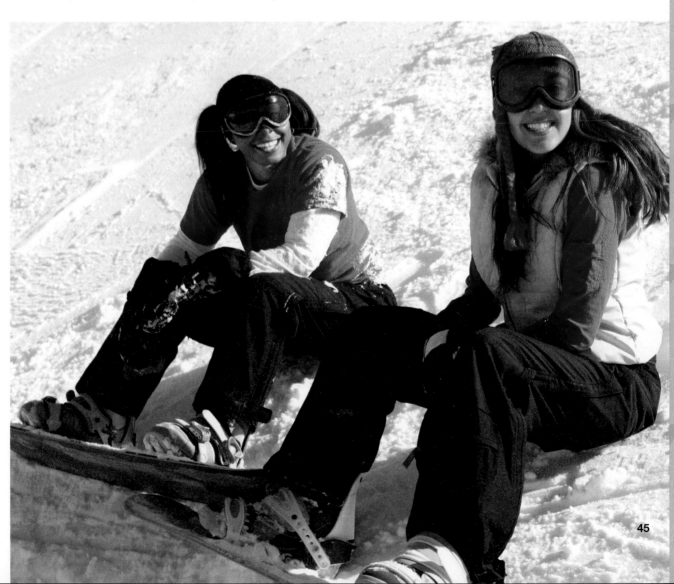

Proper preparation can help make physical activity enjoyable, effective, and safe.

For people just beginning a physical activity program, adequate preparation may be the key to persistence. For those who have been regularly active for some time, sound preparation can help reduce risk of injury and make activity more enjoyable. It is hoped that a person armed with good information about preparation will become involved and stay involved in physical activity for a lifetime. For long-term maintenance, physical activity must be something that is a part of a person's normal lifestyle. Some factors that will help you prepare for and make physical activity a part of your normal routine are presented in this concept.

Factors to Consider Prior to Physical Activity

(i) FEATURE 1 **Screening before beginning regular physical activity is important to establish medical readiness.** The most recent guidelines for exercise testing and prescription of the American College of Sports Medicine (ACSM) suggest that there are two types of pre-participation screening: self-guided screening and professionally guided screening. For self-guided screening, the ACSM endorses the basic recommendation of the Surgeon General's Report on Physical Activity and Health, that "previously inactive men over age of 40 and women over age 50, and people at high risk of cardiovascular disease (CVD) should first consult a physician before embarking on a program to which they are unaccustomed."

An alternative method of self-screening involves the use of the Physical Activity Readiness Questionnaire (**PAR-Q**). This seven-item questionnaire was designed

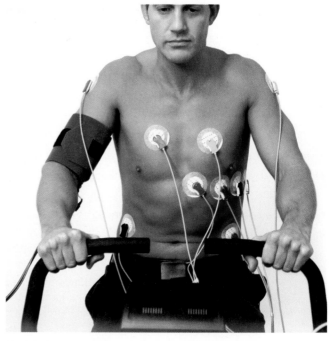

A clinical exercise test is recommended for some individuals to ensure they can exercise safely.

by the British Columbia (Canada) Ministry of Health to help people to know when it is advisable to seek medical consultation prior to beginning or altering an exercise program. The goal is to prevent unnecessary medical examinations while helping people to be reasonably assured that regular moderate physical activity is appropriate. Other self-administered surveys recommended by the ACSM include those given at a physician's office or those administered by certified health and fitness professionals (e.g., AHA/ACSM Pre-participation Screening Questionnaire). If a pre-participation questionnaire indicates the need, medical clearance is recommended. A **clinical exercise test** may also be appropriate. Those who do not identify health concerns using a self-screening questionnaire (e.g., all "no" answers on the PAR-Q) typically are cleared for moderate self-planned activity programs. For more vigorous exercise and sports, additional screening may be appropriate.

ACSM has developed additional guidelines to standardize professionally guided screening (e.g., assessments conducted by a medical doctor or certified health/fitness professional). As noted in Table 1, the ACSM divides people into three general risk categories: low, moderate, and high risk. Some of the risk factors used to identify risk categories are identifiable without professional consultation (e.g., age, family history, smoking, sedentary lifestyle),

HELP   Health is available to Everyone for a Lifetime, and it's **PERSONAL**

According to the Mayo Clinic and many other health authorities, it's best to check with your doctor before starting a new exercise program if you have previously been inactive and especially if you have certain health conditions—for example, if you have asthma, diabetes, arthritis, an untreated joint or muscle injury, or if you are overweight or obese.

Have you ever spoken to your doctor about exercise and the healthy (or not so healthy) changes you've made in your lifestyle behaviors?

Table 1 ▶ American College of Sports Medicine Risk Stratification Categories and Criteria

Stratification Category	Criteria
Low risk	People who have no heart disease symptoms and have no more than one of the risk factors listed below
Moderate risk	People without heart disease symptoms who have two or more of the risk factors listed below
High risk	People with known pulmonary or metabolic disease, OR one or more signs or symptoms in the list below

Risk Factors

Family history of heart disease; smoker; high blood pressure (hypertension); high cholesterol; abnormal blood glucose levels; obesity (high BMI, excess waist girth); sedentary lifestyle; low HDL cholesterol level; men age 45 or older; women age 55 or older

Signs and Symptoms

Chest, neck, or jaw pain from lack of oxygen to the heart; shortness of breath at rest or in mild exercise; dizziness or fainting; difficult or labored breathing when lying, sitting, or standing; ankle swelling; fast heartbeat or heart palpitations; pain in the legs from poor circulation; heart murmur; unusual fatigue or shortness of breath with usual activities

Source: American College of Sports Medicine.

Table 2 ▶ Selecting Appropriate Clothing for Activity

General Guidelines

- Avoid clothing that is too tight or that restricts movement.
- Material in contact with skin should be porous.
- Clothing should protect against wind and rain but allow for heat loss and evaporation—e.g., Gortex, Coolmax.
- Wear layers so that a layer can be removed if not needed.
- Wear socks for most activities to prevent blisters, abrasions, odor, and excessive shoe wear.
- Socks should be absorbent and fit properly.
- Do not use nonporous clothing that traps sweat to lose weight; these garments prevent evaporation and cooling.

Special Considerations

- Women should wear an exercise bra for support.
- Men should consider an athletic supporter for support.
- Wear helmets and padding for activities with risk of falling, such as biking or inline skating.
- Wear reflective clothing for night activities.
- Wear water shoes for some aquatic activities.
- Consider lace-up ankle braces to prevent injury.
- Consider a mouthpiece for basketball and other contact sports.

while others may require professional screening (e.g., blood cholesterol, blood glucose). Low-risk people who are apparently healthy are typically cleared for moderate and many forms of vigorous activity without a medical exam or an exercise test. Those with moderate risk can participate in low to moderate activity without a medical exam or exercise test; however, both are recommended before initiating vigorous programs. For those in the high-risk category, a comprehensive medical exam is necessary before starting either a moderate or high-intensity program and before taking an exercise test. For those just beginning a program or those resuming physical activity after an injury or illness, consultation with a physician is always wise, no matter what your age or medical condition.

Consideration should also be given to altering exercise patterns if you have an illness or a temporary sickness, such as a cold or the flu. The immune system and other body systems may be weaker at this time, and medicines (even over-the-counter ones) may alter responses to exercise. It is best to work back gradually to your normal routine after illness.

There is no way to be absolutely sure that you are medically sound to begin a physical activity program. Even a thorough exam by a physician cannot guarantee that a person does not have some limitations that may cause a problem during exercise. Use of the PAR-Q (see Lab 3A) and adherence to the ACSM guidelines

are advised to help minimize the risk while preventing unnecessary medical cost. However, if you are unsure about your readiness for activity, a medical exam and a clinical exercise test are the surest ways to make certain that you are ready to participate.

It is important to dress properly for physical activity. Clothing should be appropriate for the type of activity being performed and the conditions in which you are participating. As with shoes, comfort is a much more important consideration than looks. Table 2 provides guidelines for dressing for activity.

Shoes are an important consideration for safe and effective exercise. Decisions about shoes should be based on intended use (e.g., running, tennis), shoe and foot characteristics, and comfort rather than looks or cosmetics. Shoes are designed for specific activities and comfort, and performance will typically be best if you select and use them for their intended purpose. Hybrid shoes, known as "cross-trainers," can be a versatile option, but they typically don't provide the needed

PAR-Q An acronym for Physical Activity Readiness Questionnaire; designed to help determine if you are medically suited to begin an exercise program.

Clinical Exercise Test A test, typically administered on a treadmill, in which exercise is gradually increased in intensity while the heart is monitored by an EKG. Symptoms not present at rest, such as an abnormal EKG, may be present in an exercise test.

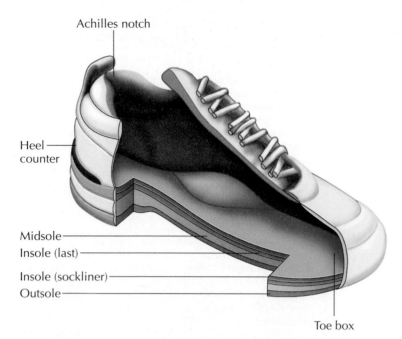

Achilles notch

Heel counter

Midsole
Insole (last)
Insole (sockliner)
Outsole

Toe box

Achilles notch: Protects tendon

Arch support: Supports arch; height and shape of arch should vary with foot characteristics

Heel counter: Provides movement control; a stiff counter helps with pronation (toes turn in) but can cause problems for those who do not pronate

Insole (last): Refers to shoe shape; curved (more flexible for those with rigid arches who pronate), straight (good for heavier or flat-footed people), or semicurved (moderate flexibility and stability)

Insole (sockliner): Removable layer for additional shock and sweat absorption; can be replaced periodically and/or customized

Material: Light, porous materials that can breathe are recommended

Midsole: Provides cushion, stability, and motion control; important for shock absorption

Outsole: Provides traction; determines shoe flexibility; type depends on intended purpose of shoe

Toe box: Should have adequate height to wiggle toes and prevent rubbing on top of toes and adequate length so toes do not contact front of shoe

Figure 1 ▶ Anatomy of an activity shoe.

features for specific activities. For example, they may lack the cushioning and support needed for running and the ankle support for activities such as basketball. Features of common activity shoes are highlighted in Figure 1.

Most shoes have very thin sockliners, but supplemental inserts can be purchased to provide more cushioning and support. Custom orthotics can also be used to correct alignment problems or minimize foot injuries (e.g., plantar fasciitis). A very important, and frequently neglected, consideration is to replace shoes after extended use. Runners typically replace shoes every 4 to 6 months (or 400 to 600 miles), even if the outer appearance of the

shoe is still good. The main functions of athletic shoes are to reduce shock from impact and protect the foot—one of the best prevention strategies for avoiding injuries is to replace your shoes on a regular basis.

It is important to keep up with advancing technology in shoes and sports equipment. Recently, two new innovations in running shoes were introduced. The first innovation is a shoe with an "all-air" sole. A "partial-air" sole has been used for several years. This feature eliminated foam from the outsole but had a midsole that included ¼ inch of foam. The Nike 360 is the first to eliminate foam completely. The shoe is lighter and uses a pocket of air from the heel to the front of the shoe based on relative need for cushioning in various parts of the shoe. The second innovation is the "smart shoe." This new shoe, made by Adidas, uses a small computer chip to automatically adjust for the runner's body weight, changes in stride caused by fatigue, terrain, and pace. The processor is lightweight but does add weight to the shoe because a battery is required. It is too early to tell how these technologies will shape the athletic shoe market. Other new shoe technologies, including running shoes containing computer chips, are described in detail in the Technology Update box.

Factors to Consider during Daily Physical Activity

There are three components of the daily activity program: the warm-up, the workout, and the cool-down. The key component of a fitness program is the daily workout. Experts agree, however, that the workout should be preceded by a warm-up and followed by a cool-down. The warm-up prepares the body for physical activity, and the cool-down returns the body to rest and

Technology Update
High-Tech Sneakers

TECH   Recently, manufacturers have made technical innovations that allow shoes to provide interesting functions. Nike and Apple have joined together to develop special shoes with sensors and a wireless system that allow the shoes to track distance and speed of running, as well as calories burned. Another company has developed shoes embedded with a global positioning system (GPS) so that the location of the runner can be determined at any time. More information is available online.

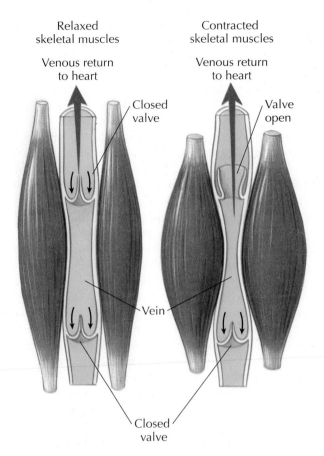

Relaxed
skeletal muscles

Venous return
to heart

Contracted
skeletal muscles

Venous return
to heart

Closed
valve

Valve
open

Vein

Closed
valve

Figure 2 ▶ Muscle contractions aid the veins in returning blood to the heart.

promotes effective recovery by aiding the return of blood from the working muscles to the heart (see Figure 2).

(i) **A warm-up is recommended prior to exercise.** The traditional **warm-up** has two

FEATURE 2 components. The first is a general aerobic and muscular endurance warm-up, and the second is a stretch warm-up. The ACSM recommends a minimum of 5 to 10 minutes of low to moderate aerobic and muscular endurance activity such as walking, slow jogging, slow swimming, slow biking, or in sports, an activity such as a layup drill in basketball. This first phase of the warm-up is intended to prepare the heart, blood vessels, muscles, and other bodily systems for more vigorous activity to follow. The ACSM indicates that the general warm-up increases body temperature and reduces the potential for after-exercise muscle soreness and stiffness, as well as allowing the body to adapt to the demand of the workout that follows. This general warm-up also decreases the risk of irregular heartbeats associated with poor coronary circulation. For those who plan moderate activities for their workout (e.g., walk, bike ride, swim), no special general warm-up is necessary since the activity itself is light to moderate in nature. Starting at a slower pace and gradually increasing intensity is recommended.

The second phase of the warm-up involves stretching the major large muscle groups, especially the muscle groups most likely to be involved in the workout that

follows. It has long been held that the stretch warm-up reduces the risk of injury, reduces the risk of delayed onset soreness, and enhances performance in sports and during a workout. Although there is little evidence that the stretch warm-up reduces delayed soreness, the evidence is mixed concerning the benefits of the stretching warm-up for injury prevention. A stretch warm-up is most likely to be beneficial to those who perform activities such as diving, gymnastics, and other similar events that require extensive range of motion. There is little evidence to indicate that stretch warm-up reduces injury in steady aerobic activities such as jogging and biking.

Evidence is also mixed concerning the effects of a stretch warm-up on performance. Some studies suggest that stretching can result in improved performance, while others suggest that strength, muscular endurance, and power performances may be decreased as a result of a static stretch warm-up. The type of warm-up appears to be a factor. Those interested in high-level performance (e.g., movements requiring great force, and fast movements) may choose a dynamic stretching warm-up that simulates the types of movements to be used in the vigorous phase of the workout or event. More details concerning dynamic stretching are provided in the concepts on flexibility (10) and performance (12).

The stretching warm-up is not intended to substitute for a regular program of stretching to build flexibility. A stretch warm-up has little immediate effect on the length of muscles and range of motion (flexibility). In other words, if you have not trained regularly to build flexibility, a warm-up will not make you flexible. Still, many recreational exercisers, who are not focused on high-level performance, may choose to do a static stretch warm-up with no negative effects and with some possible benefit. The stretch warm-up included in Lab 3B is appropriate. The ACSM recommends at least 10 minutes of stretching to increase range of movement and indicates that it can be done after the general warm-up or after the cool-down phase described later in this concept. To be effective as a complete flexibility program, the warm-up provided in Lab 3B would need to be personalized and include additional or exercises from Concept 10.

The workout is the principal component of an activity program and occurs after the warm-up and before the cool-down. The **workout**, also referred

Warm-Up Light to moderate physical activity performed before a more vigorous workout, including a general aerobic/ muscular endurance warm-up and often a stretch warm-up.

Workout The component of a total physical activity program designed to produce health, wellness, fitness, and other benefits using appropriate amounts of different types of physical activity.

to as the conditioning phase of a training session, is the component of the physical activity program that is designed to provide health and other benefits, depending on the type of activity performed (see Concept 4). Workout information, including appropriate frequency, intensity, and length of time for many types of physical activities in the physical activity pyramid (Concept 5), is included in subsequent concepts.

A cool-down after the workout promotes an effective recovery from physical activity. The ACSM recommends a 5- to 10-minute **cool-down** similar to the general warm-up (e.g., light to moderate activity) after a vigorous workout. In addition to helping reduce metabolic by-products, the general cool-down helps the cardiovascular system (heart rate and blood pressure) return to a normal state.

During physical activity, the heart pumps a large amount of blood to supply the working muscles with the oxygen necessary to keep moving. The muscles squeeze the veins (see Figure 2), which forces the blood back to the heart. Valves in the veins prevent the blood from flowing backward. As long as exercise continues, muscles move the blood back to the heart, where it is once again pumped to the body. If exercise is stopped abruptly, the blood is left in the area of the working muscles and has no way to get back to the heart. In the case of a runner, the blood pools in the legs. Because the heart has less blood to pump, blood pressure may drop. This can result in dizziness and can even cause a person to pass out. The best way to prevent this problem is to slow down gradually after exercise and keep moving until blood pressure and heart rate have returned to near resting values. This phase is especially important for those with cardiovascular risk factors or disease.

The cool-down can also include a stretching phase. The ACSM indicates that the 10-plus minutes recommended for stretching can be performed after the workout or after the general warm-up. Stretching the muscles after the workout can help relieve muscle spasms in fatigued muscles, and stretching is more effective in building flexibility when the muscles are warm. To be effective, as a complete flexibility program, stretching performed in a cool-down would need to be personalized and include exercises for all muscle groups (see Concept 10).

Physical Activity in the Heat and Cold

(i) FEATURE 3 **Physical activity in hot and humid environments challenges the body's heat loss mechanisms.** During vigorous activity, the body produces heat, which must be dissipated to regulate body temperature. The body has several ways to dissipate heat. *Conduction* is the transfer of heat from a hot body to a cold body. *Convection* is the transfer of heat

through the air or any other medium. Fans and wind can facilitate heat loss by convection and help regulate temperature. The primary method of cooling is through *evaporation* of sweat. The chemical process involved in evaporation transfers heat from the body and reduces the body temperature. When conditions are humid, the effectiveness of evaporation is reduced, since the air is already saturated with moisture. This is why it is difficult to regulate body temperature when conditions are hot and humid.

Heat-related illness can occur if proper hydration is not maintained. Maximum sweat rates during physical activity in the heat can approach 1–2 liters per hour. If this fluid is not replaced, **dehydration** can occur. If dehydration is not corrected with water or other fluid-replacement drinks, it becomes increasingly difficult for the body to maintain normal body temperatures. At some point, the rate of sweating decreases as the body begins to conserve its remaining water. It shunts blood to the skin to transfer excess heat directly to the environment, but this is less effective than evaporation. **Hyperthermia** and associated heat-related problems can result (see Table 3).

One way to monitor the amount of fluid loss is to monitor the color of your urine. The American College of Sports Medicine indicates that clear (almost colorless) urine produced in large volumes indicates that you are hydrated. As water in the body is reduced, the urine becomes more concentrated and is a darker yellow color. This indicates dehydration and a need for fluid replacement. Dietary supplements that contain amphetamine derivatives and/or creatine may contribute to undetected dehydration among some individuals.

Acclimatization improves the body's tolerance in the heat. Individuals with good fitness will respond better to activity in the heat than individuals with poor fitness. With regular exposure, the body adapts to the heat. The majority of the adaptation to hot environments occurs in 7 to 14 days, but complete acclimatization can take up to 30 days. As you adapt to the heat, your body becomes conditioned to sweat earlier, to sweat more profusely, and to distribute the sweat more effectively around

Table 3 ▶ Types of Heat-Related Problems

Problem	Symptoms	Severity
Heat cramps	Muscle cramps, especially in muscles most used in exercise	Least severe
Heat exhaustion	Muscle cramps, weakness, dizziness, headache, nausea, clammy skin, paleness	Moderately severe
Heatstroke	Hot, flushed skin; dry skin (lack of sweating); dizziness; fast pulse; unconsciousness; high temperature	Extremely severe

Table 4 ▶ Heat Index Values (Apparent Temperatures)

To read the table, find air temperature on the top; then find the humidity on the left. Find the heat index where the columns meet.

Relative Humidity (%)	Air Temperature (Degrees F)										
	70	75	80	85	90	95	100	105	110	115	120
100	72	80	91	108	132						
95	71	79	89	105	128						
90	71	79	88	102	122						
85	71	78	87	99	117	141					
80	71	78	86	97	113	136					
75	70	77	86	95	109	130					
70	70	77	85	93	106	124	144				
65	70	76	83	91	102	119	138				
60	70	76	82	90	100	114	132	149			
55	69	75	81	89	98	110	126	142			
50	69	75	81	88	96	107	120	135	150		
45	68	74	80	87	95	104	115	129	143		
40	68	74	79	86	93	101	110	123	137	151	
35	67	73	79	85	91	98	107	118	130	143	
30	67	73	78	84	90	96	104	113	123	135	148
25	66	72	77	83	88	94	101	109	117	127	139
20	66	72	77	82	87	93	99	105	112	120	130
15	65	71	76	81	86	91	97	102	108	115	123
10	65	70	75	80	85	90	95	100	105	111	116
5	64	69	74	79	84	88	93	97	102	107	111
0	64	69	73	78	83	87	91	95	99	103	107

"Apparent Temperatures" (Heat Index)

■ = Extreme danger zone
■ = Danger zone
■ = Extreme caution zone
■ = Caution zone
□ = Safe

Source: Data from National Oceanic and Atmospheric Administration.

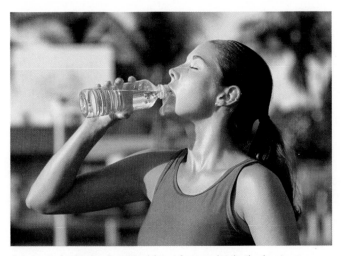

Adequate hydration is critical for safe exercise in the heat.

the body, and the composition of sweat is altered. This process makes it easier for your body to maintain a safe body temperature.

Precautions should be taken when doing physical activity in hot and humid environments. The **heat index** (also referred to as apparent temperature) combines temperature and humidity to help you determine when an environment is safe for activity. The combination of high temperature and humidity presents the greatest risk of heat-related problems in exercise. Physical activity is safe when the apparent temperature is below 80°F (26.7°C). Table 4 shows the increasing risk of exercise at progressively higher apparent temperatures.

Consider the following guidelines for performing exercise in the heat and humidity.

Cool-Down Light to moderate activity done after a workout to help the body recover; often consisting of the same exercises used in the warm-up.

Dehydration Excessive loss of water from the body, usually through perspiration, urination, or evaporation.

Hyperthermia Excessively high body temperature caused by excessive heat production or impaired heat loss capacity. Heatstroke is a hyperthermic condition.

Heat Index An index based on a combination of temperature and humidity that is used to determine if it is dangerous to perform physical activity in hot, humid weather (also called apparent temperature).

- Limit or cancel activity if the apparent temperature reaches the danger zone (see Table 4).
- Drink fluids before, during, and after activity. Guidelines suggest about 2 cups before activity and about 1 cup for each 15–20 minutes during activity. After activity, drink about 2 cups for each pound of weight lost. The thirst mechanism lags behind the body's actual need for fluid, so drink even if you don't feel thirsty. Fluid-replacement beverages (e.g., Gatorade, Powerade) are designed to provide added energy (from carbohydrates) without impeding hydration. If you choose to use one of these beverages, select one that contains electrolytes and no more than 4 to 8 percent carbohydrates.
- Avoid extreme fluid intake. Drinking too much water can cause a condition called **hyponatremia,** sometimes referred to as "water intoxication." It occurs when you drink too much water, resulting in the dilution of the electrolytes in the blood; interestingly, it has symptoms similar to those of dehydration. If left untreated, it can result in loss of consciousness and even death.
- Gradually expose yourself to physical activity in hot and humid environments to facilitate acclimatization.
- With extreme care, experienced exercisers who have become acclimatized to the heat may be able to perform at higher apparent temperatures than those who are less experienced. However, care should be used by all people who perform physical activity in hot and humid environments.
- Dress properly for exercise in the heat and humidity. Wear white or light colors that reflect rather than absorb heat. Select wickable clothes instead of cotton to aid evaporative cooling. Rubber, plastic, or other nonporous clothing is especially dangerous. A porous hat or cap can help when exercising in direct sunlight.
- Watch for signs of heat stress (see Table 3). If signs are present, stop immediately, get out of the heat, remove excess clothing, and drink cool water. Seek medical attention if symptoms progress. Consider cold water immersion for heat stroke.

Physical activity in exceptionally cold and windy weather can be dangerous. Activity in the cold presents the opposite problems as exercise in the heat. In the cold, the primary goal is to retain the body's heat and avoid **hypothermia** and frostbite. Early signs of hypothermia include shivering and cold extremities caused by blood shunted to the body core to conserve heat. As the core temperature continues to drop, heart rate, respiration, and reflexes are depressed. Subsequently, cognitive functions decrease, speech and movement become impaired, and bizarre behavior may occur. Frostbite results from water crystallizing in the tissues, causing cell destruction.

When doing activity in cold, wet, and windy weather, precautions should be taken. A combination of cold and wind (windchill) poses the greatest danger for cold-related problems during exercise. Research conducted in Canada, in cooperation with the U.S. National Weather Service, produced tables for determining **windchill factor** and the time of exposure necessary to get frostbite (see Table 5). The old method of

Table 5 ▶ Windchill Factor Chart

Actual Temperature Reading (Degrees F)	Estimated Wind Speed (mph)									Minutes to Frostbite
	Calm	5	10	15	20	25	30	35	40	
40	40	36	34	32	30	29	28	27	27	
30	30	25	21	19	17	16	15	14	13	
20	20	13	9	6	4	3	1	0	-1	
10	10	1	-4	-7	-9	-11	-12	-14	-15	
0	0	-11	-16	-19	-22	-24	-26	-27	-29	30
-10	-10	-22	-28	-32	-35	-37	-39	-41	-43	10
-20	-20	-34	-41	-45	-48	-51	-53	-55	-57	5
-30	-30	-46	-53	-58	-61	-64	-67	-69	-71	
-40	-40	-57	-66	-71	-74	-78	-80	-82	-84	

Source: National Weather Service.

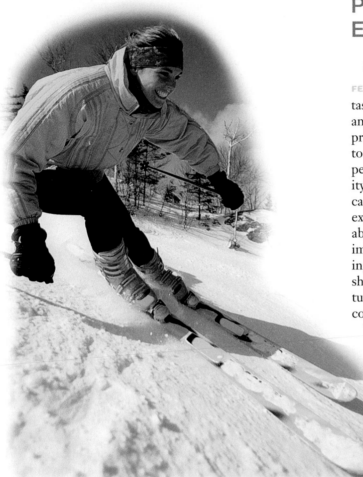

Wind, cold, and altitude present some additional challenges for winter exercise.

measurement overestimated the impact of cold weather. Consider the following guidelines for performing physical activity in cold and wind:

- Limit or cancel activity if the windchill factor reaches the danger zone (see Table 5).
- Dress properly. Wear light clothing in several layers rather than one heavy garment. The layer of clothing closest to the body should transfer (wick) moisture away from the skin to a second, more absorbent layer. Polypropylene and capilene are examples of wickable fabrics. A porous windbreaker keeps wind from cooling the body and allows the release of body heat. The hands, feet, nose, and ears are most susceptible to frostbite, so they should be covered. Wear a hat or cap, mask, and mittens. Mittens are warmer than gloves. A light coating of petroleum jelly on exposed body parts can be helpful.
- Keep from getting wet in cold weather. If you get wet because of unavoidable circumstances, seek a warm dry place to dry out.

Physical Activity in Other Environments

ⓘ **High altitude may limit performance and require adaptation of normal physical**
FEATURE 4 **activity.** The ability to do vigorous physical tasks is diminished as altitude increases. Breathing rate and heart rates are more elevated at high altitude. With proper acclimation (gradual exposure), the body adjusts to the lower oxygen pressure found at high altitude, and performance improves. Nevertheless, performance ability at high altitudes, especially for activities requiring cardiovascular fitness, is usually less than would be expected at sea level. At extremely high altitudes, the ability to perform vigorous physical activity may be impossible without an extra oxygen supply. When moving from sea level to a high altitude, vigorous exercise should be done with caution. Acclimation to high altitudes requires a minimum of 2 weeks and may not be complete for several months. Care should be taken to drink adequate water at high altitude.

Exposure to air pollution should be limited. Various pollutants can cause poor performance and, in some cases, health problems. Ozone, a pollutant produced primarily by the sun's reaction to car exhaust, can cause symptoms, including headache, coughing, and eye irritation. Similar symptoms result from exposure to carbon monoxide, a tasteless and odorless gas, caused by combustion of oil, gasoline, and/or cigarette smoke. Most news media in metropolitan areas now provide updates on ozone and carbon monoxide levels in their weather reports. When levels of these pollutants reach moderate levels, some people may need to modify their exercise. When levels are high, some may need to postpone exercise. Exercisers wishing to avoid ozone and carbon monoxide may want to exercise indoors early in the morning or later in the evening. It is wise to avoid areas with a high concentration of traffic.

Hyponatremia A condition caused by excess water intake, sometimes referred to as "water intoxication," that can cause loss of electrolytes, leading to serious medical complications.

Hypothermia Excessively low body temperature (less than 95°F), characterized by uncontrollable shivering, loss of coordination, and mental confusion.

Windchill Factor An index that uses air temperature and wind speed to determine the chilling effect of the environment on humans.

Pollens from certain plants may cause allergic reactions for certain people. Some people are allergic to dust or other particulates in the air. Weather reports of pollens and particulates may help exercisers determine the best times for their activities and when to avoid vigorous activities.

Soreness and Injury

ⓘ
FEATURE 5
Understanding soreness can help you persist in physical activity and avoid problems. A common experience for many exercisers is a certain degree of muscle soreness that occurs 24–48 hours after intense exercise. This soreness, termed delayed-onset muscle soreness **(DOMS),** typically occurs when muscles are exercised at levels beyond their normal use. Some people mistakenly believe that lactic acid is the cause of muscle soreness. Lactic acid (a by-product of anaerobic metabolism) is produced during vigorous exercise, but levels return to normal within 30 minutes after exercise, while DOMS occurs 24 hours after exercise. DOMS is caused by microscopic muscle tears that result from the excessive loads on the muscles. Soreness is not a normal part of the body's response to exercise but occurs if an individual violates the principle of progression and does more exercise than the body is prepared for. While it may be uncomfortable to some, it has no long-term consequences and does not predispose one to muscle injury. To reduce the likelihood of DOMS, it is important to progress your program gradually. See Web information for more details.

The most common injuries incurred in physical activity are sprains and strains. A strain occurs when the fibers in a muscle are injured. Common activity-related injuries are hamstring strains that occur after a vigorous sprint. Other commonly strained muscles include the muscles in the front of the thigh, the low back, and the calf.

A sprain is an injury to a ligament—the connective tissue that connects bones to bones. The most common sprain is to the ankle; frequently, the ankle is rolled to the outside (inversion) when jumping or running. Other common sprains are to the knee, the shoulder, and the wrist.

Tendonitis is an inflammation of the tendon; it is most often a result of overuse rather than trauma. Tendonitis can be painful but often does not swell to the extent that sprains do. For this reason, elevation and compression are not as effective as ice and rest. Information about other common injuries is included on the Web, but a physician should be consulted for an appropriate diagnosis.

Being able to treat minor injuries will help reduce their negative effects. Minor injuries, such as muscle strains and sprains, are common to those who are persistent in their exercise. If a serious injury should occur or if symptoms persist, it is important to get immediate medical attention. However, for minor injuries, following the **RICE** formula will help you reduce the pain and speed recovery. In this acronym, *R* stands for *rest.* Muscle sprains and strains heal best if the injured area is rested. Rest helps you avoid further damage to the muscle. *I* stands for *ice.* The quick application of cold (ice or ice water) to a minor injury minimizes swelling and speeds recovery. Cold should be applied to as large a surface area as possible (soaking is best). If ice is used, it should be wrapped to avoid direct contact with the skin. Apply cold for 20 minutes, three times a day, allowing 1 hour between applications. *C* stands for *compression.* Wrapping or compressing the injured area also helps minimize swelling and speeds recovery. Elastic bandages or elastic socks are good for applying compression. Care should be taken to avoid wrapping an injury too tightly because this can result in loss of circulation to the area. *E* stands for *elevation.* Keeping the injured area elevated (above the level of the heart) is effective in minimizing swelling. If pain or swelling does not diminish after 24 to 48 hours, or if there is any doubt about the seriousness of an injury, seek medical help. Some experts recommend adding a *P* to RICE (PRICE) to indicate that *prevention* (P) is as important as treatment of injuries. Building strength and flexibility, warming up, beginning gradually when starting a new activity, and wearing protective equipment, such as lace-up ankle braces, are simple methods of prevention.

Taking over-the-counter pain remedies can help reduce the pain of muscle strains and sprains. Aspirin and ibuprofen (e.g., Excedrin, Motrin) have anti-inflammatory properties. However, acetaminophen (e.g., Tylenol) does not. It may reduce the pain but will not reduce inflammation.

Muscle cramps can be relieved by statically stretching a muscle. Muscle cramps are pains in the large muscles that result when the muscles contract vigorously for a continued period of time. Muscle cramps are usually not considered to be an injury, but they are painful and may seem like an injury. They are usually short in duration and can often be relieved with proper treatment. Cramps can result from lack of fluid replacement (dehydration), from fatigue, and from a blow directly to a muscle. Static stretching can help relieve some cramps. For example, the calf muscle, which often cramps among runners and other sports participants, can be relieved using the calf stretcher exercise, which is part of the warm-up in this concept.

Attitudes about Physical Activity

Knowing the most common reasons for inactivity can help you avoid sedentary living. Most people want to be active but find many barriers get in the way.

Table 6 ▶ Common Reasons People Give for Not Being Active

Reason	Description	Strategy for Change
I don't have the time.	This is the number 1 reason people give for not exercising. Invariably, those who feel they don't have time know they should do more exercise. They say they plan to do more in the future when "things are less hectic." Young people say they will have more time to exercise in the future. Older people say they wish they had taken the time to be active when they were younger.	Planning a daily schedule can help you find the time for activity and avoid wasting time on things that are less important. Learning the facts in the concepts that follow will help you see the importance of activity and how you can include it in your schedule with a minimum of effort and with time efficiency.
It's too inconvenient.	Many who avoid physical activity do so because it is inconvenient. They are procrastinators. Specific reasons for procrastinating include "It makes me sweaty" and "It messes up my hair."	If you have to travel more than 10 minutes to do activity or if you do not have easy access to equipment, you will avoid activity. Locating facilities and finding a time when you can shower is important.
I just don't enjoy it.	Many do not find activity to be enjoyable or invigorating. These people may assume that all forms of activity have to be strenuous and fatiguing.	There are many activities to choose from. If you don't enjoy vigorous activity, try more moderate forms of activity, such as walking.
I'm no good at physical activity.	"People might laugh at me," "Sports make me nervous," and "I am not good at physical activities" are reasons some people give for not being active. Some people lack confidence in their own abilities. This may be because of past experiences in physical education or sports.	With properly selected activities, even those who have never enjoyed exercise can get hooked. Building skills can help, as can changing your way of thinking. Avoiding comparisons with others can help you feel successful.
I am not fit, so I avoid activity.	Some people avoid exercise because of health reasons. Some who are unfit lack energy. Starting slowly can build fitness gradually and help you realize that you can do it.	There are good medical reasons for not doing activity, but many people with problems can benefit from exercise if it is properly designed. If necessary, get help adapting activity to meet your needs.
I have no place to be active, especially in bad weather.	Regular activity is more convenient if facilities are easy to reach and the weather is good. Opportunities have increased considerably in recent years. Some of the most popular activities require little equipment, can be done in or near home, and are inexpensive.	If you cannot find a place, if it is not safe, or if it is too expensive, consider using low-cost equipment at home, such as rubber bands or calisthenics. Lifestyle activity can be done by anyone at almost any time.
I am too old.	As people grow older, many begin to feel that activity is something they cannot do. For most people, this is simply not true! Properly planned exercise for older adults is not only safe but also has many health benefits—e.g., longer life, fewer illnesses, an improved sense of well-being, and optimal functioning.	Older people who are just beginning activity should start slowly. Lifestyle activities are a good choice. Setting realistic goals can help, as can learning to do resistance training and flexibility exercises.

The most common reasons given by people who do not do regular physical activity are listed in Table 6. Experts consider many of these attitudes to be barriers that can be overcome. In fact, a key self-management skill that predicts long-term behavior change is the ability to overcome barriers. The strategies in Table 6 can help inactive people become more active.

Knowing the reasons people give for being active can help you adopt positive attitudes toward activity. To enhance the promotion of physical activity in society, many researchers have sought to determine why some people choose to be active and others do not.

The most common reasons for physical activity are highlighted in Table 7. The table also offers strategies for changing behaviors.

DOMS An acronym for delayed-onset muscle soreness, a common malady that follows relatively vigorous activity, especially among beginners.

RICE An acronym for rest, ice, compression, and elevation; a method of treating minor injuries.

Table 7 ▶ Common Reasons for Doing Regular Physical Activity

Reason	Description	Strategy for Change
I do activity for my health, wellness, and fitness.	Surveys show this is the number 1 reason for doing regular physical activity. Unfortunately, many adults say that a "doctor's order to exercise" would be the most likely reason to get them to begin a program. For some, however, waiting for a doctor's order may be too late.	Gaining information contained in this book will help you see the value of regular physical activity. Performing the self-assessments in the various concepts will help you determine the areas in which you need personal improvement.
I do activity to improve my appearance.	In our society, looking good is highly valued; thus, physical attractiveness is a major reason people participate in regular exercise. Regular activity can contribute to looking your best.	Some people have failed in past attempts to change their appearance through activity. Setting realistic goals and avoiding comparisons with others can help you be more successful.
I do activity because I enjoy it.	A majority of adults say that enjoyment is of paramount importance in deciding to be active. Statements include experiencing the "peak experience," the "runner's high," or "spinning free." The sense of fun, well-being, and general enjoyment associated with physical activity is well documented.	People who do not enjoy activity often lack performance skills or feel that they are not competent in activity. Improving skills with practice, setting realistic goals, and adopting a new way of thinking can help you be successful and enjoy activities.
I do activity because it relaxes me.	Relaxation and release from tension rank high as reasons people do regular activity. It is known that activity in the form of sports and games provides a catharsis, or outlet, for the frustrations of daily activities. Regular exercise can help reduce depression and anxiety.	Activities such as walking, jogging, or cycling are ways of getting some quiet time away from the job or the stresses of daily living. In a later concept, you will learn about exercises that you can do to reduce stress.
I like the challenge and sense of personal accomplishment I get from physical activity.	A sense of personal accomplishment is frequently a reason for people doing activity. In some cases, it is learning a new skill, such as racquetball or tennis; in other cases, it is running a mile or doing a certain number of crunches. The challenge of doing something you have never done before is apparently a powerful experience.	Some people get little sense of accomplishment from activity. Taking lessons to learn skills or attempting activities new to you can provide the challenge that makes activity interesting. Also, adopting a new way of thinking allows you to focus on the task rather than on competition with others.
I like the social involvement I get from physical activities.	"Why am I physically active?" "It is a good way to spend time with members of my family." "It is a good way to spend time with close friends." "Being part of the team is satisfying." Activity settings can also provide an opportunity for making new friends.	If you find activity to be socially unrewarding, you may have to find activities that you, your family, or your friends enjoy. Taking lessons together can help. Also, finding a friend with similar skills can help. Focus on the activity rather than the outcome.
Competition is the main reason I enjoy physical activity.	"The thrill of victory" and "sports competition" are two reasons given for being active. For many, the competitive experience is very satisfying.	Some people simply do not enjoy competing. If this is the case for you, select noncompetitive individual activities.
Physical activity helps me feel good about myself.	For many people, participation in physical activity is an important part of their identity. They feel better about themselves when they are regularly participating.	Physical activity is something that is self-determined and within your control. Participation can help you feel good about yourself, build your confidence, and increase your self-esteem.
Physical activity provides opportunities to get fresh air.	Being outside and experiencing nature are reasons that some people give for being physically active.	Many activities provide opportunities to be outside. If this is an important reason for you, seek out parks and outdoor settings for your activities.

In the News

National Physical Activity Plan

In May 2010 a new National Physical Activity was launched. Coordinated by the CDC and the Prevention Research Center of the University of South Carolina, the plan was developed by leading experts from a variety of health fields. The national plan organizational group (www.physicalactivityplan.org) indicates that "A comprehensive plan for promoting physical activity in the American population would provide the framework to support a broad and comprehensive national effort to increase physical activity throughout the population." More information is available online.

▶▶ Strategies for Action

Screening for risks can help make activity safer. Athletes in competitive sports often undergo pre-participation physical examinations to screen for potential cardiac arrhythmias or conditions known to increase risks during exercise. Recreational athletes may not take the same precautions. The best advice is to get a physical prior to beginning serious training. This is especially critical if you have a family history of heart problems. Lab 3A will help you determine if you should consult a physician.

A proper warm-up and cool-down can make activity more effective and more enjoyable. A proper warm-up can prepare your body for activity and a gradual cool-down can improve recovery. Lab 3B provides a sample flexibility-based warm-up and cool-down routine that may be helpful. Determine what works best for your needs.

Assess your attitudes concerning physical activity. When preparing for physical activity, assessing your attitudes can be helpful. Active people generally have more positive attitudes than negative ones. This is referred to as a "positive balance of attitudes." The questionnaire in Lab 3C gives you the opportunity to assess your balance of attitudes. If you have a "negative balance" score, you can analyze your attitudes and determine how you can change them to view activity more favorably.

Be prepared for emergencies. To be prepared for physical activity, you also need to be prepared for emergencies. This concept has highlighted risks associated with different environmental conditions. Consider potential risks prior to exercise and be prepared (see position statements in Web Resources). Having a cell phone with you, when possible, during exercise is a good idea.

It is also important to know basic first aid and to be prepared to give CPR if needed. Guidelines from the American Heart Association have been revised to increase the likelihood that bystanders might give help. The most important change is a shift from mouth-to-mouth resuscitation to chest compressions. Proper certification is recommended, but the guidelines were revised to get more people to help, even when not certified (some CPR is better than no CPR). If a person is unresponsive, call for help and begin chest compressions immediately at a rate of 100–120 per minute. Continue compression until help arrives. Automatic defibrillators are now available in many public places, including fitness centers. Information on CPR guidelines and automatic defibrillators is available on the Web.

Web Resources

Additional websites with information related to Concept 3 are available at the associated Web link.

ACSM and ACSM/AHA Position Statements

ACSM/AHA. 2007. Exercise and Acute Cardiovascular Events.

ACSM. 2007. Exertional Heat Illness during Training and Competition.

ACSM. 2007. Exercise and Fluid Replacement.

ACSM. 2006. Prevention of Cold Injuries during Exercise. www.acsm-msse.org/pt/re/msse/positionstandards.htm

ACSM's Fit Society Page www.acsm.org/health+fitness/fit_society.htm

ACSM's Health and Fitness Journal www.acsm.org/publications/health_fitness_journal.htm

American Red Cross (AED information) www.redcross.org

Med Watch www.fda.gov/medwatch

National Athletic Trainers Association www.nata.org

Suggested Readings

Selected readings and references are listed on the next page. A more comprehensive list is available at the associated Web link.

ACSM. 2010. *ACSM's Guidelines for Exercise Testing and Prescription.* 8th ed. Philadelphia: Lippincott, Williams & Wilkins.

ACSM. 2010. *ACSM's Resource Manual for Guidelines for Exercise Testing and Prescription.* 6th ed. Philadelphia: Lippincott, Williams & Wilkins.

Baker, L. B., and W. L. Kenney. 2007. Exercising in the heat and sun. *President's Council on Physical Fitness and Sports Research Digest* 8(2):1–8.

Barwood, M. J., Thelwell, R. C., and M. J. Tipton. 2008. Psychological skills training improves exercise performance in the heat. *Medicine and Science in Sports and Exercise* 40(2): 387–396.

Bernardot, D. 2007. Timing of energy and fluid intake. *ACSM's Health and Fitness Journal* 11(4):13–19.

Fradkin, A., et al. 2009. Warm-up and physical performance: What is the relationship? A systematic review with meta analysis (abstract). *Medicine and Science in Sports and Exercise* 41(5 Supplement):151–152.

Lowry, R., et al. 2007. Physical activity–related injury and body mass index among U.S. high school students. *Journal of Physical Activity and Health* 4(3): 225–342.

Mayo Clinic. 2008. Sports injuries A–Z. Available at **www.mayoclinic.com/health/sportsinjuries/SM00108.**

Perberdy, M. A., and J. P. Ornato. 2008. Progress in resuscitation: An evolution, not a revolution. *Journal of the American Medical Asssociation* 299(10):1188–1190.

Rea, T. D., et al. 2010. CPR with chest compression alone or with rescue breathing. *New England Journal of Medicine* 363(5): 423–433.

Stover, B., and B. Murray. 2007. Drink up: Science of hydration. *ACSM's Health and Fitness Journal* 11(3): 7–12.

Thacker, S. B., et al. 2004. The impact of stretching on sports injury risk: A systematic review of the literature. *Medicine and Science in Sports and Exercise* 36(3):371–378.

Volpe, S. L. 2007. A nutritionist's view: Sodium and fluid needs in athletes. *ACSM's Health and Fitness Journal* 11(1): 32.

Lab 3A Readiness for Physical Activity

Name	**Section**	**Date**

Purpose: To help you determine your physical readiness for participation in a program of regular exercise

Procedures

1. Read the directions on the "PAR-Q & You" on page 60.
2. Answer each of the seven questions on the form.
3. If you answered "yes" to one or more of the questions, follow the directions just below the PAR-Q questions regarding medical consultation.
4. If you answered "no" to all seven questions, follow the directions at the lower left-hand corner of the PAR-Q.
5. Answer the five questions about physical readiness for sports or vigorous training in Chart 1 below.
6. Record your score below and answer the question in the Conclusions and Implications section.

Results

Chart 1 ▶ Physical Readiness for Sports or Vigorous Training

Answer the PAR-Q before using this chart. If your answer to any of these questions is "yes," you should consult with your personal physician by telephone or in person to determine if you have a potential problem with sports or vigorous training.

Yes   No

☐ ☒ 1. Do you plan to participate on an organized team that will play intense competitive sports (e.g., varsity team, professional team)?

☐ ☒ 2. If you plan to participate in a collision sport (even on a less organized basis), such as football, boxing, rugby, or ice hockey, have you been knocked unconscious more than one time?

☐ ☒ 3. Do you currently have symptoms from a previous muscle injury?

☐ ☒ 4. Do you currently have symptoms from a previous back injury, or do you experience back pain as a result of involvement in physical activity?

☐ ☒ 5. Do you have any other symptoms during physical activity that give you reason to be concerned about your health?

Determine your PAR-Q score. Place an X over the circle that includes the number of "yes" answers that you had for the PAR-Q (see page 60).

⊗(0) (1) (2) (3) (4) (5) (6) (7)

Determine your readiness for sports or rigorous training (see Chart 1 above). Place an X over the number of "yes" answers that you had for the Physical Readiness for Sports or Vigorous Training chart.

⊗(0) (1) (2) (3) (4) (5)

Conclusions and Implications: In several sentences, discuss your readiness for physical activity. Base your comments on your questionnaire results and the types of physical activities you plan to perform in the future.

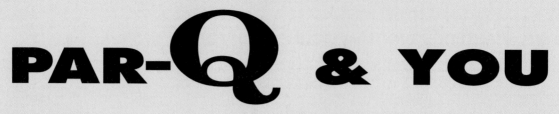

PAR-Q & YOU

Regular physical activity is fun and healthy, and increasingly more people are starting to become more active every day. Being more active is very safe for most people. However, some people should check with their doctor before they start becoming much more physically active.

If you are planning to become much more physically active than you are now, start by answering the seven questions in the box below. If you are between the ages of fifteen and sixty-nine, the PAR-Q will tell you if you should check with your doctor before you start. If you are over sixty-nine years of age, and you are not used to being very active, check with your doctor.

Common sense is your best guide when you answer these questions. Please read the questions carefully and answer each one honestly: check YES or NO.

YES	NO	
☐	☐	1. Has your doctor ever said that you have a heart condition <u>and</u> that you should only do physical activity recommended by a doctor?
☐	☐	2. Do you feel pain in your chest when you do physical activity?
☐	☐	3. In the past month, have you had chest pain when you were not doing physical activity?
☐	☐	4. Do you lose your balance because of dizziness or do you ever lose consciousness?
☐	☐	5. Do you have a bone or joint problem that could be made worse by a change in your physical activity?
☐	☐	6. Is your doctor currently prescribing drugs (for example, water pills) for your blood pressure or heart condition?
☐	☐	7. Do you know of <u>any other reason</u> you should not do physical activity?

If you answered

Yes

YES to one or more questions

Talk with your doctor by phone or in person BEFORE you start becoming much more physically active or BEFORE you have a fitness appraisal. Tell your doctor about the PAR-Q and which questions you answered YES.

- You may be able to do any activity you want—as long as you start slowly and build up gradually. Or you may need to restrict your activities to those that are safe for you. Talk with your doctor about the kinds of activities you wish to participate in and follow his or her advice.
- Find out which community programs are safe and helpful for you.

No

NO to all questions

If you answered NO honestly to <u>all</u> PAR-Q questions, you can be reasonably sure that you can

- Start becoming much more physically active—begin slowly and build up gradually. This is the safest and easiest way to go.
- Take part in a fitness appraisal—this is an excellent way to determine your basic fitness so that you can plan the best way for you to live actively.

DELAY BECOMING MUCH MORE ACTIVE:

- If you are not feeling well because of a temporary illness, such as a cold or a fever—wait until you feel better or
- If you are or may be pregnant—talk to your doctor before you start becoming more active.

Please note: If your health changes so that you then answer YES to any of the above questions, tell your fitness or health professional. Ask whether you should change your physical activity plan.

<u>Informed Use of the PAR-Q</u>: The Canadian Society for Exercise Physiology, Health Canada, and their agents assume no liability for persons who undertake physical activity, and if in doubt after completing this questionnaire, consult your doctor prior to physical activity.

You are encouraged to copy the PAR-Q but only if you use the entire form

*Developed by the British Columbia Ministry of Health.
Produced by the British Columbia Ministry of Health and the Department of National Health & Welfare

Physical Activity Readiness
Questionnaire • PAR-Q
(revised 2002)

Note: It is important that you answer all questions honestly. The PAR-Q is a scientifically and medically researched pre-exercise selection device. It complements exercise programs, exercise testing procedures, and the liability considerations attendant with such programs and testing procedures. PAR-Q, like any other pre-exercise screening device, will misclassify a small percentage of prospective participants, but no pre-exercise screening method can entirely avoid this problem.

Lab 3B The Warm-Up and Cool-Down

FWGTJQ

Name

Purpose: To familiarize you with a sample group of warm-up and cool-down exercises

Procedures

1. Perform a 2- to 5-minute cardiovascular warm-up (walk, jog, slow jump rope, swim).
2. Perform the exercises in Chart 1, including the alternative exercises, on the back of this lab page three times each. Hold the stretch for 15 to 30 seconds.
3. Complete the Results section below and answer the questions in the Conclusions and Implications section.

Results: In the following, put an X over the circle that represents the amount of tightness you felt when performing each of the stretching warm-up and cool-down exercises. Tightness indicates that you may have shortness of a specific muscle group and that stretching exercises at times other than the warm-up or cool-down are needed.

Amount of Tightness

	None	Moderate	Severe
Calf stretch	◯	◯	◯
Hamstring stretch	◯	◯	◯
Leg hug	◯	◯	◯
Sitting side stretch	◯	◯	◯
Zipper	◯	◯	◯

Alternative Exercises

	None	Moderate	Severe
Side stretch	◯	◯	◯
One-leg stretch	◯	◯	◯
Hip and thigh stretch	◯	◯	◯

Conclusions and Implications: In several sentences, discuss the warm-up and cool-down. Include in the discussion your feelings about the adequacy of the warm-up and cool-down for you personally. Those who plan to do vigorous sports will need to supplement this group of exercises.

Chart 1 ▶ Sample warm-up and cool-down exercises

The exercises shown here can be used before a moderate workout as a warm-up or after a workout as a cool-down. Perform these exercises slowly, preferably after completing a cardiovascular warm-up. Do not bounce. Hold each stretch for at least 15–30 seconds. Perform each exercise at least once and up to three times. Other stretching exercises are presented in the concept on flexibility, and they can be used in a warm-up or cool-down.

Cardiovascular Exercise

Before you perform a vigorous workout, walk or jog slowly for 2 minutes or more. After exercise, do the same. Do this portion of the warm-up prior to muscle stretching.

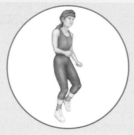

Calf Stretcher

This exercise stretches the calf muscles (gastrocnemius and soleus). Face a wall with your feet 2 or 3 feet away. Step forward on your left foot to allow both hands to touch the wall. Keep the heel of your right foot on the ground, toe turned in slightly, knee straight, and buttocks tucked in. Lean forward by bending your front knee and arms and allowing your head to move nearer the wall. Hold. Repeat with the other leg.

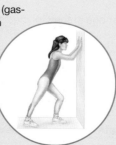

Hamstring Stretcher

This exercise stretches the muscles of the back of the upper leg (hamstrings) as well as those of the hip, knee, and ankle. Lie on your back. Bring the right knee to your chest and grasp the toes with the right hand. Place the left hand on the back of the right thigh. Pull the knee toward the chest, push the heel toward the ceiling, and pull the toes toward the shin. Attempt to straighten the knee. Stretch and hold. Repeat with the other leg.

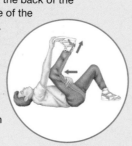

Leg Hug

This exercise stretches the hip and back extensor muscles. Lie on your back. Bend one leg and grasp your thigh under the knee. Hug it to your chest. Keep the other leg straight and on the floor. Hold. Repeat with the opposite leg.

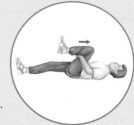

Seated Side Stretch

This exercise stretches the muscles of the trunk. Begin in a seated position with the legs crossed. Stretch the left arm over the head to the right. Bend at the waist (to right), reaching as far as possible to the left with the right arm. Hold. Do not let the trunk rotate. Repeat to the opposite side. For less stretch, the overhead arm may be bent. This exercise can be done in the standing position but is less effective.

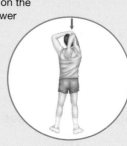

Zipper

This exercise stretches the muscle on the back of the arm (triceps) and the lower chest muscles (pecs). Lift the right arm and reach behind the head and down the spine (as if pulling up a zipper). With the left hand, push down on the right elbow and hold. Reverse arm position and repeat.

ALTERNATE EXERCISES

Because of location (wet or hard surface), you may choose to substitute exercises that do not require you to lie down. The side stretch (standing) can be substituted for the seated side stretch, the one-leg stretch (standing) for the hamstring stretch, and the hip and thigh stretch for the leg hug (does not stretch the same muscles).

Side Stretch

This exercise stretches the trunk lateral flexors. Stand with feet shoulder-width apart. Stretch left arm overhead to right. Bend to right at waist reaching as far as possible with left arm; reach as far as possible with right arm. Hold. Do not let trunk rotate or lower back arch. Repeat on opposite side. Note: This exercise is made more effective if a weight is held down at the side in the hand opposite the side being stretched. More stretch will occur if the hip on the stretched side is dropped and most of the weight is borne by the opposite foot.

Hip and Thigh Stretch

This exercise stretches the hip (iliopsoas) and thigh muscles (quadriceps) and is useful for people with lordosis and back problems. Place right knee directly above right ankle and stretch left leg backward so knee touches floor. If necessary, place hands on floor for balance.
1. Tilt the pelvis backward by tucking in the abdomen and flattening the back.
2. Then shift the weight forward until a stretch is felt on the front of the thigh: hold. Repeat on opposite side. Caution: Do not bend front knee more than 90 degrees.

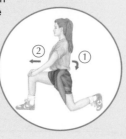

One-Leg Stretch

This exercise stretches the lower back muscles. Stand with one foot on a bench, keeping both legs straight. Contract the hamstrings and gluteals by pressing down on bench with the heel for three seconds; then relax and bend the trunk forward, toward the knee. Hold for 10–15 seconds. Return to starting position and repeat with opposite leg. As flexibility improves, the arms can be used to pull the chest toward the legs. Do not allow either knee to lock. This exercise is useful in relief of backache and correction of swayback.

Lab 3C Physical Activity Attitude Questionnaire

Name	**Section** **Date**

Purpose: To evaluate your feelings about physical activity and to determine the specific reasons you do or do not participate in regular physical activity

Directions: The term *physical activity* in the following statements refers to all kinds of activities, including sports, formal exercises, and informal activities, such as jogging and cycling. Make an X over the circle that best represents your answer to each question.

	Strongly Disagree	Disagree	Undecided	Agree	Strongly Agree	Item Score	Attitude Score
1. I should do physical activity regularly for my health.	1	2	3	4	⊗5	5	Health and Fitness Score
2. Doing regular physical activity is good for my fitness and wellness.	1	2	3	4	⊗5	5	+ = 10
3. Regular exercise helps me look my best.	1	2	3	4	⊗5	5	Appearance Score
4. I feel more physically attractive when I do regular physical activity.	1	2	3	4	⊗5	5	+ = 10
5. One of the main reasons I do regular physical activity is that it is fun.	1	2	3	4	⊗5	5	Enjoyment Score
6. The most enjoyable part of my day is when I am exercising or doing a sport.	1	2	3	⊗4	5	4	+ = 9
7. Taking part in physical activity helps me relax.	1	2	3	4	⊗5	5	Relaxation Score
8. Physical activity helps me get away from the pressures of daily living.	1	2	3	4	⊗5	5	+ = 10
9. The challenge of physical training is one reason I do physical activity.	1	2	3	4	⊗5	5	Challenge Score
10. I like to see if I can master sports and activities that are new to me.	1	2	3	⊗4	5	4	+ = 9
11. I like to do physical activity that involves other people.	1	2	3	4	⊗5	5	Social Score
12. Exercise offers me the opportunity to meet other people.	1	2	3	4	⊗5	5	+ = 10
13. Competition is a good way to make physical activity fun.	1	2	3	4	⊗5	5	Competition Score
14. I like to see how my physical abilities compare with those of others.	1	2	3	4	⊗5	5	+ = 10
15. When I do regular exercise, I feel better than when I don't.	1	2	3	4	⊗5	5	Feeling Good Score
16. My ability to do physical activity is something that makes me proud.	1	2	3	4	⊗5	5	+ = 10
17. I like to do outdoor activities.	1	2	3	4	⊗5	5	Outdoor Score
18. Experiencing nature is something I look forward to when exercising.	1	2	3	4	⊗5	5	+ = 10

Procedures

1. Read and answer each question in the questionnaire.
2. Write the number in the circle of your answer in the box labeled "Item Score."
3. Add scores for each pair of scores and record in the "Attitude Score" box.
4. Record each attitude score and a rating for each score (use Rating Chart) in the chart below.
5. Record the number of good and excellent scores in the box provided. Use the score in the box to determine your rating using the Balance of Feelings Rating Chart.

Results: Record your results as indicated in the Procedures section.

Physical Activity Attitude Questionnaire Results

Attitude	Score	Rating
Health and fitness	10	Excellent
Appearance	10	Excellent
Enjoyment	9	Excellent
Relaxation	10	Excellent
Challenge	9	Excellent
Social	10	Excellent
Competition	10	Excellent
Feeling good	10	Excellent
Outdoor	10	Excellent

How many good or excellent scores do you have?

9
Balance of Feeling Score

Having 5 or more in the box above indicates that you have a positive balance of feelings (more positive than negative attitudes).

Attitude Rating Chart

Rating Category	Attitude Score
Excellent	9–10
Good	7–8
Fair	5–6
Poor	3–4
Very poor	2

Balance of Feelings Rating Chart

Excellent	6–9
Good	5
Fair	4
Poor	2–3
Very poor	0–1

In a few sentences, discuss your "balance of feelings" rating. Having more positive than negative scores (positive balance of feelings) increases the probability of being active. Include comments on whether you think your ratings suggest that you will be active or inactive and whether your ratings are really indicative of your feelings. Do you think that the scores on which you were rated poor or very poor might be reasons you would avoid physical activity? Explain.

The Health Benefits of Physical Activity

Health Objectives for the Year 2020

- Attain high-quality, longer lives free of preventable disease, injury, and premature death.
- Increase percentage of adolescents and adults who meet national guidelines for aerobic and muscle fitness activities.
- Increase overall cardiovascular health, reduce heart disease, stroke, high blood pressure, and high blood cholesterol, increase screening, increase awareness, and increase emergency treatment by professionals or bystanders.
- Reduce cancer incidence, cancer death rates, increase patient longevity, increase quality of life of survivors, and increase screening.
- Reduce diabetes incidence and death rates, increase screening, education, and care.
- Reduce depression and increase screening for depression and mental health.
- Increase percentage of population having a healthy weight, increase screening and counseling.
- Reduce osteoporosis (related hip fractures), pain of arthritis, and limitations from chronic back pain.
- Increase percentage of college students receiving risk factor information.
- Decrease activity limitations, especially in older adults and disabled.
- Increase percentage of physicians who counsel or educate patients about exercise.

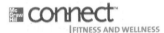 **connect** | FITNESS AND WELLNESS **http://connect.mcgraw-hill.com**

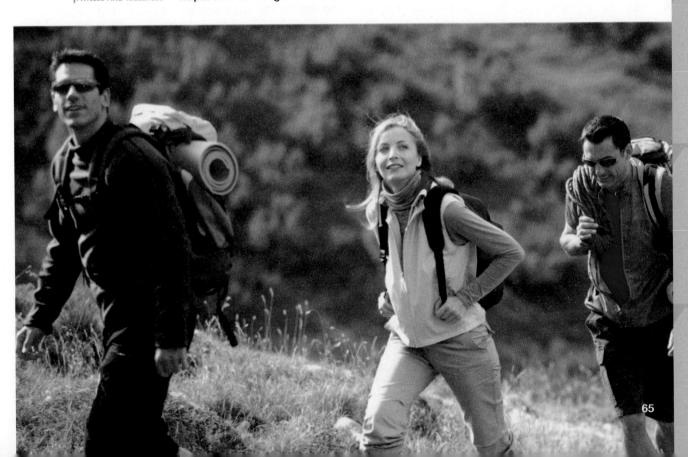

Physical activity and good physical fitness can reduce risk of illness and contribute to optimal health and wellness.

The *Surgeon General's Report on Physical Activity and Health* was an especially important document that informed the general public of the risks of sedentary living and the health benefits of physical activity. Since that document was published, much more evidence has accumulated supporting the benefits of an active lifestyle. The first chapter of ACSM's new *Guidelines for Exercise Testing and Prescription* and Chapter 2 of the 2008 *Physical Activity Guidelines for Americans* are devoted to the benefits and risks associated with physical activity. Both *Healthy People 2020 and Achieving Health for All* (Canada) highlight the importance of regular physical activity for improving population health in the 21st century. This concept summarizes the health benefits of regular physical activity and good fitness.

Physical Activity and Hypokinetic Diseases

Regular physical activity and good fitness can promote good health, help prevent disease, and be a part of disease treatment. There are three major ways in which regular physical activity and good fitness can contribute to optimal health and wellness. First, they can aid in disease/illness prevention. There is considerable evidence that the risk of **hypokinetic diseases or conditions** can be greatly reduced among people who do regular physical activity and achieve good physical fitness. Virtually all **chronic diseases** that plague society are considered to be hypokinetic, though some relate more to inactivity than others. Nearly three-quarters of all deaths among those 18 and older are a result of chronic diseases. Leading public health

officials have suggested that physical activity reduces the risk for several of these diseases. Physical activity provides benefits on multiple conditions and may offer the most promising public health solution controlling such chronic disease, much as immunization controls infectious diseases.

Second, physical activity and fitness can be significant contributors to disease/illness treatment. Even with the best disease prevention practices, some people will become ill. Regular exercise and good fitness have been shown to be effective in alleviating symptoms and aiding rehabilitation after illness for such hypokinetic conditions as diabetes, heart disease, and back pain.

Finally, physical activity and fitness are methods of health and wellness promotion. They contribute to quality living associated with wellness, the positive component of good health. In the process, they aid in meeting many of the nation's health goals.

 Too many adults suffer from hypokinetic disease, and the economic cost is high. In FEATURE 1 1961, Kraus and Raab coined the term *hypokinetic disease* to describe health problems associated with lack of physical activity. They showed how sedentary living, or as they called it, "take it easy" living, contributes to the leading killer diseases in our society.

A public advocacy group has recently coined the term **sedentary death syndrome (SeDS)** to describe inactive living and associated hypokinetic disease risk factors. They indicate that SeDS is responsible for the epidemic of chronic disease in our society and resulting increases in health costs. In the next few years, expenditures for health care are expected to account for one-fifth of all spending in the United States.

 In the News

The Surgeon General's Vision for a Healthy and Fit Nation

The Office of the Surgeon General (OSG), a unit of the U.S. Department of Health and NEWS Human Services, has four principal priorities: disease prevention, elimination of health disparities, public health preparedness, and improvement of health literacy. The current Surgeon General, Dr.

Regina Benjamin, recently announced the publication of the *Surgeon General's Vision for a Healthy and Fit Nation* (**www.surgeongeneral.gov**). This report focuses on "helping Americans lead healthier lives through better nutrition and regular physical activity." Combating overweight and obesity through healthy choices is a major goal. More information about the Surgeon General's vision is available at the associated Web link.

Regular physical activity over a lifetime may overcome the effects of inherited risk. Some people with a family history of disease may conclude they can do nothing because their heredity works against them. There is no doubt that heredity significantly affects risk for early death from hypokinetic diseases. New studies of twins, however, suggest that active people are less likely to die early than inactive people with similar genes. This suggests that long-term adherence to physical activity can overcome other risk factors, such as heredity.

Hypokinetic diseases and conditions have many causes. Regular physical activity and good physical fitness are only two of the preventive factors associated with the conditions described in this concept as hypokinetic diseases. Other healthy lifestyle factors, such as nutrition and stress management, cannot be overlooked.

Physical Activity and Cardiovascular Diseases

The various types of cardiovascular disease are the leading killers in automated societies. There are many forms of **cardiovascular disease (CVD).** Some are classified as **coronary heart disease (CHD)** because they affect the heart muscle and the blood vessels that supply the heart. **Coronary occlusion** (heart attack) is a type of CHD. **Atherosclerosis** and **arteriosclerosis** are two conditions that increase risk for heart attack and are considered to be types of CHD. **Angina pectoris** (chest or arm pain), which occurs when the oxygen supply to the heart muscle is diminished, is sometimes considered to be a type of CHD, though it is really a symptom of poor circulation.

Hypertension (high blood pressure), **stroke** (brain attack), **peripheral vascular disease,** and **congestive heart failure** are other forms of CVD. Inactivity relates in some way to each of these types of disease.

In the United States, CVD accounts for more than 34 percent of all deaths. More than 81 million people currently have one or more forms of CVD. Men are more likely to suffer from heart disease than women, although the differences have narrowed in recent years. African American, Hispanic, and Native American populations are at higher than normal risk. Heart disease and stroke death rates are similar in the United States, Canada, Great Britain, Australia, and other automated societies.

There is a wealth of statistical evidence that physical inactivity is a primary risk factor for CHD. Much of the research relating inactivity to heart disease has come from occupational studies that show a high incidence of

heart disease in people involved only in sedentary work. Even with the limitations inherent in these types of studies, the findings of more and more occupational studies present convincing evidence that the inactive individual

Hypokinetic Diseases or Conditions *Hypo-* means "under" or "too little" and *-kinetic* means "movement" or "activity." Thus, *hypokinetic* means "too little activity." A hypokinetic disease or condition is associated with lack of physical activity or too little regular exercise. Examples include heart disease, low back pain, and Type II diabetes.

Chronic Diseases Diseases or illnesses associated with lifestyle or environmental factors, as opposed to infectious diseases; hypokinetic diseases are considered to be chronic diseases.

Sedentary Death Syndrome (SeDS) A group of symptoms associated with sedentary living, including low health-related fitness (low cardiovascular fitness and weak muscles), low bone density, and the presence of metabolic syndrome (poor metabolic fitness).

Cardiovascular Disease (CVD) A broad classification of diseases of the heart and blood vessels that includes CHD, high blood pressure, stroke, and peripheral vascular disease.

Coronary Heart Disease (CHD) Diseases of the heart muscle and the blood vessels that supply it with oxygen, including heart attack.

Coronary Occlusion The blocking of the coronary blood vessels; sometimes called heart attack.

Atherosclerosis The deposition of materials along the arterial walls; a type of arteriosclerosis.

Arteriosclerosis Hardening of the arteries due to conditions that cause the arterial walls to become thick, hard, and nonelastic.

Angina Pectoris Chest or arm pain resulting from reduced oxygen supply to the heart muscle.

Hypertension High blood pressure; excessive pressure against the walls of the arteries that can damage the heart, kidneys, and other organs of the body.

Stroke A condition in which the brain, or part of the brain, receives insufficient oxygen as a result of diminished blood supply; sometimes called apoplexy or cerebrovascular accident (CVA).

Peripheral Vascular Disease A lack of oxygen supply to the working muscles and tissues of the arms and legs, resulting from decreased blood flow.

Congestive Heart Failure The inability of the heart muscle to pump the blood at a life-sustaining rate.

has an increased risk for coronary heart disease. A study summarizing all of the important occupational studies shows a 90 percent reduced risk for coronary heart disease for those in active versus inactive occupations.

The American Heart Association, after carefully examining the research literature, elevated sedentary living from a secondary to a primary risk factor, comparable to high blood pressure, high blood cholesterol, obesity, and cigarette smoke. The reason for this change is that inactivity increases risk in multiple ways and large numbers of adults are sedentary and vulnerable to these risks. After reviewing hundreds of studies on exercise and heart disease, the *Surgeon General's Report on Physical Activity and Health* concluded that "physical inactivity is causally linked to atherosclerosis and coronary heart disease."

Physical Activity and the Healthy Heart

Regular exercise increases the heart muscle's ability to pump oxygen-rich blood. A fit heart muscle can handle extra demands placed on it. Through regular exercise, the heart muscle gets stronger, contracts more forcefully, and therefore pumps more blood with each beat. The heart is just like any other muscle—it must be exercised regularly to stay fit. The fit heart also has open, clear arteries free of atherosclerosis (see Figure 1).

The "normal" resting heart rate is said to be 72 beats per minute (bpm). However, resting rates of 50 to 85 bpm are common. People who regularly do physical activity

typically have lower resting heart rates than people who do no regular activity. Some endurance athletes have heart rates in the 30 and 40 bpm range, which is considered healthy or normal. Although resting heart rate is *not* considered to be a good measure of health or fitness, decreases in individual heart rate following training reflect positive adaptations. Low heart rates in response to a standard amount of physical activity *are* a good indicator of fitness. The bicycle and step tests presented later in this book use your heart rate response to a standard amount of exercise to estimate your cardiovascular fitness.

Physical Activity and Atherosclerosis

Atherosclerosis, which begins early in life, is implicated in many cardiovascular diseases. Atherosclerosis is a condition that contributes to heart attack, stroke, hypertension, angina pectoris, and peripheral vascular disease. Deposits on the walls of arteries restrict blood flow and oxygen supply to the tissues. Atherosclerosis of the coronary arteries, the vessels that supply the heart muscle with oxygen, is particularly harmful. If these arteries become narrowed, the blood supply to the heart muscle is diminished, and angina pectoris may occur. Atherosclerosis increases the risk of heart attack because a fibrous clot is more likely to obstruct a narrowed artery than a healthy, open one.

Current theory suggests that atherosclerosis begins when damage occurs to the cells of the inner wall, or intima, of the artery (see Figure 2). Substances associated

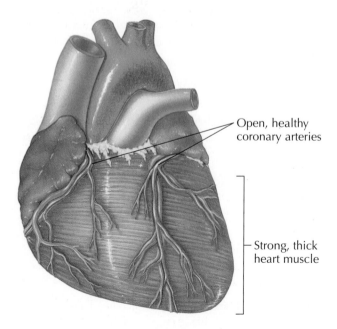

Figure 1 ▶ The fit heart muscle.

Open, healthy coronary arteries

Strong, thick heart muscle

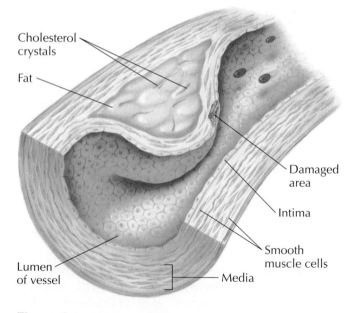

Figure 2 ▶ Atherosclerosis.

Cholesterol crystals

Fat

Damaged area

Intima

Smooth muscle cells

Media

Lumen of vessel

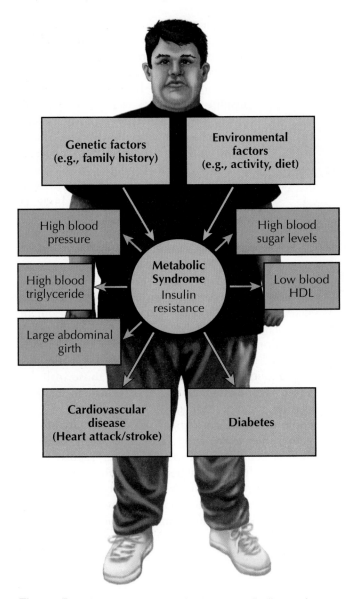

Figure 5 ▶ Mechanism and effects of metabolic syndrome.

is better at predicting heart disease than metabolic syndrome alone, but metabolic syndrome is a better predictor of diabetes. Lab 4A at the end of the concept can be used by those who do not have the necessary metabolic syndrome measures, though having a metabolic fitness assessment is advised periodically, especially as you grow older.

Many factors in addition to healthy lifestyle have led to a significant reduction in cardiovascular disease deaths in recent years. The focus of this book is on healthy lifestyle changes. While lifestyle changes such as being active, eating well, managing stress, and abstaining from tobacco use are important in the prevention and treatment of cardiovascular diseases, a variety of other factors have contributed to the recent decrease in deaths associated with the diseases. Heart disease is

still the leading killer of both men and women. In the late 1990s deaths exceeded one million per year, but the most recent statistics indicate that 810,000 die annually from heart diseases. Over the last decade death rates from heart disease have decreased by more than 29 percent. Some of the reasons for that decline, other than healthy lifestyle change, include earlier and better detection (e.g., exercise tests, angiograms, CT scans) and better emergency care. Improved medications for lowering blood fat levels (e.g., blood thinners, including aspirin), and lowering blood pressure levels have also played a role. Improved and less invasive surgical methods (e.g., angioplasty, stents) and improvements in postcoronary care have also contributed to reducing death rates.

Physical Activity and Other Hypokinetic Conditions

Physical activity reduces the risk of some forms of cancer. According to the American Cancer Society (ACS), cancer is a group of many different conditions characterized by abnormal, uncontrolled cell growth. As illustrated in Figure 6, the abnormal cells divide, forming **malignant tumors (carcinomas).** If the abnormal cells reach the blood, they can spread, causing tumors elsewhere in the body. **Benign tumors** are generally not considered to be cancerous because their growth is restricted to a specific area of the body by a protective membrane. The first editions of this book did not include any form of cancer as a hypokinetic disease. We now know, however, that overall death rates from some types of cancer are lower among active people than those who are sedentary. These cancers are described in Table 3 with possible reasons for the cancer/inactivity link. The entries in Table 3 are listed in order based on the strength of evidence supporting the cancer/inactivity link.

As indicated in Concept 1, cancer is a leading cause of death. In the United States cancer causes more than 560,000 deaths annually. However, the five-year survival rate for people diagnosed with cancer is up 50 percent over the past three decades. Many factors are responsible, including early diagnosis and improved medical treatments. Healthy lifestyles can also play a role. The American Cancer Society (ACS) recently released guidelines that highlight the importance of regular physical activity and a healthy diet in preventing cancer and

Malignant Tumors (carcinomas) An uncontrolled and dangerous growth capable of spreading to other areas; a cancerous tumor.

Benign Tumors An abnormal growth of tissue confined to a particular area; not considered to be cancer.

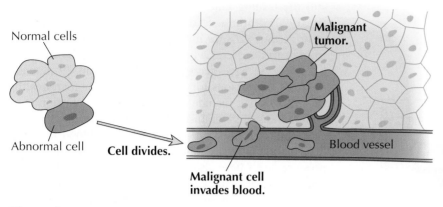

Figure 6 ▶ The spread of cancer (metastasis).

Table 3 ▶ Physical Activity and Cancer

Cancer Type	Effect of Physical Activity
Colon	Exercise speeds movement of food and cancer-causing substances through the digestive system, and reduces prostaglandins (substances linked to cancer in the colon).
Breast	Exercise decreases the amount of exposure of breast tissue to circulating estrogen. Lower body fat is also associated with lower estrogen levels. Early life activity is deemed important for both reasons. Fatigue from therapy is reduced by exercise.
Rectal	Similar to colon cancer, exercise leads to more regular bowel movements and reduces "transit time."
Prostate	Fatigue from therapy is reduced by exercise. Regular exercise, especially vigorous exercise, may reduce death rate.

early death associated with it. Physical activity is also considered to be important to the wellness of the cancer patient. Patients can benefit from activity in many ways, including improved quality of life, physical functioning, and self-esteem, as well as less dependence on others, reduced risk for other diseases, and reduced fatigue from disease or disease therapy. The ACS and the Lance Armstrong Foundation (www.Livestrong.org) are two good sources of information about cancer and cancer treatments.

 Physical activity plays a role in the management and treatment of Type II FEATURE 7 **diabetes.** Diabetes mellitus (diabetes) is a group of disorders that results when there is too much sugar in the blood. It occurs when the body does not make enough **insulin** or when the body is not able to use insulin effectively.

Type I diabetes, or insulin-dependent diabetes, accounts for a relatively small number of the diabetes cases and is not considered to be a hypokinetic condition. Type II diabetes (often not insulin-dependent) was formerly called "adult-onset diabetes." Reports indicate more cases of Type II diabetes among children than in the past, in part because of better record keeping but also because childhood diabetes is associated with increases in obesity and high body fat among children in recent years.

Diabetes is the seventh leading cause of death among people over 40. It accounts for at least 10 percent of all short-term hospital stays and has a major impact on health-care costs in Western society. According to the American Diabetes Association (ADA), there are nearly 24 million people in the United States with diabetes (7.8 percent of the population). Unfortunately, 5.7 million of those don't know it. An estimated additional 57 million are prediabetic; they have metabolic profiles characteristic of those with diabetes (see Web Resources, ADA, or Canadian Diabetes Association, for more statistics).

People who perform regular physical activity are less likely to suffer from Type II diabetes than sedentary people. For people with Type II diabetes, regular physical activity can help reduce body fatness, decrease **insulin resistance,** improve **insulin sensitivity,** and improve the body's ability to clear sugar from the blood in a reasonable time. With sound nutritional habits and proper medication, physical activity can be useful in the management of both types of diabetes.

 Regular physical activity is important to maintaining bone density and decreasing FEATURE 8 **risk for osteoporosis.** As noted in Concept 1, some experts consider bone integrity to be a health-related component of physical fitness. Bone density cannot be self-assessed. It is measured using a dual X-ray absorptiometry (DXA) machine, an expensive and sophisticated form of X-ray machine that can also be used to measure body fatness (see Technology Update in Concept 13). Healthy bones are dense and strong. When bones lose calcium and become less dense, they become porous and are at risk for fracture. The bones of young children are not especially dense, but during adolescence (see Figure 7) bone density increases to a level higher than at any other time in life (peak bone density). Though bone density often begins to decrease in young adulthood, it is not until older adulthood that bone loss becomes dramatic. As illustrated in Figure 7, many older adults have lost enough bone density to have a condition called **osteoporosis** (when bone density

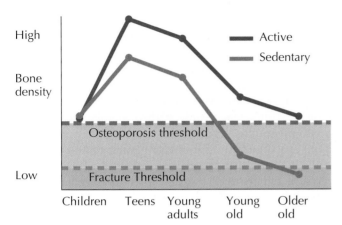

Figure 7 ► Changes in bone density with age.

• Talk to your health-care provider about bone health.
• When appropriate, have a bone density test and take medication. There is no cure for osteoporosis, but the FDA has approved a variety of treatments for osteoporosis to help reduce bone loss over time. When appropriate, a physician may prescribe FDA-approved medications such as raloxifene (sold as Evista), alendronate (sold as Fosomax), or other approved drugs. Hormone treatments such as thyroid-based Calcitonin treatments and estrogen are approved. Estrogen replacement therapy (ERT), also known as hormone replacement treatment (HRT), can reduce risk of osteoporosis among postmenopausal women, but may increase risk for cancer and other diseases. Medical consultation based on individual factors is recommended.

drops below the osteoporosis threshold). Some will have crossed the fracture threshold, putting them at risk for fractures, especially to the hip, vertebrae, and other "soft" or "spongy" bones of the skeletal system. Active people have a higher peak bone mass and are more resistant to osteoporosis (see blue line in Figure 7) than sedentary people (see red line in Figure 7).

Women, especially postmenopausal women, have a higher risk of osteoporosis than men, but it is a disease of both sexes. Figure 7 reflects bone density status for both men and women, but note that males typically have a higher peak bone mass than females, and for this reason, males can lose more bone density over time without reaching the osteoporosis or fracture threshold. More women reach the osteoporosis and fracture thresholds at earlier ages than men. Other risk factors for osteoporosis are northern European ancestry, smoking, caffeine use, alcohol use, current or previous eating disorders, early menstruation, low dietary calcium intake, low body fat, amenorrhea, and extended bed rest.

The National Osteoporosis Foundation (NOF) recommends five steps to bone health and osteoporosis prevention:

• Get daily recommended amounts of calcium and vitamin D. Eat a diet rich in both nutrients. Exposure to the sun provides a source of vitamin D. The NOF recommends 1,000 mg of calcium daily for people under 50, and 1,200 mg for those over 50. Adults under age 50 need 400–800 IU of vitamin D, and adults over 50 need 800–1,000 units. If you have difficulty getting enough of these nutrients from food or sunlight, a supplement may be indicated. It is recommended that you discuss this with your health-care provider.
• Engage in regular weight-bearing exercise. Weight-bearing exercise (e.g., walking, dancing, jogging) and resistance training are good choices. The load bearing and pull of muscles build bone density.
• Avoid smoking and excessive alcohol.

Active people who possess good muscle fitness are less likely to have back and musculoskeletal problems than are inactive, unfit people. Because few people die from it, back pain does not receive the attention given to such medical problems as heart disease and cancer. But back pain is considered to be the second leading medical complaint in the United States, second only to headaches. Only the common cold and the flu cause more days lost from work. At some point in our lives, approximately 80 percent of all adults experience back pain that limits their ability to function normally. In National Safety Council data, the back was the most frequently injured of all body parts, and the injury rate was double that of any other part of the body.

Many years ago, medical doctors began to associate back problems with the lack of physical fitness. It is now known that the great majority of back ailments are the result of poor muscle strength, low levels of endurance, and poor flexibility. Tests on patients with back problems show weakness and lack of flexibility in key muscle groups.

Though lack of fitness is probably the leading reason for back pain in Western society, many other factors increase the risk of back ailments, including poor

Insulin A hormone secreted by the pancreas that regulates levels of sugar in the blood.

Insulin Resistance A condition that occurs when insulin becomes ineffective or less effective than necessary to regulate sugar levels in the blood.

Insulin Sensitivity A person with insulin resistance (see previous definition) is said to have decreased insulin sensitivity. The body's cells are not sensitive to insulin, so they resist it and sugar levels are not regulated effectively.

Osteoporosis A condition associated with low bone density and subsequent bone fragility, leading to high risk for fracture.

posture, improper lifting and work habits, heredity, and disease states such as scoliosis and arthritis.

Physical activity is important in maintaining a healthy body weight and avoiding the numerous health conditions associated with obesity. National studies indicate that more than two-thirds of adults are overweight and more than one-third are obese (32.2 percent of men and 35.5% of women). Nearly a third of children are either overweight or obese. From 1950 through 1980, obesity (15 percent) and overweight were fairly stable but increased dramatically from 1980 to the present. In the past few years the rate of increase in overweight and obesity has not been as dramatic as during the previous decade (see Figure 8). Obesity is not a disease state in itself but is a hypokinetic condition associated with a multitude of far-reaching complications. Research has shown that fat people who are fit are not at especially high risk for early death. However, when high body fatness is accompanied by low cardiovascular and low metabolic fitness, risk for early death increases substantially. Obesity contributes to sedentary death syndrome, described earlier in this concept. For more information on obesity see Concept 13 or go to this Web link: www.cdc.gov/obesity/index.html.

Physical activity reduces the risk and severity of a variety of common emotional/mental health disorders. Such disorders can be considered hypokinetic conditions. Some emotional/mental health conditions are prevalent in modern society. Nearly half of adult Americans will report having a mental health disorder at some point in life. A recent summary of studies revealed that there are several emotional/mental disorders associated with inactive lifestyles.

Depression is a stress-related condition experienced by many adults. Thirty-three percent of inactive adults report that they often feel depressed. For some, depression is a serious disorder that physical activity alone will not cure; however, research indicates that activity, combined with other forms of therapy, can be effective.

Anxiety is an emotional condition characterized by worry, self-doubt, and apprehension. More than a few studies have shown that symptoms of anxiety can be reduced by regular activity. Low-fit people who do regular aerobic activity seem to benefit the most. In one study, one-third of active people felt that regular activity helped them cope better with life's pressures.

Physical activity is also associated with better and more restful sleep. People with insomnia (the inability to sleep) seem to benefit from regular activity if it is not done too vigorously right before going to bed. A recent study indicates that 52 percent of the population feel that physical activity helps them sleep better. Regular aerobic activity is associated with reduced brain activation, which can result in greater ability to relax or fall asleep.

Even more common than depression and insomnia is the condition called Type A behavior. Type A personalities are stress-prone individuals with a greater than normal incidence of diseases. A Type A person is tense, overcompetitive, and worried about meeting schedules. Apparently, all Type A personalities are not equally stressed. It has been suggested that aggressive Type A personalities are most likely to be prone to negative consequences of stress. Regular physical activity can benefit the Type A person, especially the aggressive Type A. Noncompetitive activities are best for this personality type.

A final benefit of regular exercise is increased self-esteem. Improvements in fitness, appearance, and the ability to perform new tasks can improve self-confidence and self-esteem.

Physical activity can help the immune system fight illness. Until recently, infectious disease and other diseases of the immune system were not considered to be hypokinetic. Recent evidence indicates that regular moderate to vigorous activity can actually aid the immune system in fighting disease. Each of us is born with an "innate immune system," which includes anatomical and physiological barriers, such as skin, mucous membranes, body temperature, and chemical mediators that help prevent and resist disease. We also develop an "acquired immune system" in the form of special disease-fighting cells that help us resist disease. Figure 9 shows a J-shaped curve that illustrates the benefits of exercise to acquired immune function. Sedentary people have more risk than those who do moderate activity, but with very high and sustained vigorous activity, such as extended high performance training, immune system function actually decreases.

Regular moderate and reasonable amounts of vigorous activity have been shown to reduce incidence of colds and days of sickness from infection. The immune system benefit may extend to other immune system disorders as well. There is evidence that regular physical activity can enhance treatment effectiveness and improve quality of life for those with HIV/AIDS. However, as Figure 9 indicates, too much exercise may cause problems rather than solve them.

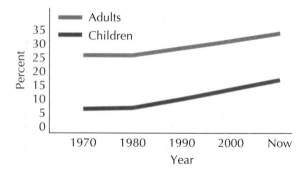

Figure 8 ► Incidence of obesity.
Source: National Center for Health Statistics.

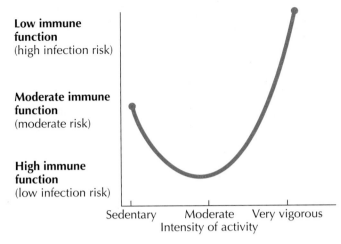

Figure 9 ▶ Physical activity and immune function.

Physical activity during pregnancy can benefit both the mother and the child. In the not too distant past, exercise during pregnancy was discouraged. Over the years, evidence has accumulated to indicate that appropriate exercise (including resistance training and moderate to vigorous aerobic exercise) by pregnant women can help prevent excess weight gain, help retain pre-pregnancy fitness levels, and result in shorter, less complicated labor. Physical activity does not cause damage to the baby or miscarriage and may help the baby developmentally.

Pregnant women are nearly twice as likely to be sedentary (fail to meet current activity guidelines) than other women in spite of the fact that guidelines from the American College of Obstetricians and Gynecologists (www.acog.org) indicate that most women should meet national guidelines as described later in this book. More intense exercise (including some forms of competitive activity) is appropriate in many cases but should be done with "close medical supervision."

Regular physical activity can have positive effects on some nonhypokinetic conditions. The following nonhypokinetic conditions can benefit from physical activity:

- *Arthritis.* Many, if not most, arthritics are in a deconditioned state resulting from a lack of activity. The traditional advice that arthritics should avoid physical activity is now being modified in view of the findings that carefully prescribed exercise has a variety of benefits. Common problems for both those with rheumatoid arthritis (RA) and osteoarthritis (OA) are decreased strength, loss of range of motion, and poor cardiovascular endurance. Well-planned exercise, designed to meet the needs of the specific type of arthritis of the individual, can be beneficial in preventing and treating impairments, enhancing function, and enhancing general fitness and well-being.

- *Asthma.* Asthmatics often have physical activity limitations. New evidence suggests that with proper management activity can be part of their daily life. In fact, when done properly, activity can reduce airway reactivity and medication use. Because exercise can trigger bronchial constriction, it is important to choose appropriate types of activity and to use inhaled medications to prevent bronchial constriction caused by exercise or other triggers, such as cold weather. Asthmatics should avoid cold weather exercise.

- *Premenstrual syndrome (PMS).* PMS, a mixture of physical and emotional symptoms that occurs prior to menstruation, has many causes. However, current evidence suggests that changes in lifestyle, including regular exercise, may be effective in relieving PMS symptoms.

- *Other conditions.* Low- to moderate-intensity aerobic activity and resistance training are currently being prescribed for some people who have chronic pain (persistent pain without relief) and/or fibromyalgia (chronic muscle pain). Evidence also suggests that active people have a 30 percent less chance of having gallstones than inactive people, and activity may decrease risk of impotence.

Physical Activity and Aging

Regular physical activity can improve fitness and functioning among older adults. Approximately 30 percent of adults age 70 and over have difficulty with one or more activities of daily living. Women have more limitations than men, and low-income groups have more limitations than higher-income groups. Nearly one-half of these adults also get no assistance in coping with their limitations.

The inability to function effectively as you grow older is associated with lack of fitness and inactive lifestyles. This loss of function is sometimes referred to as "acquired aging," as opposed to "time-dependent" aging. Because so many people experience limitations in daily activities and find it difficult to get assistance, it is especially important for older people to stay active and fit. In Africa, Asia, and South America, where older adults maintain an active lifestyle, individuals do not acquire many of the characteristics commonly associated with aging in North America.

In general, older adults are much less active than younger adults. Losses in muscle fitness are associated with loss of balance, greater risk of falling, and less ability to function independently. Studies also show that exercise can enhance cognitive functioning and perhaps reduce risk for dementia. Though the amount of activity performed must be adapted as people grow older, fitness benefits discussed in the next section and throughout this book apply to people of all ages.

Regular physical activity can compress illness into a shorter period of our life. An important national health goal is to increase the years of healthy life. Living longer is important, but being able to function effectively during all years of life is equally—if not more—important. *Compression of illness,* also called compression of morbidity, refers to shortening the total number of years that illnesses and disabilities occur. Healthy lifestyles, including regular physical activity, have been shown to compress illness and increase years of effective functioning. Inactive people not only have a shorter life span, but have more years of illness and disability than active people.

Recent evidence indicates that Alzheimer's disease and dementia are hypokinetic conditions. More than a few studies indicate that factors relating to heart health also contribute to brain health. The studies indicate that physical and challenging mental activities are especially important among the lifestyle factors involved in maintaining brain health and preventing Alzheimer's disease and dementia. An increasing number of studies point to the value of physical activity in preventing cognitive decline function and reducing risk of developing Alzheimer's and dementia. Although additional research is needed, this is important news for physicians and public health officials looking for ways to reduce the prevalence of Alzheimer's disease. Approximately 5.3 million people in the United States have Alzheimer's, and the prevalence is expected to increase in the future as people live longer. The direct and indirect costs associated with Alzheimer's in the United States are estimated to be $148 billion annually.

Physical Activity, Health, and Wellness

Good health-related physical fitness and regular physical activity contribute to optimal wellness. Regular physical activity and good fitness not only help prevent illness (see Table 4) and disease but also promote quality of life and wellness. Good health-related physical fitness can help you look good, feel good, and enjoy life. Specific benefits of wellness associated with good fitness are the following:

* *Good physical fitness can help an individual work effectively and efficiently.* A person who can resist fatigue, muscle soreness, back problems, and other symptoms associated with poor health-related fitness is capable of working productively and having energy left over at the end of the day. Employees involved with fitness programs at work report an improved sense of well-being. Employers indicate that absenteeism decreases by up to 50 percent among program participants.

People with good skill-related fitness may be more effective and efficient in performing certain jobs.

* *Good physical fitness can help an individual enjoy leisure time.* A person who is lean, has no back problems, does not have high blood pressure, and has reasonable skills in a lifetime of sports is more likely to get involved and stay regularly involved in leisure-time activities than one who does not have these characteristics. Enjoying your leisure time may not add years to your life but can add life to your years.

* *Good physical fitness is essential to effective living.* Although the need for each component of physical fitness is specific to each individual, every person requires enough fitness to perform normal daily activities without undue fatigue. Whether it be walking, performing household chores, or merely feeling good and enjoying the simple things in life without pain or fear of injury, good fitness is important to all people.

* *Physical fitness is the basis for dynamic and creative activity.* Though the following quotation by former President John F. Kennedy is more than 40 years old, it clearly points out the importance of physical fitness:

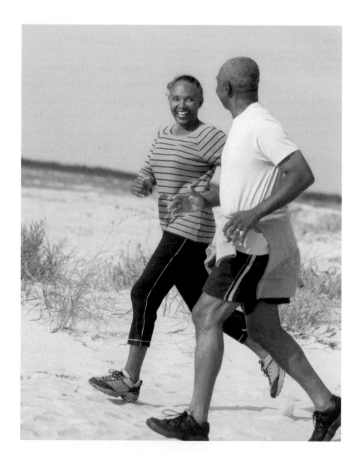

Regular physical activity promotes healthy aging and high quality of life.

Table 4 ▶ Health and Wellness Benefits of Physical Activity and Fitness

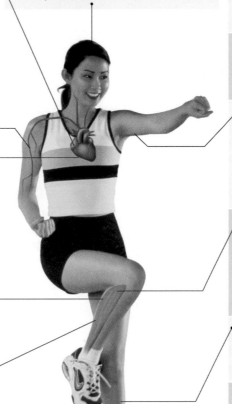

Improved Cardiovascular Health
- Stronger heart muscle fitness and health
- Lower heart rate
- Better electric stability of heart
- Decreased sympathetic control of heart
- Increased O_2 to brain
- Reduced blood fat, including low-density lipoproteins (LDLs)
- Increased protective high-density lipoproteins (HDLs)
- Delayed development of atherosclerosis
- Increased work capacity
- Improved peripheral circulation
- Improved coronary circulation
- Resistance to "emotional storm"
- Reduced risk for heart attack
- Reduced risk for stroke
- Reduced risk for hypertension
- Greater chance of surviving a heart attack
- Increased oxygen-carrying capacity of the blood

Improved Strength and Muscular Endurance
- Greater work efficiency
- Less chance for muscle injury
- Reduced risk for low back problems
- Improved performance in sports
- Quicker recovery after hard work
- Improved ability to meet emergencies

Resistance to Fatigue
- Ability to enjoy leisure
- Improved quality of life
- Improved ability to meet some stressors

Other Health Benefits
- Decreased diabetes risk
- Quality of life for diabetics
- Improved metabolic fitness
- Extended life
- Decrease in dysfunctional years
- Aids for some people who have arthritis, PMS, asthma, chronic pain, fibromyalgia, or impotence
- Improved immune system

Enhanced Mental Health and Function
- Relief of depression
- Improved sleep habits
- Fewer stress symptoms
- Ability to enjoy leisure and work
- Improved brain function

Improved Wellness
- Improved quality of life
- Leisure-time enjoyment
- Improved work capacity
- Ability to meet emergencies
- Improved creative capacity

Opportunity for Successful Experience and Social Interactions
- Improved self-concept
- Opportunity to recognize and accept personal limitations
- Improved sense of well-being
- Enjoyment of life and fun
- Improved quality of life

Improved Appearance
- Better figure/physique
- Better posture
- Fat control

Greater Lean Body Mass and Less Body Fat
- Greater work efficiency
- Less susceptibility to disease
- Improved appearance
- Less incidence of self-concept problems related to obesity

Improved Flexibility
- Greater work efficiency
- Less chance of muscle injury
- Less chance of joint injury
- Decreased chance of developing low back problems
- Improved sports performance

Bone Development
- Greater peak bone density
- Less chance of developing osteoporosis

Reduced Cancer Risk
- Reduced risk for colon and breast cancer
- Possible reduced risk for rectal and prostate cancers

Reduced Effect of Acquired Aging
- Improved ability to function in daily life
- Better short-term memory
- Fewer illnesses
- Greater mobility
- Greater independence
- Greater ability to operate an automobile
- Lower risk for dementia

"The relationship between the soundness of the body and the activity of the mind is subtle and complex. Much is not yet understood, but we know what the Greeks knew: that intelligence and skill can only function at the peak of their capacity when the body is healthy and strong, and that hardy spirits and tough minds usually inhabit sound bodies. Physical fitness is the basis of all activities in our society; if our bodies grow soft and inactive, if we fail to encourage physical development and prowess, we will undermine our capacity for thought, for work, and for the use of those skills vital to an expanding and complex America."

Health is available to EVERYONE for a Lifetime, and it's Personal

The benefits associated with regular physical activity are enormous and have been well documented—but participation in exercise and physical activity still remains low. According to the National Center for Health Statistics, only 30% of adults engage in regular leisure-time physical activity.

Health, United States 2009 http://www.cdc.gov/nchs/hus.htm

Why do you think people, in general, don't feel that physical activity is valuable enough to make time for in their lives?

President Kennedy's belief that activity and fitness are associated with intellectual functioning has now been backed up with research. A recent research summary suggests that, though modest, the effect of activity and fitness on intellectual functioning is positive. One study shows activity to foster new brain cell growth. Time taken to be active during the day has been shown to help children learn more, even though less time is spent in intellectual pursuits.

- *Good physical fitness may help you function safely and assist you in meeting unexpected emergencies.* Emergencies are never expected, but, when they do arise, they often demand performance that requires good fitness. For example, flood victims may need to fill sandbags for hours without rest, and accident victims may be required to walk or run long distances for help. Also, good fitness is required for such simple tasks as safely changing a spare tire or loading a moving van without injury.

(i) **Physical activity is a major part of most employee health promotion programs.**
FEATURE 9 Companies have come to understand the importance of promoting healthy lifestyles among their employees. Work-site health promotion programs typically use a broad focus on promoting a variety of healthy lifestyles, but physical activity is considered the mainstay of most programs. To facilitate active lifestyles in employees, many companies build their own fitness centers inside the workplace or provide free or reduced-cost memberships for employees. Work-site programs that promote activity can reduce risk factors in employees and help companies control the high cost of health care. Studies have consistently documented that the cost of these programs more than offsets the expense. Companies that offer comprehensive programs frequently save more than $4 for each dollar invested. The expansion of work-site health programs is viewed as

Table 5 ▶ Hypokinetic Disease Risk Factors

Factors That Cannot Be Altered

1. *Age.* As you grow older, your risk of contracting hypokinetic diseases increases. For example, the risk for heart disease is approximately three times as great after 60 as before. The risk of back pain is considerably greater after 40.
2. *Heredity.* People who have a family history of hypokinetic disease are more likely to develop a hypokinetic condition, such as heart disease, hypertension, back problems, obesity, high blood lipid levels, and other problems. African Americans are 45 percent more likely to have high blood pressure than Caucasians; therefore, they suffer strokes at an earlier age with more severe consequences.
3. *Gender.* Men have a higher incidence of many hypokinetic conditions than women. However, differences between men and women have decreased recently. This is especially true for heart disease, the leading cause of death for both men and women. Postmenopausal women have a higher heart disease risk than premenopausal women.

Factors That Can Be Altered

4. *Regular physical activity.* As noted throughout this book, regular exercise can help reduce the risk for hypokinetic disease.
5. *Diet.* A clear association exists between hypokinetic disease and certain types of diets. The excessive intake of saturated fats, such as animal fats, is linked to atherosclerosis and other forms of heart disease. Excessive salt in the diet is associated with high blood pressure.
6. *Stress.* People who are subject to excessive stress are predisposed to various hypokinetic diseases, including heart disease and back pain. Statistics indicate that hypokinetic conditions are common among those in certain high-stress jobs and those having Type A personality profiles.
7. *Tobacco use.* Smokers have five times the risk of heart attack as nonsmokers. Most striking is the difference in risk between older women smokers and nonsmokers. Tobacco use is also associated with the increased risk for high blood pressure, cancer, and several other medical conditions. Apparently, the more you use, the greater the risk. Stopping tobacco use even after many years can significantly reduce the hypokinetic disease risk.
8. *Body (fatness).* Having too much body fat is a primary risk factor for heart disease and is a risk factor for other hypokinetic conditions as well. For example, loss of fat can result in relief from symptoms of Type II diabetes, can reduce problems associated with certain types of back pain, and can reduce the risks of surgery.
9. *Blood lipids, blood glucose, and blood pressure levels.* High scores on these factors are associated with health problems, such as heart disease and diabetes. Risk increases considerably when several of these measures are high.
10. *Diseases.* People who have one hypokinetic disease are more likely to develop a second or even a third condition. For example, if you have diabetes,* your risk of having a heart attack or stroke increases dramatically. Although you may not be entirely able to alter the extent to which you develop certain diseases and conditions, reducing your risk and following your doctor's advice can improve your odds significantly.

*Some types of diabetes cannot be altered.

a critical public health priority and one of the most promising approaches for controlling health-care costs. See associated Web link for additional information.

Too much activity can lead to hyperkinetic conditions. The information presented in this concept points out the health benefits of physical activity performed in appropriate amounts. When done in excess or incorrectly, physical activity can result in **hyperkinetic conditions.** The most common hyperkinetic condition is overuse injury to muscles, connective tissue, and bones. Recently, anorexia nervosa and body neurosis have been identified as conditions associated with inappropriate amounts of physical activity. These conditions will be discussed in the concept on performance.

Physical activity is now recognized as effective "medicine" for prevention of chronic disease. For some time, exercise has been prescribed for patients recovering from heart attacks and for a variety of other conditions (e.g., high blood pressure, metabolic syndrome). The American College of Sports Medicine (ACSM) has initiated a program called "Exercise Is Medicine (EIM)" designed to "encourage primary care physicians, and other health care providers, to include exercise when designing treatment plans for patients." The program is endorsed by the American Medical Association and now has a dedicated staff and Web page (www.exerciseismedicine.org). EIM provides information

to the general public, health-care providers, health and fitness professionals, and the media.

 There are many positive lifestyles that can reduce the risk for disease and FEATURE 10 **promote health and wellness.** Inactivity, poor nutrition, smoking, and inability to cope with stress are all risk factors associated with various diseases (see Table 5). Changing these risk factors can dramatically reduce the risk for chronic diseases. It is important to recognize that three risk factors (age, heredity, and gender) are not within your control.

However, by adopting healthy lifestyles, you can take control over the preventable disease risks. For example, controlling body fatness reduces the risk for diabetes, hypertension, and back problems. Altering your diet can reduce the chances of developing high levels of blood lipids and reduce the risk for atherosclerosis. Being active and adopting healthy lifestyles is a proactive approach to health and wellness. While reducing risk can alter the probability of disease, it does not assure disease immunity.

Hyperkinetic Conditions Diseases/illnesses or health conditions caused, or contributed to, by too much physical activity.

 Strategies for Action

A self-assessment of risk factors can help you modify your lifestyle to reduce risk for heart disease. The Heart Disease Risk Factor Questionnaire in Lab 4A will help you assess your personal risk for heart disease. Although the questionnaire is educationally useful in making you aware of risk factors, it is not a substitute for a regular medical exam. A medical exam that includes an assessment of blood lipids as described in this concept is recommended. This will allow you to use more sophisticated and accurate risk factor assessments, such as the Framingham Risk Score.

It is never too early to start being active to improve health. Many of the studies presented in

this concept indicate that being "active for a lifetime" prevents health problems. College-aged students have been known to comment, "I'm young; I don't have these health problems," or "I'll worry about these problems when I get older." But the best evidence indicates that what you do early in life has much to do with your current health, as well as your health later in life. It is never too early to begin. Subsequent concepts in this book cover the different components of health-related fitness and the type and amount of activity needed to improve these components. The lab activities in each of these concepts and the culminating lab activity at the end of this book are designed to help you begin planning *now* for lifelong physical activity.

Web Resources

Additional websites with information related to Concept 4 are available at the associated Web link.

Alzheimer's Association **www.alz.org**

American Cancer Society **www.cancer.org**

American College of Obstetricians and Gynecologists **www.acog.org**

American Diabetes Association **www.diabetes.org**

American Heart Association **www.americanheart.org**

American Lung Association **www.lungusa.org**

Arthritis Foundation **www.arthritis.org**

Canadian Diabetes Association **www.diabetes.ca**

Centers for Disease Control and Prevention **www.cdc.gov**

Exercise Is Medicine **www.exerciseismedicine.org**

Healthy People 2010 **www.health.gov/healthypeople**

Lance Armstrong Foundation **www.livestrong.org**

National Heart Lung and Blood Institute Your Guide to Lowering High Blood Pressure **www.nhlbi.nih.gov/hbp/index.html**

National Osteoporosis Foundation **www.nof.org**

National Stroke Association **www.stroke.org**

Surgeon General **www.surgeongeneral.gov**

Worksite Wellness Information **http://healthproject.stanford .edu/koop/work.html**

United States Physical Activity Guidelines **http://www.health .gov/paguidelines/**

Suggested Readings

Selected readings and references are listed below. A more comprehensive list is available at the associated Web icon.

ACSM. 2010. *ACSM's Guidelines for Exercise Testing and Prescription.* 8th ed. Philadelphia: Lippincott, Williams & Wilkins, Chapter 1.

American Cancer Society. 2009. *Cancer Facts and Figures 2009.* Atlanta: ACS. Available at **www.cancer.org/docroot/home/ index.asp?level=0**

Baker, L. D., et al. 2010 Effects of aerobic exercise on middle cognitive impairment. *Archives of Neurology* 67(1): 71–79.

Brady, J. F. 2009. Exercising and the brain. *ACSM's Health and Fitness Journal* 13(2):27–31.

Chodzko-Zajko, W. J., et al., 2009. Exercise and physical activity for older adults. *Medicine & Science in Sports & Exercise* 41(7):1510–1530.

Churilla, J. R. 2009. The metabolic syndrome: The crucial role of exercise prescription and diet. *ACSM's Health and Fitness Journal* 13(2):27–31.

Flegal, K. M. 2010. Prevalence and trends in obesity among US adults. *Journal of the American Medical Association* 303(3):235–241.

Geda, Y. E., et al. 2010. Physical exercise, aging, and mild cognitive impairment. *Archives of Neurology* 67(1): 80–86.

Ogden, C. L., et al. 2010. Prevalence of high body mass index in U.S. children and adolescents. *Journal of the American Medical Association* 303(3): 242–249.

Rosenberg, R. N. Exercised against dementia. *Archives of Neurology* 66(3): 311–312.

Rowland, T. W. 2009. Exercise and cardiovascular health in children: A new paradigm on the horizon? *Pediatric Exercise Science* 21(3): 249–256.

Sorace, P., et al. 2010. Peripheral arterial disease. *ACSM's Health and Fitness Journal* 14(1): 16–22.

Surgeon General's Vision for a Healthy and Fit Nation. 2010. Available at **www.surgeongeneral.gov**

Tangka, F. K., et al. 2010. Cancer treatment costs in the United States. *Cancer.* Published online May 10, 2010, **www.canceronlinejournal.com**

U.S. Department of Health and Human Services. 2008. *2008 Physical Activity Guidelines for Americans.* Washington, DC: USDHHS. Available at **www.health.gov/paguidelines**

Walther, C., et al. 2004. The effect of exercise training on endothelial function in cardiovascular diseases in humans. *Exercise and Sport Sciences Reviews* 32:129–134.

Lab 4A Assessing Heart Disease Risk Factors

Name			Section		Date

Purpose: To assess your risk of developing coronary heart disease. See page 84 for directions.

Heart Disease Risk Factor Questionnaire
Risk Points

	1	2	3	4	Score
Unalterable Factors					
1. How old are you?	30 or less	31–40	41–54	55+	
2. Do you have a history of heart disease in your family?	None	Grandparent with heart disease	Parent with heart disease	More than one with heart disease	
3. What is your gender?	Female		Male		
				Total Unalterable Risk Score	
Alterable Factors					
4. Do you get regular physical activity?	4–5 days a week	3 days a week	Fewer than 3 days a week	No	
5. Do you have a high-fat diet?	No	Slightly high in fat	Above normal in fat	Eat a lot of meat and fried and fatty foods	
6. Are you under much stress?	Less than normal	Normal	Slightly above normal	Quite high	
7. Do you use tobacco?	No	Cigar or pipe	Less than 1/2 pack a day or use smokeless tobacco	More than 1/2 pack a day	
8. What is your percentage of body fat?*	F = 17–28% M = 10–20%	29–31% 21–23%	32–35% 24–30%	35+% 30+%	
9. What is the systolic number in your blood pressure?	120	121–140	141–160	160+	
10. Do you have other diseases?	No	Ulcer	Diabetes**	Both	

Extra Points: Add points for as many of the following test results as you have available: 1 point for CRP above 3, 1 point for homocysteine above 100, 3 points for LDL above 130, 3 points for TC/HDL-C above 4. If only total cholesterol is available, add 1 point for a score of 200–240 or 3 points for scores above 240.

Total Alterable Risk Score	
Extra Points	
Grand Total Risk Score	

Adapted from *CAD Risk Assessor,* William J. Stone. Reprinted by permission.

*If unknown, estimate your body fat percentage or see Lab 13A.

**Diabetes is a risk factor that is often not alterable.

Procedures

1. Complete the 10 questions and the extra points, if available, on the Heart Disease Risk Factor Questionnaire by circling the answer that is most appropriate for *you* (see front of this lab).
2. Look at the top of the column for each of your answers. In the box provided at the right of each question, write down the number of risk points for that answer.
3. Determine your unalterable risk score by adding the risk points for questions 1, 2, and 3.
4. Determine your alterable risk score by adding the risk points for questions 4 through 10.
5. Determine your total heart disease risk score by adding the scores obtained in steps 3 and 4.
6. Look up your risk ratings on the Heart Disease Risk Rating Scale and record them in the Results section. Answer the questions in the Conclusions and Implications section.

Results: Write your risk scores and risk ratings in the appropriate boxes below.

Heart Disease Risk Scores and Ratings

	Score	Rating
Unalterable risk		
Alterable risk		
Total heart disease risk		

Heart Disease Risk Rating Chart

Rating	Unalterable Score	Alterable Score	Total Score
Very high	9 or more	21 or more	31 or more
High	7–8	15–20	26–30
Average	5–6	11–14	16–25
Low	4 or less	10 or less	15 or less

Conclusions and Implications: The higher your score on the Heart Disease Risk Factor Questionnaire, the greater your heart disease risk. In several sentences, discuss your risk for heart disease. Which of the risk factors do you need to control to reduce your risk for heart disease? Why?

How Much Physical Activity Is Enough?

Health Objectives for the Year 2020

- Reduce proportion of adults who do no leisure-time activity.
- Increase proportion of adults who meet guidelines for aerobic activity.
- Increase proportion of adults who meet guidelines for muscle fitness activity.
- Increase access to employee-based exercise facilities and programs.
- Increase proportion of trips made by walking.
- Increase counseling about physical activity by physicians.
- Increase proportion of youth who meet guidelines for TV viewing and computer use (overuse is 2 hours a day or more).
- Increase proportion of youth who get daily physical education in school.
- Increase proportion of youth who get recess in school.
- Increase schools with activity spaces that can be used in non-school hours.

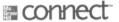

|FITNESS AND WELLNESS http://connect.mcgraw-hill.com

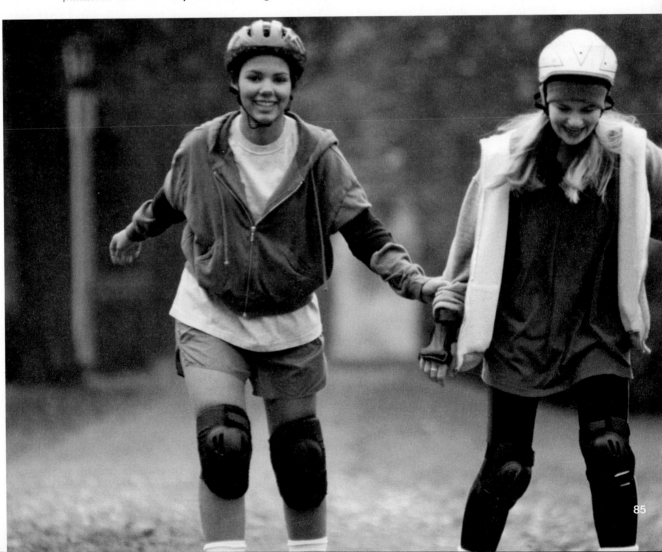

There is a minimal and an optimal amount of physical activity necessary for developing and maintaining good health, wellness, and fitness.

Physical activity is a behavior that leads to fitness, health, and wellness. For physical activity to have an optimal effect, the appropriate amount of activity must be performed. This concept describes the basic principles of physical activity. You will learn about the FITT formula, as well as key concepts such as "threshold of training" and "target zones." Use the physical activity pyramid to help understand and remember physical activity guidelines for different types of activities.

The Principles of Physical Activity

Overload is necessary to achieve the health, wellness, and fitness benefits of physical activity. The **overload principle,** the most basic of all physical activity principles, indicates that doing "more than normal" is necessary if benefits are to occur. In order for a muscle (including the heart muscle) to get stronger, it must be overloaded, or worked against a load greater than normal. To increase flexibility, a muscle must be stretched longer than is normal. To increase muscular endurance, muscles must be exposed to sustained exercise for a longer than normal period. The health benefits associated with metabolic fitness seem to require less overload than for health-related fitness improvement, but overload is required, just the same.

Increase physical activity progressively for safe and effective results. The **principle of progression** indicates that overload should occur in a gradual progression rather than in major bursts. Failure to adhere to this principle can result in excess soreness or injury. Although some tightness or fatigue is common after exercise, it is not necessary to feel sore in order to improve. Training is most effective when the sessions become progressively more challenging over time.

The benefits of physical activity are specific to the form of activity performed. The **principle of specificity** states that to benefit from physical activity you must overload specifically for that benefit. For example, strength-building exercises may do little for developing cardiovascular fitness, and stretching exercises may do little for altering body composition or metabolic fitness.

Overload is also specific to each body part. If you exercise the legs, you build fitness of the legs. If you exercise the arms, you build fitness of the arms. Some gymnasts, for example, have good upper body development but poor leg development, whereas some soccer players have well-developed legs but lack upper body development.

Specificity is important in designing your warm-up, workout, and cool-down programs for specific activities. Training is most effective when it closely resembles the activity for which you are preparing. For example, if your goal is to improve performance in putting the shot, it is not enough to strengthen the arm muscles. You should train using exercises that require overload of all muscles used and that require motions similar to those used in putting the shot.

The benefits achieved from overload last only as long as overload continues. The **principle of reversibility** is the overload principle in reverse. To put it simply, if you don't use it, you lose it. Some people have the mistaken impression that if they achieve a health or fitness benefit it will last forever. This, of course, is not true. There is evidence that you can maintain health benefits with less physical activity than it took to achieve them. Still, if you do not adhere to regular physical activity, any benefits attained will gradually erode.

In general, the more physical activity you do, the more benefits you receive. Just as there is a correct dosage of medicine for treatment of illness, there is a correct dosage of physical activity for promoting health benefits and the development of physical fitness. Though there are some exceptions, a considerable amount of research has demonstrated that benefits from physical activity follow a **dose-response relationship**—the more physical activity you perform, the more benefits you gain.

Figure 1 illustrates the overall pattern of the dose-response relationship. The red bar indicates the high risk for hypokinetic disease and early death for those who are inactive. A modest increase in physical activity, such as the 30 minutes of moderate activity recommended in the new activity guidelines, results in a substantial decrease in risk and early death (green bar). Additional activity (blue bar) has extra benefits, but the benefits are not as great as those that come from making the change from being inactive to doing some activity. As the black bar indicates, very high levels of activity produce little additional health benefit.

As you learned in Concept 4, and as will be pointed out in the concepts that follow, the "dose" of activity necessary to get one benefit is not the same as the "dose" for another. For example, changes in cholesterol levels resulting from physical activity may change at a different rate than changes in blood pressure. Many benefits in health, wellness, and fitness are obtained with moderate amounts of activity, so the key is to be at least active enough to obtain these benefits.

The rate of improvement levels off as you become more fit, and at some point maintenance is an appropriate goal. In physical fitness, more is not always better. As the principle of progression indicates, beginners will benefit most from small doses of activity. For them, doing too much too soon is a bad idea. Also, the **principle of diminished returns** indicates that as you get fitter and fitter you may not get as big a benefit for each additional amount of activity that you perform. When improvements become more difficult and performance levels off, maintenance may become most important. In some cases, excessive amounts of activity can be counterproductive.

Health, wellness, and fitness benefits occur as you increase your physical activity. But understand that if you keep increasing physical activity by equal increments, each additional amount of activity will yield less benefit.

At some point, improvements will plateau and if activity is overdone, may actually decrease.

Rest is needed to allow the body to adapt to exercise. The **principle of rest and recovery** indicates that you should allow time for recuperation after overload. Proper rest is needed within intense periods of activity, and appropriate rest is needed between training sessions. Rest provides time for the body to adapt to the stimulus provided during the workout. Failure to take sufficient rest can lead to overuse injuries, fatigue, and reduced performance. For recreational exercisers, rest generally implies taking a day off between bouts of exercise or alternating hard and easy days of exercise.

All people benefit from physical activity, but the benefits are unique for each person. Heredity, age, gender, ethnicity, lifestyles, current fitness and health

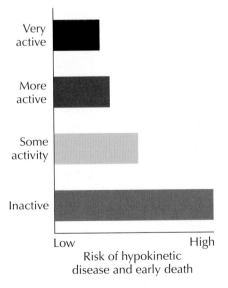

Very active

More active

Some activity

Inactive

Low   High
Risk of hypokinetic
disease and early death

Figure 1 ▶ Decrease in risk with increase in dose of activity.

Overload Principle The basic principle that specifies that you must perform physical activity in greater than normal amounts (overload) to get an improvement in physical fitness or health benefits.

Principle of Progression The corollary of the overload principle that indicates the need to gradually increase overload to achieve optimal benefits.

Principle of Specificity The corollary of the overload principle that indicates a need for a specific type of exercise to improve each fitness component or fitness of a specific part of the body.

Principle of Reversibility The corollary of the overload principle that indicates that disuse or inactivity results in loss of benefits achieved as a result of overload.

Dose-Response Relationship A term adopted from medicine. With medicine, it is important to know what response (benefit) will occur from taking a specific dose. When studying physical activity, it is important to know what dose provides the best response (most benefits). The contents of this book are designed to help you choose the best doses of activity for the responses (benefits) you desire.

Principle of Diminished Returns The corollary of the overload principle indicating that the more benefits you gain as a result of activity, the harder additional benefits are to achieve.

Principle of Rest and Recovery The corollary of the overload principle that indicates that adequate rest is needed to allow the body to adapt to and recover from exercise.

In the News

Increase in Participation in Physical Activity

As noted earlier in this concept, the percentage of Americans meeting standards for moderate and vigorous physical activity has increased over the last decade. It is difficult to determine the specific factors that have contributed to the trends. Some of the effect is likely due to greater public awareness of the health benefits of physical activity. However, environmental changes and the availability of worksite wellness programs in many corporations are also likely contributors to the positive trends. Regardless of the cause, the results are encouraging since they indicate that change is possible! Over the past 15–20 years there has been a concerted effort by state health agencies, educational institutions, non-profit agencies, state and national organizations and many health-related foundations to promote physical activity in society. Additional detail on the documented changes in activity levels are available at the associated Web link.

status, and a variety of other factors make each person unique at any point in time. The **principle of individuality** indicates that the benefits of physical activity vary from individual to individual based on each person's unique characteristics.

The FITT Formula

The acronyms FITT and FIT help you remember important variables for applying the overload principle and its corollaries. For physical activity to be effective, each type of activity must be done with enough frequency, with enough intensity, and for a long enough time. The first letters from four words spell **FITT** and can be considered as the formula for achieving health, wellness, and fitness benefits.

Frequency (how often)—Physical activity must be performed regularly to be effective. The number of days a person does activity in a week determines frequency. Most benefits require at least 3 days and up to 6 days of activity per week, but frequency ultimately depends on the specific activity and the benefit desired.

Intensity (how hard)—Physical activity must be intense enough to require more exertion (overload) than normal to produce benefits. The method for determining appropriate intensity varies with the desired benefit. For example, metabolic fitness and associated health benefits require only moderate intensity; cardiovascular fitness for high-level performance requires vigorous activity that elevates the heart rate well above normal.

Time (how long)—Physical activity must be done for an adequate length of time to be effective. The length of the activity session depends on the type of activity and the expected benefit.

Type (kind of activity)—The benefits derived depend on the type of activity performed. Each activity has a different frequency, intensity, and time. For example, moderate activity must be done at least 5 days a week, while muscle fitness activity may be done as few as 2 days a week.

When determining the formula for each type of activity, the shorter acronym (FIT) can be used because you have already determined the activity type. In the following section, you will learn more about the **FIT** formula for each activity in the physical activity pyramid. In subsequent concepts, each formula is described in greater detail.

"Threshold of training" and "target zone" help you use the FIT formula. The **threshold of training** is the minimum amount of activity (frequency, intensity, and time) necessary to produce benefits. Depending on the benefit expected, slightly more than normal activity may not be enough to promote health, wellness, or fitness benefits. The **target zone** begins at the threshold of training and stops at the point where the activity becomes counterproductive. Figure 2 illustrates the threshold of training and target zone concepts.

Some people incorrectly associate threshold of training and target zones with only cardiovascular fitness. As the principle of specificity suggests, each component of fitness, including metabolic fitness, has its own FIT formula and its own threshold and target zone. The target and threshold levels for **health benefits** are different from those for achieving **performance benefits** associated with high levels of physical fitness.

It takes time for activity to produce health, wellness, and fitness benefits, even when the FIT formula is properly applied. Sometimes people beginning a physical activity

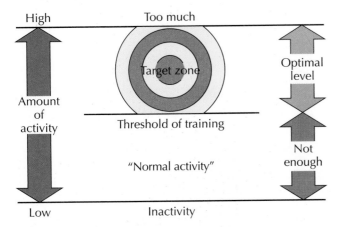

Figure 2 ► Physical activity target zone.

The Physical Activity Pyramid

The physical activity pyramid classifies activities by type and associated benefits. The **physical activity pyramid** (see Figure 3) is a good way to illustrate the different types of activities and how each contributes to the development of health, wellness, and physical fitness. The pyramid depicts five different steps, each one representing a different type of activity. Key concepts illustrated by the physical activity pyramid include the following:

- Each type of activity has its own FIT formula and unique health, wellness, and physical fitness benefits.
- The different types of physical activity can be combined to meet activity guidelines.
- Extended periods of inactivity can be harmful to your health.
- Eating well (sound nutrition) is an important companion behavior to physical activity (see color bands at right in Figure 3).

program expect to see immediate results. They expect to see large losses in body fat or great increases in muscle strength in a few days. Evidence shows, however, that improvements in health-related physical fitness and the associated health benefits take several weeks to become apparent. Though some people report psychological benefits, such as "feeling better" and a "sense of personal accomplishment" almost immediately after beginning regular exercise, the physiological changes take considerably longer to be realized. Proper preparation for physical activity includes learning not to expect too much too soon and not to do too much too soon. Attempts to get fit fast will probably be counterproductive, resulting in soreness and even injury. The key is to start slowly, stay with it, and enjoy yourself. Benefits will come to those who persist.

(i) **Many organizations have developed physical activity guidelines based on** FEATURE 2 **sound principles.** To help the general public determine the appropriate FIT formula for each type of physical activity, various organizations have developed guidelines. The earliest guidelines were developed by ACSM. Over the years, guidelines have also been developed by the American Heart Association (AHA), the Office of the Surgeon General (OSG), the Institute of Medicine (IOM), the U.S. Department of Health and Human Services (DHHS), and the Centers for Disease Control and Prevention (CDC). The FITT formula used in this book is based on information from several of these sources, most prominently the ACSM's new guidelines for exercise prescription published in 2010 and the DHHS national physical activity guidelines published in 2008. Details of guidelines from various organizations are provided at the associated Web link.

Principle of Individuality The corollary of the overload principle that indicates that overload provides unique benefits to each individual based on the unique characteristics of that person.

FITT, FIT A formula used to describe the frequency, intensity, time, and type of physical activity necessary to produce benefits. When the type of activity has been determined, the second *T* is dropped and the shorter acronym FIT is used.

Threshold of Training The minimum amount of physical activity that will produce health and fitness benefits.

Target Zone The amounts of physical activity that produce optimal health and fitness benefits.

Health Benefits The results of physical activity that provide protection from hypokinetic disease or early death.

Performance Benefits The results of physical activity that improve physical fitness and physical performance capabilities.

Physical Activity Pyramid A pyramid that illustrates how different types of activities contribute to the development of health and physical fitness. Activities lower in the pyramid require more frequent participation, whereas activities higher in the pyramid require less frequency.

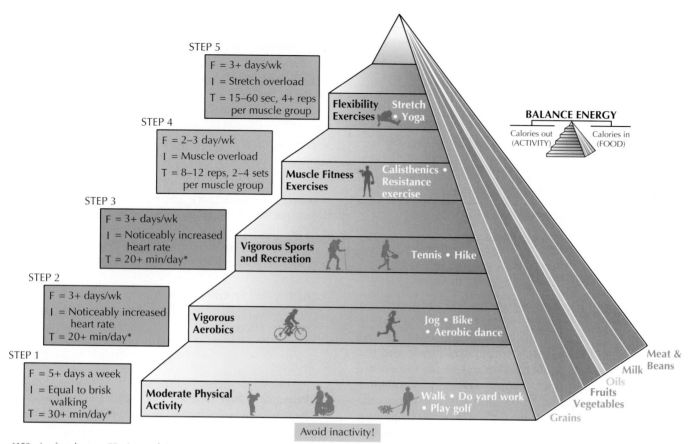

Figure 3 ► The physical activity pyramid.

Each of the five steps of the physical activity pyramid are discussed in greater detail in the paragraphs that follow as well as in Concepts 6, 8, 9, and 10.

Inactivity can be hazardous to your health. The five steps in the physical activity pyramid illustrate the different types of physical activity (Figure 3). New evidence suggests that minimizing inactivity may be just as important as being active. For children, the physical activity guidelines published by the National Association for Sport and Physical Education (NASPE) recommend periods of inactivity should not exceed 2 hours at a time. One goal of Healthy People 2020 is to reduce the proportion of youth who are inactive for long periods of time (defined as viewing television and videos or playing computer games more than 2 hours a day).

It is interesting that *Healthy People 2020* does not have a goal for reducing inactivity for adults, inasmuch as many adults sit for many hours each day. A recent editorial in the *British Journal of Sports Medicine* suggests that sitting for hours provides "harmful signals" to the body's systems. Another study of 17,000 Canadians showed that those who sit more have higher rates of chronic disease and death than those who sit less, independent of the amount of activity they performed. Yet another study showed that among adults the death rates from all causes are significantly related to the amount of television a person watches. Surveys indicate that people in Western cultures spend more than half of their time sitting, often in front of a television or a computer.

Although regular physical activity from the five steps of the physical activity pyramid (see Figure 3) is recommended, evidence is accumulating that even "sub-threshold"

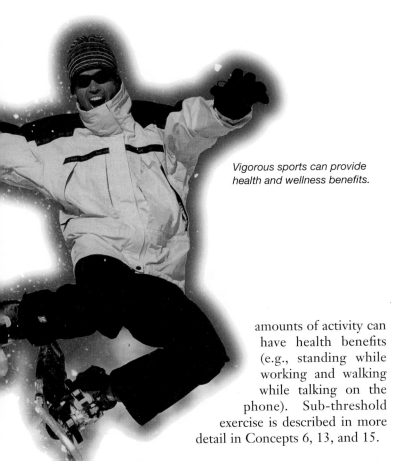

Vigorous sports can provide health and wellness benefits.

amounts of activity can have health benefits (e.g., standing while working and walking while talking on the phone). Sub-threshold exercise is described in more detail in Concepts 6, 13, and 15.

Moderate activities are at the base of the pyramid because they provide many benefits for modest amounts of effort. **Moderate aerobic activity** equal in intensity to brisk walking results in significant health benefits. Moderate aerobic physical activities are depicted in step 1 of the physical activity pyramid (see Figure 3). Moderate aerobic activities, such as walking to and from work, climbing the stairs rather than taking an elevator, or doing brisk housework, when done as part of the normal daily routine are often referred to as lifestyle physical activities. Moderate activities that are not part of the normal daily routine, such as taking a walk or a bike ride, can also be planned specifically to increase activity levels.

Studies have demonstrated that individuals with active jobs have reduced risks for many chronic conditions. Individuals who use active commuting (biking or walking) to get to work or to run errands have also been found to have better health profiles. The regular accumulation of activity as a part of one's lifestyle is sufficient to promote positive improvements in metabolic fitness, and these improvements can positively impact health. Additional activity from the other layers of the pyramid are strongly recommended, and additional benefits occur

from involvement in these activities. Moderate activity can be viewed as the baseline, or minimal, activity that should be performed. A summary of the FIT formula for moderate activity is illustrated in step 1 of Figure 3. The summary is based on the National Physical Activity Guidelines for Americans and the ACSM exercise prescription guidelines.

Vigorous aerobic activity is at the second step of the pyramid. **Vigorous aerobic activities** (step 2) are of greater intensity than moderate activities (step 1). The greater intensity results in significantly higher heart rates and higher oxygen consumption. Because of its greater intensity, vigorous aerobics can be performed as few as 3 days a week and are especially good for building cardiovascular fitness and helping to control body fatness. Examples of vigorous aerobic activities, sometimes referred to as active aerobics, are jogging, biking, and aerobic dance. Vigorous aerobic activities can provide metabolic fitness and health benefits similar to moderate activities and can be performed instead of, or in combination with, moderate activities to meet national activity guidelines.

Vigorous sports and recreation activities are at the third step of the pyramid. **Vigorous sports and recreation** are activities of similar intensity to vigorous aerobics. Some sports, such as golf and bowling, can be classified as moderate aerobic activities because they are of a lower intensity. Vigorous sports and recreation activities (see Figure 3, step 3) can be performed instead of, or in combination with, vigorous aerobic activities or moderate activities, to meet national activity guidelines.

Muscle fitness exercises are at the fourth step of the pyramid. There are muscle fitness benefits from many different activities, including vocational activities

Moderate Aerobic Activities In this book, aerobic activities equal in intensity to a brisk walk are referred to as moderate activities (see step 1 of the activity pyramid).

Vigorous Aerobic Activities In this book, vigorous aerobic activities are those that elevate the heart rate and are greater in intensity than a brisk walk (see step 2 of the activity pyramid).

Vigorous Sports and Recreation In this book, these are sports such as soccer and volleyball or recreational activities such as hiking that elevate the heart rate and are of greater intensity than a brisk walk.

that require lifting, active sports such as gymnastics and wrestling, and recreational activities such as rock climbing. The muscle fitness activities included at step 4 of the pyramid are those that are planned specifically to build strength and muscular endurance, such as resistance training and calisthenics. The many health and performance benefits of muscle fitness exercises are described in Concept 9. A general description of the FIT formula for muscle fitness exercises is included in Figure 3 (step 4).

Flexibility exercises are included at the fifth step of the pyramid. There are flexibility benefits from many different activities, including sports such as gymnastics and diving. The flexibility exercises included at step 5 of the pyramid are those that are planned specifically to build flexibility, such as stretching exercises and yoga. The many benefits of flexibility exercises are described in Concept 10. A general description of the FIT formula for flexibility exercises is included in Figure 3 (step 5).

The physical activity pyramid provides information for maintaining a healthy body composition. Weight management requires that energy intake be matched by energy expenditure. The FIT formula boxes in the physical activity pyramid provide general information about the amounts of activity (energy expenditure) necessary for general health and fitness benefits. But these amounts may not be enough for weight management (or weight loss). New physical activity guidelines suggest that 45–60 minutes of daily moderate activity may be necessary (as opposed to 30 minutes).

The color bands at the right of the activity pyramid depict the various food groups from MyPyramid (see small diagram at lower right of Figure 3). Balancing energy intake from food (colored bars at right) with energy expenditure (colored activity steps) is essential to weight management. Eating well is also important to good health and fitness, independent of benefits to weight control. More information about MyPyramid and energy balance is included in Concepts 14 and 15.

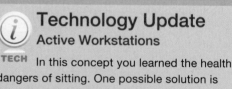 **Some important factors should be considered when using the physical activity pyramid.** The physical activity pyramid is a useful model for describing different types of activity and their benefits. The pyramid is also useful in summarizing the FIT formula for each of the benefits of activity. However, as the American College of Sports Medicine pointed out, physical activity guidelines "cannot be implemented in an overly rigid fashion and recommendations presented should be used with careful

FEATURE 3

ⓘ Technology Update
Active Workstations

TECH   In this concept you learned the health dangers of sitting. One possible solution is to work while standing or moving. Schools in Illinois have used standing desks to get people moving. They also use exercise balls as chairs because they require the muscles to work to stay balanced. Dr. James Levine at the Mayo Clinic advocates using a treadmill to move while working (Treadmill Desk). Scientists at the Cooper Institute in Dallas have used similar devices to encourage activity in the workplace. In Phoenix, a company called TrekDesk sells desks that allow multitasking. More details are available on the Web.

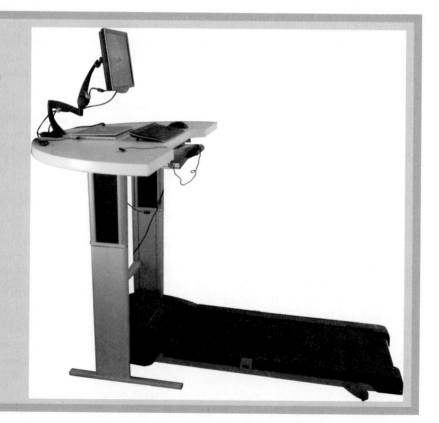

attention to the goals of the individual." The following guidelines for using the pyramid should also be considered:

- *No single activity provides all of the benefits.* Many people have asked the question "What is the perfect form of physical activity?" It is evident that there is no single activity that can provide all of the health, wellness, and fitness benefits. For optimal benefits to occur, it is desirable to perform activities from all levels of the pyramid because each type of activity has different benefits.

- *Something is better than nothing.* Some people may say, "I just don't have time to do all of the activities in the pyramid." This could lead some to throw up their hands in despair, concluding, "I just won't do anything at all." Evidence indicates that something is better than nothing. If you do nothing or feel that you can't do it all, performing moderate activity is a good place to start. Additional activities from different steps of the pyramid can be added as time allows.

- *Activities from steps 2 and 3 can be used instead of, or in combination with, those from step 1 to achieve health and fitness benefits.* While more people typically perform moderate activities (step 1), many prefer more vigorous activities from steps 2 and 3 of the pyramid. Both provide health benefits and the two can be combined to meet activity guidelines. More information on combining moderate and vigorous activities is provided in Concept 8.

- *Activities from steps 4 and 5 are useful even if you are limited in performing activities at other levels.* Though flexibility and muscle fitness exercises do not produce all of the benefits associated with step 1 and step 2 activities, they will produce benefits even if you are unable to perform as much activity from other levels as you like.

- *Good planning will allow you to schedule activities from all steps in a reasonable amount of time.* In subsequent concepts, you will learn more about each level of the pyramid, as well as more information about planning a total physical activity program.

- *Specific activity recommendations exist for youth.* Children are different from adults, and they have different needs for activity. The National Association for Sports and Physical Education (NASPE) and the CDC have developed activity recommendations specific to children. According to these guidelines, children should accumulate at least 60 minutes, and up to several hours, of age-appropriate physical activity on most, if not all, days of the week. This daily accumulation should include participation in a variety of age-appropriate activities (both moderate and vigorous)

with the majority of the time being spent in intermittent activity. The guidelines also recommend minimizing periods of inactivity (periods of 2 or more hours). Adults play a major role in shaping children's activity patterns. Helping children meet these guidelines may help reduce the prevalence of inactive and overweight adults in future years. The comprehensive Physical Activity Guidelines for Americans also recommends 60+ minutes of activity for youth each day. Both documents recommend daily muscle fitness and flexibility exercises. For more information see the associated Web feature.

- *Specific guidelines exist for older adults.* New activity guidelines are now available for adults 65 and older. The guidelines are similar to those for younger adults but differ in some important ways. Recommendations are included for flexibility and balance, and the guidelines for intensity of aerobic activity take into account the older adult's activity level. These guidelines will be described in greater detail later in this book.

Physical Activity Patterns

The proportion of adults meeting national health goals varies with activity type and gender. National health goals have been established for each type of activity illustrated in the physical activity pyramid. The percentages of adults 18 and over meeting the national goals for moderate and vigorous activity are presented in Table 1. Adults who did either moderate activity 5 days a week for at least 30 minutes a day OR vigorous activity for 3 days a week for at least 20 minutes a day met the guideline. The survey was conducted before the announcement of the most recent

FEATURE 4

Table 1 ▶ Percentages of Adults Who Meet National Activity Goals for Moderate or Vigorous Aerobic Physical Activity

	Male	Female	All
General Population	37	33	35
Age	18–24	24–65	65–74
	42.9	36	35
Ethnicity	White[a]	Hispanic[b]	Black[c]
	38.3	28.4	29.1
Other			

Source: Center for Disease Control and Prevention.

[a]Non-Hispanic. [b]Hispanic/Latino. [c]African American

Table 2 ▶ Percentage of Adults Who Meet National Activity Goals by Gender, Age, Income, Ethnicity, and Disability

	Gender		
	Male	**Female**	**All**
Moderate	16	13	14
Vigorous	25	22	23
Muscle fitness	27	23	19
Flexibility	29	31	30
	Age		
	18–24	**25–44**	**45–65**
Moderate	14	16	13
Vigorous	28[a]	28[a]	22
Muscle fitness	19	27	23
Flexibility	30	29	31
	Income		
	Low	**Medium**	**High**
Moderate	11	14	17
Vigorous	16	20	25
Muscle fitness	18	22	36
Flexibility	— — —	— — —	— — —

	Ethnicity			
	White[b]	**Hispanic[c]**	**Black[d]**	**Asian[e]**
Moderate	16	10	10	23
Vigorous	24	17	19	20
Muscle fitness	28	21	30	28
Flexibility	31	22	26	34

	Disability	
	With	**Without**
Moderate	12	16
Vigorous	13	25
Muscle fitness	14	20
Flexibility	29	31

Source: National Health Interview Survey.
Values represent percentages of adults who reach national goals for each of four types of activity and percentages of adults who get no leisure activity.
[a]Data available for 18–44, same statistic used for both.
[b]Non-Hispanic. [c]Hispanic/Latino. [d]African American. [e]Or Pacific Islander.

guidelines and did not include people who combined moderate and vigorous activity. The percentages of adults meeting muscle fitness exercise and flexibility exercise goals are presented in Table 2. The good news is that the numbers in Table 1 show higher percentages of adults meeting activity goals than in the past. Currently 35 percent of adults meet the national goal for aerobic activity, up from 30 percent 10 years earlier. The not so good news is that more than 50 percent of adults do the minimum amount of activity necessary for gaining the health and fitness benefits of aerobic exercise. Fewer adults meet guidelines for muscle fitness and flexibility exercise than for moderate or vigorous activity.

The proportion of people meeting national health goals varies based on age. Children are the most active group in Western society. During adolescence, activity starts to decrease, but teens still do more activity than young adults. Activity levels of all types decrease from young adulthood to ages 65 and over (see Tables 1 and 2).

The proportion of adults meeting national health goals varies based on income, education, and disability status. People at or near poverty levels are more than twice as likely to be totally inactive during leisure time, compared with those with high income. Low-income people are much less likely to meet national health goals for activity than middle- to high-income people. High school dropouts are three times more likely to be totally inactive than college graduates and meet national activity goals less frequently. Adults with one or more physical disabilities have a high probability of being inactive. Minority groups have high rates of inactivity, and as illustrated in Tables 1 and 2, White non-Hispanic people are more likely to meet national activity goals than Hispanic and Black Americans. While no information was provided in the most recent survey for Asian Americans, previous surveys indicate that they are similar in activity levels to White non-Hispanics.

Physical Fitness Standards

(i) **Health-based criterion-referenced standards are recommended for rating your fitness.** This concept has focused on the amount of physical activity necessary to get health and fitness benefits. Another question to be answered is "How much physical fitness is enough?" Most experts recommend **health-based criterion-referenced standards** to rate your current fitness. These standards

FEATURE 5

Health-Based Criterion-Referenced Standards
The amount of a specific type of fitness necessary to gain a health or wellness benefit.

Health is available to **EVERYONE** for a Lifetime, and it's Personal

According to national physical activity guidelines (CDC) adults should get a minimum of 150 minutes of moderate activity each week (e.g., 30 minutes five days a week). Vigorous activity of 75 minutes (or more) per week can substitute for moderate activity.

Do you think 150 minutes of moderate activity or 75 minutes of vigorous activity per week is a realistic goal for most people?

are based on how much fitness is needed for good health. Other standards use norms or percentiles that compare a person's fitness against a reference population. Knowing how you compare with other people is not that important. In fact, such comparisons have been shown to be discouraging to many people. Determining if your fitness is adequate to enhance your health and wellness is more relevant.

In this book, the health-related standard is referred to as the *good fitness zone* (see Table 3). With reasonable amounts of physical activity, most people should be able to improve their fitness enough to make it into this range. For personal reasons, some may wish to aim for a higher level, referred to as the *high performance zone*.

Table 3 ▶ The Four Fitness Zones

High-Performance Zone

It is not necessary to reach this level to experience good health benefits. Achievement of high performance scores has more to do with performance than it does with good health. In some cases, extreme fitness scores can increase health risk—e.g., very low body fatness.

Good Fitness Zone

If you reach the good fitness zone, you have enough of a specific fitness component to help reduce health risk. However, even reaching the good fitness zone may not result in optimal health benefits for inactive people.

Marginal Zone

Marginal scores indicate that some improvement is in order, but you are nearing minimal health standards set by experts.

Low-Fit Zone

If you score low in fitness, you are probably less fit than you should be for your own good health and wellness.

Attaining this level does not provide many additional health benefits but may be important for those interested in performance. The *low fit zone* and the *marginal zone* are levels of fitness that are not sufficient for optimal health benefits. If you score in these ranges, you should try to improve your level of fitness.

 Strategies for Action

A self-assessment of your current activity at each level of the pyramid can help you determine future activity goals. Lab 5A provides you with the opportunity to assess your physical activity at each level of the pyramid. Lab 5B offers a general assessment of fitness. Later you will develop a program of activity, and these assessments will provide a basis for program planning.

Self-assessments of physical fitness can help you prepare a fitness profile that can be used in program planning. In the concepts that follow, you will learn to perform a variety of self-assessments of fitness and will learn the scores that are necessary on these assessments to reach the good fitness zone as described in Table 3. In the meantime, you can complete Lab 5B. This lab will help you understand the nature of each part of fitness and estimate your current fitness level for each type of fitness. When you complete the more accurate self-assessments later in the book, you will be able to determine the accuracy of your estimates.

Web Resources

Additional websites with information related to Concept 5 are available at the associated Web link.

Centers for Disease Control and Prevention (CDC) **www.cdc.gov**
Health Canada **www.healthcanada.ca**

Healthy People 2020 **www.healthypeople.gov/HP2020**
Let's Move **www.letsmove.gov**
Morbidity and Mortality Weekly Reports **www.cdc.gov/mmwr**
Physical Activity Guidelines for Americans **www.health.gov/paguidelines**

Suggested Readings

REFERENCES   Selected readings and references are listed below. A more comprehensive list is available at the associated Web link.

ACSM. 2010. *ACSM's Guidelines for Exercise Testing and Prescription.* 8th ed. Philadelphia: Lippincott, Williams & Wilkins.

Barnes, P. M., et al. 2009. Early release of selected estimates based on data from the January–June 2009. *National Health Interview Survey.* National Center for Health Statistics. Available at **www.cdc.gov/nchs/nhis/released200912 .htm#7**

Bassett, D. R., P. Freedson, and S. Kozey. 2010. Medical hazards of prolonged sitting. *Exercise and Sport Sciences Reviews* 38(3):101–102.

Blair, S. N. 2009. Physical inactivity: The biggest public health problem of the 21st century. *British Journal of Sports Medicine* 43(1):1–2.

Centers for Disease Control and Prevention. 2007. Prevalence of regular physical activity among adults— United States. *Morbidity and Mortality Weekly Reports* 56(46):1209–1212.

Corbin, C. B. 2009. Helping clients understand national physical activity guidelines. *ACSM's Health and Fitness Journal* 13(5):17–22.

Dunstan, D. W., et al. 2010. Television viewing time and mortality. *Circulation* 121(3):384–391.

Edmunds, J., et al. 2009. Helping your clients and patients take ownership over their exercise. *ACSM's Health and Fitness Journal* 13(1):20–25.

Ekblom-Bak, E., et al. 2010. Are we facing a new paradigm of inactivity physiology? *British Journal of Sports Medicine* 10:1136.

Hance, B. J. and M. Moore. 2009. Climbing out of negativity and up to the top of Mount Lasting Change. *ACSM's Health and Fitness Journal* 13(4):27–32.

Owen, N., et al. 2010. Too much sitting: The population health science of sedentary behavior. *Exercise and Sport Sciences Reviews* 38(3):105–113.

Pescatello, L. S., et al. 2009. A preview of ACSM's guidelines for exercise testing and prescription: Eighth edition. *ACSM's Health and Fitness Journal* 13(4):23–26.

Pleis, J. R. and B. W. Ward. 2009. Summary health statistics for U. S. Adults: National Health Interview Survey. *Vital Health Statistics* 10(242):74–75.

Pekmezi, D., et al. 2009. Evaluating and enhancing self-efficacy in physical activity. *ACSM's Health and Fitness Journal* 14(1):8–15.

Rodgers, W. M. and C. C. Loitz. 2009. The role of motivation in behavior change. *ACSM's Health and Fitness Journal* 13(2):16–21.

White, S. M., et al. 2010. Leading a physically active lifestyle: Effective individual behavior change strategies. *ACSM's Health and Fitness Journal* 14(1):8–15.

United States Department of Health and Human Services. 2008. *2008 Physical Activity Guidelines for Americans.* Washington: USDHHS. Available at: **www.health.gov /paguidelines**

Lab 5A Self-Assessment of Physical Activity

Name	**Section**	**Date**

Purpose: To estimate your current levels of physical activity from each category of the physical activity pyramid

Procedures

1. Place an X over the circle that characterizes your participation in each category in the pyramid. Place an X over one circle below the yellow box at the bottom of the pyramid to indicate days of inactivity.

2. Determine if you met the national goal for each type of activity. Place an X over the "yes" circle if you met the goal in each area (see Results). In the results section of the chart on the next page, place an X over the "yes" circle if you meet the goal in each area or an X over the "no" circle if you do not meet the goal.

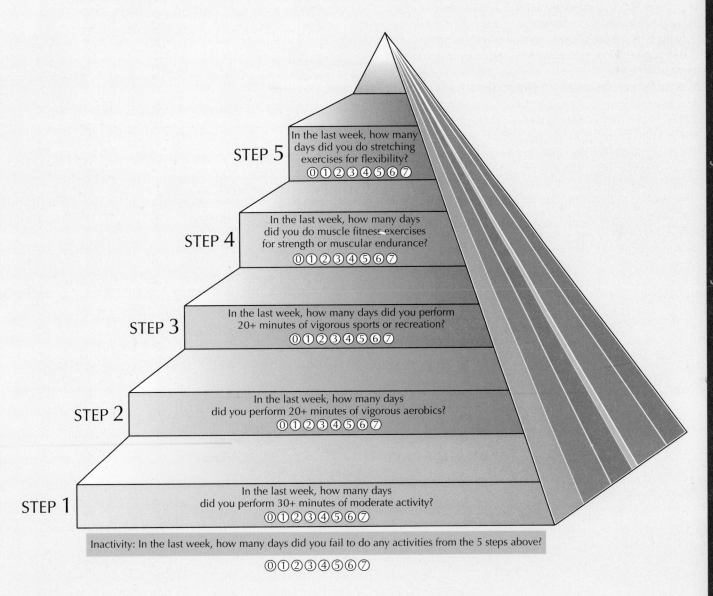

STEP 5 — In the last week, how many days did you do stretching exercises for flexibility? ⓪①②③④⑤⑥⑦

STEP 4 — In the last week, how many days did you do muscle fitness exercises for strength or muscular endurance? ⓪①②③④⑤⑥⑦

STEP 3 — In the last week, how many days did you perform 20+ minutes of vigorous sports or recreation? ⓪①②③④⑤⑥⑦

STEP 2 — In the last week, how many days did you perform 20+ minutes of vigorous aerobics? ⓪①②③④⑤⑥⑦

STEP 1 — In the last week, how many days did you perform 30+ minutes of moderate activity? ⓪①②③④⑤⑥⑦

Inactivity: In the last week, how many days did you fail to do any activities from the 5 steps above? ⓪①②③④⑤⑥⑦

Results

Activity Type	Level	National Goal	Did You Meet the National Health Goal?	
Moderate activity	1	5 days or more	Yes	No
Vigorous activity	2 and 3	3 days or more	Yes	No
Muscle fitness	4	2 days or more	Yes	No
Flexibility exercises	5	3 days or more	Yes	No
Inactivity	4	Avoid total inactivity	Yes	No

Conclusions and Implications: In the space below, write a brief paper describing your current physical activity patterns. Do you meet the national health goals in all areas? If not, in what types of activity from the pyramid do you need to improve? Are the answers you gave for the past week typical of your regular activity patterns? If you meet all national health goals, explain why you think this is so. Do you think that meeting the goals in the pyramid on the previous page indicates good activity patterns for you?

Write your physical activity assessment paper in the space below.

Lab 5B Estimating Your Fitness

Name		Section	Date

Purpose: To help you better understand each of the 11 components of health-related and skill-related physical fitness and to help you estimate your current levels of physical fitness

Special Note: The activities performed in the lab are *not intended as valid tests of physical fitness.* It is hoped that completing the activities will help you better understand each component of fitness and help you estimate your current fitness levels. You should not rely primarily on the results of the activities to make your estimates. Rather, you should rely on previous fitness tests you have taken and your own best judgment of your current fitness. Later in this book, you will learn how to perform accurate assessments of each fitness component and determine the accuracy of your estimates.

Procedures

1. Warm up. Perform each of the activities described in Chart 1 on page 100. Cool down.
2. Use past fitness test performances and your own judgment to estimate your current levels for each of the health-related and skill-related physical fitness parts. Low fitness = improvement definitely needed, marginal fitness = some improvement necessary, good fitness = adequate for healthy daily living.
3. Place an X in the appropriate circle for your fitness estimate in the Results section.

Results

Fitness Component	Low Fitness	Marginal Fitness	Good Fitness
Body composition	◯	◯	◯
Cardiovascular fitness	◯	◯	◯
Flexibility	◯	◯	◯
Muscular endurance	◯	◯	◯
Strength	◯	◯	◯
Agility	◯	◯	◯
Balance	◯	◯	◯
Coordination	◯	◯	◯
Power	◯	◯	◯
Reaction time	◯	◯	◯
Speed	◯	◯	◯

Conclusions and Implications: In several sentences, discuss the information you used to make your estimates of physical fitness. How confident are you that these estimates are accurate?

Directions: Attempt each of the activities in Chart 1. Place an X in the circle next to each component of physical fitness to indicate that you have attempted the activity.

Chart 1 ▶ Physical Fitness Activities

Balance

1. *One-foot balance.* Stand on one foot; press up so that the weight is on the ball of the foot with the heel off the floor. Hold the hands and the other leg straight out in front for 10 seconds.

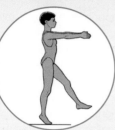

Power

2. *Standing long jump.* Stand with the toes behind a line. Using no run or hop step, jump as far as possible. Men must jump their height plus 6 inches. Women must jump their height only.

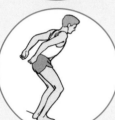

Agility

3. *Paper ball pickup.* Place two wadded paper balls on the floor 5 feet away. Run until both feet cross the line, pick up the first ball, and return both feet behind the starting line. Repeat with the second ball. Finish in 5 seconds.

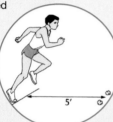
5'

Reaction Time

4. *Paper drop.* Have a partner hold a sheet of notebook paper so that the side edge is between your thumb and index finger, about the width of your hand from the top of the page. When your partner drops the paper, catch it before it slips through the thumb and finger. Do not lower your hand to catch the paper.

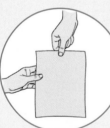

Speed

5. *Double-heel click.* With the feet apart, jump up and tap the heels together twice before you hit the ground. You must land with your feet at least 3 inches apart.

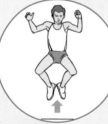

Coordination

6. *Paper ball bounce.* Wad up a sheet of notebook paper into a ball. Bounce the ball back and forth between the right and left hands. Keep the hands open and palms up. Bounce the ball three times with each hand (six times total), alternating hands for each bounce.

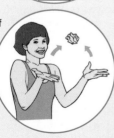

Cardiovascular Fitness

7. *Run in place.* Run in place for 1½ minutes (120 steps per minute). Rest for 1 minute and count the heart rate for 30 seconds. A heart rate of 60 (for 30 sec.) or lower passes. A step is counted each time the right foot hits the floor.

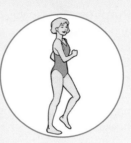

Flexibility

8. *Backsaver toe touch.* Sit on the floor with one foot against a wall. Bend the other knee. Bend forward at the hips. After three warm-up trials, reach forward and touch your closed fists to the wall. Bend forward slowly; do not bounce. Repeat with the other leg straight. Pass if fists touch the wall with each leg straight.

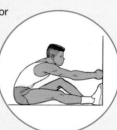

Body Composition

9. *The pinch.* Have a partner pinch a fold of fat on the back of your upper arm (body fatness), halfway between the tip of the elbow and the tip of the shoulder.

Men: no greater than 3/4 inch

Women: no greater than 1 inch

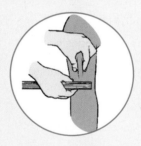

Strength

10. *Push-up.* Lie face down on the floor. Place the hands under the shoulders. Keeping the legs and body straight, press off the floor until the arms are fully extended. Women repeat once; men, three times.

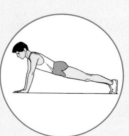

Muscular Endurance

11. *Side leg raise.* Lie on the floor on your side. Lift your leg up and to the side of the body until your feet are 24 to 36 inches apart. Keep the knee and pelvis facing forward. Do not rotate so that the knees face the ceiling. Perform 10 with each leg.

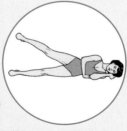

week outlined in Table 3, but it is easier to accomplish. If you fail to meet the 30-minute guideline on one day, you can make it up on another and still meet the guideline. Vigorous-intensity activity can also be substituted to meet the weekly targets. According to the DHHS guidelines, each minute of vigorous activity counts as 2 minutes of moderate. Therefore, the guideline can also be met by performing 75 minutes of vigorous activity instead of 150 minutes of moderate activity.

(i) **FEATURE 5** **Energy expenditure from can be used to monitor moderate physical activity.** As shown in Table 3, an energy expenditure of between 150 and 300 kcal/day from physical activity is sufficient for meeting physical activity guidelines. While not as simple as tracking time, calories expended from physical activity can be estimated if the approximate MET value of the activity is known. The energy cost of resting energy expenditure (1 MET) is approximately 1 calorie per kilogram of body weight per hour (1 kcal/kg/ hour). An activity such as walking (4 mph) requires an energy expenditure of about 4 METs, or 4 kcal/kg/hour. A 150 lb. person (~70 kg) walking for an hour would expend about 280 kcal (4 kcal/kg/hour × 70 kg × 1 hr.). Note that a 30-minute walk would burn approximately 150 calories and satisfy the guideline.

Many commercial pieces of fitness equipment provide energy expenditure estimates. The devices use an estimated MET level based on the selected intensity or a measured heart rate (if a heart rate sensor is used). The timer on the machine then tracks the time of the workout, and this allows calories to be estimated during the workout. The estimate will only be somewhat accurate if the machine also obtained a body weight value from you during the setup process. If this wasn't obtained, the calorie estimates are probably based on some reference value of weight and therefore may not be accurate. Table 4 lists estimated METs for different activities, along with calorie estimates (per hour of exercise) for people of different body weights. This table can help you learn how to track the number of calories you expend while performing physical activity. Additional information about calculating energy expenditure from physical activity is available at the associated Web link.

(i) **FEATURE 6** **Many people use pedometers to monitor daily activity levels.** Digital pedometers are a popular self-monitoring tool used to track physical activity patterns. They provide information about the number of steps a person takes. Stride length and weight can be entered into most pedometers to provide estimates of distance traveled and/or

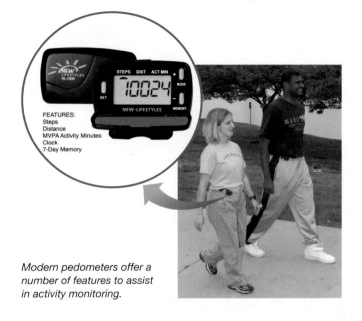

Modern pedometers offer a number of features to assist in activity monitoring.

calories burned. Some newer pedometers include timers, which track the total amount of time spent moving; some allow step information to be stored over a series of days.

Pedometers provide a helpful reminder about the importance of being active during the day. They also are useful for tracking activity patterns over a series of days. The interest in and popularity of pedometers has resulted in media stories promoting the standard of 10,000 steps as the level of activity needed for good health. This standard was originally developed in Japan, where pedometers were popularized before gaining popularity elsewhere in the world. Experts have warned against using an absolute step count standard, such as 10,000 steps for all people. It will likely be too hard for

 Health is available to Everyone for a Lifetime, and it's **PERSONAL**

According to the American Council on Exercise, many people have an "all-or-nothing" approach to physical activity; believing that exercise must be hard, long, and uncomfortable for it to be beneficial. Finding moderately intense exercises that you enjoy and a routine you can maintain over time may be more beneficial, because you will be more likely to stick with something you take pleasure in.

Is taking an "all-or-nothing" approach to physical activity keeping you from your health goals?

Table 4 ▶ Calories Expended in Lifestyle Physical Activities

Activity Classification / Description	METs[a]	Calories Used per Hour for Different Body Weights					
		100 lb. (45 kg)	120 lb. (55 kg)	150 lb. (70 kg)	180 lb. (82 kg)	200 lb. (91 kg)	220 lb. (100 kg)
Gardening Activities							
Gardening (general)	5.0	227	273	341	409	455	502
Mowing lawn (hand mower)	6.0	273	327	409	491	545	599
Mowing lawn (power mower)	4.5	205	245	307	368	409	450
Raking leaves	4.0	182	218	273	327	364	401
Shoveling snow	6.0	273	327	409	491	545	599
Home Activities							
Child care	3.5	159	191	239	286	318	350
Cleaning, washing dishes	2.5	114	136	170	205	227	249
Cooking / food preparation	2.5	114	136	170	205	227	249
Home / auto repair	3.0	136	164	205	245	273	301
Painting	4.5	205	245	307	368	409	450
Strolling with child	2.5	114	136	170	205	227	249
Sweeping / vacuuming	2.5	114	136	170	205	227	249
Washing / waxing car	4.5	205	245	307	368	409	450
Leisure Activities							
Bocci ball / croquet	2.5	114	136	170	205	227	249
Bowling	3.0	136	164	205	245	273	301
Canoeing	5.0	227	273	341	409	455	501
Cross-country skiing (leisure)	7.0	318	382	477	573	636	699
Cycling (<10 mph)	4.0	182	218	273	327	364	401
Cycling (12–14 mph)	8.0	364	436	545	655	727	799
Dancing (social)	4.5	205	245	307	368	409	450
Fishing	4.0	182	218	273	327	364	401
Golf (riding)	3.5	159	191	239	286	318	350
Golf (walking)	5.5	250	300	375	450	500	550
Horseback riding	4.0	182	218	273	327	364	401
Swimming (leisure)	6.0	273	327	409	491	545	599
Table tennis	4.0	182	218	273	327	364	401
Walking (3.5 mph)	3.8	173	207	259	311	346	387
Occupational Activities							
Bricklaying / masonry	7.0	318	382	477	573	636	699
Carpentry	3.5	159	191	239	286	318	350
Construction	5.5	250	300	375	450	500	550
Electrical work / plumbing	3.5	159	191	239	286	318	350
Digging	7.0	318	382	477	573	636	699
Farming	5.5	250	300	375	450	500	550
Store clerk	3.5	159	191	239	286	318	350
Waiter / waitress	4.0	182	218	273	327	364	401

Note: MET values and caloric estimates are based on values listed in *The Compendium of Physical Activities* (see Suggested Readings).

[a]Based on values of those with "good fitness" ratings.

Technology Update
Physical Activity Monitoring Devices

TECH Many high-tech devices are now available for monitoring moderate activity. Some of the more expensive devices can be used to monitor vigorous activity. Pedometers are inexpensive and easy to use. The least expensive keep track of steps, and the more expensive allow you to keep track of minutes in activity as well as the number of 10-minute bouts performed each day. Accelerometers, about the size of a pedometer, track movement and allow you to monitor both moderate and vigorous activity. One new GPS device, which you wear on your wrist, allows you to determine where you are at any time and how far you have walked. More details on different high-tech monitoring devices are available at the associated Web link.

Table 5 ▶ Activity Classification for Pedometer Step Counts in Healthy Adults

Category		Steps/Day
Sedentary		< 5000
Low active		5,000–7,500
Somewhat active	Threshold	7,500–9,999
Active	Target Zone	10,000–12,500
Very active		> 12,500

Source: Based on values from Tudor-Locke.

some and not hard enough for others based on current activity patterns.

Studies on large numbers of people provide data to help classify people into activity categories based on step counts (see Table 5), but actual step goals should vary from individual to individual. The approach most frequently recommended is to first wear the pedometer for 1 week to establish a baseline step count (average steps per day). Once this has been done, setting a goal of increasing steps per day by 1,000 to 3,000 steps per day is recommended. Keeping records of daily step counts will help you determine if you are meeting your goal. Setting a goal that you are likely to meet will help you find success. As you meet your goal, you can increase your step counts gradually.

Pedometers do have some limitations as indicators of total physical activity. A person with longer legs will accumulate fewer steps over the same distance than someone with shorter strides (due to a longer stride length). A person running will also accumulate fewer steps over the same distance than a person who walks. There is considerable variability in the quality (and accuracy) of commercial pedometers, so it is important to consider this when purchasing one.

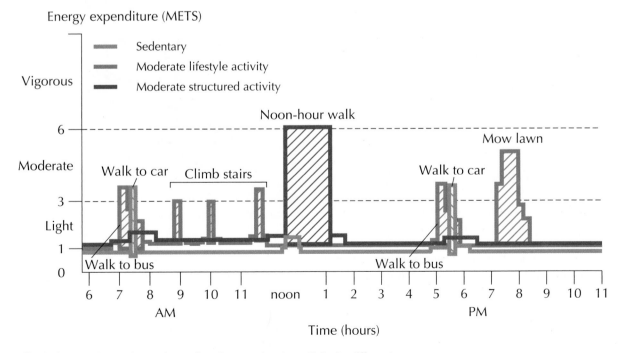

Figure 2 ▶ Comparison of people performing moderate activity in different ways.

A variety of methods can be used to accumulate moderate physical activity for health benefits. For many people, finding 30 minutes or longer for continuous physical activity may be difficult, especially on very busy days. The physical activity guidelines emphasize that moderate activity can be accumulated throughout the day. Figure 2 illustrates the activity profiles for three different people. The red line profiles a person who is inactive except for brief walks from the car to the office in the morning and from the office to the car in the evening. This person is sedentary and does not meet the moderate activity guidelines. Because some activity is better than none, the brief walks are better than no activity at all. The blue line represents a person who is sedentary most of the day but meets the moderate activity guideline by taking a long walk during the noon hour. The green line represents the activity of a person who meets the moderate activity standard in multiple bouts, including lifestyle activities such as walking to and from work, walking to lunch, climbing the stairs, and mowing the lawn. You can accumulate activity using the method that you prefer as long as you meet the guidelines outlined in Table 2.

Moderate Activity and the Environment

The sedentary nature of our society is due in part to environmental factors. Many people would like to be more active, but they may not live in an area conducive to activity. Studies have demonstrated that the extent of urban sprawl is associated with population levels of physical inactivity and obesity. Researchers have also determined that certain characteristics of an environment can make it more or less "walkable." Research shows that walking is more likely when the weather is warm, but factors such as availability of sidewalks, good lighting, safe neighborhoods, and aesthetic surroundings are the key factors in making an area walkable. America's most walkable neighborhoods have now been ranked using a walkscore. You can learn more about what makes a city walkable and where your city ranks at www.walkscore.com. Currently San Francisco ranks first and Jacksonville last of the 40 cities in the survey. In Lab 6B you will evaluate the walkability of your community based on some of these characteristics.

ⓘ **Changes in the environment can often promote lifestyle physical activity.** Studies

FEATURE 7 showing associations between physical activity and the **"built environment"** are important,

but inherent limitations in research designs have made it difficult to determine if there is a cause-effect association. It is possible, for example, that active people choose to move to environments with less sprawl and more access to parks and green spaces. Recent research, however, has demonstrated that *changes* in the environment can lead to changes in population levels of physical activity. Other studies have reported significant increases in levels of physical activity following a community-based awareness program. This type of evidence has been important because it indicates that our environment does contribute to our physical activity patterns. The results also help justify expenses to make communities more walkable. One organization called Active Living by Design (**www.activelivingbydesign.org**) is dedicated to promoting more active environments in society. The vision is for neighborhoods that allow physical activity to be built into a person's normal routine (going to the store, visiting friends) and communities with integrated biking paths and walking paths. These concepts are consistent with other recommendations for urban planning (e.g., Smart Growth Movement). Additional information about environmental issues related to lifestyle activity can be found on the book's online resources.

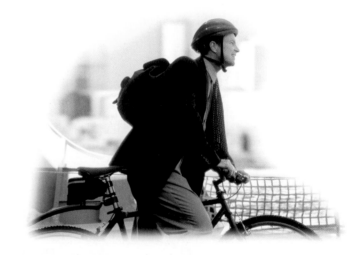

Bike commuting is an effective way to add physical activity to your day.

Built Environment A term used to describe aspects of our created physical environment (e.g., buildings, roads).

Consider personal strategies for increasing lifestyle activity. While the environment has an impact on population levels of physical activity, it does not determine individual behavior. People are autonomous beings and can make decisions about where they go and what they do. The key is to take stock of your lifestyle and your environment and determine ways to integrate more activity into your daily routine. One activity that is often overlooked is commuting to work or school on foot or by bike. In addition to providing beneficial amounts of physical activity, this can save time, gas, and money. Studies show that providing environments that make it easy and safe to commute on foot or by bike results in improvements in fitness of the local populations. The benefits to the individual, the environment, and to society as a whole are significant. Review the associated Web material for additional information about the benefits of active commuting.

 Strategies for Action

A regular plan of moderate physical activity is a good place to start. Moderate physical activity is something that virtually anyone can do. In Lab 6A, you can set moderate physical activity goals and plan a 1-week lifestyle physical activity program. In the plan, you can indicate the moderate activities you plan to do on all or most days of the week. For some, this plan may be the main component of a lifetime plan. For others, it may be only a beginning that leads to the selection of activities from other levels of the physical activity pyramid. Even the most active people should consider regular moderate physical activity because it is a type of activity that can be done throughout life.

Self-monitoring moderate physical activity can help you stick with it. Self-monitoring is a self-management skill that can be valuable in encouraging long-term activity adherence. A self-monitoring chart is provided in Lab 6A to help you keep a log of moderate activities (or step counts) you perform during a 1-week period. This is a short-term record sheet. Charts like this can be copied to make a log book for long-term activity self-monitoring.

Because environmental factors have an influence on our moderate physical activity patterns, it is important to become sensitive to different aspects of your environment. In Lab 6B, you will conduct an evaluation of the walkability of your community and an evaluation of community resources available for physical activity. The purpose of this lab is to increase your awareness of the importance of active environments for promoting physical activity. Becoming an advocate for physical activity in your community is a great way to help promote local change.

Web Resources

 Additional websites with information related to Concept 6 are available at the associated Web link.

America On the Move **www.americaonthemove.org**
Compendium of Physical Activities **http://prevention.sph .sc.edu/tools/compendium.htm**
National Coalition for Promoting Physical Activity **www.ncppa.org**
Public Broadcasting System/America's Walking Homepage **www.pbs.org/americaswalking**
Walkable Cities (walkscores) **www.walkscore.com**

Walking Cities Book Series (guides to major cities) **http://www.globepequot.com/globepequot/index.cfm**

Suggested Readings

Selected readings and references are listed on the next page. A more comprehensive list is available at the associated Web link.

ACSM. 2010. *ACSM's Guidelines for Exercise Testing and Prescription.* 8th ed. Philadelphia: Lippincott, Williams & Wilkins, Chapters 2 and 7.
Ainsworth, B. E. 2000. Compendium of physical activities: An update of activity codes and MET intensities.

Medicine and Science in Sports and Exercise 32 (Suppl):S498–S516.

Chaloupka, F. J., et al. 2010. The association between community physical activity settings and youth physical activity, obesity, and body mass index. *Journal of Adolescent Health*. Published online June 10, 2010, **www .jahonline.org**

Coogan, P. F., et al. 2009. Prospective study of urban form and physical activity in the black women's health study. *Archives of Internal Medicine* 170(9):1105–1117.

Fenton, M. 2008. *A Complete Guide to Walking for Health, Weight Loss and Fitness*. Guilford, CT: The Lyons Press.

Mowen, A., and A. Kaczynski. 2008. The potential of parks and recreation in addressing physical activity and fitness. *President's Council on Physical Fitness and Sports Research Digest* 9(1):1–8.

Newman, M. A. 2009. Monthly variation in physical activity levels in postmenopausal women. *Medicine and Science in Sports and Exercise* 41(2): 32–327.

Owen, N., et al. 2010. Too much sitting: The population health science of sedentary behavior. *Exercise and Sport Sciences Reviews* 38(3): 105–113.

Zhu, W. 2008. Promoting physical activity using technology. *President's Council on Physical Fitness and Sports Research Digest* 9(3):1–8.

Lab 6A Setting Goals for Moderate Physical Activity and Self-Monitoring (Logging) Program

Name		Section	Date

Purpose: To set moderate activity goals and to self-monitor (log) physical activity.

Procedures

1. Read the five stages of change questions below. Place a check by the stage that best represents your current moderate physical activity level. If you are at stages 1–3 (precontemplation, contemplation, or preparation), you may want to set goals below the threshold of 30 minutes per day to get started. Those at the action or maintenance stage should consider goals of 30 minutes or more per day.
2. Determine moderate activity goals for each day of a 1-week period. In the columns (Chart 1) under the heading "Moderate Activity Goals," record the total minutes per day that you expect to perform **OR** the total steps per day that you expect to perform. Record the specific date for each day of the week in the "Date" column.
3. The goals should be realistic for you, but try to set goals that would meet current physical activity guidelines. If you choose step goals, you will need a pedometer. Use Table 5 to help you to choose daily step goals.
4. If you choose minutes per day as your goals, use Chart 2 to keep track of the number of minutes of activity that you perform on each day of the 7-day period. Record the number of minutes for each bout of activity of at least 10 minutes in length performed during each day (Chart 2). Determine a total number of minutes for the day and record this total in the last column of Chart 2 and in the "Minutes Performed" column of Chart 1.
5. If you choose steps per day as your goals, determine the total steps per day accumulated on the pedometer and record that number of steps in the "Steps Performed" column for each day of the week (Chart 1).
6. Answer the questions in the Conclusions and Implications section (use full sentences for your answers).

Determine your stage for moderate physical activity. Check only the stage that represents your current moderate activity level.

☐ Precontemplation: I do not meet moderate activity guidelines and have not been thinking about starting.

☐ Contemplation: I do not do moderate activity guidelines but have been thinking about starting.

☐ Preparation: I am planning to start doing regular moderate activity to meet guidelines.

☐ Action: I do moderate activity, but I am not as regular as I should be.

☐ Maintenance: I regularly meet national goals for moderate activity.

Chart 1 ▶ Moderate Physical Activity Goals and Summary Performance Log

Select a goal for each day in a 1-week plan. Keep a log of the activities performed to determine if your goals are met.

	Date:	Moderate Activity Goals		Summary Performance Log	
		Minutes/day	Steps/day	Minutes Performed	Steps Performed
Day 1					
Day 2					
Day 3					
Day 4					
Day 5					
Day 6					
Day 7					

Chart 2 ▶ **Moderate Physical Activity Log (Daily Minutes Performed)**

For those who choose minutes per day as goals, write the number of minutes for each bout of moderate activity performed each day. Record a daily total (total minutes of moderate activity per day) in the "Daily Total" column. Record daily totals in Chart 1.

	Date	Bout 1	Bout 2	Bout 3	Bout 4	Bout 5	Daily Total
			Moderate Activity Bouts of 10 Minutes or More				
Day 1							
Day 2							
Day 3							
Day 4							
Day 5							
Day 6							
Day 7							

Did you meet your moderate activity goals for at least 5 days of the week? (Yes) (No)

Do you think you can consistently meet your moderate activity goals? (Yes) (No)

What activities did you perform most often when doing moderate activity?
List most common activities in the spaces below.

Conclusions and Interpretations

1. Do you feel that you will use moderate physical activity as a regular part of your lifetime physical activity plan, either now or in the future? Use several sentences to explain your answer.

2. Did setting goals and logging activity make you more aware of your daily moderate physical activity patterns? Explain why or why not.

Cardiovascular Fitness

Health Objectives for the Year 2020

- Increase proportion of adults who meet guidelines for moderate to vigorous aerobic activity.
- Increase overall cardiovascular health, reduce heart disease, stroke, high blood pressure, and high blood cholesterol, increase screening, and increase emergency treatment by professionals or bystanders.
- Increase percentage of college students receiving risk factor information.
- Increase counseling about physical activity by physicians.
- Increase weight control efforts and activity levels of adults with high LDL.
- Increase young adult awareness of CHD signs and symptoms.
- Attain high-quality, longer lives free of preventable disease, injury, and premature death.

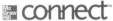 **connect** |FITNESS AND WELLNESS http://connect.mcgraw-hill.com

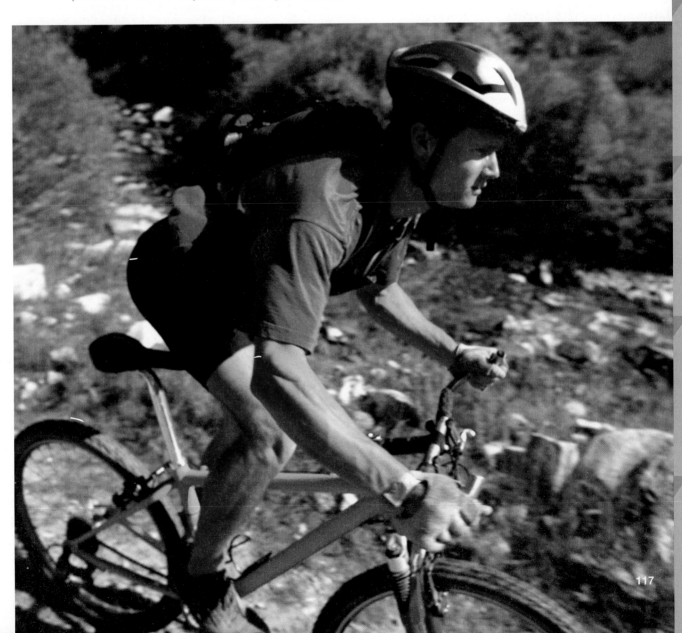

Cardiovascular fitness is probably the most important aspect of physical fitness because it has a major impact on health and greatly influences physical performance.

Cardiovascular fitness is generally considered to be the most important aspect of physical fitness. Those who possess reasonable amounts of fitness have a decreased risk for heart disease, reduced risk for premature death, and improved quality of life. Regular cardiovascular exercise promotes fitness and provides additional health and wellness benefits that extend well beyond reducing risks for disease. This concept describes the function of the cardiovascular system and explains how to determine the appropriate intensity of exercise needed to promote cardiovascular fitness.

Elements of Cardiovascular Fitness

There are several synonyms for the term cardiovascular fitness. Cardiovascular fitness is sometimes referred to as *cardiovascular endurance* because a person who possesses this type of fitness can persist in physical activity for long periods without undue fatigue. It has been referred to as *cardiorespiratory fitness* because it requires delivery and utilization of oxygen, which is only possible if the circulatory and respiratory systems are capable of these functions.

The term *aerobic fitness* has also been synonymous with *cardiovascular fitness* because **aerobic capacity** is considered to be the best indicator of cardiovascular fitness, and aerobic physical activity is the preferred method for achieving it. Regardless of the words used to describe it, cardiovascular fitness is complex because it requires fitness of several body systems.

Good cardiovascular fitness requires a fit heart muscle. The heart is a powerful muscle that pumps blood through the body. The heart of a normal individual beats reflexively about 40 million times a year. In a single day, the heart pumps over 4,000 gallons of blood through the body. To keep the cardiovascular system working effectively, it is crucial to have a strong and fit heart.

Like other muscles in the body, the heart becomes stronger if it is exercised. With regular exercise, the size and strength of the heart increase, and it can pump more blood with each beat. This allows the heart to accomplish the same amount of work with fewer beats. Typical resting heart rate (RHR) values are around 70–80 beats per minute, but a highly trained endurance athlete may have a resting heart rate in the 40s or 50s. There is some individual variability in RHR, but a decrease in your RHR with training indicates clear improvements in cardiovascular fitness.

Good cardiovascular fitness requires a fit vascular system. The heart has four chambers, which pump and receive blood in a rhythmical fashion to maintain good circulation (see Figure 1). Blood containing a high concentration of oxygen is pumped by the left ventricle through the aorta (a major artery), where it is carried to the tissues. Blood flows through a sequence of arteries to capillaries and to veins. Veins carry the blood containing lesser amounts of oxygen back to the right side of the heart, first to the atrium and then to the ventricle. The right ventricle pumps the blood to the lungs. In the lungs, the blood picks up oxygen (O_2), and carbon dioxide (CO_2) is removed. From the lungs, the oxygenated blood travels back to the heart, first to the left atrium and then to the left ventricle. The process then repeats itself. A dense network of arteries distributes the oxygenated blood to the muscles, tissues, and organs (see Figure 2 on p. 120).

Healthy arteries are elastic, are free of obstruction, and expand to permit the flow of blood. Muscle layers line the arteries and control the size of the arterial opening upon the impulse from nerve fibers. Unfit arteries may have a reduced internal diameter (atherosclerosis) because of deposits on the interior of their walls, or they may have hardened, nonelastic walls (arteriosclerosis).

Fit coronary arteries are especially important to good health. The blood in the four chambers of the heart does not directly nourish the heart. Rather, numerous small arteries within the heart muscle provide for coronary circulation. Poor coronary circulation precipitated by unhealthy arteries can be the cause of a heart attack.

Deoxygenated blood flows back to the heart through a series of veins. The veins are intertwined in the skeletal muscle, and this allows normal muscle action to facilitate the return of blood to the heart. When a muscle is contracted, the vein is squeezed, and this pushes the blood back to the heart. Small valves in the veins prevent the backward flow of the blood, but defects in the valves can lead to pooling of blood in the veins. A common condition, known as varicose veins, is associated with the pooling of blood in the leg. Regular physical activity helps reduce pooling of blood in the veins and helps keep the valves of the veins healthy.

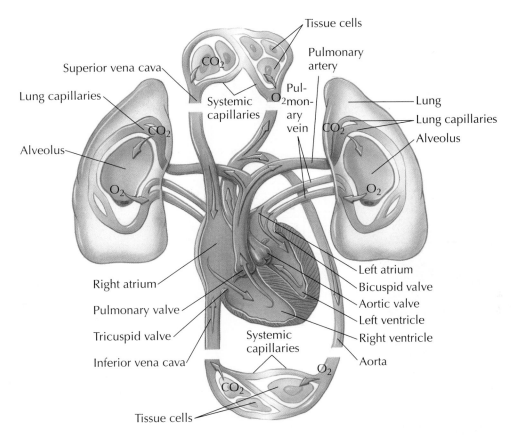

Figure 1 ▶ Cardiovascular system.

Capillaries are the transfer stations where oxygen and fuel are released, and waste products, such as carbon dioxide, are removed from the tissues. The veins receive the blood from the capillaries for the return trip to the heart.

Good cardiovascular fitness requires healthy blood and a fit respiratory system. The process of taking in oxygen (through the mouth and nose) and delivering it to the lungs, where it is picked up by the blood, is called external respiration. External respiration requires fit lungs as well as blood with adequate **hemoglobin.** Hemoglobin carries oxygen through the bloodstream. Lack of hemoglobin reduces oxygen-carrying capacity— a condition known as **anemia.**

Delivering oxygen to the tissues from the blood is called internal respiration. Internal respiration requires an adequate number of healthy capillaries. In addition to delivering oxygen to the tissues, these systems remove carbon dioxide. Good cardiovascular fitness requires fitness of both the external and internal respiratory systems.

Cardiovascular fitness requires fit muscle tissue capable of using oxygen. Once the oxygen is delivered, the muscle tissues must be able to use oxygen to sustain physical performance (see Figure 2e). Physical activity that promotes cardiovascular fitness stimulates changes in muscle fibers that make them more effective in using oxygen. Outstanding distance runners have high numbers of well-conditioned muscle fibers that can readily use oxygen to produce energy for sustained running. Training in other activities would elicit similar adaptations in the specific muscles used in those activities.

During exercise the performance and function of the cardiovascular system is maximized. During exercise, a number of changes occur to increase the availability of oxygen to the muscles (see Table 1). Breathing rate and heart rate increase, allowing the body to take in more oxygen and distribute it more quickly. Activation of the sympathetic nervous system leads to a redistribution of the blood flow, so that more of it gets shunted

Aerobic Capacity A measure of aerobic or cardiovascular fitness.

Hemoglobin The oxygen-carrying protein (molecule) of red blood cells.

Anemia A condition in which hemoglobin and the blood's oxygen-carrying capacity are below normal.

Major Blood Vessels

Cardiovascular Fitness Characteristics

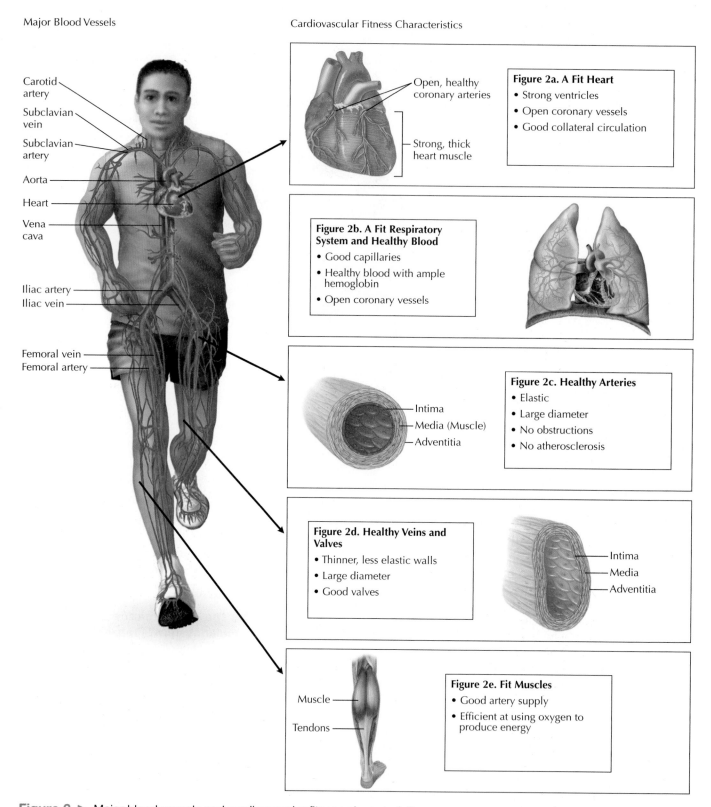

Figure 2a. A Fit Heart
- Strong ventricles
- Open coronary vessels
- Good collateral circulation

Open, healthy coronary arteries

Strong, thick heart muscle

Figure 2b. A Fit Respiratory System and Healthy Blood
- Good capillaries
- Healthy blood with ample hemoglobin
- Open coronary vessels

Figure 2c. Healthy Arteries
- Elastic
- Large diameter
- No obstructions
- No atherosclerosis

Intima
Media (Muscle)
Adventitia

Figure 2d. Healthy Veins and Valves
- Thinner, less elastic walls
- Large diameter
- Good valves

Intima
Media
Adventitia

Figure 2e. Fit Muscles
- Good artery supply
- Efficient at using oxygen to produce energy

Muscle
Tendons

Carotid artery
Subclavian vein
Subclavian artery
Aorta
Heart
Vena cava
Iliac artery
Iliac vein
Femoral vein
Femoral artery

Figure 2 ► Major blood vessels and cardiovascular fitness characteristics.

Table 1 ▶ Changes in Cardiovascular Function between Rest and Exercise for a Person with Good Cardiovascular Fitness

		Rest	Maximal Exercise
Lungs	Breathing Rate (# / Minute)	12	30
Heart	Heart Rate (Beats / Minute)	70	190–200
	Stroke Volume (mL / Beat)	75	150
	Cardiac Output[a] (L / Minute)	5.2	28.5
Arteries	Blood Flow Distribution (%)	20%	70%
Muscle	Oxygen Extraction (%)	5%	20%
System	$\dot{V}O_2$ (mL/kg/min.)[b]	3.5	60

[a] Cardiac output = heart rate × stroke volume.
[b] $\dot{V}O_2$ = oxygen consumption = CO × oxygen extraction.

to the working skeletal muscle. During rest, the muscles get about 20 percent of the available blood flow, but this increases to about 70 percent during vigorous exercise. Within the muscles, a larger percentage of the available oxygen is also extracted from the muscles during exercise. Collectively, these changes help provide the muscles with the oxygen needed to maintain aerobic metabolism (visit the book's website for a related activity).

ⓘ **FEATURE 1 Cardiovascular fitness is often evaluated using an indicator known as maximum oxygen uptake, or $\dot{V}O_2$ max.** A person's **maximum oxygen uptake ($\dot{V}O_2$ max)**, commonly referred to as aerobic capacity, is determined in a laboratory by measuring how much oxygen a person can use in maximal exercise. The test is usually done on a treadmill using specialized gas analyzers to measure oxygen use. The treadmill speed and grade are gradually increased, and when the exercise becomes very hard, oxygen use reaches its maximum. The test is a good indicator of overall cardiovascular fitness because you cannot take in and use a lot of oxygen if you do not have good fitness throughout the cardiovascular system (heart, blood vessels, blood, respiratory system, and muscles).

Elite endurance athletes can extract 5 or 6 liters of oxygen per minute from the environment, and this high aerobic capacity is what allows them to maintain high speeds in both training and competition without becoming excessively tired. In comparison, an average person typically extracts about 2 to 3 liters per minute. $\dot{V}O_2$ max is typically adjusted to account for a person's body size because bigger people may have higher scores due to their larger size. Values are reported in milliliters (mL) of oxygen (O_2) per kilogram (kg) of body weight per minute (mL/kg/min.).

A number of field tests have been developed to provide estimates of maximum aerobic capacity (see Lab Resource Materials). These tests are developed and validated based on comparisons with laboratory protocols that directly measure the amount of oxygen that is consumed.

Cardiovascular Fitness and Health Benefits

ⓘ **FEATURE 2 Good cardiovascular fitness reduces risk for heart disease, other hypokinetic conditions, and early death.** Numerous studies over the past 30–40 years have confirmed that good cardiovascular fitness is associated with a reduced risk for heart disease as well as a number of other chronic, hypokinetic conditions. Recent studies have further strengthened the evidence. A review of 33 studies involving nearly 200,000 people showed that people with low fitness have had a 70 percent higher death rate from all causes and a 56 percent higher death rate from heart diseases than people of intermediate fitness. The consensus is that low-fit individuals are three to six times more likely to develop symptoms of metabolic syndrome or diabetes than high-fit individuals. While the specific amount of fitness needed to reduce risks varies by condition and population, evidence clearly supports the need for at least a moderate level of fitness. As shown in Figure 3, there are dramatic reductions in risk in moving from the low fitness category to the moderate fitness category for both males and females. In terms of longevity, studies suggest that individuals with moderate fitness will live 5–6 years longer than low-fit individuals.

The risk for low cardiovascular fitness is independent of other risk factors. Physical activity has been shown to have beneficial effects on some other established heart disease risk factors, such as cholesterol,

Maximum Oxygen Uptake ($\dot{V}O_2$ max) A laboratory measure held to be the best measure of cardiovascular fitness. Commonly referred to as $\dot{V}O_2$ max, or the volume ($\dot{V}$) of oxygen used when a person reaches his or her maximum (max) ability to supply it during exercise.

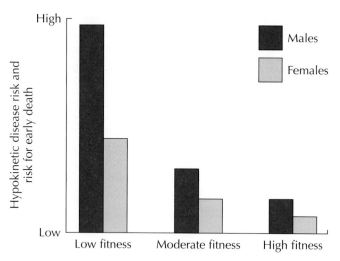

Figure 3 ▶ Risk reduction associated with cardiovascular fitness.
Source: Adapted from Blair et al.

blood pressure, and body fat. It is important to note that the beneficial effects of cardiovascular fitness on risk for heart disease and early death are considered to be independent of these other effects. This means that active/fit people would still have lower health risks even if their cholesterol, blood pressure, and body fat levels were identical to a matched set of inactive/unfit people. This evidence contributed to the labeling of physical inactivity as a major, independent risk factor for heart disease. The risk associated with physical inactivity is as large as (or larger than) risks associated with any of the other established risk factors.

Good fitness provides protection against the health risks associated with obesity. FEATURE 3 Some people think they cannot be fit if they are overweight or overfat. It is now known that appropriate physical activity can build cardiovascular fitness in all types of people, including those with excess body fat. In fact, having good cardiovascular fitness greatly reduces risk for those who are overweight. Poor cardiovascular fitness, on the other hand, increases risk for both lean and overfat people. The greatest risk is among people who are unfit and overfat.

Recent studies have helped explain how physical activity protects against risks from overweight/obesity. Individuals with higher levels of activity (and/or higher levels of fitness) have been shown to have lower levels of abdominal body fatness, even after correcting for differences in body mass index. In other words, individuals can be about the same size (i.e., similar weight for a given height), but active/fit individuals tend to have lower levels of abdominal body fat. The beneficial effects of physical activity are due, in part, to the ability

of physical activity to help reduce levels of abdominal body fat.

Good cardiovascular fitness enhances the ability to perform various tasks, improves the ability to function, and is associated with a feeling of well-being. Moving out of the low fitness zone is of obvious importance to disease risk reduction. Achieving the good zone on tests further reduces disease and early death risk and promotes optimal wellness benefits, and a position statement by the American College of Sports Medicine shows an improved ability to function among older adults. Other wellness benefits include the ability to enjoy leisure activities and meet emergency situations, as well as the health and wellness benefits described earlier in this book. Cardiovascular fitness in the high-performance zone enhances the ability to perform in certain athletic events and in occupations that require high performance levels (e.g., firefighters).

The FIT Formula for Cardiovascular Fitness

A FIT formula specifies how much moderate to vigorous physical activity is needed to improve cardiovascular fitness. As we have seen, evidence clearly shows that moderate physical activity has many health and wellness benefits. For people with low fitness, moderate activity has cardiovascular fitness benefits. Moderate activity can help move a person from low to marginal cardiovascular fitness and help the person progress toward performing more vigorous activity. For people who are fit, more vigorous activity from steps 2 and 3 in the physical activity pyramid is necessary to produce cardiovascular fitness increases. Steps 2 (vigorous aerobics) and 3 (vigorous sports and recreation) in the pyramid are highlighted because these activities are the

HELP   Health is available for Everyone for a **LIFETIME,** and it's Personal

Physical activity patterns tend to vary with difference phases of life. Those who felt out of place in school team sports may find themselves enjoying solo workouts at the gym in college or adulthood. On the other hand, people who are used to being active may not be able to find time to exercise, at least for a while, when they are adjusting to new family obligations.

How have your physical activity patterns changed over the years, and what future changes do to you anticipate?

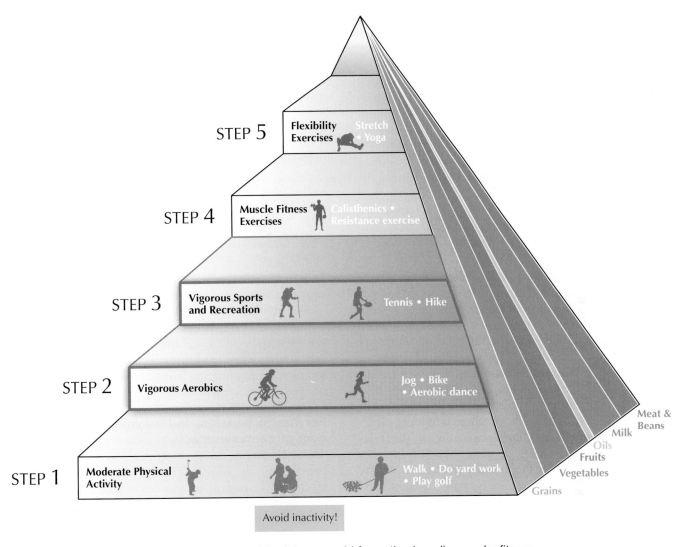

Figure 4 ▶ Select activities from steps 2 and 3 of the pyramid for optimal cardiovascular fitness.

most beneficial for those with good cardiovascular fitness (See Figure 4).

The FIT formula for cardiovascular fitness varies for people of different activity levels. Adaptations to physical activity are based on the overload principle and the principle of progression. It is important to provide an appropriate challenge to the cardiovascular system (overload), but the challenge should be progressive, increasing gradually as fitness improves. Table 2 presents the FIT formulas for people of five different fitness and activity levels. While the *frequency* of exercise is similar for the different levels, the *intensity* and amount of *time* spent in activity vary considerably.

Cardiovascular fitness can be developed by exercising 3 to 5 days per week. Unlike less intense moderate physical activities, the types of activities that promote cardiovascular fitness may be done as few as 3 days a week. Additional benefits occur with added days of activity; however, vigorous physical activity has been shown to increase risk for orthopedic injury if done too frequently. The ACSM recommends 5 days as the upper limit. However, healthy people who are fit and regularly active, and have no evidence of joint problems or injuries, may train up to 6 days a week. Most experts agree that at least 1 day off a week is beneficial. Use Table 2 to determine the appropriate *frequency of exercise* for you based on your current activity and fitness level. It would be wise to complete the fitness assessments at the end of this concept before making your decision.

Because individuals vary in their level of fitness, the appropriate intensity of exercise needed to maintain or improve fitness also varies. Like all dimensions of fitness, adaptations to cardiovascular fitness are based on the overload principle. When the body is regularly challenged, it essentially adapts to make the same

Table 2 ▶ FIT Formula for Cardiovascular Fitness for People of Different Fitness and Activity Levels

Fitness Level	Very Low	Low	Marginal	Good	High Performance
Activity Level	Sedentary	Some LM	Sporadic MV	Reg. MV	Habitual MV
Frequency (days per week)	3–5	3–5	3–5	3–5	3–5
Intensity					
Heart Rate Reserve (HRR)	30–40%	40–55%	55–70%	65–80%	70–85%
Max. Heart Rate (max HR)	57–67%	64–74%	74–84%	80–91%	84–94%
Relative Perceived Exertion (RPE)	12–13	12–13	13–14	13–15	14–16
Time (minutes per day)	20–30	30–60	30–90	30–90	30–90

amount of exercise easier on itself. Therefore, fit people need to exercise at a higher intensity to provide a sufficient challenge. The relative intensity of a given bout of exercise can be directly determined if you have a measure of your **oxygen uptake reserve V(O₂R)** and the actual oxygen cost of a given activity. You would simply calculate what percentage of oxygen consumption the task requires, compared with your maximal capacity. Because these values cannot be calculated without special equipment, other indicators of relative intensity are more commonly used.

Heart rate provides a good indicator of the relative challenge presented by a given bout of exercise. Therefore, guidelines for the intensity of physical activity to build cardiovascular fitness are typically based on percentages of **heart rate reserve (HRR)** or maximal heart rate (maxHR). Current guidelines as outlined in Table 2 specify different intensity levels based on current fitness and activity levels. Calculations of HRR and maxHR will be described in detail later, but the general range for HRR is 30 to 85 percent and for maxHR, 57 to 94 percent.

Ratings of perceived exertion (RPE) have also been shown to be useful in assessing the intensity of aerobic physical activity. The RPE scale ranges from 6 (very very light) to 20 (very very hard), with 1-point increments in between. If the values are multiplied by 10, the RPE values loosely correspond to HR values (e.g., 60 = rest HR and 200 = maxHR). Details will be provided later, but the target zone for aerobic activity is from 12 to 16 (see Table 2).

Regardless of what method is used, the important point is that lower intensities provide a cardiovascular fitness benefit for low-fit sedentary people, but higher intensities are needed for more fit people. Use Table 2 to determine the appropriate *intensity of exercise* based on your current activity and fitness level.

The amount of time for building cardiovascular fitness is based on minutes of activity per day. National (DHHS) physical activity guidelines recommend 150 minutes of moderate activity per week or 75 minutes of vigorous activity per week (or a combination of minutes from moderate and vigorous activity). These numbers are based on the minimum number of minutes for health benefits and were not designed with the principal goal of building cardiovascular fitness. For those who want cardiovascular fitness improvements, minutes per day ranging from 20 to 90 are recommended on 3 to 5 days a week.

For health benefits, the minimum length of one bout of continuous activity should be 10 minutes. Three 10-minute bouts of activity would provide similar benefits to one 30-minute session. However, for those interested in improving cardiovascular fitness into the high-performance zone for endurance activities (e.g., distance running, swimming, biking) and high-level sports, longer bouts of activity are necessary (see Concept 12). Use Table 2 to determine the appropriate *length of time* for daily exercise for you based on your current activity and fitness level.

Threshold and Target Zones for Intensity of Activity to Build Cardiovascular Fitness

There is a minimum intensity and an optimal intensity range for activity designed to develop cardiovascular fitness. As noted earlier, monitoring heart rate and making ratings of perceived exertion are the most practical methods of determining the intensity of activity necessary to build cardiovascular fitness. The threshold of training (minimum intensity) and the target zone (optimal intensity range) can be determined using either of the two heart rate monitoring methods (HRR or maxHR). The target zone using these two methods is referred to as *target heart rate zone*. Ratings of perceived exertion (RPE) can also be used to define the target zone

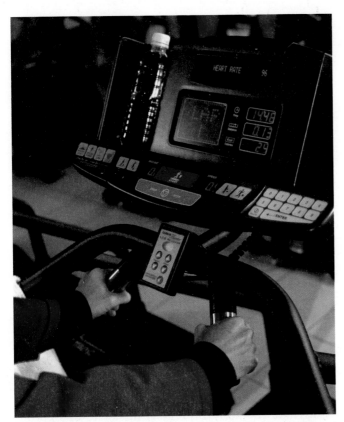

Many exercise machines have built-in heart rate monitors to help gauge exercise intensity.

Table 3 ▶ Calculating Target Heart Rate Zones with the Percentage of Heart Rate Reserve Method

Calculating Maximal Heart Rate

Maximal heart rate	$= 208 - (.7 \times age)$
	$= 208 - (.7 \times 22)$
	$= \underline{208 - 15.4}$
	193

Calculating Heart Rate Reserve

Maximal heart rate	193 bpm
Minus resting heart rate	−68 bpm
Equals heart rate reserve (HRR)	125 bpm

Calculating Threshold Heart Rate

HRR	125 bpm
× 65%	× .65
Equals	81 bpm
Plus resting heart rate	+68 bpm
Equals threshold heart rate	149 bpm

Calculating Upper Limit Heart Rate

HRR	125 bpm
× 80%	× .80
Equals	100 bpm
Plus resting heart rate	+68 bpm
Equals upper limit heart rate	168 bpm

for exercise intensity. This section provides details of using these methods.

You must determine your maximal heart rate to use the HRR or maxHR methods of determining exercise intensity. Calculations of threshold and target zone heart rates require an estimate of your maximal heart rate. Your maxHR is the highest heart rate attained in maximal exercise. It could be determined using an electrocardiogram while exercising to exhaustion; however, using a formula is easier for most people. Until recently, a simple formula has been used (220 − age = maxHR). Although this formula gives a general estimate, recent research has found that it tends to overpredict for young people (ages 20 to 40) and underpredict for those over 40. Based on extensive research, several new formulas have been developed. The ACSM uses the formula, maxHR = 206.9 − (.67 × age). In this book, we use the previously developed formula: maxHR = 208 − (.7 × age). Calculations made at a variety of ages show little, if any differences between the formulas, so we use the one that makes calculations the easiest (it limits use of fractions). Table 3 illustrates the calculations for determining maxHR for a 22-year-old.

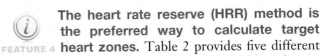 **The heart rate reserve (HRR) method is the preferred way to calculate target heart zones.** Table 2 provides five different intensity ranges for activity designed to build cardiovascular fitness. After you have assessed your fitness using fitness tests (see Lab Resource Materials and Lab 7B), determine which of the five intensity ranges is best for you based on your current activity and fitness. A new formula for women is also available (206 × [.88 × age]). Table 3 provides a worked example for calculating heart

Oxygen Uptake Reserve ($\dot{V}O_2R$) The difference between maximum oxygen uptake and resting oxygen uptake. A percentage of this value is often used to determine appropriate intensities for physical activities.

Heart Rate Reserve (HRR) The difference between maximum heart rate (highest heart rate in vigorous activity) and resting heart rate (lowest heart rate at rest).

Ratings of Perceived Exertion (RPE) The assessment of the intensity of exercise based on how the participant feels; a subjective assessment of effort.

In the News

Heredity and Cardiovascular Fitness

(i) NEWS As we have seen, many factors contribute to health, wellness, and fitness. One factor over which you have little control is heredity. For years we have known that all people do not respond equally to regular exercise, even when it is done using the correct FIT formula. A recent study published in the *Journal of Applied Physiology* found that about 80 to 85 percent of 423 men and women who participated in a cardiovascular fitness program saw improvements in cardiovascular fitness over a period of 20 weeks. However, 15 to 20 percent of the participants showed little fitness improvement. The researchers found that a genetic profile predicted which people would get the most improvement from exercise.

This study prompted more than a few articles in newspapers and reports on television throughout the United States. Some suggested that this was evidence that exercise is of little value to some people. The researchers who conducted the study suggest that exercise is of value to all, noting that exercise has many benefits in addition to increases in cardiovascular fitness. Even those who do not respond with big gains in CV fitness can have changes in blood pressure, blood sugar, heart rate, and other biological markers. More information about heredity and fitness is available at the associated Web link.

---

rate target zones using the HRR method. The example is for a 22-year-old with good cardiovascular fitness, who does regular moderate-to-vigorous physical activity and who has a resting heart rate of 68 beats per minute. The target heart rate zone for this hypothetical person is 65 to 80 percent.

To determine the threshold of training (minimum heart rate for building cardiovascular fitness) for the hypothetical 22-year-old, use 65 percent of the working heart rate, and then add that value to the resting heart rate. To determine the upper limit of the target zone, use 80 percent of the working heart rate and add that value to the resting heart rate. Because target zone heart rates vary for people of different fitness and activity levels and because resting and maximal heart rates vary, each person will have a unique range of heart rates defining the target heart rate zone. Somewhat paradoxically, fitter individuals (with a lower resting HR) will tend to have lower target heart zones than less fit individuals (see Figure 5). The range is lower because the HRR is larger. Charts with target heart rate zones for each of the five fitness and activity levels described in Table 2 are provided at the associated Web link.

The percentage of maximum heart rate method is an alternative way to calculate target heart rate zones. The percentage of maxHR method is simpler to use than the HRR method, but it is not as accurate. This procedure takes maximal heart rate into account but does not factor in individual differences in resting heart rate. People with a typical resting HR of 60 to 70 bpm will tend to get similar values with both methods, but the percentage of maxHR method tends to be less accurate for people with high or low resting heart rates.

To use the percentage of maxHR method, first find your maximum HR with the formula (maxHR = 208 − (.7 × age). Then multiply your maxHR by the appropriate percentages from Table 2. For a person with good fitness and who performs regular moderate-to-vigorous activity, the percentages would be 80 to 91 percent. The maxHR for our hypothetical 22-year-old is 193, so the target heart rate zone would be 154 to 176 using this method (.80 × 193 = 154 and .91 × 193 = 176). As illustrated in Table 3, this procedure yields somewhat similar but higher values for the maxHR method than for the HRR method. The differences between the two methods vary for people of different ages, resting heart rates, and fitness/activity levels. The percentage of maxHR method is considered an acceptable alternative method, but the HRR method is more precise. Charts with calculated target heart rate zones are provided in the associated web features to make it easier to see the

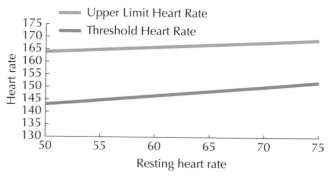

Figure 5 ▶ Effect of different resting heart rate values on target heart range (values assume an age of 22 and a range of 65–80 percent HRR).

general ranges for different resting and maximal heart rate values (based on age). Threshold and target zone heart rates should be used as general guidelines for cardiovascular exercise. You should check your resting heart rate and learn to calculate your target heart range based on the HRR method. It is important to understand how to make the calculations, since the process explains the relationships.

The target heart ranges should be used as just that, a general target to try for during your exercise session. By bringing your heart rate above the threshold and into the target zone, you will provide an optimal challenge to your cardiovascular system and maintain/improve your cardiovascular fitness. Guidelines for heart rate monitoring are provided in the next section.

Ratings of perceived exertion can be used to monitor the intensity of physical activity. The ACSM suggests that people experienced in physical activity can use RPE to determine if they are exercising in the target zone (see Table 4). Ratings of perceived exertion have been shown to correlate well with $\dot{V}O_2R$ and HRR. For this reason, RPE can be used to estimate exercise intensity among those who have learned to use the RPE rating categories. This avoids the need to stop and count heart rate during exercise. A rating of 12 is equal to threshold, and a rating of 16 is equal to the upper limit of the target zone. With practice, most people can recognize when they are in the target zone using ratings of perceived exertion.

Guidelines for Heart Rate and Exercise Monitoring

Learning to count heart rate can help you monitor the intensity of your physical activity. To determine the intensity of physical activity for building cardiovascular fitness, you need to know how to count your pulse. Each time the heart beats, it pumps blood into the arteries. The surge of blood causes a pulse, which can be felt by holding a finger against an artery. The major arteries that are easy to locate and are frequently used for pulse counts are the radial just below the base of the thumb on the wrist (see Figure 6) and the carotid on either side of the Adam's apple (see Figure 7). Counting the pulse at the carotid is the most popular procedure, probably because the carotid pulse is easy to locate. The radial pulse is a bit harder to find because of the many tendons near the wrist, but it works better for some people.

To count the pulse rate, simply place the fingertips (index and middle finger) over the artery at the wrist or

Table 4 ▶ Ratings of Perceived Exertion (RPE)	
Rating	**Description**
6	
7	Very, very light
8	
9	Very light
10	
11	Fairly light
12	
13	Somewhat hard
14	
15	Hard
16	
17	Very hard
18	
19	Very, very hard
20	

Source: Data from Borg.

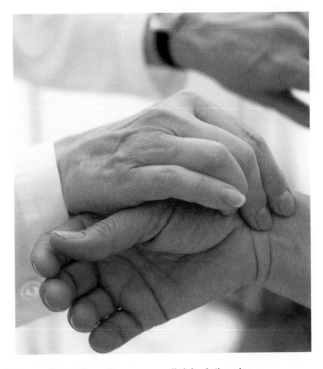

Figure 6 ▶ Counting your radial (wrist) pulse.

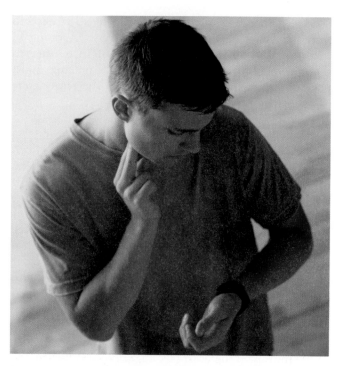

Figure 7 ▶ Counting your carotid (neck) pulse.

neck location. Move the fingers around until a strong pulse can be felt. Press gently so as not to cut off the blood flow through the artery. Counting the pulse with the thumb is *not* recommended because the thumb has a relatively strong pulse of its own, and it could be confusing when counting another person's pulse.

Technology Update
New Technology in Activity Monitoring

TECH   A variety of technologies have been developed to make it easier to monitor vital signs and responses to exercise. Heart rate monitors have made it possible for individuals to monitor heart rate during exercise but new tools make it easier to track fitness and health data over time. Applications are also available to facilitate communication with physicians. An iPod application called Health Vitals Tracker allows you to send health data such as blood sugar level and blood pressure directly to your health care provider. Another iPod application called iStethoscope allows you to send heart sounds directly to your doctor. The Mayo Clinic recently released a new (free) iPod application called (Mayo Clinic Symptom Checker) that enables people to get answers and advice when experiencing a variety of symptoms. It is designed to help people manage acute problems and provides guidance on practicing self-care at home, as well as insights into when additional care is needed. More information is available at the associated web icon.

Counting heart rates during exercise presents some additional challenges. To obtain accurate exercise heart rate values, it is best to count heart beats or pulses while moving; however, this is difficult during most activities.

The most practical method is to count the pulse immediately after exercise. During physical activity, the heart rate increases, but immediately after exercise, it begins to slow and return to normal. In fact, the heart rate has already slowed considerably within 1 minute after activity ceases. Therefore, you must locate the pulse quickly and count the rate for a short period in order to obtain accurate results. For best results, keep moving while quickly locating the pulse; then stop and take a 15-second count. Multiply the number of pulses by 4 to convert heart rate to beats per minute.

You can also count the pulse for 10 seconds and multiply by 6, or count the pulse for 6 seconds and multiply by 10 to estimate a 1-minute heart rate. The latter method allows you to calculate heart rates easily by adding 0 to the 6-second count. However, short-duration pulse counts increase the chance of error because a miscount of 1 beat is multiplied by 6 or 10 beats rather than by 4 beats.

The pulse rate should be counted after regular activity, not after a sudden burst. Some runners sprint the last few yards of their daily run and then count their pulse. Such a burst of exercise will elevate the heart rate considerably. This gives a false picture of the actual exercise heart rate. Everyone should learn to determine resting heart rate accurately and to estimate exercise heart rate by quickly and accurately making pulse counts after activity (see Lab 7A).

Declines in resting heart rate and exercise heart rate signal improvements in cardiovascular fitness. As described in this concept, the heart beats to provide the body (and working muscles) with oxygen. Oxygen is used to produce energy using aerobic metabolism. During rest, the heart can beat relatively slowly to provide sufficient oxygen to the body. During exercise, the demand for energy increases, so the body increases heart rate (and respiration) to help distribute more oxygen to the body. Changes in resting heart rate and exercise heart rate provide good indicators of improvements in fitness because they indicate that the heart can pump fewer times to provide the same amount of blood flow to the body. A fit individual has a stronger heart and can pump more blood with each beat.

A comparison of resting and exercise heart rates for three hypothetical individuals performing the same bout of exercise is shown in Figure 8. The column labeled "A" shows the response of an unfit person. This person has a high resting heart rate of 90, and this increases to 160 during the exercise. This intensity would feel pretty hard, so an RPE would likely be about 17. Compare this response to the results for a moderately or highly fit

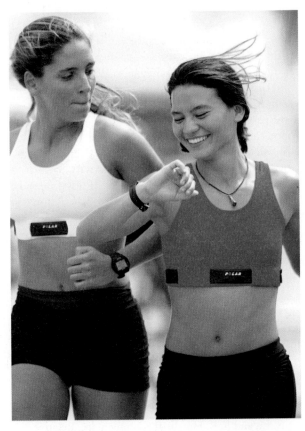

Heart rate monitors provide an effective way to track heart rate during exercise.

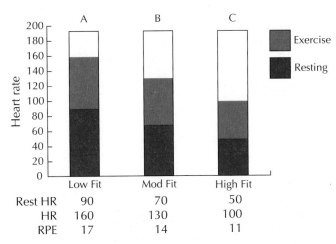

	A	B	C
	Low Fit	Mod Fit	High Fit
Rest HR	90	70	50
HR	160	130	100
RPE	17	14	11

Figure 8 ▶ Comparison of resting and exercise heart for three 22-year-old individuals (maxHR = 193) with different levels of fitness (A = low fitness, B = moderate fitness, C = high fitness).

person. Both have a lower resting heart rate and a lower exercise heart rate, so exercise is easier and can be maintained more easily.

Heart rate monitors can help monitor the intensity and duration of cardiovascular exercise. Heart rate monitors have been used for years by competitive endurance athletes to monitor their training programs.

Athletes learn what their heart rate is for certain paces and know how hard they can push to optimize their performance in a race. Technological advances have continued to enhance the utility of these devices, and the costs of the devices are now within the reach of many recreational exercisers.

The watch (receiver), typically worn on the wrist, receives a signal from a transmitter attached to a strap worn around the chest. Basic units display heart rate only, whereas more advanced models have alarms to indicate time spent in target zones and software that allows the heart rate signals to be downloaded and processed on a personal computer. The software can automatically track time spent in different target zones and allow users to see a graphical display of how hard they exercised. The immediate feedback on heart rate during exercise and the ability to log workouts over time may help some individuals maintain interest in their exercise program.

▶ Strategies for Action

(i) **An important step in taking action to develop and maintain cardiovascular FEATURE 5 fitness is assessing your current status.** For an activity program to be most effective, it should be based on personal needs. Some type of testing is necessary to determine your personal need for cardiovascular fitness. As noted earlier, the best measure of cardiovascular fitness is a laboratory assessment of $\dot{V}O_2$ max, but this is not possible for most people. To provide alternatives, researchers have developed other tests that give reasonable estimates. Commonly used tests are the step test, the

swim test, the 12-minute run, the Astrand-Ryhming bicycle test, and the walking test. These tests are developed based on comparisons with measured $\dot{V}O_2$ max and are good general indicators of cardiovascular fitness. In Lab 7B you will be able to compare estimates from several tests.

The self-assessment you choose depends on your current fitness and activity levels, the availability of equipment, and other factors. The walking test is probably best for those at beginning levels because more vigorous forms of activity may cause discomfort and may discourage future participation. The step test is somewhat less vigorous than the running test and takes only a few minutes to complete. The bicycle test is also submaximal or relatively moderate in intensity. It is quite accurate but requires more equipment than the other tests and requires more expertise. You may need help from a fitness expert to do this test properly. The swim test is especially useful to those with musculoskeletal problems and other disabilities. The running test is the most vigorous and for this reason may not be best for beginners. On the other hand, more advanced exercisers with high levels of motivation may prefer this test.

Results on the walking, running, and swimming tests are greatly influenced by the motivation of the test taker. If the test taker does not try hard, fitness results are underestimated. The bicycle and step tests are influenced less by motivation because one must exercise at a specified workload and at a regular pace. Because heart rate can be influenced by emotional factors, by exercise prior to the test, and other factors, tests using heart rate can sometimes give incorrect results. It is important to do your self-assessments when you are relatively free from stress and are rested.

Prior to performing any of these, be sure that you are physically and medically ready. Prepare yourself by doing some regular physical activity for 3 to 6 weeks before actually taking the tests. If possible, take more than one test and use the summary of your test results to make a final assessment of your cardiovascular fitness. In Lab 7B, you will have the opportunity to self-assess your cardiovascular fitness using one or more tests. A nonexercise estimate of cardiovascular fitness is also provided for comparison. Although this self-report tool has limitations, it is increasingly being used as a screening tool in physicians' offices to determine if patients have risks associated with poor fitness.

Web Resources

Additional websites with information related to Concept 7 are available at the associated Web link.

American College of Sports Medicine **www.acsm.org**
American Health Association **www.americanheart.org**
The Cooper Institute **www.cooperinst.org**
President's Challenge **http://presidentschallenge.org/home _adults.aspx**
Fitnessgram Youth Fitness Test **www.fitnessgram.net**

Suggested Readings

Selected readings and references are listed below. A more comprehensive list is available at the associated Web link.

ACSM. 2010. *ACSM's Guidelines for Exercise Testing and Prescription.* 8th ed. Philadelphia: Lippincott, Williams & Wilkins, Chapters 4 and 7.

Ding, E. L., and F. B. Hu. 2010. Commentary: Relative importance of diet vs physical activity for health. *International Journal of Epidemiology* 39(1):209–211.

Gulati, M., et al. Heart rate response to exercise stress testing in asymptomatic women. The St. James Women Take Heart Project. *Circulation.* Published online June 28, 2010, **http://circ.ahajournals.org**

Heroux, M., et al. 2010. Dietary patterns and the risk of mortality: Impact of cardiorespiratory fitness. *International Journal of Epidemiology* 39(1):197–209.

Kodama, S., et al. 2009. Cardiorespiratory fitness as a quantitative predictor of all-cause mortality and cardiovascular events in healthy men and women: A Meta-analysis. *Journal of the American Medical Association* 301(19):2024–2035.

Rubin, R. Exercise won't boost endurance for 1 in 5. *USA Today.* **www.usatoday.com/news/health/2010-02-04 -exercise_N.htm**

Lab Resource Materials: Evaluating Cardiovascular Fitness

The Walking Test

- Warm up; then walk 1 mile as fast as you can without straining. Record your time to the nearest second.

- Immediately after the walk, count your heart rate for 15 seconds; then multiply by 4 to get a 1-minute heart rate. Record your heart rate.

- Use your walking time and your postexercise heart rate to determine your rating using Chart 1.

Chart 1 ▶ Walking Ratings for Males and Females

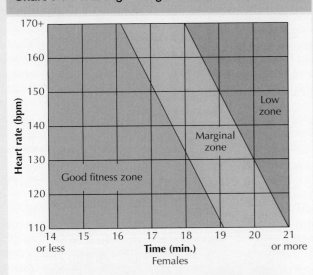

Females

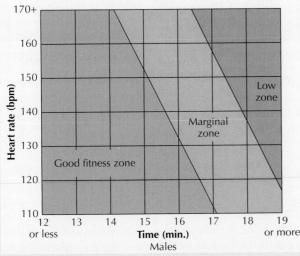

Males

Source: James M. Rippe, M.D.

The ratings in Chart 1 are for ages 20 to 29. They provide reasonable ratings for people of all ages.

Note: The walking test is not a good indicator of high performance; the running and bicycle tests are recommended.

Step Test

- Step up and down on a 12-inch bench for 3 minutes at a rate of 24 steps per minute. One step consists of 4 beats—that is, "up with the left foot, up with the right foot, down with the left foot, down with the right foot."

- Immediately after the exercise, sit down on the bench and relax. Don't talk.

- Locate your pulse or have someone locate it for you.

- Five seconds after the exercise ends, begin counting your pulse. Count the pulse for 60 seconds.

- Your score is your 60-second heart rate. Locate your score and your rating on Chart 2.

Chart 2 ▶ Step Test Rating Chart

Classification	60-Second Heart Rate
High-performance zone	84 or less
Good fitness zone	85–95
Marginal zone	96–119
Low zone	120 and above

Source: Kasch and Boyer.

As you grow older, you will want to continue to score well on this rating chart. Because your maximal heart rate decreases as you age, you should be able to score well if you exercise regularly.

The Astrand-Ryhming Bicycle Test

- Ride a stationary bicycle ergometer for 6 minutes at a rate of 50 pedal cycles per minute (one push with each foot per cycle). Cool down after the test.

- Set the bicycle at a workload between 300 and 1,200 kpm. For less fit or smaller people, a setting in the range of 300 to 600 is appropriate. Larger or fitter people will need to use a setting of 750 to 1,200. The workload should be enough to elevate the heart rate to at least 125 bpm but no more than 170 bpm during the ride. The ideal range is 140–150 bpm.

- During the sixth minute of the ride (if the heart rate is in the correct range—see previous step), count the heart rate for the entire sixth minute. The carotid or radial pulse may be used.

- Use Chart 3 (males) or 4 (females) to determine your predicted oxygen uptake score in liters per minute. Locate your heart rate for the sixth minute of the ride in the left column and the work rate in kp·m/min. across the top. The number in the chart where the heart rate and work rate intersect represents your predicted O_2 uptake in liters per minute. The bicycle you use must allow you to easily and accurately determine the work rate in kp·m/min.

- Ratings are typically assigned based on milliliters per kilogram of body weight per minute. To convert your score to milliliters per kilogram per minute (mL/kg/min.), the first step is to multiply your score from Chart 3 or 4 by 1,000. This converts your score from liters to milliliters. Then divide your weight in pounds by 2.2. This converts your weight to kilograms. Then divide your score in milliliters by your weight in kilograms. This gives you your score in mL/kg/min.

- Example: An oxygen uptake score of 3.5 liters is equal to a 3,500-milliliter score (3.5 × 1,000). If the person with this score weighed 150 pounds, his or her weight in kilograms would be 68.18 kilograms (150 divided by 2.2). The person's oxygen uptake would be 51.3 mL/kg/min. (3,500 divided by 68.18).

- Use your score in mL/kg/min. to determine your rating (Chart 5).

Chart 3 ▶ Determining Oxygen Uptake Using the Bicycle Test—Men (Liters O_2/min.)

Heart Rate	Work Rate (kp·m/min.)				Heart Rate	Work Rate (kp·m/min.)					Heart Rate	Work Rate (kp·m/min.)				
	450	600	900	1,200		450	600	900	1,200	1,500		450	600	900	1,200	1,500
123	3.3	3.4	4.6	6.0	139	2.5	2.6	3.6	4.8	6.0	155	2.0	2.2	3.0	4.0	5.0
124	3.3	3.3	4.5	6.0	140	2.5	2.6	3.6	4.8	6.0	156	1.9	2.2	2.9	4.0	5.0
125	3.2	3.2	4.4	5.9	141	2.4	2.6	3.5	4.7	5.9	157	1.9	2.1	2.9	3.9	4.9
126	3.1	3.2	4.4	5.8	142	2.4	2.5	3.5	4.6	5.8	158	1.8	2.1	2.9	3.9	4.9
127	3.0	3.1	4.3	5.7	143	2.4	2.5	3.4	4.6	5.7	159	1.8	2.1	2.8	3.8	4.8
128	3.0	3.1	4.2	5.6	144	2.3	2.5	3.4	4.5	5.7	160	1.8	2.1	2.8	3.8	4.8
129	2.9	3.0	4.2	5.6	145	2.3	2.4	3.4	4.5	5.6	161	1.7	2.0	2.8	3.7	4.7
130	2.9	3.0	4.1	5.5	146	2.3	2.4	3.3	4.4	5.6	162	1.7	2.0	2.8	3.7	4.6
131	2.8	2.9	4.0	5.4	147	2.3	2.4	3.3	4.4	5.5	163	1.7	2.0	2.8	3.7	4.6
132	2.8	2.9	4.0	5.3	148	2.2	2.4	3.2	4.3	5.4	164	1.6	2.0	2.7	3.6	4.5
133	2.7	2.8	3.9	5.3	149	2.2	2.3	3.2	4.3	5.4	165	1.6	1.9	2.7	3.6	4.5
134	2.7	2.8	3.9	5.2	150	2.2	2.3	3.2	4.2	5.3	166	1.6	1.9	2.7	3.6	4.5
135	2.7	2.8	3.8	5.1	151	2.2	2.3	3.1	4.2	5.2	167	1.5	1.9	2.6	3.5	4.4
136	2.6	2.7	3.8	5.0	152	2.1	2.3	3.1	4.1	5.2	168	1.5	1.9	2.6	3.5	4.4
137	2.6	2.7	3.7	5.0	153	2.1	2.2	3.0	4.1	5.1	169	1.5	1.9	2.6	3.5	4.3
138	2.5	2.7	3.7	4.9	154	2.0	2.2	3.0	4.0	5.1	170	1.4	1.8	2.6	3.4	4.3

Chart 4 ▶ Determining Oxygen Uptake Using the Bicycle Test—Women (Liters O_2/min.)

Heart Rate	Work Rate (kp·m/min.)					Heart Rate	Work Rate (kp·m/min.)					Heart Rate	Work Rate (kp·m/min.)			
	300	450	600	750	900		300	450	600	750	900		400	600	750	900
123	2.4	3.1	3.9	4.6	5.1	139	1.8	2.4	2.9	3.5	4.0	155	1.9	2.4	2.8	3.2
124	2.4	3.1	3.8	4.5	5.1	140	1.8	2.4	2.8	3.4	4.0	156	1.9	2.4	2.8	3.2
125	2.3	3.0	3.7	4.4	5.0	141	1.8	2.3	2.8	3.4	3.9	157	1.8	2.3	2.7	3.2
126	2.3	3.0	3.6	4.3	5.0	142	1.7	2.3	2.8	3.3	3.9	158	1.8	2.3	2.7	3.1
127	2.2	2.9	3.5	4.2	4.8	143	1.7	2.2	2.7	3.3	3.8	159	1.8	2.3	2.7	3.1
128	2.2	2.8	3.5	4.2	4.8	144	1.7	2.2	2.7	3.2	3.8	160	1.8	2.2	2.6	3.0
129	2.2	2.8	3.4	4.1	4.8	145	1.6	2.2	2.7	3.2	3.7	161	1.8	2.2	2.6	3.0
130	2.1	2.7	3.4	4.0	4.7	146	1.6	2.2	2.6	3.2	3.7	162	1.8	2.2	2.6	3.0
131	2.1	2.7	3.4	4.0	4.6	147	1.6	2.1	2.6	3.1	3.6	163	1.7	2.2	2.5	2.9
132	2.0	2.7	3.3	3.9	4.6	148	1.6	2.1	2.6	3.1	3.6	164	1.7	2.1	2.5	2.9
133	2.0	2.6	3.2	3.8	4.5	149	1.5	2.1	2.6	3.0	3.5	165	1.7	2.1	2.5	2.9
134	2.0	2.6	3.2	3.8	4.4	150	1.5	2.0	2.5	3.0	3.5	166	1.7	2.1	2.5	2.8
135	2.0	2.6	3.1	3.7	4.4	151	1.5	2.0	2.5	3.0	3.4	167	1.6	2.0	2.4	2.8
136	1.9	2.5	3.1	3.6	4.3	152	1.4	2.0	2.5	2.9	3.4	168	1.6	2.0	2.4	2.8
137	1.9	2.5	3.0	3.6	4.2	153	1.4	2.0	2.4	2.9	3.3	169	1.6	2.0	2.4	2.8
138	1.8	2.4	3.0	3.5	4.2	154	1.4	2.0	2.4	2.8	3.3	170	1.6	2.0	2.4	2.7

Chart 5 ▶ Bicycle Test Rating Scale (mL/O$_2$/kg/min.)

Women					
Age	17–26	27–39	40–49	50–59	60–69
High-performance zone	46+	40+	38+	35+	32+
Good fitness zone	36–45	33–39	30–37	28–34	24–31
Marginal zone	30–35	28–32	24–29	21–27	18–23
Low zone	<30	<28	<24	<21	<18

Men					
Age	17–26	27–39	40–49	50–59	60–69
High-performance zone	50+	46+	42+	39+	35+
Good fitness zone	43–49	35–45	32–41	29–38	26–34
Marginal zone	35–42	30–34	27–31	25–28	22–25
Low zone	<35	<30	<27	<25	<22

The 12-Minute Run Test

- Locate an area where a specific distance is already marked, such as a school track or football field, or measure a specific distance using a bicycle or automobile odometer.
- Use a stopwatch or wristwatch to accurately time a 12-minute period.
- For best results, warm up prior to the test; then run at a steady pace for the entire 12 minutes (cool down after the tests).
- Determine the distance you can run in 12 minutes in fractions of a mile. Depending upon your age, locate your score and rating in Chart 6.

Chart 6 ▶ Twelve-Minute Run Test Rating Chart

Classification—Men	Men (Age)							
	17–26		27–39		40–49		50+	
	Miles	Km	Miles	Km	Miles	Km	Miles	Km
High-performance zone	1.80+	2.90+	1.60+	2.60+	1.50+	2.40+	1.40+	2.25+
Good fitness zone	1.55–1.79	2.50–2.89	1.45–1.59	2.35–2.59	1.40–1.49	2.25–2.39	1.25–1.39	2.00–2.24
Marginal zone	1.35–1.54	2.20–2.49	1.30–1.44	2.10–2.34	1.25–1.39	2.00–2.24	1.10–1.24	1.75–1.99
Low zone	<1.35	<2.20	<1.30	<2.10	<1.25	<2.00	<1.1	<1.75

Classification—Women	Women (Age)							
	17–26		27–39		40–49		50+	
	Miles	Km	Miles	Km	Miles	Km	Miles	Km
High-performance zone	1.45+	2.35+	1.35+	2.20+	1.25+	2.00+	1.15+	1.85+
Good fitness zone	1.25–1.44	2.00–2.34	2.20–1.34	1.95–2.19	1.15–1.24	1.85–1.99	1.05–1.14	1.70–1.84
Marginal zone	1.15–1.24	1.85–1.99	1.05–1.19	1.70–1.94	1.00–1.14	1.60–1.84	.95–1.04	1.55–1.69
Low zone	<1.15	<1.85	<1.05	<1.70	<1.00	<1.60	<.95	<1.55

Source: Based on data from Cooper.

The 12-minute Swim Test

- Locate a swimming area with premeasured distances, preferably 20 yards or longer.
- After a warm-up, swim as far as possible in 12 minutes using the stroke of your choice.

- For best results, have a partner keep track of your time and distance. A degree of swimming competence is a prerequisite for this test.
- Determine your score and rating using Chart 7.

Chart 7 ▶ Twelve-Minute Swim Rating Chart

	Men (Age)							
	17–26		27–39		40–49		50+	
Classification—Men	Yards	Meters	Yards	Meters	Yards	Meters	Yards	Meters
High-performance zone	700+	650+	650+	600+	600+	550+	550+	500+
Good fitness zone	600–699	550–649	550–649	500–599	500–599	475–549	450–549	425–499
Marginal zone	500–599	450–549	450–459	400–499	400–499	375–475	350–449	325–424
Low zone	Below 500	Below 450	Below 450	Below 400	Below 400	Below 375	Below 350	Below 325

	Women (Age)							
	17–26		27–39		40–49		50+	
Classification—Women	Yards	Meters	Yards	Meters	Yards	Meters	Yards	Meters
High-performance zone	600+	550+	550+	500+	500+	450+	450+	400+
Good fitness zone	500–599	450–549	450–549	400–499	400–499	375–449	350–449	325–400
Marginal zone	400–499	350–449	350–449	325–399	300–399	275–375	250–349	225–324
Low zone	Below 400	Below 350	Below 350	Below 325	Below 300	Below 275	Below 250	Below 225

Source: Based on data from Cooper.

Chart 8 ▶ Non-Exercise Fitness Assessment Rating Chart

Rating	Score
Needs Improvement	1–4
Marginal	5–9
Good Conditioning	10–13
Highly Conditioned	13+

Lab 7B Evaluating Cardiovascular Fitness

Name		**Section**	**Date**

Purpose: To acquaint you with several methods for evaluating cardiovascular fitness and to help you evaluate and rate your own cardiovascular fitness

Procedure

1. Perform one or more of the four cardiovascular fitness tests and determine your ratings using the information in the Lab Resource Materials.
2. Perform each of the four steps for the Non-Exercise Estimate of Cardiovascular Fitness using the information on the back of this page. Learning this technique will allow you to estimate your fitness when you are injured or for some other reason cannot do a performance test.

Results

1. Record the information from your cardiovascular fitness test(s) in the spaces provided.
2. After you have completed the four steps for the Non-Exercise Estimate of Cardiovascular Fitness, use Chart 8 in Lab resource materials (page 134) to determine your fitness rating.

Walking Test

Time ___ minutes

Heart rate ___ bpm

Rating ___ (see Chart 1, page 131)

Bicycle Test

Workload ___ kpm

Heart rate ___ bpm

Weight ___ pounds

Weight in kg* ___

mL/O$_2$/kg ___

Rating ___ (see Chart 5, page 133)

Non-Exercise Test

Score ___

Rating ___ (see Chart 8, page 134)

*Weight in lb. ÷ 2.2.

Step Test

Heart rate ___ bpm

Rating ___ (see Chart 2, page 131)

12-Minute Run

Distance ___ miles

Rating ___ (see Chart 6, page 133)

12-Minute Swim Test

Distance ___ yards

Rating ___ (see Chart 7, page 134)

Non-Exercise Cardiovascular Fitness Rating

Record your scores and do the calculations to determine scores for A to E below.

- Look up your activity score on Chart 1 (below). Record score in box A. [_____] (A)

- Record your gender (female = 0/male = 1) _____ × 2.77 = [_____] (B)

- Determine your resting heart rate (Lab 7A), record here _____ × 0.03 = [_____] (C)

- Calculate your BMI (see Lab 13B), record here _____ × 0.17 = [_____] (D)

- Record your age in years. _____ × 0.10 = [_____] (E)

Use the following formula to calculate your score. Use Chart 8 on page 134 to get your rating.

18.07 + A + B − C − D − E = Estimated Cardiovascular Fitness (METs)

18.07 + [__] + [__] − [__] − [__] − [__] = [_____]

Chart 1 ▶ Self-Reported Activity Score (for Step 1 Above)	
Activity Score	**Choose the Score That Best Describes Your Physical Activity Level**
0.00	I am inactive or do little activity other than usual daily activities.
0.32	I regularly (> 5 d/wk) participate in physical activities requiring low levels of exertion that result in slight increases in breathing and heart rate for at least **10 minutes** at a time.
1.06	I participate in aerobic exercises such as brisk walking, jogging, or running, cycling, swimming, or vigorous sports at a comfortable pace, or activities requiring similar levels of exertion for **20–60 minutes per week.**
1.76	I participate in aerobic exercises such as brisk walking, jogging, or running at a comfortable pace, or other activities requiring similar levels of exertion for **1–3 hours per week.**
3.03	I participate in aerobic exercises such as brisk walking, jogging, or running at a comfortable pace, or other activities requiring similar levels of exertion for **over 3 hours per week.**

Conclusions and Implications

1. In several sentences, explain why you selected the tests you selected. Discuss your current level of cardiovascular fitness and steps you will need to take to maintain or improve it. Comment on the effectiveness of the tests you selected.

[ ]

2. In several sentences, explain your results from the non-exercise assessment by comparing the results with the other test(s). Did the self-report version classify you into the same fitness category? Try to explain any differences you noted.

[ ]

Vigorous Aerobics, Sports, and Recreational Activities

Health Goals for the Year 2020

- Increase proportion of adults who meet guidelines for moderate to vigorous aerobic activity.

- Reduce proportion of adults who do no leisure-time activity.

- Increase access to employee-based exercise facilities and programs.

- Create social and physical environments that promote good health for all.

- Attain high-quality, longer lives free of preventable disease, injury, and premature death.

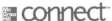 **connect** | FITNESS AND WELLNESS   http://connect.mcgraw-hill.com

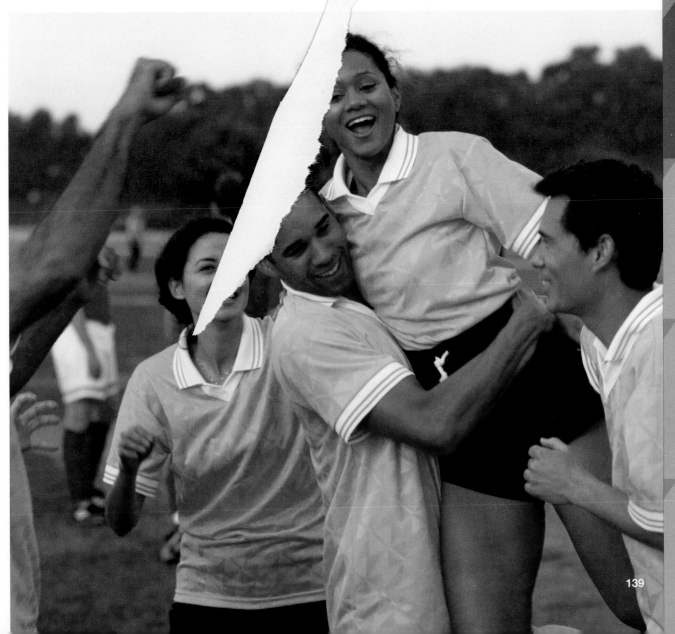

Vigorous physical activity, including vigorous aerobics, sports, and recreational activities, promotes health, fitness, and enhanced performance.

In Concept 6, you learned the many values of moderate physical activity. In this concept, you learn the value of vigorous physical activity as depicted in steps 2 and 3 of the physical activity pyramid (see Figure 1). The threshold of training and target zones described in Concept 7 for building cardiovascular fitness help define the nature of vigorous physical activity. Except for those with low fitness or those who are sedentary, activities intense enough to build cardiovascular fitness are considered to be vigorous in nature.

Three different types of vigorous physical activity are described, including vigorous aerobics, vigorous sports, and vigorous recreational activities. In the past, vigorous physical activity was recommended for people who wanted to build cardiovascular fitness and for enhancing performance, but it was not included as a method of meeting the national physical activity guidelines. The new activity guidelines explicitly include vigorous physical activity. In other words, people can choose moderate activity or vigorous activity to meet the guidelines,

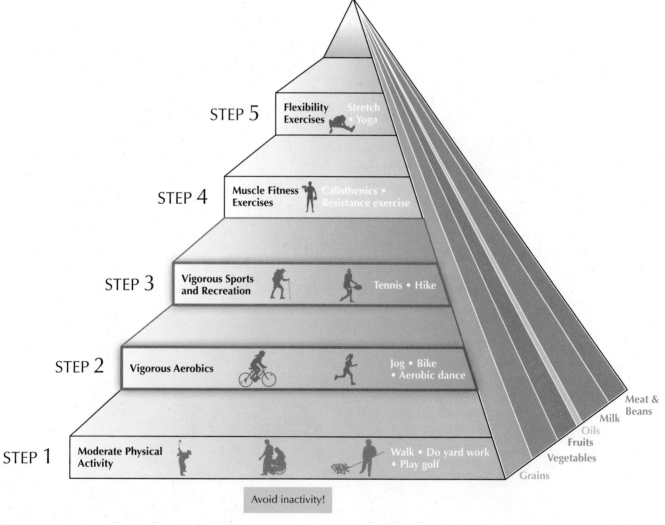

Figure 1 ▶ Vigorous aerobics, sports, and recreational activities are included at the second and third steps of the physical activity pyramid.

depending on the activities of preference. The ACSM/AHA also indicate that moderate and vigorous physical activities can be combined to meet the guidelines.

Physical Activity Pyramid: Step 2

A variety of popular vigorous *aerobic* activities are included at step 2 of the pyramid. The word aerobics literally means "with oxygen." Aerobic activity is generally defined as activity that is rhythmical, uses the large muscles, and is performed in a continuous manner. Many activities meet these criteria, including walking, doing housework, and performing many other light to moderate physical activities.

Dr. Ken Cooper of the Cooper Institute in Dallas popularized the term aerobics in his book, *Aerobics*, published in 1968. His book featured **vigorous aerobic activities** such as those in step 2 of the physical activity pyramid (see Figure 1). The activities included in step 2 of the pyramid are aerobic activities that are at least 6 METs (6 times more intense than resting) and significantly elevate the heart rate. Examples include jogging, aerobic dance, and cycling. These vigorous forms of aerobics are among the most popular leisure-time activities performed by adults.

An advantage of these vigorous aerobic activities is that they provide a good cardiovascular workout in a short time and can often be done by oneself. A disadvantage (or barrier) for some people is that they are generally more vigorous and fast paced than other forms of activity. The more vigorous nature is the most likely explanation for the age-related patterns that exist for participation in vigorous aerobic activity. Young adults are far more likely to participate in vigorous aerobic activity than are older adults. Most statistics report three- to fivefold differences in participation rates for young adults and older adults (40 to 60). The declining interest in vigorous activity for older adults is a concern to public health officials only if older adults fail to substitute moderate physical activity when they discontinue more vigorous activity.

Vigorous sports and recreation at step 3 of the pyramid can provide the same benefits as vigorous aerobic activities. Vigorous sports are not always continuous in nature as are many vigorous aerobic activities such as jogging, swimming, or cycling. Examples of vigorous sports include basketball, racquetball, soccer, and hockey. These activities involve intermittent activity with bursts of activity and short periods of rest but typically are at an intensity that provides benefits similar to vigorous aerobic activities. Swimming and cycling are also popular activities that can be considered sports. However, most people do these activities noncompetitively, so they are

considered as vigorous aerobics in this book. Sports such as golf, bowling, and billiards/pool are aerobic but are light to moderate in intensity. For this reason, they are classified as moderate physical activities.

Activities such as hiking, boating, fishing, horseback riding, and other such outdoor activities are generally classified as recreation. Because many of these activities can be performed at intensities suitable for building cardiovascular fitness, some can be categorized as **vigorous recreational activities**. Hiking, skiing, kayaking, canoeing, hunting, and rock climbing are examples of vigorous recreation activities that typically involve a considerable amount of activity. Recreation activities such as fishing and boating are typically done at lower intensities and can be considered as moderate activities.

Physical activities at step 2 of the pyramid produce improvements in cardiovascular fitness and health in addition to those produced by moderate physical activities. Participation in moderate activity provides important health benefits, but vigorous aerobic activity results in additional health benefits. The many benefits of vigorous activity are described in Table 1. The same benefits (see Concept 4) provided by moderate activity result for people who choose vigorous physical activity instead. Additional benefits, such as improved cardiovascular fitness, improved performance, and added health benefits, occur for those who do vigorous activity. The key is performing vigorous activity at least 3 days a week for 20 minutes at the appropriate target intensity. People who perform both moderate and vigorous activity, or who do vigorous activity above the minimum, get additional benefits. The ACSM/AHA guidelines indicate that "physical activity above the recommended minimum provides even greater health benefits" than meeting only minimum standards. The guidelines further indicate that "the point of maximum benefits for most health

Vigorous Aerobic Activities Aerobic activities of an intensity at least six times that of resting (6 METs), commonly defined as activities with enough intensity to produce improvements in cardiovascular fitness.

Vigorous Sports Sports are competitive activities that have an organized set of rules, along with winners and losers. Vigorous sports are those of similar intensity to vigorous aerobic activities.

Vigorous Recreational Activities Recreational activities are those that are done during leisure time that do not meet the characteristics of sports. Vigorous recreational activities are of similar intensity to vigorous aerobics.

Table 1 ▶ Benefits of Vigorous Physical Activity*
• Vigorous activity meets national guidelines for reducing risk of chronic disease and early death.
• Vigorous activity provides disease risk reduction in addition to moderate activity alone (even when calorie expenditure is the same).
• Vigorous activity provides disease risk reduction in addition to moderate activity when done in addition to moderate physical activity.
• Vigorous activity improves cardiovascular fitness.
• Vigorous activity enhances ability to perform activities that require good cardiovascular fitness.

*Benefits depend on regular participation (at least 3 days a week) and appropriate intensity and duration (at least 20 minutes at target intensity).

benefits has not yet been established . . . but exceeding the minimum recommendation further reduces the risk of inactivity-related chronic disease."

 Moderate and vigorous physical activity can be combined to meet national guidelines. National guidelines specify the total amount of activity that should be performed rather than having separate recommendations for moderate and vigorous activity. This approach helps people incorporate both moderate and vigorous activity into their lifestyle. The guidelines are based on tracking the total "MET-minutes" of physical activity performed. Because vigorous activity is performed at higher intensities (higher MET values), it makes a larger contribution to total activity than moderate-intensity activity performed for the same time. To determine MET-minutes, you multiply the MET value of an activity by the number of minutes that you perform it. For example, if a person walked for 10 minutes at 4 mph (4 METs), the MET-minutes would be 40 (4 METs × 10 minutes). If the person also jogged for 20 minutes at 5 mph (8 METs), the MET-minutes for jogging would be 160 (8 METs × 20 minutes); the total MET-minutes for the day would be 200.

To meet the new physical activity guidelines, a person must accumulate a total of 450 to 750 MET-minutes per week. Beginners start at 450 and gradually work toward the 750 MET-minute goals. More fit people can start at a higher level. Activity should be done at least 3 days a week when this combined method is used, even though the MET-minute standard could be met with large amounts of activity performed on 1 or 2 days. Bouts of activity must be at least 10 minutes in length to be counted toward the recommendation. MET values for a variety of moderate activities are included in Concept 6 (Table 4) on page 108. A complete list of the MET values for a variety of activities can be found at http://prevention.sph.sc.edu/tools/compendium.htm. In

Lab 8C you will learn more about how to combine moderate and vigorous activity to meet national goals.

Not all activities at level 2 and 3 of the pyramid are equally safe. Sports medicine experts indicate that certain types of physical activities are more likely than others to result in injury. Walking and low-impact dance aerobics are among the least risky activities. Skating, an aerobic activity, is the most risky, followed by basketball and competitive sports. Among the most popular aerobic activities, running has the greatest risk, with cycling, high-impact dance aerobics, and step aerobics having moderate risk for injury. Swimming and water aerobics are among those least likely to cause injuries because they do not involve impact, falling, or collision. In general, activities that require high-volume training (aerobics and jogging), collision (football, basketball, and softball), falling (biking, skating, cheerleading, and gymnastics), the use of specialized equipment that can fail (biking), and repetitive movements that stress the joints (tennis and high-impact aerobics) increase risk for injury. These statistics point out the importance of using proper safety equipment, proper performance techniques, and proper training techniques.

Rates of participation in vigorous activity decrease with age. A study on a representative sample of college students from 119 schools found declines in participation between high school and college. Approximately 48 percent of college students met the recommended criteria for vigorous physical activity, a sharp decline from the percentage of the same students who met the criteria when they were in high school. Participation in high school athletics was associated with higher participation rates in vigorous activity in college. A concern to public health researchers is the decline in participation with age in college and the lower levels of participation for college students over the age of 25. The trends are consistent with a study on a representative sample of U.S. adults, which showed clear differences in the types of individuals likely to participate in vigorous activity. Participation was higher among males than females and higher among

 Health is available to Everyone for a **LIFETIME**, and it's Personal

Great-grandmother Morjorie Newlin started weight training when she was 72. At 86, she was the world's oldest competing female body builder. Ernestine Shepherd started exercising at 53, became a certified personal trainer, and at 73 was running 80 miles a week and could bench press 150 pounds.

What types of activities do you hope to be doing 30, 40, or 50 years from now?

younger respondents than older ones. There were also higher rates for individuals with higher education and higher income levels.

Many students presume they will be able to establish regular exercise habits once they finish college, but results from these studies suggest that regular involvement in vigorous physical activity is important for establishing a lifelong pattern.

Vigorous Aerobic Activities

A variety of vigorous aerobic activities are available for meeting individual needs and interests. Because there are so many choices, many beginning exercisers want to know which type of aerobic exercise is best. The best form of exercise is clearly whatever form you enjoy and will do regularly. Some people tend to be very consistent in performing their favorite form of activity, while others stay active by participating in a variety of activities. Seasonal differences are also common with physical activity participation. Many people choose to remain indoors during very hot or very cold weather and perform outdoor activities when temperatures are more moderate.

The charts in Figure 2 show the frequency of participation in a variety of vigorous aerobic activities. These data were compiled from the recent Sporting Goods Manufacturers Association (SGMA) survey, a nationally representative survey designed to track trends in the fitness and sports industry. While the survey is designed primarily for marketing purposes, it provides valuable information about activity interests in the United States. A recent 2010 report (conducted in partnership with the Physical Activity Council) evaluated participation in 117 sports fitness and recreation activities. The results indicated that 77% of Americans age 6 and over took part in at least one activity. A separate report (Tracking the Fitness Movement) provided detailed trends for 28 different activities. Increases in participation rates were evident in 17 activities. Participation rates were up for aerobic exercise equipment such as elliptical motion trainers (up 4.9% in the last year), treadmills (up 4.1%), and stationary cycling (up 2.0%). Increases were also evident for class-oriented activities such as high impact aerobics (up 8.1%), low impact aerobics (up 6.3%), and step aerobics (up 4.5%). Participation in running has increased by 6.7% and various forms of resistance exercise continue to increase in popularity.

Vigorous aerobic activities are often rhythmical and typically involve the large muscle groups of the legs. The rhythmical nature of aerobic activity allows it to be performed continuously and in a controlled manner. The activation of a large muscle mass is important in providing an appropriate challenge to the cardiovascular system. Descriptions of the most common individual forms of aerobic activity are provided below in order of their popularity (see also Figure 2).

Walking

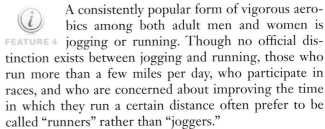

Walking is generally considered as a moderate physical activity and is effective in promoting metabolic fitness and overall health. If cardiovascular fitness is desired, walking must be done intensely enough to elevate the heart rate to target zone levels. For elderly and unfit individuals, walking often provides an intensity sufficient to maintain or improve cardiovascular fitness. For younger and more fit individuals, walking needs to be quite brisk to enhance cardiovascular fitness.

As shown in Figure 2, a large segment of the population has embraced fitness walking as their predominant conditioning activity. Over 10 million women and 6 million men report walking for exercise more than 100 days a year. Of those who walk, not all walk in bouts long enough to meet national activity guidelines. A recent survey of thousands of adults found that nearly twice as many people who walked enough to meet national guidelines walked for leisure as compared to walking for transportation.

Jogging/Running

A consistently popular form of vigorous aerobics among both adult men and women is jogging or running. Though no official distinction exists between jogging and running, those who run more than a few miles per day, who participate in races, and who are concerned about improving the time in which they run a certain distance often prefer to be called "runners" rather than "joggers."

The popularity of jogging and running declined during the 1990s, but trends show progressive increases in participation rates since 2000. Over 25 million Americans report jogging/running for exercise; approximately 10 million (about 6 million males and 4 million females) report running regularly. A major advantage of running is that it requires little equipment and can be done almost anywhere.

Swimming

Swimming is a popular recreational activity, but a relatively small percentage of Americans are considered to be regular fitness swimmers. According to the SGMA survey, nearly 100 million people report participating in "recreational swimming." The number of people that report regular fitness swimming is only about 2.5 million, but this figure is increasing. A 7 percent increase in swimming among women occurred over the past 5 years.

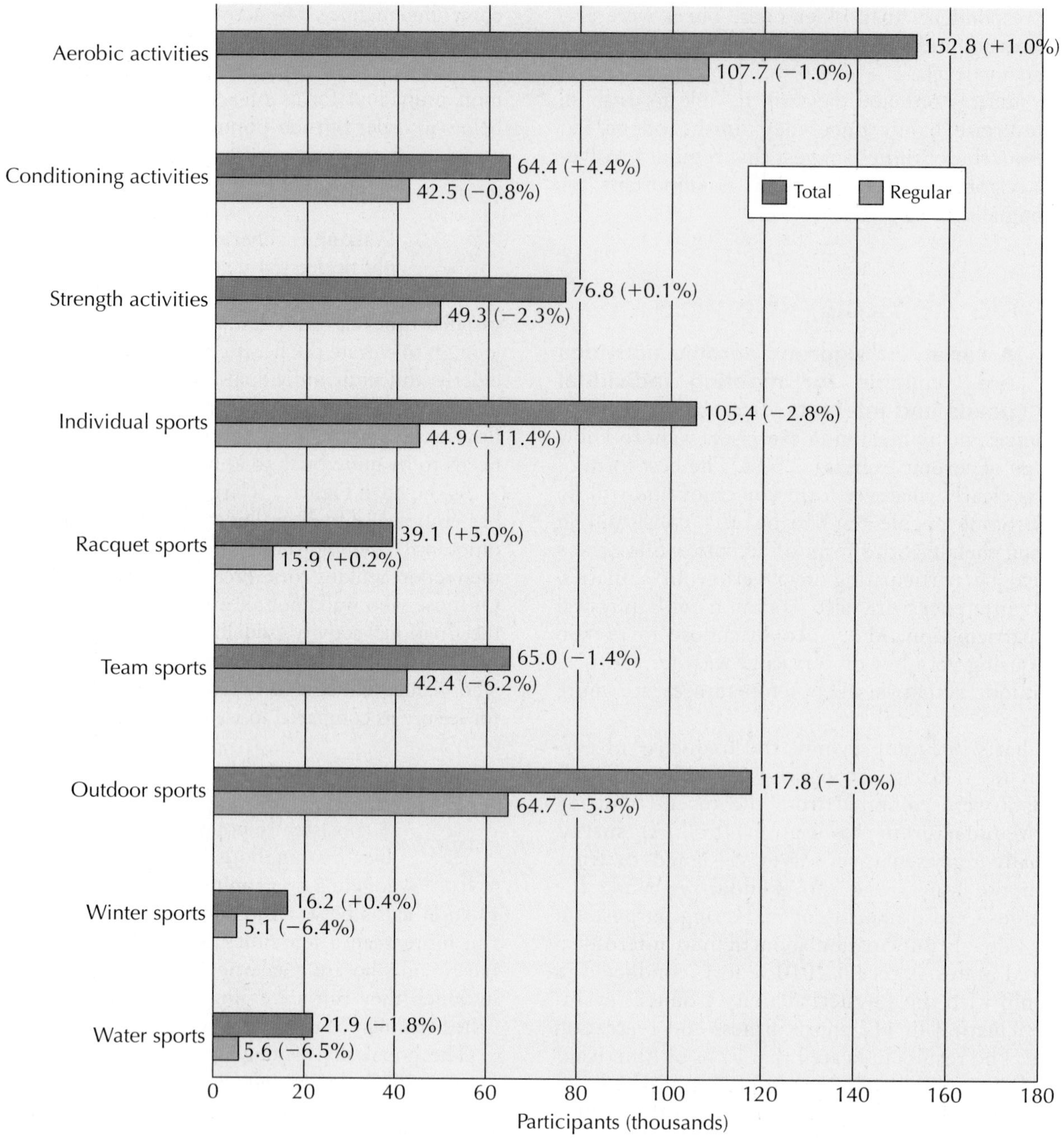

Figure 2 ▶ Participation rates and rates of change for various physical activities in the United States. Total refers to the total number of participants (in millions) that reported doing the activity. Regular refers to number of consistent or regular participants (in millions). Values in parentheses reflect 1 year changes in popularity (percent change).

(Data based on Sporting Good Manufacturer Association (SGMA))

Because it requires considerable skill to move efficiently through the water, many individuals are not able to swim long enough to benefit. Even highly trained athletes can be exhausted after a few hundred yards if they do not have good skills. For those who do swim, it can be an excellent form of physical activity to promote cardiovascular fitness. Because of the water environment and the non-weight-bearing status, the heart rate response to swimming is typically lower for the same intensity of exercise. The heart rate does not increase as rapidly in response to swimming, so target heart rates should be set about 5 to 10 beats lower than for other aerobic activities.

Bicycling

(i) Bicycling can be an excellent vigorous aerobic activity, but it requires a properly fitted bike,
FEATURE 6   as well as safety equipment, such as a helmet and light if done after dark. There are different types of bikes to fit the needs and interests of the rider. Road bikes are most common, but mountain bikes are becoming increasingly popular. Many people appreciate having a versatile bike suitable for different conditions and select a "city bike," which has upright handlebars but more durable wheels and tires for more rugged conditions.

Cycling is more efficient than running and some other aerobic activities because of the mechanical efficiency of the bicycle. Cycling on the level at 5 mph is about three times less intense than running the same speed. It would take a pace of 13 mph to expend a similar number of calories, compared with running at 5 mph. The speed of cycling will give you an indicator of intensity, but this can be influenced by hills and wind. A better indicator of intensity is heart rate or a rating of perceived exertion (RPE). Because biking may involve periods of coasting, it may need to be performed for longer periods of time than jogging to get the same benefit.

According to the SGMA survey, an estimated 50 million Americans report riding their bike for recreation. A smaller number (15 million) report frequent recreational bike riding, and a still smaller segment of the population (about 2 million) can be classified as a regular fitness bicyclist. One of the strategies recommended by the CDC for reducing obesity is to increase the infrastructure supporting bicycling (e.g., bike paths, safe bike routes, bike racks).

Cross-Country Skiing

In most colder climates, cross-country skiing is one of the more popular forms of aerobic activity. Of course, this activity requires snow and specialized equipment. Because it involves both the arms and legs in a coordinated movement, cross-country skiing is one of the most effective types of cardiovascular fitness exercises. The downside is that it requires some degree of skill to perform the movements correctly. There are two main

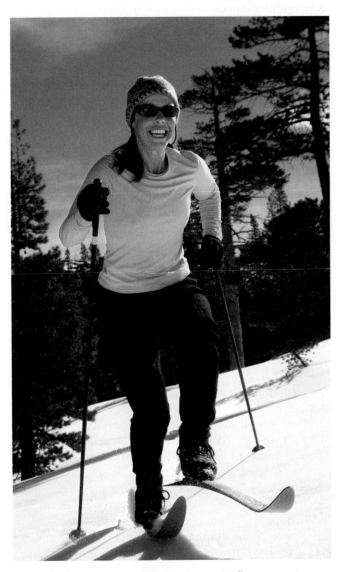

Vigorous physical activity builds cardiovascular fitness.

(i) **Technology Update**
Technology for Vigorously Active People

TECH   Adidas has developed two devices, the miCoach Zone and the miCoach Pacer. The Zone includes a chest strip containing heart rate sensors that send signals to a wristwatch (similar to other heart rate monitoring devices). The Pacer includes the chest strap with sensors as well as a stride sensor and monitor. It works with an MP3 device, allowing you to receive audible coaching while running. Recreational bikers may be interested in the Shake sound generator made by Tunebug, which attaches to an MP3 device such as an iPod and is mounted on a rider's helmet. It is thought to be safer than using an MP3 player with earbuds because it does not play directly into the ear. The Shake can also be mounted on snowboard helmets. G-Tech Backpacks made by Goodhope Bags are high-tech backpacks. Among the many options are battery-operated speakers, iPod connection, strap containing controls for all devices, solar panel power source, and keyboard for texting. More information is available at the associated website.

types of cross-country skiing: classic, or diagonal stride, and skating. Each requires a different type of ski and technique.

Inline Skating

Because of the speed and freedom of movement, inline skating has become a popular aerobic activity. Technological advances in equipment have made it much safer, though injury rates are still high compared with other aerobic activities. Because of the injury risk, precautions should be taken. Special equipment is recommended, including a helmet, knee and elbow pads, wrist supporters, and hand protectors. Some degree of skill is necessary to perform skating safely and effectively, so it is wise to practice in a controlled environment before taking to the streets.

Many types of vigorous aerobics can be done in group settings. Although most vigorous aerobics can be done individually, many people prefer the social interactions and challenge of group exercise classes. Many fitness centers and community recreation centers offer group exercise classes.

An advantage of group exercise classes is that there is a social component, which helps to increase motivation and promote consistency. A disadvantage is that all participants are generally guided through the same exercise. A vigorous routine can cause unfit people to overextend themselves, while an easy routine may not be intense enough for experienced exercisers. A well-trained group exercise leader can help participants adjust the exercise to their own level and ability. Check the qualifications of the exercise leader to be sure that he or she is certified to lead group exercise. Descriptions of the most common group aerobic activities follow.

Dance and Step Aerobics

Dance aerobics is a choreographed series of dance steps and exercises done to music. A variety of forms of dance aerobics are available for different interests and abilities. "Low-impact" aerobics were developed to reduce the risk for injury or soreness. In this form, one foot stays on the floor at all times. Low-impact is an especially wise choice for beginners or older exercisers. Traditional "high-impact" is still common in many settings. In this form, both feet leave the ground simultaneously for a good part of the routine. It is recommended only for advanced exercisers. Even for these people, high-impact aerobics can increase risk for injuries. A hybrid aerobic dance format known as "hi-lo" is gaining in popularity. This form integrates the two types of impact to provide a more balanced routine. The use of alternating sequences

moderates the risks associated with both types and is considered to reflect movements more typical of the activities of daily living. Step aerobics, also known as bench stepping and step training, is an adaptation of dance aerobics. In this activity, the performer steps up and down on a bench when performing various dance steps. In most cases, step aerobics is considered to be low impact, but higher in intensity than many forms of dance aerobics.

There are many variations of aerobic dance or rhythmic aerobic exercise. Jazzercize is one of the more long lasting and well known forms. Other currently popular forms of rhythmical aerobics include Zumba™ (Latin Rhythms), Hip-Hop Aerobics, as well as Line Dancing and Dance done to computers, such as DanceDance Revolution.

Martial Arts Exercise

A variety of martial arts have become popular vigorous aerobic activities. In addition to traditional martial arts, such as karate and tae kwon do, a number of other alternative formats have been developed, including kickboxing, aerobic boxing, cardio-karate, box-fitness, and tae-bo. These activities involve intermittent bouts of high-intensity movements and lower-intensity recovery

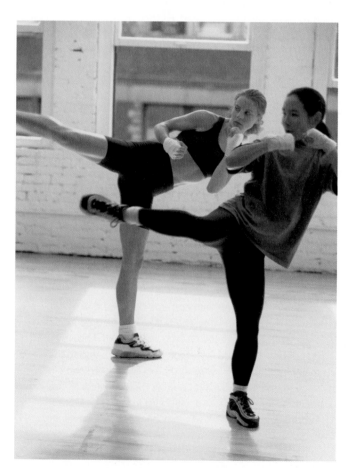

Kickboxing and martial arts are popular ways to stay in shape.

phases. Because martial arts involve a lot of arm work, they can be effective in promoting good overall fitness. Some activities are more intense than others, so consider the alternatives to find the best fit for you. Good instruction is critical for this form of activity, so look for appropriate certifications and credentials before choosing a facility or setting. Many of the disciplines involve a number of contraindicated movements that may increase risk for injury, so it is important to be aware of the risks and minimize your use of bad movements (see Concept 11). If contact is involved, be sure you are matched with a person of similar size and ability.

Spinning

Spinning is a type of stationary cycling typically performed in a group. A group leader typically instructs participants on what pace, gear, and/or cadence to use. In most cases, the routines involve intermittent bursts of high-intensity intervals followed by spinning at lower resistance to recover. The instructor may help riders simulate hill climbing or extended sprints to simulate competitive biking conditions. Although the class relates most directly to cycling, the format has appealed to a broader set of fitness enthusiasts who just enjoy the challenge it provides. Spinning was named as one of the 20 worldwide fitness trends in 2010.

Water Exercise

Swimming is not the only activity done in the water. Water walking and water exercise are two popular alternatives to swimming. Although these activities can be done alone, they are typically conducted in group settings to provide access to pools and certified instructors trained in water safety. Water aerobics are especially good for people with arthritis or other musculoskeletal problems and for people relatively high in body fat. The body's buoyancy in water assists the participant and reduces injury risk. The resistance of the water provides an overload that helps the activity promote health and cardiovascular benefits. Exercises done in shallow water are low in impact, and deeper-water exercises are considered to be higher-impact activities. An advantage of water walking and water exercise is that neither requires the ability to swim. Many classes include activities designed to promote flexibility and muscle fitness development, as well as cardiovascular benefits. Many injured athletes use water activity as a way to rehabilitate from injuries without losing too much fitness.

There has been an increasing trend in the use of cardiovascular exercise machines. While some forms of vigorous aerobic activities have leveled off in recent years, the use of cardiovascular exercise machines has increased primarily because of the increased availability of home equipment and in commercial fitness centers. Treadmills are the most commonly used exercise machine, followed by stationary bikes and stair climbers. However, trends within the fitness industry change quickly. Elliptical trainers have increased in popularity, and this has led to corresponding reductions in the use of other equipment, such as rowing machines and ski machines. Use of these machines can be fun and interesting initially, but that interest may decrease with repeated use. Many people enjoy using different machines to provide some degree of cross training and to have more variety in their program.

Many new features have been developed to enhance interest and ease of use. Most newer machines feature feedback systems, which provide continuous readouts of total exercise time, distance traveled, target and goal intensity, and estimates of calories burned. Most models also include modes that provide built-in warm-up and cool-down phases or a series of predetermined intervals with varying intensities. Some devices have built-in heart rate monitors to allow more precise monitoring of exercise intensity.

There is considerable competition within fitness clubs to offer the latest technology in exercise machines. Some clubs have personalized key systems, which automatically track personal preferences and settings and record time spent on each machine. This information can then be downloaded onto computers for automatic logging. Other fitness clubs have installed video monitors for individual pieces of equipment so that you can watch TV programs or view interactive displays that allow you to compete against a virtual or real opponent. These features provide additional feedback that may enhance motivation or provide for a customized experience. Visit the online learning center for comparisons of new aerobic exercise machines.

Vigorous aerobics can be done either continuously or intermittently. We generally think of vigorous aerobics as being continuous. Jogging, swimming, and cycling at a steady pace for long periods are classic examples. Experts have shown that aerobic exercise can be done intermittently as well as continuously. Both **continuous** and **intermittent aerobic activities** can build cardiovascular fitness. For example, studies have shown that three 10-minute exercise sessions in the

Continuous Aerobic Activities Aerobic activities that are slow enough to be sustained for relatively long periods without frequent rest periods.

Intermittent Aerobic Activities Aerobic activities, relatively high in intensity, alternated with frequent rest periods.

target zone are as effective as one 30-minute exercise session. Still, experts recommend bouts of 20 to 60 minutes in length, with several 10- to 15-minute bouts being an acceptable alternative when longer sessions are not possible.

Vigorous Sport Activities

Some sports are more vigorous than others. Some sports require many muscles from different parts of the body and are more vigorous than those that involve fewer muscles. Some are of high intensity and others are less intense. When done vigorously, tennis and basketball involve many different muscle groups and are high in intensity. Soccer involves many muscle groups and is high in intensity but does not emphasize the use of the arms. Golf, on the other hand, is less intense and relies more on skill and technique. The action in basketball, tennis, and soccer involves bursts of activity followed by rest but requires persistent, vigorous activity over a relatively long time. Golf requires little vigorous activity. Sports that have characteristics similar to those of basketball, tennis, and soccer have benefits like those of vigorous aerobic activities. Of course, any sport can be more or less active, depending on how you perform it. Shooting baskets or even playing half-court basketball is not as vigorous as playing a full-court game.

The most popular sports share characteristics that contribute to their popularity. The most popular sports are often considered to be lifetime sports because they can be done at any age. The characteristics that make these sports appropriate for lifelong participation probably contribute significantly to their popularity. Often, the popular sports are adapted so people without

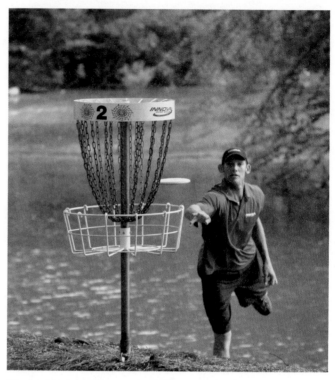

Disc golf is a popular sports activity.

exceptional skill can play them. For example, bowling uses a handicap system to allow people with a wide range of abilities to compete. Slow-pitch softball is much more popular than fast-pitch softball or baseball because it allows people of all abilities to play successfully.

One of the primary reasons sports participation is so popular is that sports provide a challenge. For the greatest enjoyment, the challenge of the activity should be balanced by the person's skill in the sport. If you choose to play against a person with lesser skill, you will not be

In the News

Injuries—Issues and Solutions

Injuries in vigorous exercise are more common than in more moderate forms of activity. Research results show that overuse injuries are among the most common. Activities that involve repetitive movements (overuse), such as aerobic dance and running, put exercisers at risk. Recently, head trauma injuries in sports have been highlighted because of repeated concussions among football players, but head injuries are also common in soccer and recreational activities such as skateboarding and snowboarding. Recently the National Athletic Trainers Association published *Guidelines for Parents to Provide a*

Safe Environment for Youth Athletes. Although these guidelines are for youth, many apply to adults in activity and are useful to parents and future parents.

Injuries are not limited to activities played in the gym or on the field. According to the Consumer Products Safety Commission, more than 1,500 people each year report visiting the emergency room as a result of injuries that occur while using aerobic exercise and resistance exercise machines. These are only the reported cases, so injuries are probably much higher. Follow instructions for properly using machines and practice at low speeds before using faster speeds, especially on devices such as treadmills.

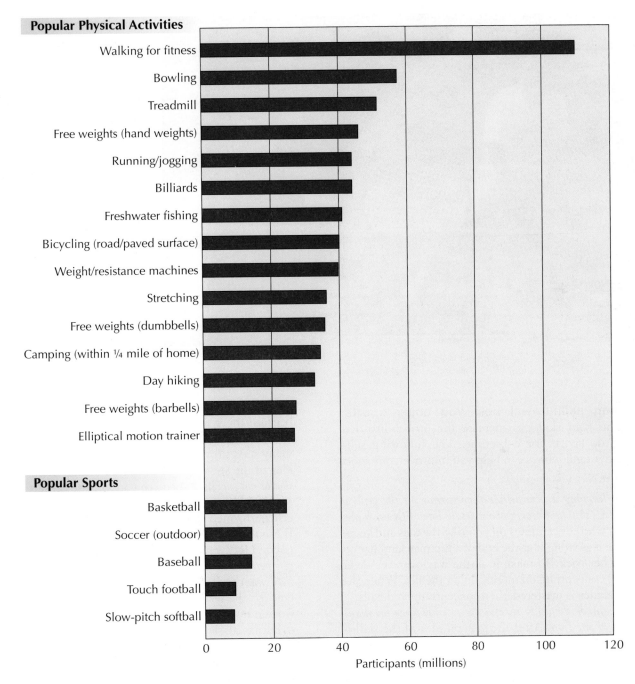

Figure 3 ▶ Top 15 participation activities and top 5 participation sports in the United States.
(Data based on Sporting Good Manufacturer Association (SGMA) Survey in 2010)

challenged. On the other hand, if you lack skill or your opponent has considerably more skill, the activity will be frustrating. For optimal challenge and enjoyment, the skills of a given sport should be learned before competing. Likewise, choose an opponent who has a similar skill level.

Data from the Sporting Goods Manufacturers Association's annual survey (2010 edition) provide a useful way to examine the relative popularity of different physical activities. The results suggest that consumers are motivated by fitness as nine of the top 15 activities

are fitness related activities (see Figure 3). The trend toward efficient (value oriented) activities was attributed in part to the weak economy as consumers seemed to favor accessible, low-cost and "efficient" sports and fitness options. Sports were surveyed separately and basketball was by far the most popular, with soccer and baseball both similar in participation. Among sports, tennis had the largest and most consistent growth trajectory with increases in participation of 40% since 2000.

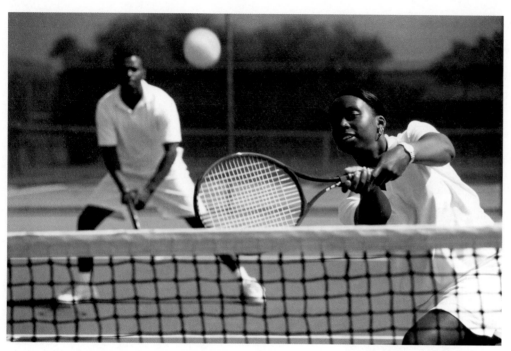
Learning new skills can be challenging but rewarding.

Becoming skillful will help you enjoy sports. Improving your skill can increase the probability that you will do sports for a lifetime. The following self-management guidelines can help you improve your sport performance:

- *When learning a new activity, concentrate on the general idea of the skill first; worry about details later.* For example, a diver who concentrates on pointing the toes and keeping the legs straight at the end of a flip may land flat on his or her back. To make it all the way over, the diver should concentrate on merely doing the flip. When the general idea is mastered, then concentrate on details.

- *The beginner should be careful not to emphasize too many details at one time.* After the general idea of the skill is acquired, the learner can begin to focus on the details, one or two at a time. Concentration on too many details at one time may result in **paralysis by analysis.** For example, a golfer who is told to keep the head down, the left arm straight, and the knees bent cannot possibly concentrate on all of these details at once. As a result, neither the details nor the general idea of the golf swing is performed properly.

- *Once the general idea of a skill is learned, a skill analysis of the performance may be helpful.* Be careful not to overanalyze; it may be helpful to have a knowledgeable person help you locate strengths and weaknesses. Movies and videotapes of skilled performances can be helpful to learners.

- *In the early stages of learning a lifetime sport or physical activity, it is not wise to engage in competition.* Beginners who compete are likely to concentrate on beating their opponent rather than on learning a skill properly. For example, in bowling, the beginner may abandon the newly learned hook ball in favor of the sure-thing straight ball. This may make the person more successful immediately, but is not likely to improve the person's bowling skills for the future.

- *To be performed well, sports skills must be overlearned.* Often, when you learn a new activity, you begin to play the game immediately. The best way to learn a skill is to overlearn it, or practice it until it becomes habit. Frequently, games do not allow you to overlearn skills. For example, during a tennis match is not a good time to learn how to serve because there may be only a few opportunities to do so. For the beginner, it is much more productive to hit many serves (overlearn) with a friend until the general idea of the serve is well learned. Further, the beginner *should not* sacrifice speed to concentrate on serving for accuracy. Accuracy will come with practice of a properly performed skill.

- *When unlearning an old (incorrect) skill and learning a new (correct) skill, a person's performance may get worse before it gets better.* For example, a golfer with a baseball swing may want to learn the correct golf swing. It is important for the learner to understand that the score may worsen during the relearning stage. As the new skill is overlearned, skill will improve, as will the golf score.

- *Mental practice may aid skill learning.* Mental practice (imagining the performance of a skill) may benefit performance, especially if the performer has had previous experience in the skill. Mental practice can be especially useful in sports when the performer cannot participate regularly because of weather, business, or lack of time.

- *For beginners, practicing in front of other people may be detrimental to learning a skill.* An audience may inhibit the beginner's learning of a new sports skill. This is especially true if the learner feels that his or her performance is being evaluated by someone in the audience.

- *There is no substitute for good instruction.* Getting good instruction, especially at the beginning level, will help you learn skills faster and better. Instruction will help you apply these rules and use practice more effectively.

Vigorous Recreation Activities

Vigorous recreation can provide important health benefits and contribute to high quality of life. Activities that you do in your free time for personal enjoyment or to "re-create" yourself are considered to be recreation activities. Recreation activities that exceed threshold intensity for cardiovascular fitness are considered to be vigorous. They are more vigorous than recreation activities such as fishing, bowling and golf, which are typically classified as lifestyle or moderate-level activities (step 1 in the pyramid).

Many of the vigorous aerobic activities, such as cycling, jogging, and skiing, could easily be classified in the vigorous recreation as well as in the vigorous aerobics section. Also, many of the sports described in a later section of this concept can be considered as vigorous recreation activities. The distinction depends somewhat on how the individual views the activities. Some people may view recreation as what they do for fun, but it can also contribute to a healthy lifestyle.

Vigorous recreation is popular, but participation rates in the population generally vary over time. Vigorous recreation provides ways to experience new things, to socialize, and to obtain important health benefits. Participation rates for some common recreation activities are highlighted in Figure 3. As indicated in the table, some activities seem to gain participants, while others lose them.

Outdoor recreation activities (e.g., hiking, fishing, camping, and mountain biking) typically have a strong core of dedicated participants who have been participating for a long time. There are fewer new participants, but the changes over time are generally pretty small. Other recreation activities vary widely in participation rates over time due to changing interests and demographics.

Extreme sports have become popularized through the X Games and other media outlets, and there have been corresponding trends for participation in these activities in recent years. As shown in Figure 2, activities such as surfing, snowboarding, and skateboarding have had some of the highest increases in reported participation. Other activities highlighted in the SGMA survey with strong growth over the past 10–15 years are mountain biking (68 percent growth rate), kayaking (80 percent growth rate), and wakeboarding (50 percent growth rate).

Paralysis by Analysis An overanalysis of skill behavior. This occurs when more information is supplied than a performer can use or when concentration on too many details results in interference with performance.

Self-Promoting Activities Activities that do not require a high level of skill to be successful.

Cross Training A term used to describe the performance of a variety of activities to meet exercise goals (e.g., performing a variety of activities from different steps of the physical activity pyramid).

 Strategies for Action

You can take steps to become successful in physical activity. You can use self-management skills to enjoy activities at the second and third steps of the pyramid:

- *Select self-promoting activities.* **Self-promoting activities** require relatively little skill and can be done in a way that avoids comparison with other people. They allow you to set your own standards of success and can be done individually or in small groups that are suited to your personal needs. Examples include wheelchair distance events, jogging, resistance training, swimming, bicycling, and dance exercise.

- *Find activities that you enjoy.* There is no best form of activity! The key for long-term exercise adherence is to find exercises that you enjoy and that fit into your lifestyle. Sports are a common form of activity for younger people, but other aerobic and recreational activities have become more common among adults. This is partially because of changing interests, but also because of changing opportunities and lifestyles. In Lab 8A, you will evaluate predisposing, enabling, and reinforcing factors that may help you identify the types of activity that are best suited to you.

- *Self-monitor your activity to help you stick with your plan.* Self-monitoring is a self-management skill that can be valuable in encouraging long-term activity adherence. A self-monitoring chart is provided in Lab 8B to help you plan and log the activities you perform in a 1-week period. This is a short-term record sheet, but you can copy it and make a log book for long-term self-monitoring.

- *Consider combining moderate and vigorous physical activity to meet activity guidelines.* **Cross training** is a term used to describe the performance of a variety of activities to meet exercise goals. For example, on different days you can do a moderate activity such as walking, a vigorous aerobic activity such as jogging on a treadmill, a vigorous sport such as tennis, and a vigorous recreational activity such as mountain biking. As discussed on page 141, the ACSM has developed a system for combining different forms of activity from the activity pyramid. Lab 8C will help you learn and use this MET-minute system.

- *Improve your performance skills and technique.* Consider taking lessons and practice the skills you want to learn. Also, work to try to improve your technique. Better skills and better technique can make exercise more enjoyable (and safer).

Web Resources

Additional websites with information related to Concept 8 are available at the associated Web link.

American Council on Exercise **www.acefitness.org**
Disabled Sports USA **www.dsusa.org**
National Academy of Podiatric Sports Medicine
www.aapsm.org
National Athletic Trainers Association **www.nata.org**
National Center on Physical Activity and Disability
www.ncpad.org and www.ncpad.org/newsletter
President's Council on Physical Fitness and Sports
www.fitness.gov
Special Olympics International **www.specialolympics.org**
Sporting Goods Manufacturers Association **www.sgma.com**
US Product Safety Commission **www.cpsc.gov**
X Sports **www.expn.com**

Suggested Readings

Selected readings and references are listed below. A more comprehensive list is available at the associated Web link.

ACSM. 2010. *ACSM's Guidelines for Exercise Testing and Prescription.* 8th ed. Philadelphia: Lippincott, Williams & Wilkins.

Berg, K. 2010. Sports and games: Fitness, function and fun. *ACSM's Health and Fitness Journal* 14(2):9–15.

Bishop, J. G. 2010. *Fitness Through Aerobics.* 8th ed. San Francisco: Benjamin Cummings.

Cooper, K. H. 1982. *The Aerobics Program for Total Well-Being.* New York: M. Evans.

Dong-Chul, D., and M. Torabi. 2007. Differences in vigorous and moderate physical activity by gender, race/ethnicity, age, education and income among U.S. adults. *American Journal of Health Education* 38(3):122–129.

Kahn, L. K., et al. 2009. Recommended community strategies and measurements to prevent obesity in the United States. *Morbidity and Mortality Weekly Reports* 58(RR07):1–26.

Kruger, J., et al. 2009. Prevalence of transportation and leisure walking among U.S. adults. *Preventive Medicine* 47(3): 329–334.

Magill, R. A. 2010. *Motor Learning and Control: Concepts and Applications.* 8th ed. New York: McGraw-Hill.

Montgomery, J. and M. Chambers. 2009. *Mastering Swimming.* Champaign, IL: Human Kinetics.

Pappas-Baun, M. 2008. *Fantastic Water Workouts.* Champaign, IL: Human Kinetics.

Schurman, C., and D. Schurman. 2009. *The Outdoor Athlete.* Champaign, IL: Human Kinetics.

Thompson, W. R. 2009. Worldwide survey reveals fitness trends for 2010. *ACSM's Health and Fitness Journal* 13(6):9–16.

Lab 8B Planning and Logging Participation in Vigorous Physical Activity

Name	Section	Date

Purpose: To set 1-week vigorous physical activity goals, to prepare a plan, and to self-monitor progress in your 1-week vigorous aerobics, vigorous sports, and recreation plan

Procedures

1. Consider your current stage of change for vigorous activity using the questions provided below. Read the five stages of change questions below and place a check by the stage that best represents your current vigorous physical activity level.
2. Determine vigorous activity (active aerobics, active sports, or active recreation) goals for each day of a 1-week period. In the columns (Chart 1) under the heading "Vigorous Activity Goals," record the total minutes per day that you expect to perform. Record the specific date for each day of the week in the "Date" column and the activity or activities that you expect to perform in the "Activity" column.
3. Only bouts of 10 minutes or longer should be considered when selecting your daily minutes goals. The daily goals should be at least 20 minutes a day in the target zone for vigorous activity for at least 3 days of the week.
4. Use Chart 2 to keep track of the number of minutes of activity that you perform on each day of the 7-day period. Record the number of minutes for each bout of activity of at least 10 minutes in length performed during each day in Chart 2. Determine a total number of minutes for the day and record this total in the last column of Chart 2 and in the "minutes performed" column of Chart 1.
5. After completing Charts 1 and 2, answer the questions and complete the Conclusions and Implications section (use full sentences for your answers).

Determine your stage for vigorous physical activity. Check only the stage that represents your current vigorous activity level.

☐ Precontemplation. I do not meet vigorous activity guidelines and have not been thinking about starting.

☐ Contemplation. I do not do vigorous activity guidelines but have been thinking about starting.

☐ Preparation. I am planning to start doing regular vigorous activity to meet guidelines.

☐ Action. I do vigorous activity, but I am not as regular as I should be.

☐ Maintenance. I regularly meet national goals for vigorous activity.

Results

Chart 1 ▶ Vigorous Physical Activity Goals and Summary Performance Log

Select a goal for each day in a 1-week plan. Keep a log of the activities performed to determine if your goals are met (see Chart 2), and record total minutes performed in the chart below.

	Date:	Vigorous Activity Goals		Summary Performance Log Total Minutes Peformed/Day
		Minutes/Day	Activity	
Day 1				
Day 2				
Day 3				
Day 4				
Day 5				
Day 6				
Day 7				

Chart 2 ▶ Vigorous Physical Activity Log (Daily Minutes Performed)

Record the number of minutes for each bout of vigorous activities performed each day. Add the minutes in each column for the day and record a daily total (total minutes of vigorous activity per day) in the "Daily Total" column. Record your daily totals in the last column of Chart 1.

	Date	Vigorous Activity Bouts of 10 Minutes or More					Daily Total
		Bout 1	Bout 2	Bout 3	Bout 4	Bout 5	
Day 1							
Day 2							
Day 3							
Day 4							
Day 5							
Day 6							
Day 7							

Did you meet your vigorous activity goals for at least 3 days of the week?   (Yes)   (No)

Do you think that you can consistently meet your vigorous activity goals?   (Yes)   (No)

What activities did you perform most often when doing vigorous activity?
List the most common activities that you performed in the spaces below.

Vigorous Aerobics   Vigorous Sports   Vigorous Recreation

_____   _____   _____

_____   _____   _____

_____   _____   _____

Conclusions and Interpretations

Are the activities that you listed above ones that you think you will perform regularly in the future?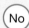

Did setting goals and logging activity make you more aware of your daily vigorous physical activity patterns? Explain why or why not.

Lab 8C Combining Moderate and Vigorous Physical Activity

Name	**Section**	**Date**

Purpose: To learn about MET-minutes and how to combine moderate and vigorous physical activity to meet physical activity guidelines and goals.

Procedures

1. National guidelines recommend at least 150 minutes of moderate or 75 minutes of vigorous physical activity as the minimum amount per week. The guidelines indicate that you can combine the two forms to meet your activity goal. When combining moderate and vigorous activity MET-minutes are used. The minimum goal for beginners is 450 MET-minutes and 750 MET-minutes is the minimum goal for a reasonably fit and active person. Consider this information as you complete the rest of this lab.

2. In Chart 1 below list several moderate activities and several vigorous activities for each day of one week. Next to the activities indicate the number of minutes you plan to perform each day activity. Be sure to choose both moderate and vigorous activities.

3. Use the information in Chart 2 to determine a MET value for each activity or use the compendium of activities website to determine values for those not listed in Chart 2. Record the MET value in the space provided for each activity.

4. Multiply the MET values for each activity by the number of minutes you plan to perform each activity to determine MET-minutes for each activity.

5. Total the MET-minute columns for both moderate and vigorous activities to be performed during the week.

6. Answer the questions in the Conclusions and Implications Section.

Results

Chart 1 ▶ Moderate and vigorous activity plan for one week

| Day | Date | Moderate Activity | | | | Vigorous Activity | | |
		Activity	Min	METs	MET-min.	Activity	METS	MET-min.
1								
2								
3								
4								
5								
6								
7								
Totals						+		=

Total MET-minutes for the Week

Did you meet the 450 MET-minute recommended minimum for beginners?   (Yes)   (No)

Did you meet the 750 MET-minute recommended minimum for beginners?   (Yes)   (No)

Which is your most likely weekly activity plan most likely to include?

☐ Moderate activity only

☐ Vigorous activity only

☐ Both moderate and vigorous activity

Chart 2 ▶ MET Values for Selected Moderate and Vigorous Physical Activities

Moderate Activities	METs	Vigorous Activities	METs
Vacuuming/Mopping	3.0	Shoveling Snow	6.0
Walking (3 mph)	3.0	Walking (4.5 mph)	6.3
Bowling	3.0	Aerobic Dance	6.5
Child Care	3.5	Bricklaying	7.0
Golf (riding)	3.5	Cross-Country Skiing (leisure)	7.0
Biking (10 mph flat)	4.0	Soccer (leisure)	7.0
Fishing and Walking	4.0	Basketball (game)	8.0
Raking Leaves	4.0	Biking (12–17 mph)	8.0
Table Tennis	4.0	Hiking Terrain (pack)	8.0
Volleyball (non-comp.)	4.0	Jogging (5 mph)	8.0
Waitress	4.0	Tennis (singles)	8.0
Ballroom (social)	4.5	Volleyball (games)	8.0
Basketball (shooting)	4.5	Step Aerobics	8.5
Mowing Lawn (power)	4.5	Digging Ditches	8.5
Painting	4.5	Cross-Country Skiing (fast-5–7 mph)	9.0
Tennis Doubles	5.0	Swimming Laps (varies with strokes)	9.0
Walking (4 mph)	5.0	Jogging (6 mph)	10.0
Construction	5.5	Racquetball (games)	10.0
Farming	5.5	Soccer (competitive)	10.0
Golf (walking)	5.5	Running (11.5 mph)	11.5
Softball (games)	5.5	Handball (games)	12.0
Swimming (leisure)	5.5		

MET values based on the Compendium of Physical Activities (available at **http://prevention.sph.sc.edu/tools/docs/documents_compendium.pdf**).

Conclusions and Implications: In the space provided below discuss the MET-minute method of combining activities to meet goals. Do you think that this method will be useful to you? Explain why or why not using full sentences.

Muscle Fitness and Resistance Exercise

Health Objectives for the Year 2020

- Increase proportion of people who regularly perform muscle fitness exercises.
- Reduce sports and recreation injuries.
- Reduce percentage of adults who do no leisure-time activity.
- Increase access to employee-based exercise facilities and programs.
- Reduce osteoporosis and hip fractures among older adults.
- Reduce activity limitations due to chronic back pain.

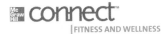 connect

| FITNESS AND WELLNESS   http://connect.mcgraw-hill.com

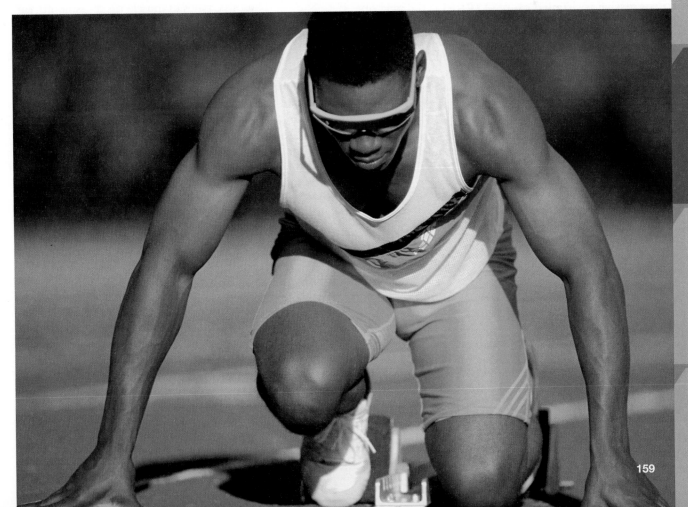

Progressive resistance exercise promotes muscle fitness that permits efficient and effective movement, contributes to ease and economy of muscular effort, promotes successful performance, and lowers susceptibility to some types of injuries, musculoskeletal problems, and some illnesses.

There are two components of muscle fitness: strength and muscular endurance. Strength is the amount of force you can produce with a single maximal effort of a muscle group. Muscular endurance is the capacity of the skeletal muscles or group of muscles to continue contracting over a long period of time. You need both strength and muscular endurance to increase work capacity, to decrease chance of injury, to prevent poor posture and back pain, to improve athletic performance, and to prepare for emergencies.

Muscle power (strength × speed) is a skill-related component of fitness that requires strength. Accordingly, power is enhanced through resistance training. It is most important for those interested in high-level sports performance. For this reason power is discussed in Concept 12.

Progressive resistance exercise (PRE) is the type of physical activity done with the intent of improving muscle fitness. *Weight training* and *progressive resistance training (PRT)* are often used as synonyms for *PRE*, but they should not be confused with the various competitive events related to resistance exercise. Weight lifting is a competitive sport that involves two lifts: the snatch and the clean and jerk. Powerlifting, also a competitive sport, includes three lifts: the bench press, the squat, and the dead lift. Bodybuilding is a competition in which participants are judged on the

size and **definition** of their muscles. Participants in these competitive events rely on highly specialized forms of PRE to optimize their training. Individuals interested in general muscular fitness also rely on PRE but do not need to follow the same routines or regimens to achieve good results. This concept covers the scientific basis of muscular fitness and provides guidelines and principles that can be used to establish an appropriate PRE program.

Factors Influencing Strength and Muscular Endurance

There are three types of muscle tissue. The three types of muscle tissue—smooth, cardiac, and skeletal—have different structures and functions. Smooth muscle tissue consists of long, spindle-shaped fibers, with each fiber containing only one nucleus. The fibers are involuntary and are located in the walls of the esophagus, stomach, and intestines, where they move food and waste products through the digestive tract. Cardiac muscle tissue is also involuntary and, as its name implies, is found only in the heart. These fibers contract in response to demands on the cardiovascular system. The heart muscle contracts at a slow, steady rate at rest but contracts more frequently and forcefully during physical activity. Skeletal muscle tissues consist of long, cylindrical, multinucleated fibers. They provide the force needed to move the skeletal system and can be controlled voluntarily.

Leverage is an important mechanical principle that influences strength. The body uses a system of levers to produce movement. Muscles are connected to bones via tendons, and some muscles (referred to as "primary movers") cross over a particular joint to produce movement. The movement occurs because when a muscle contracts it physically shortens and pulls the two bones connected by the joint together. Figure 1 shows the two heads of the biceps muscle inserting on the forearm. When the muscle contracts, the forearm is pulled up toward the upper arm (elbow flexion). A person with long arms and legs has a mechanical advantage in most movements, since the force that is exerted can act over a longer distance. Although

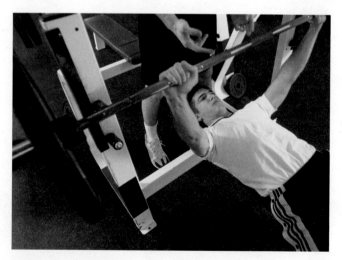

Progressive resistance exercises are methods of training designed to build muscle fitness.

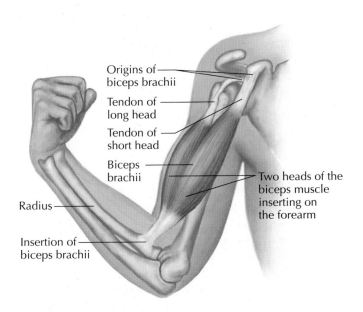

Figure 1 ► Muscle action on body levers.

it is not possible to change the length of your limbs, it is possible to learn to use your muscles more effectively. The ability of elite golfers, to hit a golf ball 350 yards, for example, is due primarily to the ability to generate torque and power rather than due to strength.

Skeletal muscle tissue consists of different types of fibers that respond and adapt differently to training. Three distinct types of muscle fibers are slow-twitch (Type I), fast-twitch (Type IIb), and intermediate (Type IIa). The slow-twitch fibers are generally red in color and are well suited to produce energy with aerobic metabolism. Slow-twitch fibers generate less tension but are more resistant to fatigue. Endurance training leads to adaptations in the slow-twitch fibers that allow them to produce energy more efficiently and to better resist fatigue. Fast-twitch fibers are generally white in color and are well suited to produce energy with anaerobic processes. They generate greater tension than slow-twitch fibers, but they fatigue more quickly. These fibers are particularly well suited to fast, high-force activities, such as explosive weight-lifting movements, sprinting, and jumping. Resistance exercise enhances strength primarily by increasing the size (muscle **hypertrophy**) of fast-twitch fibers, but cellular adaptations also take place to enhance various metabolic properties. Intermediate fibers have biochemical and physiological properties that are between those of the slow-twitch and fast-twitch fibers. A distinct property of these intermediate fibers is that they are highly adaptable, depending on the type of training that is performed.

An example of fast-twitch muscle fiber in animals is the white meat in the flying muscles of a chicken. The chicken is heavy and must exert a powerful force to fly a few feet up to a perch. A wild duck that flies for hundreds of miles has dark meat (slow-twitch fibers) in the flying muscles for better endurance.

People who want large muscles will use PRE designed to build strength (fast-twitch fibers). People who want to be able to persist in activities for a long period of time without fatigue will want to use PRE programs designed to build muscular endurance (slow-twitch fibers).

Muscular endurance and strength are part of the same continuum. Though strength and muscular endurance are developed in different ways, they are part of the same continuum. **Absolute strength** is the maximal force that can be exerted at one time, while **absolute endurance** reflects the ability to sustain a submaximal force over an extended period of time. Most activities rely on various combinations of strength and endurance. For this reason, it is important to have sufficient amounts of strength and endurance. Studies show that a person who is strength-trained will fatigue as much as four times faster than a person who is endurance-trained. However, there is a modest correlation between strength and endurance. A person who trains for strength will develop some endurance, and a person who trains for endurance will develop some strength.

Genetics, gender, and age affect muscle fitness performance. Each person inherits a certain percentage of fast-twitch and slow-twitch muscle fibers. This allocation influences the potential a person has for muscle fitness activities. Individuals with a larger percentage of fast-twitch fibers will generally increase muscle size and strength more readily than individuals endowed with a larger percentage of slow-twitch fibers. People with a larger percentage of slow-twitch fibers have greater potential for muscular endurance performance. Regardless of genetics, all people can improve their strength and muscular endurance with proper training.

Progressive Resistance Exercise (PRE) The type of physical activity done with the intent of improving muscle fitness.

Definition The detailed external appearance of a muscle.

Hypertrophy Increase in the size of muscles as a result of strength training; increase in bulk.

Absolute Strength The maximum amount of force one can exert—e.g., the maximum number of pounds or kilograms that can be lifted on one attempt.

Absolute Endurance Muscular endurance measured by the maximum number of repetitions one can perform against a given resistance—e.g., the number of times you can bench press 50 pounds.

Women have smaller amounts of the anabolic hormone testosterone and, therefore, have less muscle mass than men. Because of this, women typically have 60 to 85 percent of the absolute strength of men. When expressed relative to lean body weight, women have **relative strength** similar to that of men. For example, a 150-pound female who lifts 150 pounds has relative strength equivalent to that of a 250-pound male who lifts 250 pounds, even though she has less absolute strength. Absolute muscular endurance is also greater for males, but the difference again is negated if **relative muscular endurance** is considered. Relative strength and endurance are better indicators of muscle fitness, since they take into account differences in size and muscle mass, but, for some activities, absolute strength and endurance are more important.

Maximum strength is usually reached in the 20s and typically declines with age. Though muscular endurance declines with age, it is not as dramatic as decreases in strength. As people grow older, regardless of gender, strength and muscular endurance are better among people who train than people who do not. This suggests that PRE is one antidote to premature aging.

Muscular endurance is related to cardiovascular endurance, but it is not the same thing. Cardiovascular endurance depends on the efficiency of the heart muscle, circulatory system, and respiratory system. It is developed with activities that stress these systems, such as running, cycling, and swimming. Muscular endurance depends on the efficiency of the local skeletal muscles and the nerves that control them. Most forms of cardiovascular exercise, such as running, require good cardiovascular and muscular endurance. For example, if your legs lack the muscular endurance to continue contracting for a sustained period of time, it will be difficult to perform well in running and other aerobic activities.

Health Benefits of Muscle Fitness and Resistance Exercise

Good muscle fitness helps prevent chronic lifestyle diseases and early death. Recent physical activity recommendations have placed considerable emphasis on muscle fitness exercises. Both the ACSM/AHA and DHHS guidelines indicate that muscle fitness exercises aid in chronic disease prevention. A separate document prepared by the American Heart Association Council on Clinical Cardiology and Council on Nutrition, Physical Activity and Metabolism notes that resistance training has benefits for younger adults, older adults, and even those with a previous history of heart disease (with proper medical supervision). Research has documented the benefits of resistance training in lowering risk for

HELP   HEALTH is available to Everyone for a Lifetime, and it's Personal

The CDC and Tufts University recently developed a program called Growing Stronger—Strength Training for Older Adults. The rationale for the program is that strength training improves muscle strength, bone density, balance, mobility, and coordination, all of which are critically important for older adults. Among young adults, however, muscular fitness tends to be poor, especially among those who watch more than 2 hours of TV a day, according to a recent study.

Is muscular fitness important for good health right now, or is it only important when you get older?

heart disease, high blood pressure, diabetes, rehabilitation from some forms of cancer, and reducing risk of metabolic syndrome. A very recent study showed that women with breast cancer experienced fewer symptoms after performing resistance training. In addition, resistance exercise can reduce risk for other conditions described in the sections that follow.

Good muscle fitness is associated with reduced risk for injury. People with good muscle fitness are less likely to suffer joint injuries (e.g., neck, knee, ankle) than those with poor muscle fitness. Weak muscles are more likely to be involuntarily overstretched than are strong muscles.

Muscle balance is important in reducing the risk for injury. Resistance training should build both **agonist** and **antagonist muscles**. For example, if you do resistance exercise to build the quadriceps muscles (front of the thigh), you should also exercise the hamstring muscles (back of the thigh). In this instance, the quadriceps are the agonist (muscle being used), and the hamstrings are the antagonist. If the quadriceps become too strong relative to the antagonist hamstring muscles, the risk for injury increases (see Figure 2).

Good muscle fitness is associated with good posture and reduced risk for back problems. When muscles in specific body regions are weak or overdeveloped, poor posture can result. Lack of fitness of the abdominal and low back muscles is particularly related to poor posture and potential back problems. Excessively strong hip flexor muscles can lead to swayback. Poor balance in muscular development can also result in postural problems. For example, the muscles on the sides of the body must be balanced to maintain an erect posture.

Good muscle fitness contributes to weight control. Regular PRE results in muscle mass increases. Muscle or lean body mass takes up less space than fat, contributing

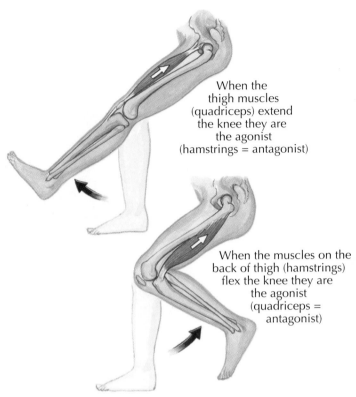

When the thigh muscles (quadriceps) extend the knee they are the agonist (hamstrings = antagonist)

When the muscles on the back of thigh (hamstrings) flex the knee they are the agonist (quadriceps = antagonist)

Figure 2 ► Agonist and antagonist muscles.

to attractive appearance. Further, muscle burns calories at rest, so extra muscle built through PRE can contribute to increased resting and basal metabolism. For each pound of muscle gained, a person can burn approximately 35 to 50 calories more per day. A typical strength training program performed at least three times a week can lead to 2 additional pounds of muscle after 8 weeks, so this can amount to an expenditure of an additional 100 calories a day, or 700 a week. Conversely, muscle mass tends to decrease with age, and this can slow metabolism by a similar amount and contribute to gradual increases in body fatness. PRE can help people retain muscle mass as they grow older.

Good muscle fitness is associated with wellness and quality of life. A person with muscle fitness is able to perform for long periods without undue fatigue. As a result, the person has energy to perform daily work efficiently and effectively and has reserve energy to enjoy leisure time. Among older people, maintenance of strength is associated with increased balance, less risk for falling, and greater ability to perform the tasks of daily living independently. Muscle fitness also contributes to looking one's best and improved athletic performance. The ACSM indicates that one of the major goals of a resistance training program should be to make activities of daily living less stressful physiologically.

Resistance exercise is associated with reduced risk for osteoporosis. Resistance exercises provide a positive stress on the bones. Together with good diet, including adequate calcium intake, this stress on the bones reduces the risk for osteoporosis. Evidence suggests that young people who do PRE develop a high bone density. As we grow older, bone mass decreases, so people who have a high bone density when they are young have a "bank account" from which to draw as they grow older. These people have bones that are less likely to fracture or be injured. Injuries to the bones, particularly the hip and back, are common among older adults. Regular PRE can reduce the risk for these conditions. Postmenopausal women are especially at risk for osteoporosis (see Concept 4).

Core strength is an important health parameter. Core strength refers to strength of the abdominal, paraspinal (back), and gluteal muscles. In the past, core muscle training has not been emphasized in PRE programs. However, there is a new emphasis on core muscle exercises because of their importance to daily life. Good core strength can help reduce back pain, prevent injuries, and improve performance in many applied tasks and sport movements. Many athletes view core strength training as an important part of their conditioning. Core strength is also important as you grow older. It promotes functional balance and may help prevent falls.

Types of Progressive Resistance Exercise

ⓘ **There are different types of PRE, and each has its advantages and disadvantages.**
FEATURE 3 The main types of PRE are isotonic, isometric, and isokinetic. These terms refer to the way in which a load or stimulus is provided to the muscles. The differences among these types of exercise are described next and are also illustrated in Figure 3. The advantages of each type are summarized in Table 1.

Relative Strength Amount of force that one can exert in relation to one's body weight or per unit of muscle cross section.

Relative Muscular Endurance Endurance measured by the maximum number of repetitions one can perform using a given percentage of absolute strength—e.g., the number of times you can lift 50 percent of your absolute strength.

Agonist Muscles Muscle group being stretched.

Antagonist Muscles Muscle group on the opposite side of the limb from the muscle group being stretched (e.g., biceps are the antagonist of triceps).

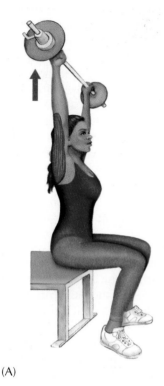

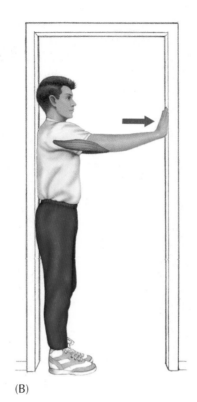

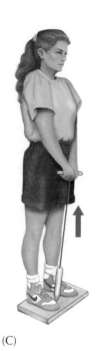

(A)   (B)   (C)

Figure 3 ► Examples of three types of muscle fitness exercises: (A) isotonic, (B) isometric, and (C) isokinetic.

Table 1 ► Advantages and Disadvantages of Isotonic, Isometric, and Isokinetic Exercises

	Advantages	**Disadvantages**
Isotonic	• Can effectively mimic movements used in sport skills • Enhance dynamic coordination • Promote gains in strength	• Do not challenge muscles through the full range of motion • Require equipment or machines • May lead to soreness
Isometric	• Can be done anywhere • Require only low-cost/little equipment • Can rehabilitate an immobilized joint	• Build strength at only one position • Cause less muscle hypertrophy • Are a poor link or transfer to sport skills
Isokinetic	• Build strength through a full range of motion • Are beneficial for rehabilitation and evaluation • Are safe and less likely to promote soreness	• Require specialized equipment • Cannot replicate natural acceleration found in sports • Are more complicated to use and cannot work all muscle groups

• **Isotonic** exercises are the most common type of PRE. When isotonic exercises are performed the muscles shorten and lengthen to cause movement. The most common types of isotonic exercises are calisthenics, resistance machine exercises, free weight exercises, and exercises using other types of resistance such as exercise bands. Isotonic exercise allows for the use of resistance through a full range of joint motion and provides an effective stimulus for muscle development.

When performing isotonic exercise, both **concentric** (shortening) and **eccentric** (lengthening)

contractions should be used. For example, in the overhead press exercise, the muscles on the back of the arms (triceps) shorten (contract concentrically) to overcome resistance or lift a weight. When the same muscles contract eccentrically, lengthening occurs, allowing a slow and controlled return of the muscle to its normal length (see Figure 3A). A workout including exclusively eccentric contractions or eccentric contractions of high intensity is not recommended because of the risk of injury and soreness associated with this type of exercise. Because isotonic exercise involves movement against a resistance, such as a resistance machine or lifting of a weight when using free weights, it is helpful for building both **dynamic strength** and **dynamic muscular endurance**. *Dynamic* refers to movement, so strength and muscular endurance that causes movement are referred to as dynamic.

- **Isometric** exercises are those in which no movement takes place while a force is exerted against an immovable object (see Figure 3B). When properly done, they are effective for developing strength and endurance, but they are not emphasized in most exercise programs because they promote **static strength** and **static endurance** by working the muscle only at the angle of the joint used in the exercise.

- **Isokinetic** exercises are isotonic-concentric muscle contractions performed on machines that keep the velocity of the movement constant through the full range of motion. Isokinetic devices essentially match the resistance to the effort of the performer, permitting maximal tension to be exerted throughout the range of motion (see Figure 3C). Isokinetic exercises are effective, but they are typically only found in sport training or rehabilitation settings.

 Plyometrics is a form of isotonic exercise that promotes athletic performance. FEATURE 4 **Plyometrics** is especially useful for athletes training for power development. High jumpers, long jumpers, and volleyball and basketball players often use this technique, which includes jumping from boxes, hopping on one foot, and engaging in similar types of activities. For most people interested primarily in the health benefits of physical activity, plyometrics is not a preferred type of exercise. In fact, it can increase risk for injury, especially among beginners. For more information on plyometrics, refer to Concept 12.

Technology Update
High-Tech, Low-Tech Muscle Fitness

TECH The different types of resistance training described in this concept range from low-tech exercises with free weights or elastic bands to high-tech training using resistance machines. One recent study shows the effectiveness of "kettlebells" as a low-tech way to build muscle fitness. Kettlebells are iron ball weights with handles. A recent high-tech innovation is the vibration board. Advocates of vibration boards suggest that performing resistance training exercises on the board increases the effectiveness of training. More details about these high- and low-tech forms of training are provided at the associated Web link.

Core training uses a variety of types of resistance training to build the core muscles of the body. Core training is not a specific type of resistance training such as isotonics, isokinetics, or isometrics. Core training can use any of these training methods, but different types of exercises are needed to selectively target the muscles that stabilize the core. These muscles tend to be shorter and deeper than the muscles involved in large movement. Inadequate development of these muscles has been shown to be a risk factor for back pain so it is important to incorporate specialized core exercises into a resistance training program. Specialized core training exercises are discussed in detail in Concept 11.

Isotonic Type of muscle contraction in which the muscle changes length, either shortening (concentrically) or lengthening (eccentrically).

Concentric Contractions Isotonic muscle contractions in which the muscle gets shorter as it contracts, such as when a joint is bent and two body parts move closer together.

Eccentric Contractions Isotonic muscle contractions in which the muscle gets longer as it contracts—that is, when a weight is gradually lowered and the contracting muscle gets longer as it gives up tension. Eccentric contractions are also called negative exercise.

Dynamic Strength A muscle's ability to exert force that results in movement. It is typically measured isotonically.

Dynamic Muscular Endurance A muscle's ability to contract and relax repeatedly. This is usually measured by the number of times (repetitions) you can perform a body movement in a given period. It is also called isotonic endurance.

Isometric Type of muscle contraction in which the muscle remains the same length. Also known as static contraction.

Static Strength A muscle's ability to exert a force without changing length; also called isometric strength.

Static Muscular Endurance A muscle's ability to remain contracted for a long period. This is usually measured by the length of time you can hold a body position.

Isokinetic Isotonic-concentric exercises done with a machine that regulates movement velocity and resistance.

Plyometrics A training technique used to develop explosive power. It consists of isotonic-concentric muscle contractions performed after a prestretch or an eccentric contraction of a muscle.

Core Training A specialized training regimen designed to improve the strength and functionality of core muscles.

FEATURE 5 **Functional balance training is a specialized form of training aimed at improving core strength and balance.** Balance tends to deteriorate with age, and this is partly due to corresponding declines in muscle strength, range of motion, and a lower ability to coordinate muscle movements. Functional balance training has been shown to help improve balance and mobility in the elderly. It is also used in rehabilitation and in specialized training regimens for sports. This type of training is typically conducted with specialized devices, such as exercise balls (Swiss balls), BOSU platforms, and balance boards. Because these devices challenge you to remain balanced, they recruit muscles that are not typically worked in most strength training regimens.

Resistance Training Equipment

Free weights are the most commonly used equipment for resistance exercise. Free weight equipment consists of weights that are typically loaded onto a barbell or a dumbbell. They have often been considered to be the domain of serious weight lifters, but recent statistics indicate they are more widely used than previously thought. According to the Sporting Goods Manufacturers Association (SGMA), over 50 million Americans use free weights with approximately 10 million classified as regular users. Factors that contribute to their popularity are their versatility, the ability to change weight in gradual increments, and the ability to modify exercises for specific muscles or movements (see Table 2). Because free weights require balance and technique, they may be more difficult for beginners to use.

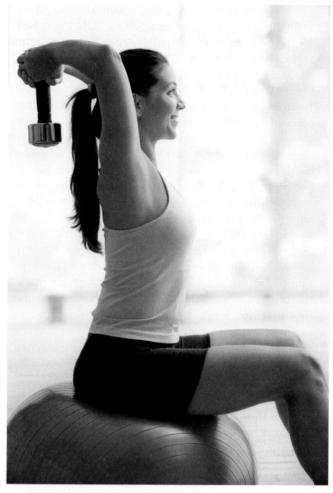

Exercise balls can be used to enhance or facilitate resistance exercises.

Table 2 ▶ Advantages (+) and Disadvantages (−) of Free Weights and Machine Weights

		Free Weights		Machine Weights
Isolation of Major Muscle Groups	−/+	Movements require balance and coordination; more muscles are used for stabilization.	+/−	Other body parts are stabilized during lift, allowing isolation, but muscle imbalances can develop.
Applications to Real-Life Situations	+	Movements can be developed to be truer to real life.	−	Movements are determined by the paths allowed on the machine.
Risk for Injury	−	There is more possibility for injury because weights can fall or drop on toes.	+	They are safer because weights cannot fall on participants.
Needs for Assistance	−	Spotters are needed for safety with some lifts.	+	No spotters are required.
Time Requirement	−	More time is needed to change weights.	+	It is easy and quick to change weights or resistance.
Number of Available Exercises	+	Unlimited number of exercises is possible.	−	Exercise options are determined by the machine.
Cost	+	They are less expensive, but good (durable) weights are still somewhat expensive.	−	They are expensive; access to a club is usually needed, since multiple machines are usually needed.
Space Requirement	+/−	Equipment can be moved, but loose weights may clutter areas.	−/+	Machines are stationary but take up large spaces.

Resistance training machines offer many advantages for overall conditioning. Resistance training machines can be effective in developing strength and muscular endurance if used properly. They can save time because, unlike free weights, the resistance can be changed easily and quickly. They may be safer because you are less likely to drop weights. A disadvantage is that the kinds of exercises that can be done on these machines are more limited than free weight exercises. They also may not promote optimal balance in muscular development, since a stronger muscle can often make up for a weaker muscle in the completion of a lift. Some machines have mechanisms that provide variable, or accommodating, resistance. These features allow the machine to provide a more appropriate resistance across the full range of motion. Recent developments in machines allow movement to take place in multiple dimensions, making it possible for independent arm/leg movements to provide a more realistic training stimulus and reduce the likelihood of creating muscle imbalances.

Many resistance training exercises can be done with little or no equipment. Calisthenics are among the most popular forms of muscle fitness exercise among adults. Calisthenics, such as curl-ups and push-ups, are suitable for people of different ability levels and can be used to improve both strength and muscular endurance. Many variations can be added to increase the difficulty of various calisthenic exercises. For example, push-ups can be made more challenging by elevating your feet. Performing regular calisthenics can help build and maintain good muscular fitness.

Other alternatives to expensive resistance training machines or commercially made free weights are homemade weights and elastic exercise bands. Homemade weights can be constructed from pieces of pipe or broom sticks and plastic milk jugs filled with water. Elastic tubes or bands available in varying strengths may be substituted for the weights and for the pulley device used in many resistance training machines to impart resistance.

In the News

Worldwide Fitness Trend for Resistance Exercise Training

Of the top 20 worldwide fitness trends from a 2010 survey, 7 are directly related to resistance training. Included among these trends are the following: strength training for both men and women, core training, special fitness training for older adults including resistance training, functional fitness training, sports-specific training, Pilates, and stability ball training. Descriptions of the various trends are available on the Web.

Progressive Resistance Exercise: How Much Is Enough?

PRE is the best type of training for muscle fitness. PRE is the most common type of training for building muscle fitness, and it is the most effective. It is sometimes referred to as progressive resistive training (PRT). The word *progressive* is used in both instances because the frequency, intensity, and length of time of muscle overload are gradually, or progressively, increased as muscle fitness increases. PREs are typically done in one to four sets, though more are used in some instances, such as for high-performance benefits. A set is a group of repetitions (reps) done in succession, followed by a rest period. For most people, a set consists of 3 to 25 reps. Rest intervals of 2 to 3 minutes are recommended between sets for those interested primarily in strength development. Shorter rest intervals (1–2 minutes) may be used for those interested primarily in muscular endurance or general muscle fitness.

The stimulus for strength is different from the stimulus for muscular endurance. The stimulus for strength is high-level exertion. Strength training should, therefore, use high resistance overload with low repetitions. The stimulus for muscular endurance is repeated contractions with short rests. Muscular endurance exercises should be performed with a relatively high number of repetitions and lower resistance. Each set should be performed to muscle fatigue, but not to muscle failure. Evidence suggests that performing to failure can result in increased injury risk and can cause muscle soreness that reduces adherence to regular training.

The graph in Figure 4 illustrates the relationship between strength and muscular endurance. Training that requires high resistance and low repetitions (top bar) results in the least gain in endurance but the greatest gain in strength. Training with moderate resistance and moderate repetitions (second bar) results in moderate gains in both strength and endurance. Training that requires a high number of repetitions and a relatively low resistance (third bar) results in small gains in strength but large increases in muscular endurance.

There are different thresholds and target zones for muscle fitness development. The amount of resistance used in a PRE program is based on a percentage of your **1 repetition maximum (1RM)**—the maximum amount of resistance you can move (or weight you can

1 Repetition Maximum (1RM) The maximum amount of resistance you can move a given number of times—for example, 1RM = maximum weight lifted one time; 6RM = maximum weight lifted six times.

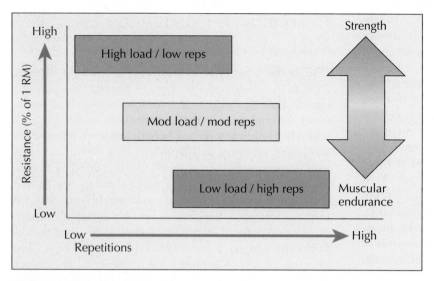

Figure 4 ▶ Comparison of muscular endurance with muscle strength by different repetitions and resistance.

lift) one time. The 1RM value provides an indicator of your maximum strength, but desired levels of resistance are determined using percentages of the 1RM value. The specific prescription depends on the program goals. For strength, the percentages typically vary 60 to 80 percent of the 1RM value, whereas for endurance the percentages vary from 20 to 50 percent, depending on current fitness level. An intensity of 60 to 70 percent is recommended for older adults. Evidence suggests that very strong people interested in high-level performance can train at 80 percent and above. Individuals interested in a combination of strength and endurance should use values ranging from 40 to 60 percent. A summary of the FIT formulas for muscular strength and muscular endurance are included in Table 3, along with guidelines for general muscle fitness.

Table 3 ▶ Threshold of Training and Fitness Target Zones for Muscular Fitness

		Threshold of Training	Fitness Target Zones
Isotonic Exercise			
Muscular Strength			
	Frequency	2 days a week for each muscle group	2–3 days per week for each muscle group
	Intensity	60% of 1RM for every repetition	60–80% of 1RM for number of reps on every set
	Time	1 set of 3–8 reps	1–4 sets of 3–12 reps
Muscular Endurance			
	Frequency	2 days per week	Every other day
	Intensity	Move 20% of 1RM	Move 20%–50% of 1RM
	Time	One set of 12 repetitions of each exercise	2–4 sets of 12–25 repetitions of each exercise
General Muscular Fitness			
	Frequency	2–3 days a week	3 days a week
	Intensity	40% of 1RM for young adults	40–60% of 1RM for young adults
		30% for adults >50 years old	30–50% for adults >50 years old
	Time	1 set of 8–12 reps for young adults	1–3 sets of 8–12 reps for young adults
		1 set of 10–15 reps for adults >50 years old	1–3 sets of 10–15 reps for adults >50
Isometric Exercise			
Static Muscular Fitness			
	Frequency	3 days per week	Every other day
	Intensity	Hold a resistance 50% of the weight you ultimately need to hold in your work or leisure activity.	Hold a resistance 50–150% of the weight you ultimately need to hold in your work or leisure activity.
	Time	Hold for lengths of time that are 50% of the time for the actual work or leisure task; repeat 10–20 times and rest 30 seconds between repetitions.	Hold for lengths of time that are 50–120% of the time for the actual work or leisure task (for longer times use fewer repetitions); rest 30–60 seconds between repetitions

A combined strength/muscle endurance program is the best choice for most individuals. Research has shown that for healthy adults most health benefits can be achieved using a combined strength/muscular endurance program. The new activity guidelines indicate that young adults can achieve significant health benefits by performing one set of 8 to 12 repetitions at least 2 days a week. For older adults (50 and older), less intense exercises performed 10 to 15 times appears to be sufficient. For both age groups, 8 to 10 basic exercises are recommended to promote good muscle fitness for the whole body. Individuals who want pure strength or high-level endurance for performance will benefit from extra sets and from more specific training protocols.

Circuit resistance training (CRT) is an effective way to build muscular endurance and cardiovascular endurance. CRT consists of the performance of high repetitions of an exercise with low to moderate resistance, progressing from one station to another, performing a different exercise at each station. The stations are usually placed in a circle to facilitate movement. CRT

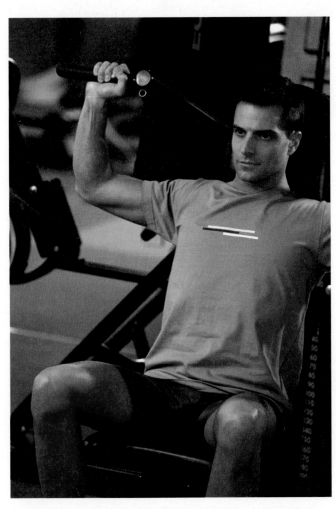

Resistance exercise can promote lean body mass and contribute to a healthy appearance.

typically uses about 20 to 25 reps against a resistance that is 30 to 40 percent of 1RM for 45 seconds. Fifteen seconds of rest is provided while changing stations. Approximately 10 exercise stations are used, and the participant repeats the circuit two to three times (sets). Because of the short rest periods, significant cardiovascular benefits have been reported in addition to muscular endurance gains.

Programs intended to slim the figure/physique should be of the muscular endurance type. Many men and women are interested in exercises designed to decrease girth measurements. High-repetition, low-resistance exercise is suitable for this because it usually brings about some strengthening and may decrease body fatness, which in turn changes body contour. Exercises do not spot-reduce fat, but they do speed up metabolism, so more calories are burned. However, if weight or fat reduction is desired, aerobic (cardiovascular) exercises are best. To increase girth, use strength exercises.

Endurance training may have a negative effect on strength and power. Some studies have shown that for athletes who rely primarily on strength and power in their sport too much endurance training can cause a loss of strength and power because of the modification of different muscle fibers. Strength and power athletes need some endurance training, but not too much, just as endurance athletes need some strength and power training, but not too much.

Training Principles for PRE

The overload principle provides the basis for PRE. For the body to adapt and improve, the muscles and systems of the body must be challenged. As noted earlier, the concept behind PRE is that the frequency, intensity, and duration of lifts are progressively increased to maintain an effective stimulus as the muscle fitness improves. It was in the area of muscle fitness development that the overload principle was first clearly outlined. Legend holds that centuries ago a Greek named Milo of Crotona became progressively stronger by repeatedly lifting his calf. As the calf grew into a bull, its weight increased, and Milo's strength increased as well. We know now that for most people, PREs are necessary if muscle fitness is to be developed and maintained. Activities from other levels of the physical activity pyramid do not provide an adequate stimulus, so specific resistance exercise is needed to improve this dimension of fitness (see Figure 5).

The muscle fitness workout should be based on the principle of progression. Many beginning resistance trainers experience soreness after the first

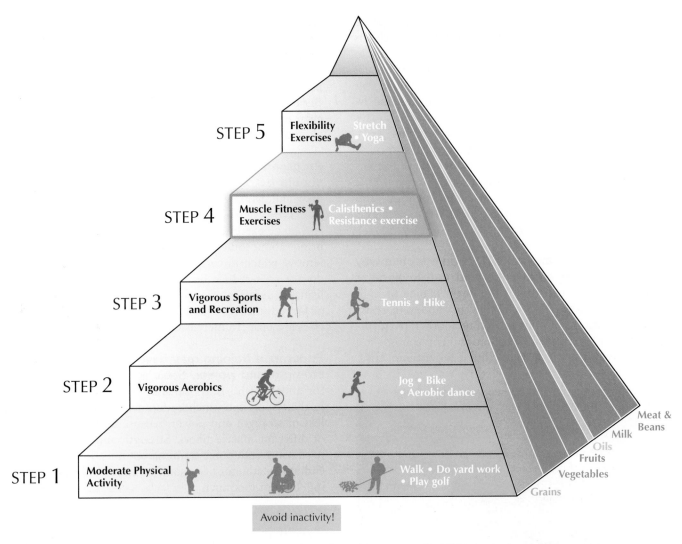

Figure 5 ► To build muscle fitness, activities should be selected from step 4 of the physical activity pyramid.

few days of training. The reason for the soreness is that the principle of progression has been violated. Soreness can occur with even modest amounts of training if the volume of training is considerably more than normal. In the first few days or weeks of training, the primary adaptations in the muscle are due to motor learning factors rather than to muscle growth. Because these adaptations occur no matter how much weight is used, it is prudent to start your program slowly with light weights. After these adaptations occur and the rate of improvement slows down, it is necessary to follow the appropriate target zone to achieve proper overload.

The most common progression used in resistance training is the double progressive system, so-called because this system periodically adjusts both the resistance and the number of repetitions of the exercise performed. For example, if you are training for strength, you may begin with three repetitions in one set. As the repetitions become easy, additional repetitions are added. When you have progressed to eight repetitions, increase the resistance and decrease the repetitions in each set back to three and begin the progression again.

The principle of specificity applies to PRE. Depending on the specific muscles you want to develop, you will use different types of resistance training programs. Factors that can be varied in your program are the type of muscle contraction (isometric or isotonic), the speed or cadence of the movement, and the amount of resistance being moved. For example, if you want strength in the elbow extensor muscles (e.g., triceps) so that you can more easily lift heavy boxes onto a shelf, you can train using isotonic contractions, at a relatively slow speed, with a relatively high resistance. If you want muscle fitness of the fingers to grip a heavy bowling ball, much of your training should be done isometrically using the fingers the same way you normally hold the ball. If you are training for a skill that requires explosive power, such as in throwing, striking, kicking, or jumping, your strength exercises should be done with less resistance and greater speed. If you are training for a skill that uses both concentric and eccentric contractions, you should perform exercises using these characteristics (e.g., plyometrics).

If you are not training for a specific task, but merely wish to develop muscle fitness for daily living, consider the advantages and disadvantages of isotonics, isometrics, and isokinetics, listed in Table 1. You may wish to use a variety of methods.

The principle of diminishing returns applies especially to resistance training. To get optimal strength gains from progressive resistance training, one or more sets of exercise repetitions are performed. Some high-level performers use as many as five sets of a particular exercise. Research indicates that most of the fitness and health benefits, however, are achieved in one set. Considerably more than 50 percent of the benefits may result in the first set, with each additional set producing less benefit. Because compliance with resistance training programs is less likely as the time needed to complete the program increases, performing one or two sets is better than performing none, especially if performing fewer sets increases adherence. There is no doubt that more sets provide greater benefits, but something is better than nothing.

The principle of rest and recovery applies especially to strength development. Progressive resistance training for strength development done every day of the week does not allow enough rest and time for recovery. Studies have shown that the greatest proportion of strength is accomplished in 2 days of training per week. Exercise done on a third day does result in additional increases, but the amount of gain is relatively small, compared with gains resulting from 2 days of training per week. For people interested in health benefits rather than performance benefits, 2 days a week saves time and may result in greater adherence to a strength training program.

For people interested in performance benefits, more frequent training may be warranted. Rotating exercises so that certain muscles are exercised on one day and other muscles are exercised the next allows for more frequent training. For example, the total-body workout can be split so that upper body exercises are performed on 2 days of the week and lower body exercises are performed on 2 different days. The ACSM recommends at least 48 hours separating exercise training sessions for the same muscle groups.

The amount of exercise necessary to maintain strength is less than the amount needed to build it. Recent evidence suggests that once strength is developed it can be maintained by performing fewer sets or exercising fewer days per week. For example, if you have performed three sets of an exercise 3 days a week to build strength, you may be able to maintain current levels of strength with one set a week. Also, you may be able to maintain strength by exercising 1 or 2 rather than 3 days per week. If schedules of fewer sets or days per week result in strength loss, frequency must be increased. Smaller muscles seem to need more frequent exercise than larger muscles.

ⓘ **There are no *(safe)* shortcuts to strength development or muscular fitness.** The use FEATURE 6 of **anabolic steroids** in sports has received considerable media attention, but it is important to understand that they are illegal and extremely dangerous (see Figure 6). A number of other dietary supplements are on the market (either legally or illegally) to capitalize on interest in muscular development and sports performance. Contrary to popular belief, they are typically ineffective or dangerous (often both):

- Prohormone nutritional supplements are marketed as testosterone "prohormones" because they are thought to lead to the production of testosterone and testosterone analogs. Examples of common ingredients in these products are dehydroepiandrosterone (DHEA), andostenedione, and androstenediol. Studies have found that these compounds did not produce anabolic or ergogenic effects, and many were found to increase the risk of negative health consequences.
- Androstenedione (andro) is a precursor of naturally occurring testosterone and estrogen. Early studies suggested that andro use did not lead to increases in

Anabolic Steroids Synthetic hormones similar to the male sex hormone testosterone. They function androgenically to stimulate male characteristics and anabolically to increase muscle mass, weight, bone maturation, and virility.

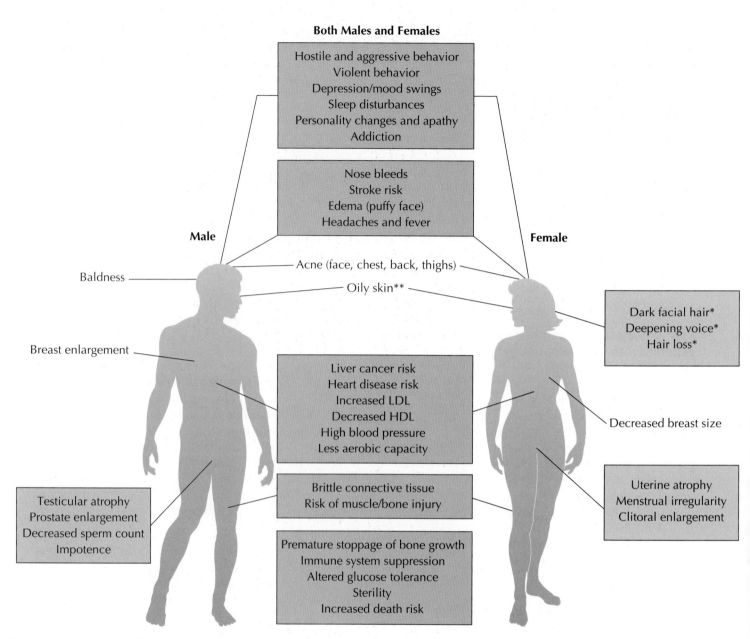

Both Males and Females

Hostile and aggressive behavior
Violent behavior
Depression/mood swings
Sleep disturbances
Personality changes and apathy
Addiction

Nose bleeds
Stroke risk
Edema (puffy face)
Headaches and fever

Male

Female

Baldness

Acne (face, chest, back, thighs)
Oily skin**

Dark facial hair*
Deepening voice*
Hair loss*

Breast enlargement

Liver cancer risk
Heart disease risk
Increased LDL
Decreased HDL
High blood pressure
Less aerobic capacity

Decreased breast size

Brittle connective tissue
Risk of muscle/bone injury

Uterine atrophy
Menstrual irregularity
Clitoral enlargement

Testicular atrophy
Prostate enlargement
Decreased sperm count
Impotence

Premature stoppage of bone growth
Immune system suppression
Altered glucose tolerance
Sterility
Increased death risk

*Among women, irreversible when use stops.
**Among women, partially reversible when use stops.

Figure 6 ▶ Adverse effects of anabolic steroids.

testosterone levels, but more recent evidence suggests that andro would probably have anabolic effects at the high doses most likely used by athletes. Andro has been found to be associated with most of the same health risks as conventional steroids and has been banned by the FDA.

- Tetrahydrogestrinone (THG) is a chemically engineered steroid that, until recently, has been undetectable by standard drug tests. It is a purely synthetic

steroid, which exhibits the same properties (and risks) of other anabolic steroids.

- Human growth hormone (HGH) is produced by the pituitary gland but is also made synthetically. Athletes often use growth hormone in combination with anabolic steroids so they can increase bone strength (the main effect of HGH) along with muscle mass. Athletes assume this will protect them from some of the bone injuries that occur among steroid users. However, these athletes are compounding their health risks, as the use of HGH only adds to the health risks of steroid use.

- Creatine is a nutrient involved in the production of energy during short-term, high-intensity exercise, such as resistance exercise. The body produces creatine naturally from foods containing protein, but some athletes take creatine supplements (usually a powder dissolved into a liquid) to increase the amounts available in the muscle. The concept behind supplementation is that additional creatine intake enhances energy production and therefore increases the body's ability to maintain force and delay fatigue. Some studies have shown improvements in athletic performance with creatine, but reviews indicate that the supplement may be effective only for athletes who are already well trained. Studies have been more consistent with regard to the performance-enhancing effects of creatine on muscle strength. It is important to recognize, though, that the benefits are due to the ability to work the muscles harder during an exercise session, not to the supplement itself. Increases in body weight may result, but this is likely due to water retention. At present, creatine usage hasn't been linked to any major health problems, but the long-term effects are unknown.

Guidelines for Safe and Effective Resistance Training

There are many fallacies, superstitions, and myths associated with resistance training. Some common misconceptions about resistance training are described in Table 4. The following are guidelines for safe and effective resistance training.

There is a proper way to perform. Although PRE offers considerable health benefits, there are also some risks if the exercises are not performed correctly or if

Table 4 ▶ Fallacies and Facts about Resistance Training

Fallacies	Facts
Resistance training will make you muscle-bound and cause you to lose flexibility.	Normal resistance training will not reduce flexibility if exercises are done through the full range of motion and with proper technique. Powerlifters who do highly specific movements have been shown to have poorer flexibility than other weight lifters.
Women will become masculine-looking if they gain strength.	Women will not become masculine-looking from resistance exercise. Women have less testosterone and do not bulk up from resistance training to the same extent as men. Women and men can make similar relative gains in strength and hypertrophy from a resistance training program, however. The greater percentage of fat in most women prevents the muscle definition possible in men and camouflages the increase in bulk.
Strength training makes you move more slowly and look uncoordinated.	Strength training, if done properly, can enhance sport-specific strength and increase power. There are no effects on coordination from having high levels of muscular fitness.
No pain, no gain.	It is not true that you have to get to the point of soreness to benefit from resistance exercise. It may be helpful to strive until you can't do a final repetition, but you should definitely stop before it is painful. Slight tightness in the muscles is common 1 to 2 days following exercise but is not necessary for adaptations.
Soreness occurs because lactic acid builds up in the muscles.	Lactic acid is produced during muscular work but is converted back into other substrates within 30 minutes after exercising. Soreness is due to microscopic tears or damage in the muscle fibers, but this damage is repaired as the body builds the muscle. Excessive soreness occurs if you violate the law of progression and do too much too soon.
Strength training can build cardiovascular fitness and flexibility.	Resistance exercise can increase heart rate, but this is due primarily to a pressure overload rather than a volume overload on the heart that occurs from endurance (aerobic) exercise. Gains in muscle mass do cause an increase in resting metabolism that can aid in controlling body fatness.
Strength training is beneficial only for young adults.	Studies have shown that people in their 80s and 90s can benefit from resistance exercise and improve their strength and endurance. Most experts would agree that resistance exercise increases in importance with age rather than decreases.

safety procedures are not followed. Before using unfamiliar equipment get instruction in proper use.

Beginners should emphasize lighter weights and progress their program gradually. When beginning a resistance training program, start with light weights so that you can learn proper technique and avoid soreness and injury. Most of the adaptations that occur in the first few months of a program are due to improvements in the body's ability to recruit muscle fibers to contract effectively and efficiently. These neural adaptations occur in response to the movement itself and not the weight that is used. Therefore, beginning lifters can achieve significant benefits from lighter weights. As experience and fitness levels improve, it is necessary to use heavier loads and more challenging sets to continually challenge the muscles.

Use proper technique to reduce the risks for injury and to isolate the intended muscles. An important consideration in resistance exercise is to complete all lifts through the full range of motion using only the intended muscle groups. A common cause of poor technique is using too heavy of a weight. If you have to jerk the weight up or use momentum to lift the weight, it is too heavy. Using heavier weights will provide a greater stimulus to your muscles only if your muscles are actually doing the work. Therefore, it is best to use a weight that you can control safely. By lifting through the full range of motion, you increase the effectiveness of the exercise and maintain good flexibility. Some safety tips are presented in Table 5.

Perform lifts in a slow, controlled manner to enhance both effectiveness and safety. Lifting at a slow cadence provides a greater stimulus to the muscles and increases strength gains. A good recommendation is to take 2 seconds on the lifting phase (concentric) and 4 seconds on the lowering (eccentric) phase.

Provide sufficient time to rest during and between workouts. The body needs time to rest in order to allow beneficial adaptations to occur. Choose an exercise sequence that alternates muscle groups so muscles have a chance to rest before another set. Lifting every other day or alternating muscle groups (if lifting more than 3 or 4 days per week) provides rest for the muscles.

Include all body parts and balance the strength of antagonistic muscle groups. A common mistake made by many beginning lifters is to perform only a few different exercises or to emphasize a few body

Table 5 ▶ How to Prevent Injury
• Warm up 10 minutes before the workout and stay warm.
• Do not hold your breath while lifting. This may cause blackout or hernia.
• Avoid hyperventilation before lifting a weight.
• Avoid dangerous or high-risk exercises.
• Progress slowly.
• Use good shoes with good traction.
• Avoid arching the back. Keep the pelvis in normal alignment.
• Keep the weight close to the body.
• Do not lift from a stoop (bent over with back rounded).
• When lifting from the floor, do not let the hips come up before the upper body.
• For bent-over rowing, lay your head on a table and bend the knees, or use one-arm rowing and support the trunk with your free hand.
• Stay in a squat as short a time as possible and do not do a full squat.
• Be sure collars on free weights are tight.
• Use a moderately slow, continuous, controlled movement and hold the final position a few seconds.
• Overload but don't overwhelm! A program that is too intense can cause injuries.
• Do not allow the weights to drop or bang.
• Do not train without medical supervision if you have a hernia, high blood pressure, a fever, an infection, recent surgery, heart disease, or back problems.
• Use chalk or a towel to keep your hands dry when handling weights.

parts. Training the biceps without working the triceps, for example, can lead to muscle imbalances that can compromise flexibility and increase risks for injury. In some cases, training must be increased in certain areas to compensate for stronger antagonist muscle groups. Many sprinters, for example, pull their hamstrings because the quadriceps are so overdeveloped that they overpower the hamstrings. The recommended ratio of quadriceps to hamstring strength is 60:40.

Customize your training program to fit your specific needs. Athletes should train muscles the way they will be used in their skill, using similar patterns, range of motion, and speed (the principle of specificity).

If you wish to develop a particular group of muscles, remember that the muscle group can be worked harder when isolated than when worked in combination with other muscle groups.

Strategies for Action

Choose exercises that build muscle fitness in the major muscle groups of the body. Table 6 (page 178) provides eight basic exercises for free weights. Table 7 (page 180) presents eight basic exercises for resistance machines. For additional options in resistance training, see the eight calisthenic exercises in Table 8 (page 182) and the eight core strength exercises in Table 9 (page 184). Since good muscular fitness in the abdominals is important, it is recommended that some abdominal or core training be performed as part of any program.

An important step in taking action for developing and maintaining muscle fitness is assessing your current status. A 1RM test of isotonic strength is described in *Lab Resource Materials.* This test allows you to determine absolute and relative strength for the arms and legs. In addition, the 1RM values can be used to help you select the appropriate resistance for your muscle fitness training program. A grip strength test of isometric strength is also provided in *Lab Resource Materials* for Lab 9A.

Three tests of muscular endurance are described in the *Lab Resource Materials* for Lab 9B. It is recommended that you perform the assessments for both strength and muscular endurance before you begin your progressive resistance training program.

Periodically reevaluate your muscle fitness using these assessments.

Many factors other than your own basic abilities affect muscle fitness test scores. If muscles are warmed up before lifting, more force can be exerted and heavier loads can be lifted. Muscle endurance performance may also be enhanced by a warm-up. Do not perform your self-assessments after vigorous exercise because that exercise can cause fatigue and result in suboptimal test results. It is appropriate to practice the techniques in the various tests on days preceding the actual testing. People who have good technique achieve better scores and are less likely to be injured when performing tests than those without good technique. It is best to perform the strength and muscular endurance tests on different days.

Keeping records of progress will help you adhere to a PRE program. Labs 9C and 9D provide activity logging sheets to help you keep records of your progress as you regularly perform PRE to build and maintain good muscle fitness. A guide to the major muscles groups is presented in Figure 7, page 176.

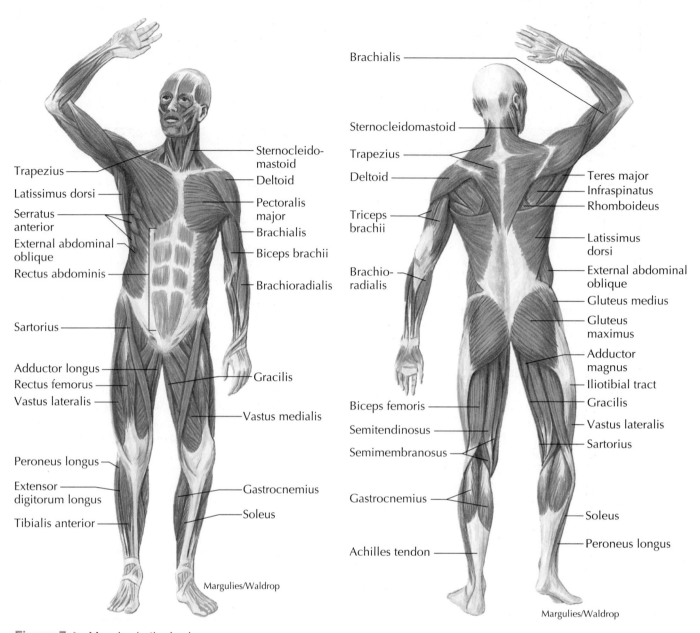

Trapezius
Latissimus dorsi
Serratus anterior
External abdominal oblique
Rectus abdominis
Sartorius
Adductor longus
Rectus femoris
Vastus lateralis
Peroneus longus
Extensor digitorum longus
Tibialis anterior

Sternocleido-mastoid
Deltoid
Pectoralis major
Brachialis
Biceps brachii
Brachioradialis
Gracilis
Vastus medialis
Gastrocnemius
Soleus

Margulies/Waldrop

Brachialis
Sternocleidomastoid
Trapezius
Deltoid
Triceps brachii
Brachio-radialis
Biceps femoris
Semitendinosus
Semimembranosus
Gastrocnemius
Achilles tendon

Teres major
Infraspinatus
Rhomboideus
Latissimus dorsi
External abdominal oblique
Gluteus medius
Gluteus maximus
Adductor magnus
Iliotibial tract
Gracilis
Vastus lateralis
Sartorius
Soleus
Peroneus longus

Margulies/Waldrop

Figure 7 ▶ Muscles in the body.

Web Resources

Additional websites with information related to Concept 9 are available at the associated Web link.

American College of Sports Medicine **www.acsm.org**

Growing Stronger: Strength Training for Older Adults
    www.cdc.gov/physicalactivity/growingstronger/index.html

National Athletic Trainers Association **www.nata.org**

National Health Interview Survey—Strength Activities
    www.cdc.gov/mmwr/preview/mmwrhtml/mm5834a6.htm

National Strength and Conditioning Association
    www.nsca-cc.org

The Physician and Sportsmedicine Online
    www.physsportsmed.com

Suggested Readings

Selected readings and references are listed below. A more comprehensive list is available at the associated Web link.

ACSM. 2010. *ACSM's Guidelines for Exercise Testing and Prescription.* 8th ed. Philadelphia: Lippincott, Williams & Wilkins, Chapter 7.

Bea, J. W., et al. 2010. Resistance training predicts 6-year body composition change in postmenopausal women. *Medicine & Science in Sports & Exercise* 42(7):1286–1295.

Baechle, T. R., and R. W. Earle. 2006. *Weight Training.* 3rd ed. Champaign, IL: Human Kinetics.

Brumitt, J. 2010. *Core Assessment and Training.* Champaign, IL: Human Kinetics.

Delavier, F. 2010. *Strength Training Anatomy.* 3rd ed. Champaign, IL: Human Kinetics.

Morbidity and Mortality Weekly Reports (MMWR). 2010. National health interview survey strength activities by 18+. *Morbidity and Mortality Weekly Reports* 58(34): 955. **www.cdc.gov/mmwr/preview/mmwrhtml/mm5834a6.htm.**

Nelson, M. E., et al. 2007. Physical activity and public health in older adults: Recommendation from the American College of Sports Medicine and the American Health Association. *Medicine and Science in Sports and Exercise* 39(8):1435–1445.

Sandler, D. 2010. *Fundamental Weight Training.* Champaign, IL: Human Kinetics.

Schmidt, K. H., et al. Weight lifting in women with breast-cancer-related lymphedema. *New England Journal of Medicine* 361(7): 664–673.

Westcott, W. 2009. ACSM strength training guidelines: Role in body composition and health enhancement. *ACSM's Health and Fitness Journal* 13(4):14–22.

Willardson, J. M. 2008. A periodized approach to core training. *ACSM's Health and Fitness Journal* 12(1):7–13.

Williams, M. A., et al. 2007. Resistance exercise in individuals with and without cardiovascular disease: 2007 update: A scientific statement from the American Heart Association Council on Clinical Cardiology and Council on Nutrition, Physical Activity, and Metabolism. *Circulation* 116(5):572–584.

Table 6 The Basic Eight for Free Weights

Table 6

1. Bench Press

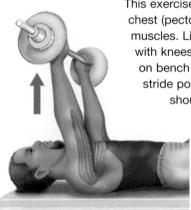

This exercise develops the chest (pectoral) and triceps muscles. Lie supine on bench with knees bent and feet flat on bench or flat on floor in stride position. Grasp bar at shoulder level. Push bar up until arms are straight. Return and repeat. Do not arch lower back. Note: Feet may be placed on floor if lower back can be kept flattened. Do not put feet on the bench if it is unstable.

Pectoralis major

Triceps

2. Overhead (Military Press)

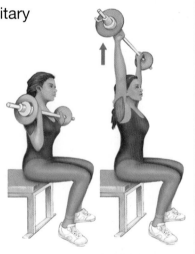

This exercise develops the muscles of the shoulders and arms. Sit erect, bend elbows, palms facing forward at chest level with hands spread (slightly more than shoulder width). Have bar touching chest; spread feet (comfortable distance). Tighten your abdominal and back muscles. Move bar to overhead position (arms straight). Lower bar to chest position. Repeat. Caution: Keep arms perpendicular and do not allow weight to move backward or wrists to bend backward. Spotters are needed.

Deltoid

3. Biceps Curl

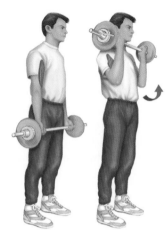

This exercise develops the muscles of the upper front part of the arms (biceps). Stand erect with back against a wall, palms forward, bar touching thighs. Spread feet in comfortable position. Tighten abdominals and back muscles. Do not lock knees. Move bar to chin, keeping body straight and elbows near the sides. Lower bar to original position. Do not allow back to arch. Repeat. Spotters are usually not needed. Variations: Use dumbbell and sit on end of bench with feet in stride position; work one arm at a time. Or use dumbbell with the palm down or thumb up to emphasize other muscles.

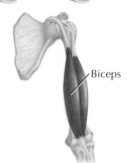

Biceps

4. Triceps Curl

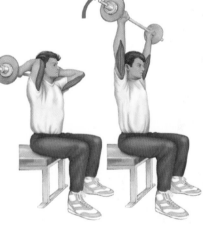

This exercise develops the muscles on the back of the upper arms (triceps). Sit erect, elbows and palms facing up, bar resting behind neck on shoulders, hands near center of bar, feet spread. Tighten abdominal and back muscles. Keep upper arms stationary. Raise weight overhead, return bar to original position. Repeat. Spotters are needed. Variation: Substitute dumbbells (one in each hand, or one held in both hands, or one in one hand at a time).

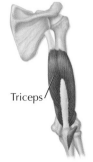

Triceps

5. Wrist Curl

This exercise develops the muscles of the fingers, wrist, and forearms. Sit astride a bench with the back of one forearm on the bench, wrist and hand hanging over the edge. Hold a dumbbell in the fingers of that hand with the palm facing forward. To develop the flexors, lift the weight by curling the fingers then the wrist through a full range of motion. Slowly lower and repeat. To strengthen the extensors, start with the palm down. Lift the weight by extending the wrist through a full range of motion. Slowly lower and repeat. Note: Both wrists may be exercised at the same time by substituting a barbell in place of the dumbbell.

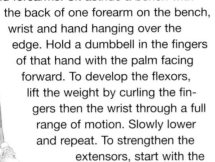

Wrist flexors

7. Half-Squat

This exercise develops the muscles of the thighs and buttocks. Stand erect, feet shoulder-width apart and turned out 45 degrees. Rest bar behind neck on shoulders. Spread hands in a comfortable position. Begin squat by first moving hips backwards, keeping back straight, eyes ahead. By moving first at the hips and then bending knees, shins will remain vertical. Bend knees to approximately 90 degrees. Pause; then stand. Repeat. Spotters are needed. Variations: Substitute dumbbell in each hand at sides.

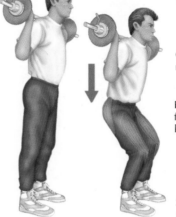

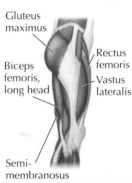

Gluteus maximus

Biceps femoris, long head

Rectus femoris

Vastus lateralis

Semi-membranosus

6. Dumbbell Rowing

This exercise develops the muscles of the upper back. It is best performed with the aid of a bench or chair for support. Grab a dumbbell with one hand and place opposite hand on the bench to support the trunk. Slowly lift the weight up until the elbow is parallel with the back. Lower the weight and repeat to complete the set. Switch hands and repeat with the opposite arm. The exercise can also be performed with one leg kneeling on the bench.

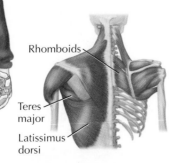

Rhomboids

Teres major

Latissimus dorsi

8. Lunge

This exercise develops the thigh and gluteal muscles. Place a barbell (with or without weight) behind your head and support with hands placed slightly wider than shoulder-width apart. In a slow and controlled motion, take a step forward and allow the leading leg to drop so that it is nearly parallel with the ground. The lower part of the leg should be nearly vertical and the back should be maintained in an upright posture. Take stride with opposite leg to return to standing posture. Repeat with other leg, remaining stationary or moving slowly in a straight line with alternating steps.

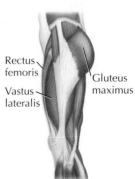

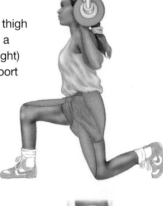

Rectus femoris

Vastus lateralis

Gluteus maximus

Table 7

Table 7 The Basic Eight for Resistance Machine Exercises

1. Chest Press

This exercise develops the chest (pectoral) and tricep muscles. Position seat height so that arm handles are directly in front of chest. Position backrest so that hands are at a comfortable distance away from the chest. Push handles forward to full extension and return to starting position in a slow and controlled manner. Repeat. Note: Machine may have a foot lever to help position, raise, and lower the weight.

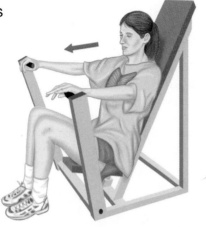

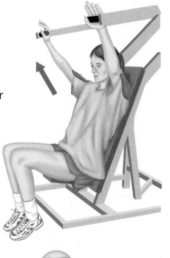

Pectoralis major

Triceps

2. Overhead Press

This exercise develops the muscles of the shoulders and arms. Position seat so that arm handles are slightly above shoulder height. Grasp handles with palms facing away and push lever up until arms are fully extended. Return to starting position and repeat. Note: Some machines may have an incline press.

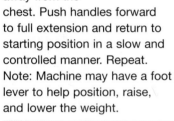

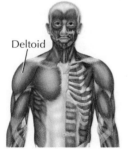

Deltoid

3. Bicep Curl

This exercise develops the elbow flexor muscles on the front of the arm, primarily the biceps. Adjust seat height so that arms are fully supported by pad when extended. Grasp handles palms up. While keeping the back straight, flex the elbow through the full range of motion.

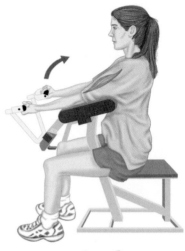

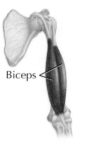

Biceps

4. Tricep Press

This exercise develops the extensor muscles on the back of the arm, primarily the triceps. Adjust seat height so that arm handles are slightly above shoulder height. Grasp handles with thumbs toward body. While keeping the back straight, extend arms fully until wrist contacts the support pad (arms straight). Return to starting position and repeat.

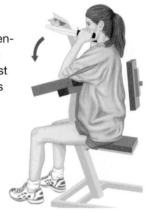

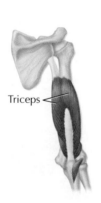

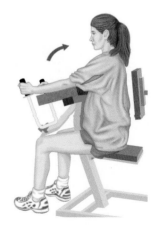

Triceps

Table 7

The Basic Eight for Resistance Machine Exercises **Table 7**

5. Lat Pull Down

This exercise primarily develops the latissimus dorsi, but the biceps, chest, and other back muscles may also be developed. Sit on the floor. Adjust seat height so that hands can just grasp bar when arms are fully extended. Grasp bar with palms facing away from you and hands shoulder-width (or wider) apart. Pull bar down to chest and return. Repeat.

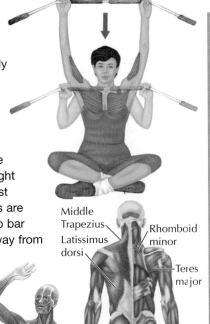

Middle Trapezius
Latissimus dorsi
Rhomboid minor
Teres major
Pectoralis major

7. Knee Extension

This exercise develops the thigh (quadriceps) muscles. Sit on end of bench with ankles hooked under padded bar. Grasp edge of table. Extend knees. Return and repeat. Alternative: Leg press (similar to half-squat).

Note: The knee extension exercise isolates the quadriceps but places greater stress on the structures of the knee than the leg press or half-squat.

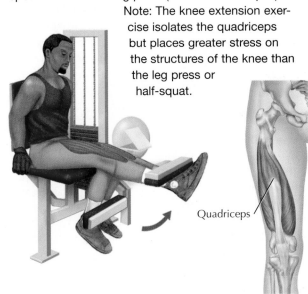

Quadriceps

6. Seated Rowing

This exercise develops the muscles of the back and shoulder. Adjust the machine so that arms are almost fully extended and parallel to the ground. Grasp handgrip with palms turned down and hands shoulder-width apart. While keeping the back straight, pull levers straight back to chest. Slowly return to starting position and repeat.

Rhomboid minor
Trapezius
Teres major
Latissimus dorsi

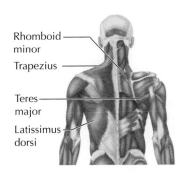

8. Hamstring Curl

This exercise develops the hamstrings (muscles on back of thigh) and other knee flexors. Lie prone on bench with ankles hooked under padded bar. Rest chin on hands or grasp bench. Flex knees as far as possible without allowing hips to raise. Return and repeat. Caution: Do not hyperextend the knees while assuming the starting position. If necessary, ask a partner to raise the pads while you place the heels under the bar.

Hamstrings

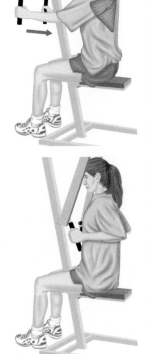

Table 8

Table 8 The Basic Eight for Calisthenics

1. Bent Knee Push-Ups and Let-Down

This exercise develops the muscles of the arms, shoulders, and chest. Lie on the floor, face down with the hands under your shoulders. Keep your body straight from the knees to the top of the head. Push up until the arms are straight. Slowly lower chest (let-down) to floor. Repeat. Variation: full push-up and let-down performed the same way except body is straight from the toes to the top of head.

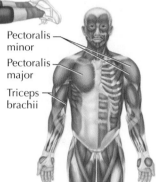

Pectoralis minor
Pectoralis major
Triceps brachii

Variation: Start from the up position and lower until the arm is bent at 90 degrees; then push up until arms are extended. Caution: Do not arch back.

2. Modified Pull-Ups

This exercise develops the muscles of the arms and shoulders. Hang (palms forward and shoulder-width apart) from a low bar (may be placed across two chairs), heels on floor, with the body straight from feet to head. Bracing the feet against a partner or fixed object is helpful. Pull up, keeping the body straight; touch the chest to the bar; then lower to the starting position. Repeat. Note: This exercise becomes more difficult as the angle of the body approaches horizontal and easier as it approaches the vertical. Variation: Perform so that the feet do not touch the floor (full pull-up). Variation: Perform with palms turned up. When palms are turned away from the face, pull-ups tend to use all the elbow flexors. With palms facing the body, the biceps are emphasized more.

Trapezius
Rhomboids
Deltoid
Teres major
Latissimus dorsi

3. Dips

This exercise develops the latissimus dorsi, deltoid, rhomboid, and tricep. Start in a fully extended position with hands grasping the bar (palms facing in). Slowly drop down until the upper part of the arm is horizontal or parallel with the floor. Extend the arms back up to the starting position and repeat. Note: Many gyms have a dip/pull-up machine with accommodating resistance that provides a variable amount of assistance to help you complete the exercise.

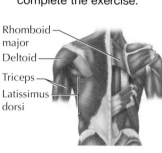

Rhomboid major
Deltoid
Triceps
Latissimus dorsi

4. Crunch (Curl-Up)

This exercise develops the upper abdominal muscles. Lie on the floor with the knees bent and the arms extended or crossed with hands on shoulders or palms on ears. If desired, legs may rest on bench to increase difficulty. For less resistance, place hands at side of body (do not put hands behind head or neck). For more resistance, move hands higher. Curl up until shoulder blades leave floor; then roll down to the starting position. Repeat. Note: Twisting the trunk on the curl-up develops the oblique abdominals.

Internal abdominal oblique
External abdominal oblique
Rectus abdominis

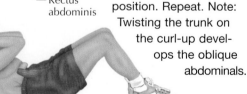

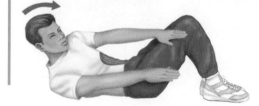

5. (Trunk) Lift

This exercise develops the muscles of the upper back and corrects round shoulders. Lie face down with hands clasped behind the neck. Pull the shoulder blades together, raising the elbows off the floor. Slowly raise the head and chest off the floor by arching the upper back. Return to the starting position; repeat. For less resistance, hands may be placed under thighs. Caution: Do not arch the lower back. Lift only until the sternum (breastbone) clears the floor. Variations: arms down at sides (easiest), hands by head, arms extended (hardest).

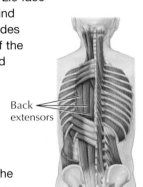

Back extensors

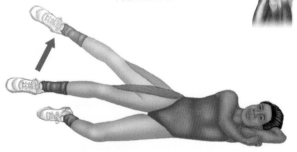

7. Lower Leg Lift

This exercise develops the muscles on the inside of thighs. Lie on the side with the upper leg (foot) supported on a bench. Note: If no bench is available, bend top leg and cross it in front of bottom leg for support. Raise the lower leg toward the ceiling. Repeat. Roll to opposite side and repeat. Keep knees pointed forward. Variation: An ankle weight may be added for greater resistance.

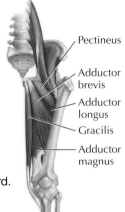

Pectineus

Adductor brevis

Adductor longus

Gracilis

Adductor magnus

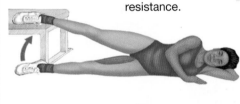

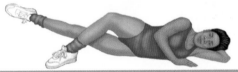

6. Side Leg Raises

This exercise develops the muscles on the outside of thighs. Lie on your side. Point knees forward. Raise the top leg 45 degrees; then return. Do the same number of repetitions with each leg. Caution: Keep knees and toes pointing forward. Variation: Ankle weights may be added for greater resistance.

Gluteus medius

Tensor fasciae latae

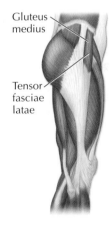

8. Alternate Leg Kneel

This exercise develops the muscles of the legs and hips. Stand tall, feet together. Take a step forward with the right foot, touching the left knee to the floor. The knees should be bent only to a 90-degree angle. Return to the starting position and

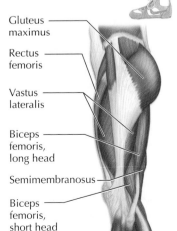

Gluteus maximus

Rectus femoris

Vastus lateralis

Biceps femoris, long head

Semimembranosus

Biceps femoris, short head

step out with the other foot. Repeat, alternating right and left. Variation: Dumbbells may be held in the hands for greater resistance.

Table 9 Exercises for Core Strength

1. Crunch (Curl-Up)

This exercise develops the upper abdominal muscles. Lie on the floor with the knees bent and the arms extended or crossed with hands on shoulders or palms on ears. If desired, legs may rest on bench to increase difficulty. For less resistance, place hands at side of body (do not put hands behind neck). For more resistance, move hands higher. Curl up until shoulder blades leave floor; then roll down to the starting position. Repeat. Note: Twisting the trunk on the curl-up develops the oblique abdominals.

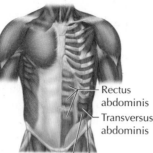

Rectus abdominis
Transversus abdominis
Internal oblique (cut)
External oblique (cut)

2. Reverse Curl

This exercise develops the lower abdominal muscles. Lie on the floor. Bend the knees, place the feet flat on the floor, and place arms at sides. Lift the knees to the chest, raising the hips off the floor. Do not let the knees go past the shoulders. Return to the starting position. Repeat.

Rectus abdominis

3. Crunch with Twist (on Bench)

This exercise strengthens the oblique abdominals and helps prevent or correct lumbar lordosis, abdominal ptosis, and backache. Lie on your back with your feet on a bench, knees bent at 90 degrees. Arms may be extended or on shoulders or hand on ears (the most difficult). Same as crunch except twist the upper trunk so the right shoulder is higher than the left. Reach toward the left knee with the right elbow. Hold. Return and repeat to the opposite side.

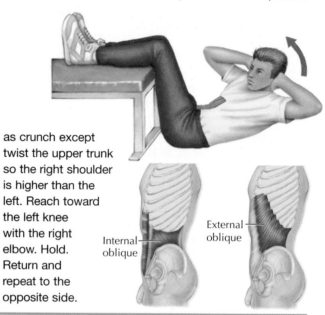

Internal oblique
External oblique

4. Sitting Tucks

This exercise strengthens the lower abdominals, increases their endurance, improves posture, and prevents backache. (This is an advanced exercise and is not recommended for people who have back pain.) Sit on floor with feet raised, arms extended for balance. Alternately bend and extend legs without letting back or feet touch floor.

Rectus abdominis

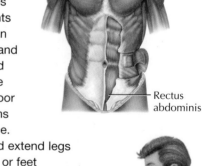

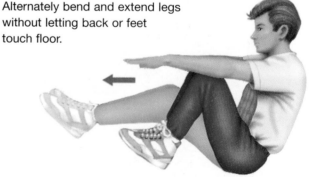

5. Hands and Knees Balance

Begin with both hands and knees placed on Bosu®. Place hands directly below shoulders and knees directly below hips. Look straight down at floor. Draw in lower abdomen. Extend one leg and raise opposite arm to a horizontal position. Keep spine in neutral position. Hold. Relax. Repeat with opposite arm and leg. Do 10 or more repetitions on each side.

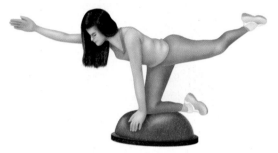

7. Side Step

Begin standing on the floor with Bosu® on your left. Step up onto the center of Bosu® with left foot. Tap right foot on top; then step back to the floor with first the right foot and then the left. Repeat for 60 seconds. Switch to the opposite side.

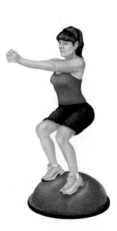

6. Marching

Stand in the middle of the Bosu® with shoulders back and lower abdomen drawn in. March in place, swinging arms in opposite directions—forward and backward—while maintaining spine in neutral position. Progress to jogging in place. Continue for 1 to 2 minutes or longer.

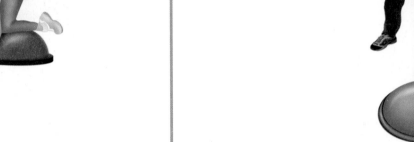

8. Squatting

Stand with feet apart on Bosu®. With knees angled outward slightly, draw abdomen in. Reach forward with hands clasped. Draw shoulder blades down and back. Squat up and down by moving hips backward and then bending knees. (Imagine the movement pattern involved in sitting back on a stool.) Repeat for 1 to 2 minutes.

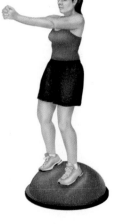

Table 10

Table 10 Strength and Muscular Endurance Self-Assessments

1. Seated Press (Chest Press)

This test can be performed using a seated press (see below) or using a bench press machine. When using the seated press, position the seat height so that arm handles are directly in front of the chest. Position backrest so that hands are at comfortable distance away from the chest. Push handles forward to full extension and return to starting position in a slow and controlled manner. Repeat. Note: Machine may have a foot lever to help position, raise, and lower the weight.

2. Leg Press

To perform this test, use a leg press machine. Typically, the beginning position is with the knees bent at right angles with the feet placed on the press machine pedals or a foot platform. Extend the legs and return to beginning position. Do not lock the knees when the legs are straightened. Typically, handles are provided. Grasp the handles with the hands when performing this test.

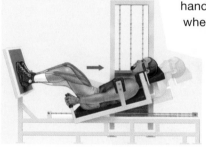

Lab Resource Materials: Muscle Fitness Tests

Evaluating Isotonic Strength: 1RM

1. Use a weight machine for the leg press and seated arm press (or bench press) for the evaluation.
2. Estimate how much weight you can lift two or three times. Be conservative; it is better to start with too little weight than too much. If you lift the weight more than 10 times, the procedure should be done again on another day when you are rested.
3. Using correct form, perform a leg press with the weight you have chosen. Perform as many times as you can up to 10.
4. Use Chart 1 to determine your 1RM for the leg press. Find the weight used in the left-hand column and then find the number of repetitions you performed across the top of the chart.
5. Your 1RM score is the value where the weight row and the repetitions column intersect.
6. Repeat this procedure for the seated arm press.
7. Record your 1RM scores for the leg press and seated arm press in the Results section.
8. Next, divide your 1RM scores by your body weight in pounds to get a "strength per pound of body weight" (str/lb./body wt.) score for each of the two exercises.
9. Finally, determine your strength rating for your upper body strength (arm press) and lower body (leg press) using Chart 2 (page 188).

Chart 1 ▶ Predicted 1RM Based on Reps-to-Fatigue

Wt.	1	2	3	4	5	6	7	8	9	10	Wt.	1	2	3	4	5	6	7	8	9	10
30	30	31	32	33	34	35	36	37	38	39	170	170	175	180	185	191	197	204	211	219	227
35	35	37	38	39	40	41	42	43	44	45	175	175	180	185	191	197	203	210	217	225	233
40	40	41	42	44	46	47	49	50	51	53	180	180	185	191	196	202	209	216	223	231	240
45	45	46	48	49	51	52	54	56	58	60	185	185	190	196	202	208	215	222	230	238	247
50	50	51	53	55	56	58	60	62	64	67	190	190	195	201	207	214	221	228	236	244	253
55	55	57	58	60	62	64	66	68	71	73	195	195	201	206	213	219	226	234	242	251	260
60	60	62	64	65	67	70	72	74	77	80	200	200	206	212	218	225	232	240	248	257	267
65	65	67	69	71	73	75	78	81	84	87	205	205	211	217	224	231	238	246	254	264	273
70	70	72	74	76	79	81	84	87	90	93	210	210	216	222	229	236	244	252	261	270	280
75	75	77	79	82	84	87	90	93	96	100	215	215	221	228	235	242	250	258	267	276	287
80	80	82	85	87	90	93	96	99	103	107	220	220	226	233	240	247	255	264	273	283	293
85	85	87	90	93	96	99	102	106	109	113	225	225	231	238	245	253	261	270	279	289	300
90	90	93	95	98	101	105	108	112	116	120	230	230	237	244	251	259	267	276	286	296	307
95	95	98	101	104	107	110	114	118	122	127	235	235	242	249	256	264	273	282	292	302	313
100	100	103	106	109	112	116	120	124	129	133	240	240	247	254	262	270	279	288	298	309	320
105	105	108	111	115	118	122	126	130	135	140	245	245	252	259	267	276	285	294	304	315	327
110	110	113	116	120	124	128	132	137	141	147	250	250	257	265	273	281	290	300	310	321	333
115	115	118	122	125	129	134	138	143	148	153	255	256	262	270	278	287	296	306	317	328	340
120	120	123	127	131	135	139	144	149	154	160	260	260	267	275	284	292	302	312	323	334	347
125	125	129	132	136	141	145	150	155	161	167	265	265	273	281	289	298	308	318	329	341	353
130	130	134	138	142	146	151	156	161	167	173	270	270	278	286	295	304	314	324	335	347	360
135	135	139	143	147	152	157	162	168	174	180	275	275	283	291	300	309	319	330	341	354	367
140	140	144	148	153	157	163	168	174	180	187	280	280	288	296	305	315	325	336	348	360	373
145	145	149	154	158	163	168	174	180	186	193	285	285	293	302	311	321	331	342	354	366	380
150	150	154	159	164	169	174	180	186	193	200	290	290	298	307	316	326	337	348	360	373	387
155	155	159	164	169	174	180	186	192	199	207	295	295	303	312	322	332	343	354	366	379	393
160	160	165	169	175	180	186	192	199	206	213	300	300	309	318	327	337	348	360	372	386	400
165	165	170	175	180	186	192	198	205	212	220	305	305	314	323	333	343	354	366	379	392	407

Source: JOPERD.

Chart 2 ▶ Fitness Classification for Relative Strength in Men and Women (1RM/Body Weight)

Age:	Leg Press			Arm Press		
	30 or Less	31–50	51+	30 or Less	31–50	51+
Ratings for Men						
High-performance zone	2.06+	1.81+	1.61+	1.26+	1.01+	.86+
Good fitness zone	1.96–2.05	1.66–1.80	1.51–1.60	1.11–1.25	.91–1.00	.76–.85
Marginal zone	1.76–1.95	1.51–1.65	1.41–1.50	.96–1.10	.86–.90	.66–.75
Low fitness zone	1.75 or less	1.50 or less	1.40 or less	.96 or less	.80 or less	.65 or less
Ratings for Women						
High-performance zone	1.61+	1.36+	1.16+	.75+	.61+	.51+
Good fitness zone	1.46–1.60	1.21–1.35	1.06–1.15	.65–.75	.56–.60	.46–.50
Marginal zone	1.31–1.45	1.11–1.20	.96–1.05	.56–.65	.51–.55	.41–.45
Low fitness zone	1.30 or less	1.10 or less	.95 or less	.55 or less	.50 or less	.40 or less

Evaluating Muscular Endurance

1. Curl-Up (Dynamic)

Sit on a mat or carpet with your legs bent more than
90 degrees so your feet remain flat on the floor (about
halfway between 90 degrees and straight). Make two
tape marks 4½ inches apart or lay a 4½-inch strip of
paper or cardboard on the floor. Lie with your arms
extended at your sides, palms down and the fingers
extended so that your fingertips touch one tape mark (or
one side of the paper or cardboard strip). Keeping your
heels in contact with the floor, curl the head and shoulders forward until your fingers reach 4½ inches (second
piece of tape or other side of strip). Lower slowly to
beginning position. Repeat one curl-up every 3 seconds.
Continue until you are unable to keep the pace of one
curl-up every 3 seconds.

   Two partners may be helpful. One stands on the
cardboard strip (to prevent movement) if one is used.
The second assures that the head returns to the floor
after each repetition.

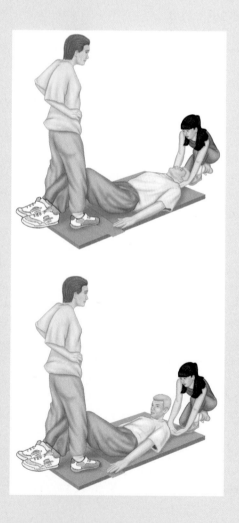

Evaluating Isometric Strength

Test: Grip Strength

Adjust a hand dynamometer to fit your hand size. Squeeze it as hard as possible. You may bend or straighten the arm, but do not touch the body with your hand, elbow, or arm. Perform with both right and left hands. *Note:* When not being tested, perform the basic eight isometric strength exercises, or squeeze and indent a new tennis ball (*after* completing the dynamometer test).

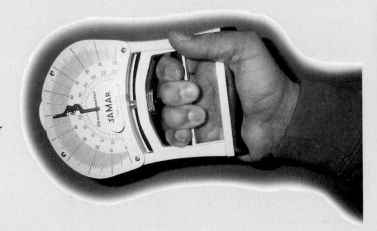

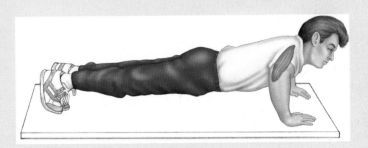

2. Ninety-Degree Push-Up (Dynamic)

Support the body in a push-up position from the toes. The hands should be just outside the shoulders, the back and legs straight, and toes tucked under. Lower the body until the upper arm is parallel to the floor or the elbow is bent at 90 degrees. The rhythm should be approximately 1 push-up every 3 seconds. Repeat as many times as possible up to 35.

3. Flexed-Arm Support (Static)

Women: Support the body in a push-up position from the knees. The hands should be outside the shoulders, the back and legs straight. Lower the body until the upper arm is parallel to the floor or the elbow is flexed at 90 degrees.

Men: Use the same procedure as for women except support the push-up position from the toes instead of the knees. (Same position as for 90-degree push-up.) Hold the 90-degree position as long as possible, up to 35 seconds.

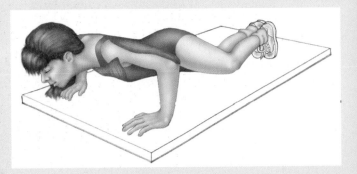

Chart 3 ▶ Isometric Strength Rating Scale (Pounds)

Classification	Left Grip	Right Grip	Total Score
Ratings for Men			
High-performance zone	125+	135+	260+
Good fitness zone	100–124	110–134	210–259
Marginal zone	90–99	95–109	185–209
Low fitness zone	<90	<95	<185
Ratings for Women			
High-performance zone	75+	85+	160+
Good fitness zone	60–74	70–84	130–159
Marginal zone	45–59	50–69	95–129
Low fitness zone	<45	<50	<95

Suitable for use by young adults between 18 and 30 years of age. After 30, an adjustment of 0.5 of 1 percent per year is appropriate because some loss of muscle tissue typically occurs as you grow older.

Chart 4 ▶ Rating Scale for Dynamic Muscular Endurance

Age:	17–26		27–39		40–49		50–59		60+	
Classification	Curl-Ups	Push-Ups	Curl-Ups	Push-Ups	Curl-Ups	Push-Ups	Curl-Ups	Push-Ups	Curl-Ups	Push-Ups
Ratings for Men										
High-performance zone	35+	29+	34+	27+	33+	26+	32+	24+	31+	22+
Good fitness zone	24–34	20–28	23–33	18–26	22–32	17–25	21–31	15–23	20–30	13–21
Marginal zone	15–23	16–19	14–22	15–17	13–21	14–16	12–20	12–14	11–19	10–12
Low fitness zone	<15	<16	<14	<15	<13	<14	<12	<12	<11	<10
Ratings for Women										
High-performance zone	25+	17+	24+	16+	23+	15+	22+	14+	21+	13+
Good fitness zone	18–24	12–16	17–23	11–15	16–22	10–14	15–21	9–13	14–20	8–12
Marginal zone	10–17	8–11	9–16	7–10	8–15	6–9	7–14	5–8	6–13	4–7
Low fitness zone	<10	<8	<9	<7	<8	<6	<7	<5	<6	<4

Chart 5 ▶ Rating Scale for Static Endurance (Flexed-Arm Support)

Classification	Score in Seconds
High-performance zone	30+
Good fitness zone	20–29
Marginal zone	10–19
Low fitness zone	10

Lab 9A Evaluating Muscle Strength: 1RM and Grip Strength

Name		**Section**	**Date**

Purpose: To evaluate your muscle strength using 1RM and to determine the best amount of resistance to use for various strength exercises

Procedures: 1RM is the maximum amount of resistance you can lift for a specific exercise. Testing yourself to determine how much you can lift only one time using traditional methods can be fatiguing and even dangerous. The procedure you will perform here allows you to estimate 1RM based on the number of times you can lift a weight that is less than 1RM.

Evaluating Strength Using Estimated 1RM

1. Use a resistance machine for the leg press and arm or bench press for the evaluation part of this lab.
2. Estimate how much weight you can lift two or three times. Be conservative; it is better to start with too little weight than too much. If you lift a weight more than 10 times, the procedure should be done again on another day when you are rested.
3. Using correct form, perform a leg press with the weight you have chosen. Perform as many times as you can up to 10.
4. Use Chart 1 in *Lab Resource Materials* to determine your 1RM for the leg press. Find the weight used in the left-hand column and then find the number of repetitions you performed across the top of the chart.
5. Your 1RM score is the value where the weight row and the repetitions column intersect.
6. Repeat this procedure for the arm or bench press using the same technique.
7. Record your 1RM scores for the leg press and bench press in the Results section.
8. Next divide your 1RM scores by your body weight in pounds to get a "strength per pound of body weight" (1RM/body weight) score for each of the two exercises.
9. Determine your strength rating for your upper body strength (arm press) and lower body (leg press) using Chart 2 in *Lab Resource Materials*. Record in the Results section. If time allows, assess 1RM for other exercises you choose to perform (see Lab 9C).
10. If a grip dynamometer is available, determine your right-hand and left-hand grip strength using the procedures in *Lab Resource Materials*. Use Chart 3 in *Lab Resource Materials* to rate your grip (isometric) strength.

Results

Arm press
(or bench press):

Wt. selected [ ]   Reps [ ]   Estimated 1RM [ ]
(Chart 1, *Lab Resource Materials*)

Strength per lb. body weight [ ]   Rating [ ]
(1RM ÷ body weight)   (Chart 2, *Lab Resource Materials*)

Leg press:

Wt. selected [ ]   Reps [ ]   Estimated 1RM [ ]
(Chart 1, *Lab Resource Materials*)

Strength per lb. body weight [ ]   Rating [ ]
(1RM ÷ body weight)   (Chart 2, *Lab Resource Materials*)

Grip strength:

Right grip score [ ]   Right grip rating [ ]

Left grip score [ ]   Left grip rating [ ]

Total score [ ]   Total rating [ ]

Seated Press (Chest Press)

This test can be performed using a seated press (see below) or using a bench press machine. When using the seated press, position the seat height so that arm handles are directly in front of the chest. Position backrest so that hands are at comfortable distance away from the chest. Push handles forward to full extension and return to starting position in a slow and controlled manner. Repeat. Note: Machine may have a foot lever to help position, raise, and lower the weight.

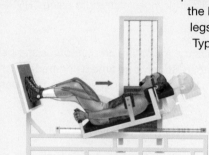

Leg Press

To perform this test, use a leg press machine. Typically, the beginning position is with the knees bent at right angles with the feet placed on the press machine pedals or a foot platform. Extend the legs and return to beginning position. Do not lock the knees when the legs are straightened. Typically, handles are provided. Grasp the handles with the hands when performing this test.

Conclusions and Implications: In several sentences, discuss your current strength, whether you believe it is adequate for good health, and whether you think that your "strength per pound of body weight" scores are representative of your true strength.

Lab 9B Evaluating Muscular Endurance

Name		Section	Date

Purpose: To evaluate the dynamic muscular endurance of two muscle groups and the static endurance of the arms and trunk muscles

Procedures

1. Perform the curl-up, push-up, and flexed-arm support tests described in *Lab Resource Materials* (pp. 188–189).
2. In Chart 1, record your test scores in the Results section. Determine and record your rating from Charts 4 and 5 in *Lab Resource Materials*.

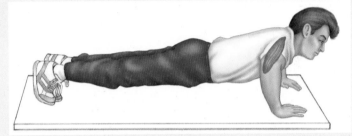

2. Ninety-degree push-up (dynamic)

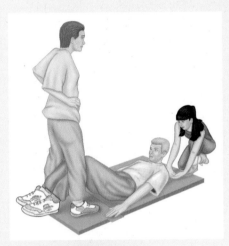

1. Curl-up (dynamic)

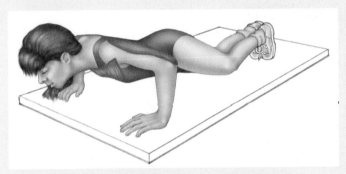

3. Flexed-arm support (static): women in knee position and men in full support position

Results

Record your scores below.

Curl-up [　　　　]　　　　Push-up [　　　　]　　　　Flexed-arm support (seconds) [　　　　]

Check your ratings in Chart 1.

Chart 1 ▶ Rating Scale for Static Endurance (Flexed-Arm Support)

	Curl-Up	Push-Up	Flexed-Arm Support
High	○	○	○
Good	○	○	○
Marginal	○	○	○
Poor	○	○	○

On which of the tests of muscular endurance did you score the lowest?

Curl-up ◯   Push-up ◯   Flexed-arm support ◯

On which of the tests of muscular endurance did you score the best?

Curl-up ◯   Push-up ◯   Flexed-arm support ◯

Conclusions and Implications: In several sentences, discuss your current level of muscular endurance and whether this level is enough to meet your health, work, and leisure-time needs in the future.

Lab 9C Planning and Logging Muscle Fitness Exercises: Free Weights or Resistance Machines

Name	**Section**	**Date**

Purpose: To set lifestyle goals for muscle fitness exercise, to prepare a muscle fitness exercise plan, and to self-monitor progress for the 1-week plan

Procedures

1. Using Chart 1, provide some background information about your experience with resistance exercise, your goals, and your plans for incorporating these exercises into your normal exercise routine.
2. In Chart 2, keep a log of your actual participation in resistance exercise. You can choose free weights, machines, or some of both. Try to do at least eight exercises on at least 2 different days and be sure to work different body parts. Also, be sure that you plan your exercise program so it fits with the goals you described in Chart 1. If you are just starting out, it is best to start with light weights and more repetitions, e.g., 12–15. For best results, take the log with you during your workout, so you can remember the weights, reps, and sets you performed.
3. Describe your experiences with your resistance exercise program. Be sure to comment on your plans for future resistance exercise.

Chart 1 ▶ Muscle Fitness Survey

1. Determine your current stage for resistance exercise. Check only the stage that represents your current activity level.

 ◯ Precontemplation. I do not meet resistance exercise guidelines and have not been thinking about starting.

 ◯ Contemplation. I do not do resistance exercises but have been thinking about starting.

 ◯ Preparation. I am planning to start doing regular resistance exercises to meet guidelines.

 ◯ Action. I do resistance exercises, but I am not as regular as I should be.

 ◯ Maintenance. I regularly meet guidelines for resistance exercises.

2. What are your primary goals for resistance exercise?

 ◯ General conditioning   ◯ Improved appearance   ◯ Other_____

 ◯ Sports training   ◯ Avoidance of back pain

3. Are you currently involved in a regular resistance exercise program?

 ◯ Yes   ◯ No

4. Describe your current program or your future goals.
 - What days and times do you lift weights (or when can you lift)?
 - Where do you lift (or where can you lift)?
 - Describe your goals (or plans for resistance exercise):

Chart 2 ▶ Muscle Fitness Exercise Log

Check the exercises you performed and the days you performed them. You can do all free weights, all machines, or some of both. List others that you added.

Exercises	Day 1 (date)			Day 2 (date)			Day 3 (date)		
	Wt.	Reps	Sets	Wt.	Reps	Sets	Wt.	Reps	Sets
Free Weight Exercises									
1 Bench press									
2 Overhead press									
3 Bicep curl									
4 Tricep curl									
5 Wrist curl									
6 Dumbbell rowing									
7 Half squat									
8 Lunge									
9									
10									
Machine Exercises									
11 Chest press									
12 Overhead press									
13 Bicep curl									
14 Tricep press									
15 Lat pull-down									
16 Seated rowing									
17 Knee extension									
18 Hamstring curl									
19									
20									

Results

Were you able to do your basic eight exercises at least 2 days in the week?   Yes ◯   No ◯

Conclusions and Implications: Do you feel that you will use muscle fitness exercises as part of your regular lifetime physical activity plan, either now or in the future? Comment on what modifications you would make in your program in the future. Use several sentences to answer.

Lab 9D Planning and Logging Muscle Fitness Exercises: Calisthenics or Core Exercises

Name		Section	Date

Purpose: To set lifestyle goals for muscle fitness exercises that can easily be performed at home, to prepare a muscle fitness exercise plan, and to self-monitor progress for a 1-week plan

Procedures

1. Using Chart 1, provide some background information about your experience with calisthenic or core exercise, your goals, and your plans for incorporating these exercises into your normal exercise routine.
2. In Chart 2, keep a log of your actual participation in these exercises. You can choose all calisthenic exercises, all core exercises, or some of both. Some of the core exercises require the use of a Bosu® balance trainer or a similar device. If you don't have access to this, you can substitute other exercises. Try to do at least eight exercises on at least 2 different days and be sure to work different body parts.
3. Describe your experiences with your resistance exercise program. Be sure to comment on your plans for future resistance exercise.

Chart 1 ▶ Muscle Fitness Survey

1. Determine your current stage for calisthenics or core exercise. Check only the stage that represents your current activity level.

   ◯ Precontemplation. I do not do calisthenics or core exercises and have not been thinking about starting.

   ◯ Contemplation. I do not do calisthenics or core exercises but have been thinking about starting.

   ◯ Preparation. I am planning to start doing calisthenics or core exercises.

   ◯ Action. I do calisthenics or core exercises, but I am not as regular as I should be.

   ◯ Maintenance. I regularly perform calisthenics or core exercises.

2. What is your level of experience with core exercises (refer to Table 9)? Check the box that best describes you.

   ◯ I have done abdominal exercises but have never done the other core exercises.

   ◯ I have done abdominal exercises and have tried core exercises with the Bosu® or similar devices.

   ◯ I regularly perform core exercises and am very experienced with the Bosu® or similar devices.

3. What are your primary reasons for doing calisthenic or core exercise?

   ◯ General conditioning

   ◯ Sports training

   ◯ Improved appearance

   ◯ Avoidance of back pain

4. Describe your current program or your present or future goals.
   • What days and times do you exercise (or when can you exercise)?
   • Where do you perform these exercises (or where can you exercise)?
   • Describe your goals/plans:

Chart 2 ▶ Muscle Fitness Exercise Log

Check the exercises you performed and the days you performed them. List others that you added.

Exercises	Day 1 (date)		Day 2 (date)		Day 3 (date)	
	Reps	Sets	Reps	Sets	Reps	Sets
Calisthenic Exercises						
1 Bent knee push-ups						
2 Modified pull-ups						
3 Dips						
4 Crunch (curl-up)						
5 Trunk lift						
6 Side leg raise						
7 Lower leg lift						
8 Alternate leg kneel						
9						
10						
Core Exercises						
11 Crunch						
12 Reverse curl						
13 Crunch with twist						
14 Sitting tucks						
15 Hands and knees balance						
16 Marching						
17 Side step						
18 Squatting						
19						
20						

Results

Were you able to do your planned exercises at least 2 days in the week?   Yes ◯   No ◯

Conclusions and Implications: Do you feel that you will use these muscle fitness exercises as part of your regular lifetime physical activity plan, either now or in the future? Discuss the exercises you feel benefited you and the ones that did not. What modifications would you make in your program for it to work better for you?

Flexibility

Health Objectives for the Year 2020

- Increase proportion of people who regularly perform exercises for flexibility.
- Reduce sports and recreation injuries.
- Reduce percentage of adults who do no leisure-time activity.
- Increase access to employee-based exercise facilities and programs.

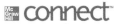 | FITNESS AND WELLNESS   http://connect.mcgraw-hill.com

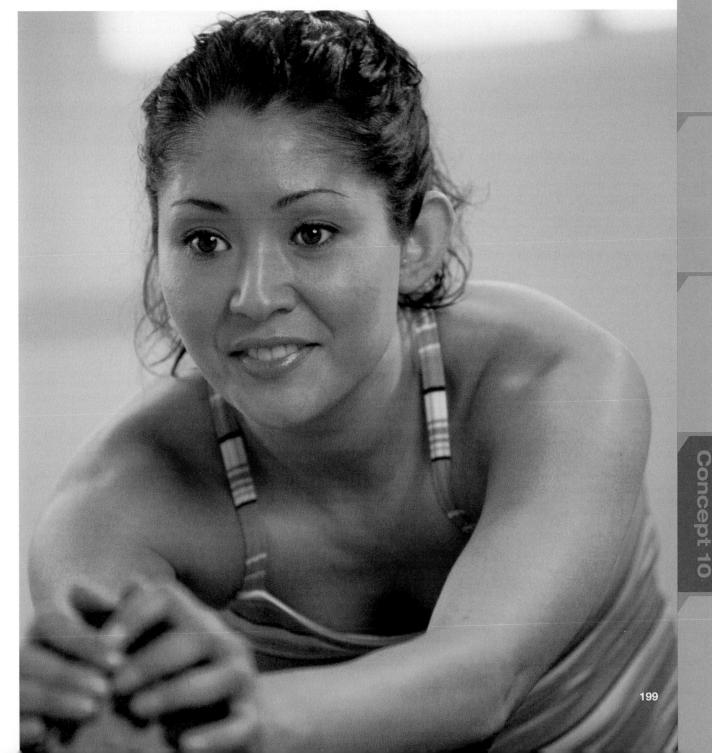

Regular stretching exercises promote flexibility—a component of fitness—that permits freedom of movement, contributes to ease and economy of muscular effort, allows for successful performance in certain activities, and provides less susceptibility to some types of injuries or musculoskeletal problems.

Flexibility refers to the amount of motion that is possible at a given joint or series of joints. A joint with limited ability to bend or straighten is said to be tight or stiff, while joints with a high degree of flexibility are referred to as loose-jointed, or hypermobile. A reasonable amount of flexibility is needed to perform efficiently and effectively in daily life, but excessive flexibility is not desirable.

This concept explains how flexibility is assessed and describes how much flexibility is needed for good health and optimal performance. Guidelines are also provided on proper stretching techniques to help you establish a program that will build good flexibility.

Flexibility Fundamentals

There are many myths and misconceptions about flexibility. Flexibility is an often-misunderstood part of health-related physical fitness. In the list that follows, some basic facts about flexibility are presented to dispel erroneous ideas.

- *Flexibility is not the same as stretching.* Flexibility is a component of health-related physical fitness. It is a state of being. Stretching is the primary technique used to improve the state of one's flexibility.
- *A stretching warm-up is not the same as a flexibility workout.* As noted in Concept 3, a stretching warm-up can be done as one part of a comprehensive warm-up. While a warm-up may have benefits, stretching before exercise is not a substitute for a regular stretching program to build flexibility. If you are not flexible and have short muscles, a single warm-up cannot make you flexible. Regular stretching is needed to see improvements in flexibility.
- *A flexibility workout should be done when adequate time is available to perform stretching exercises applying the FIT formula.* Some people perform a complete stretching program to build flexibility at the end of a workout when muscles are warm. Others perform their flexibility workout (stretching) at a time when they can concentrate specifically on building flexibility. In either case, sufficient time should be allowed to ensure that the exercises are

done correctly. Guidelines for proper stretching with sample exercises are provided later in this concept.
- Flexibility is important to health and performance. Independent from recommendations for a stretch warm-up, the ACSM recommends that at least 10 minutes be spent on each bout of exercise designed to build flexibility. The Healthy People 2020 national goals statement does not include a specific recommendation for flexibility exercises (the objective was archived), but experts note the importance of stretching for maintaining good health. Information concerning the health benefits of good flexibility is presented later in this concept.
- Flexibility is highly specific. An individual may demonstrate optimal flexibility in one region of the body while having stiffness in other joints. For example, a person may have good flexibility of the spine, hips, and legs in order to reach down and touch the toes but be unable to clasp both hands behind the back due to stiffness of the shoulder joints. The optimal amount of flexibility for a given joint depends on the specific needs of the individual. For instance, a figure skater requires a greater degree of trunk and hip flexibility for skill performance than does a hockey player. An electrician doing overhead work requires a greater degree of shoulder flexibility than does a receptionist.

Factors Influencing Flexibility

(i) **The range of motion in a joint or joints is a reflection of the flexibility at that joint.** FEATURE 1 Clinically, the **range of motion (ROM)** of a joint is the extent *and* direction of movement that is possible. The extent of movement is described by the arc through which a joint moves and is typically measured in degrees using a tool called a goniometer. The direction of movement at a specific joint is determined by the shapes of the bony surfaces that are in contact. Certain types of joints allow for greater movement than others.

Medical professionals use a specific vocabulary to describe the movement of joints. Figure 1 illustrates some of these movement terms as they relate to hip, knee, or

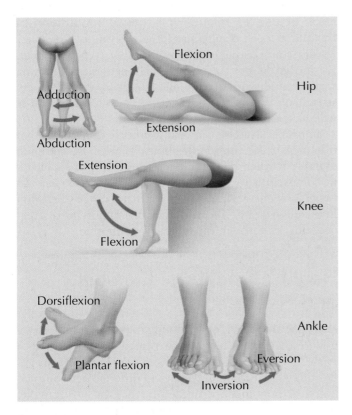

Figure 1 ▶ Ranges of joint motion.

ankle motion. Similar terms are applied in describing movement of the spine and upper body. Note that the same terms (such as *flexion/extension*) can be applied to different joints, while other terms (such as *dorsiflexion/plantar flexion*) are unique to a specific joint such as the ankle.

The shape, size, and orientation of a joint greatly influence the amount of motion available. The circular surface of the ball-and-socket joint of the hip, for example, allows for considerable mobility, including movement to the side (adduction and abduction), forward and backward (flexion and extension), and in and out (internal and external rotation). The hinge joint of the knee is more restrictive and limits movement to primarily forward and backward (flexion and extension). Motion at other joints, such as the ankle, involves the combined movements of numerous bony surfaces. A hinge-type portion permits the up and down motion of the foot (dorsiflexion and plantar flexion), while a separate planar-type joint allows the side-to-side motion (inversion and eversion) of the foot. A basic understanding of this terminology is important in understanding principles of flexibility and stretching.

Long muscle-tendon units (MTUs) are important to flexibility. The extent of movement available at a specific joint is determined by the shape of the joint, as well as by the tautness of the ligaments and the action of the muscles and tendons that cross the joint. **Ligaments** are

bands of connective tissue that connect bones together at a joint. They provide rigidity and stability to the joint capsule and restrict excessive motion at the joint. Damage to ligaments from repeated sprains can lead to excessive joint **laxity** and increase risk for injuries. **Tendons** are also made of connective tissue, but they attach muscles to bone. Having long muscles and tendons allows for greater range of motion and better flexibility. Together, the muscles and tendons are referred to as a **muscle-tendon unit (MTU)**. Muscle fibers are more extensible and elastic than tendons, but both are stretched together. In this book we will refer to muscle stretching without further mention of the MTU.

The properties of connective tissue and muscle impact flexibility. Nearly one-fourth of the body's protein is collagen, a connective tissue making up the ligaments, tendons, and noncontractile elements of muscle. Collagen has both viscous and elastic properties. Viscous tissue will lengthen permanently when a force is applied to it, much like a piece of taffy being pulled and stretched. Elastic tissue, on the other hand, returns to its original length, much like the recoil of a rubber band or spring after being stretched. Stretching must be performed for an adequate time to allow the viscous tissues to stretch and lengthen. Stretching must also be done frequently to keep elastic tissues from returning to their normal length.

Static flexibility is different from dynamic flexibility. A joint's flexibility can be described differently depending on how it is assessed. Static flexibility is the maximum range a joint can achieve under stationary conditions. An example is the hip ROM achieved during a hamstring stretch. Static flexibility is limited by passive viscous and elastic properties of the MTU. Dynamic flexibility is the maximum range a joint can achieve under active conditions. An example is the maximum height and position of a hurdler's lead leg. While it may seem logical

---

Range of Motion (ROM) The full motion possible in a joint or series of joints.

Ligaments Bands of tissue that connect bones. Unlike muscles and tendons, overstretching ligaments is not desirable.

Laxity Motion in a joint outside the normal plane for that joint, due to loose ligaments.

Tendons Fibrous bands of tissue that connect muscles to bones and facilitate movement of a joint.

Muscle-Tendon Unit (MTU) The skeletal muscles and the tendons that connect them to bones. Stretching to improve flexibility is associated with increased length of the MTU.

that dynamic flexibility would be greater than static, the opposite is true. Dynamic flexibility is affected by both passive and active elements of the MTU. The hurdler's performance depends on passive MTU extensibility as well as the ability to move against gravity, at fast speeds, and without elicitation of a stretch reflex. While good static flexibility is necessary for good dynamic flexibility, it does not ensure it. Athletes must train both static and dynamic flexibility for optimal performance.

Flexibility varies considerably across the life span. Flexibility is generally high in children but declines during adolescence because of the rapid changes in growth—essentially, the bones grow faster than the MTU. In early adulthood, the MTU catches up to the skeletal system, causing flexibility to peak in the mid- to late 20s. With increasing age, range of motion tends to decline again. Reduced flexibility is due to a loss of elasticity in the MTU and cross-linkages within collagen fibers of tendons, ligaments, and joint capsules. Over the span of their working lives, adults typically lose 3 to 4 inches of lower back flexibility as measured by the common "sit-and-reach" test. Research studies have confirmed that declines in flexibility are not as evident in individuals who maintain regular patterns of physical activity. The use of planned stretching programs has also been shown to help maintain flexibility with age.

Gender differences exist in flexibility. Girls tend to be more flexible than boys at young ages, but the gender difference decreases for adults. Greater flexibility of females is generally attributed to anatomical differences (e.g., wider hips) and hormonal influences.

Genetic factors can explain some individual variability in flexibility. In some families, the trait for loose joints is passed from generation to generation. This **hypermobility** is sometimes referred to as joint looseness. Studies show that people with this trait may be more prone to joint dislocation. There is not much research evidence, but some experts believe that those with hypermobility may also be more susceptible to athletic or dance injuries, especially to the knee, ankle, and shoulder, and may be more apt to develop premature osteoarthritis.

Dynamic flexibility is important in many sports.

Lack of use or misuse can cause reductions in flexibility. Lack of physical activity is one of the major factors contributing to poor flexibility. When muscles are moved as part of normal daily activities or during structured physical activity, the muscles and tendons get stretched. Without this regular stimulation, flexibility will decrease.

Improper exercise can lead to muscle imbalances that may negatively impact flexibility. The most common example is when body builders overdevelop their biceps in comparison to their triceps. This leads to a *muscle-bound* look characterized by a restricted range of motion in the elbow joint. To avoid this, it is important to exercise muscles through the full range of motion.

Health Benefits of Flexibility and Stretching

No ideal standard for flexibility exists. It is not known how much flexibility any one person should have in a joint. Norms are available that summarize the amount of flexibility for males and females of different ages but it is not clear how much is needed for health. For example, there is little scientific evidence to indicate that a person who can reach 2 inches past his or her toes on a sit-and-reach test is less fit than a person who can reach 8 inches past the toes. Too much flexibility could be as detrimental as too little. The standards presented in the *Lab Resource Materials* are based on the best available evidence.

Hyperflexibility of a joint may increase susceptibility to injury. An appropriate amount of flexibility is beneficial, but too much or too little flexibility can present risks. If tissues around the joints, especially ligaments, become too long from trauma of overstretching or are slack for other reasons, the integrity of the joint is compromised. Most muscles and tendons can lengthen (extensibility) and return to their normal length after appropriate stretching (elasticity). However, short, tight muscles and tendons can be easily overstretched (strained). Even

HELP HEALTH is available to Everyone for a Lifetime, and it's Personal

Although stretching before or after exercise has not been proven to significantly reduce injuries among competitive or recreational athletes, stretching and flexibility are still seen as key components in a complete physical activity program. Despite its benefits, stretching is often the first part of a workout to be dropped if time becomes an issue.

How important do you feel flexibility is to your overall level of fitness, health, and wellness?

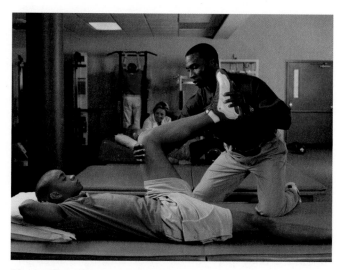

Physical therapists and athletic trainers use carefully planned stretching exercise for treatment.

more likely to be injured are the ligaments that connect bone to bone. Ligaments and the joint capsule lack the elasticity and tensile strength of the muscles and tendons. When involuntarily overstretched, they may remain in a lengthened state or become ruptured (sprained). If this occurs, the joint loses stability and is susceptible to chronic dislocation, repeated sprains, and excessive wear and tear of the joint surface. This is particularly true of weight-bearing joints, such as the hip, knee, and ankle.

Stretching is used by physical therapists to improve flexibility and to aid in rehabilitation from injuries. People of all ages, especially older adults, regularly receive treatment for musculoskeletal problems ranging from vocational and sports injuries (trauma and overuse) to disease-related problems and accidental injury. Stretching exercises are routinely recommended to regain normal range of motion, normal function, and to reduce pain. Many people with pain have reduced range of motion similar to people who have an injury. Maintaining functional range of motion in joints of the body is important for preventing problems, and regular stretching is the best way to accomplish this. Physical therapists use flexibility exercises as a form of treatment but also as a means of preventing future problems.

Adequate flexibility is necessary for achieving and maintaining optimal posture. Short and tight muscles in certain body regions can result in poor posture. Shortness of muscles of the chest and back of the neck can result in "rounded shoulders" and a "forward head" position. Tightness of the hip flexor muscles can result in excessive lordosis, or arching, of the low back.

Adequate flexibility may help prevent muscle strain and such orthopedic problems as backache. Back pain is a leading medical complaint in Western culture.

One common cause of backache is shortened lower back muscles and hip flexor muscles. Short hamstrings (muscles in the back of the leg) are also associated with lower back problems. Improving flexibility can decrease risk for back problems.

Stretching may help relieve muscle cramps and pain associated with myofascial trigger points. Many people experience some form of muscle cramping during exercise. A muscle spasm or cramp may result for various reasons, including overexertion, dehydration, and heat stress. Stretching a cramped (but not a strained) muscle will often help relieve the cramp.

Myofascial **trigger points** are less understood and typically more painful. They are characterized by taut bands within skeletal muscle that have a nodular texture. They are sensitive to touch and can produce a radiating pain in specific regions of the body when touched. Research suggests that myofascial trigger points are caused by a sustained neural spinal reflex. They are thought to develop after trauma, after overuse, or from prolonged spasm in the muscles. Stretching and direct pressure on myofascial trigger points have been shown to help relieve the pain. In contrast, nonspecific areas of soft tissue tenderness in the body (often referred to as tender points) are not as responsive to stretching.

Stretching is probably *ineffective* in preventing muscle soreness. In the past, it was suggested that stretching during a cool-down will *prevent* muscular soreness. In a controlled study, however, muscle soreness was deliberately induced in a group of subjects. When half of the group stretched immediately afterward and at intervals for 48 hours, they had as much soreness as the group who did not stretch.

Performance Benefits of Flexibility and Stretching

Good flexibility can be beneficial to one's ability to function effectively at work and in daily life. Lack of joint range of motion can negatively affect one's ability to perform tasks at work and daily activities such as driving a car. It is well documented that as people

Hypermobility Looseness or slackness in the joint and of the muscles and ligaments (soft tissue) surrounding the joint.

Trigger Points Especially irritable spots, usually tight bands or knots in a muscle or fascia (a sheath of connective tissue that binds muscles and other tissues together). Trigger points often refer pain to another area of the body.

grow older their range of motion in the neck decreases resulting in reduced ability to turn the head and effectively anticipate movements to the side and rear of the car. Reduced range of motion can also increase risk of accidents in automobiles and around the home. Regular stretching is important to everyday functioning in a variety of settings.

Good flexibility can benefit performance in sports. The longer length and reduced **stiffness** of muscles in people with good flexibility allows greater **stretch tolerance** that can lead to improved performance. For example, a diver must have flexibility to perform a pike dive, and a hurdler must have good flexibility in the back, hip, and leg to perform well. Stretching and good flexibility is most beneficial in sports that require joints to work in a large range of motion. A few examples, in addition to gymnasts and divers, are swimmers, wrestlers, and skaters.

Good flexibility and stretching has limited ability to prevent sports injuries. Stretching is widely recommended for injury prevention despite the fact that there is limited evidence to support this potential benefit. The potential reduction in risk depends on the characteristics and demands of the activity. Stretching is probably most important for injury prevention in activities that require great range of motion, such as gymnastics and diving.

Stretching Methods

Static stretching is the safest and most commonly used method of stretching. Static stretching is done slowly and held for a period of several seconds. With this type of stretch, the probability of tearing the soft tissue is low if performed properly. Static stretches can be performed with **active assistance** or with **passive assistance**. When active assistance is used, the opposing muscle group is contracted to produce a reflex relaxation **(reciprocal inhibition)** in the muscle being stretched. This enables the muscle to be more easily stretched. For example, when doing a calf stretch exercise (see Figure 2A), the muscles on the front of the shin are contracted to assist in the stretch of the muscles of the calf. However, active assistance to static stretching has one problem. It is almost impossible to produce adequate overload by simply contracting the opposing muscles.

When passive assistance (see Figure 2B, C) is used, an outside force, such as a partner, aids in the stretching. For example, in the calf stretch, passive assistance can be provided by another person, another body part (Figure 2B), or gravity (Figure 2C). This type of stretch does not create the relaxation in the muscle associated with active assisted stretch. An unrelaxed muscle cannot be stretched as far, and injury may happen. Therefore, it is best to combine the active assistance with a passive assistance when performing a static stretch. This gives the advantage of a relaxed muscle and a sufficient force to provide an overload to stretch it.

A good way to begin static stretching exercises is to stretch until tension is first felt, back off slightly and hold the position several seconds, and then gradually stretch a little farther, back off, and hold. Decrease the stretch slowly after the hold.

Ballistic stretch is an acceptable form of stretching, especially for those who plan to do sports and activities involving ballistic movements. A ballistic stretch uses momentum to produce the stretch. Momentum is produced by vigorous motion, such as flinging a body part (bobbing) or rocking it back and forth to create a bouncing movement. As with static stretching, the ballistic movement can be provided either actively or passively. For example, in the calf stretch shown in Figure 2D, E, and F, the foot is actively bounced forward by the **antagonist muscle** force or passively by an assist from another person or gravity. The forceful movement in ballistic stretching may increase risks for injury. Therefore, this form of stretching is not recommended for most people.

The inherent problem with most ballistic stretching is lack of control over the force and range of movement. Experts have begun to characterize *dynamic stretching* as a safe derivative of ballistic stretching. This form of stretching uses gradual and controlled movement of body parts up to the limit of a joint's range of motion. Stretches may involve arm or leg swings of increasing reach or increasing speed. The key is to perform the movement in a controlled manner through the normal range of motion. This approach allows dynamic stretching to be a safe and efficient means of using active stretching techniques.

Ballistic stretch has not been recommended for most people because of concerns for injury. Recent studies

Stiffness Elasticity in the MTU; measured by force needed to stretch.

Stretch Tolerance Greater stretch for the same pain level.

Active Assistance An assist to stretch from an active contraction of the opposing (antagonist) muscle.

Passive Assistance Stretch imposed on a muscle with the assistance of a force other than the opposing muscle.

Reciprocal Inhibition Reflex relaxation in stretched muscle during contraction of the antagonist.

Antagonist Muscles In this concept, *antagonist* refers to the muscle group on the opposite side of the limb from the muscle group being stretched (e.g., biceps is the antagonist of triceps).

Contrasting Three Methods of Stretching

I. Static Stretch

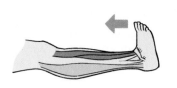
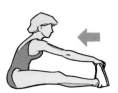
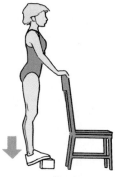

Active
A.

Passive
(Self Assisted)
B.

Passive
(Gravity Assisted)
C.

II. Ballistic Stretch

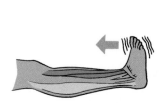
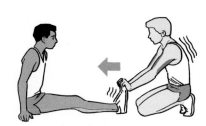
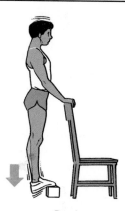

Active
D.

Passive
(Partner Assisted)
E.

Passive
(Gravity Assisted)
F.

III. PNF (CRAC) Stretch

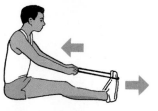
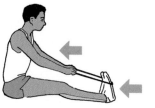

Step 1: From a lengthened position, contract calf muscles isometrically against resistance of rope or partner.
G.

Step 2: Relax calf muscles and contract dorsiflexors (shin muscles) in active stretch of calf.
H.

Step 3: Continue active contraction while rope provides passive assist.
I.

Figure 2 ▶ Examples of static, ballistic, PNF, active, and passive stretches of the calf muscles (gastronemius and soleus). Muscles shown in dark pink are the muscles being contracted. Muscles shown in light pink are those being stretched.

have cast doubt about the dangers of ballistic stretch, especially when done in a controlled manner as described above. Still, most exercise professionals prefer static stretch and PNF for those lacking in flexibility and those who are not regularly active. For relatively fit people who plan to perform sports and activities that involve ballistic movements, ballistic stretch is an appropriate alternative.

(i) **PNF techniques have proven to be most effective at improving flexibility.** PNF FEATURE 2 stretching utilizes techniques to stimulate muscles to contract more strongly (and relax more fully) in order to enhance the effectiveness of stretching. The contract-relax-antagonist-contract (CRAC) technique is the most popular. CRAC PNF involves three specific steps: (1) Move the limb so the muscle to be stretched is elongated initially; then contract it (**agonist muscle**) isometrically for several seconds (against an immovable object or the resistance of a partner); (2) relax the muscle; and (3) immediately statically stretch the muscle with the active assistance of the antagonist muscle and an assist

from a partner, gravity, or another body part. Figure 2G, H, and I provide a detailed illustration of how this technique is applied to the calf stretch. Research shows that this and other types of PNF stretch are more effective than a simple static stretch.

How Much Stretch Is Enough?

Specific efforts are needed to improve flexibility. Lifestyle and cardiovascular activity do little to develop flexibility. To build this important part of fitness, stretching exercises from step 3 of the pyramid are essential (see Figure 3).

To increase the length of a muscle, you must stretch it more than its normal length (overload) but not overstretch it. The best evidence suggests that muscles should be stretched to about 10 percent beyond their normal length to bring about an improvement in flexibility. More practical indicators of the intensity of

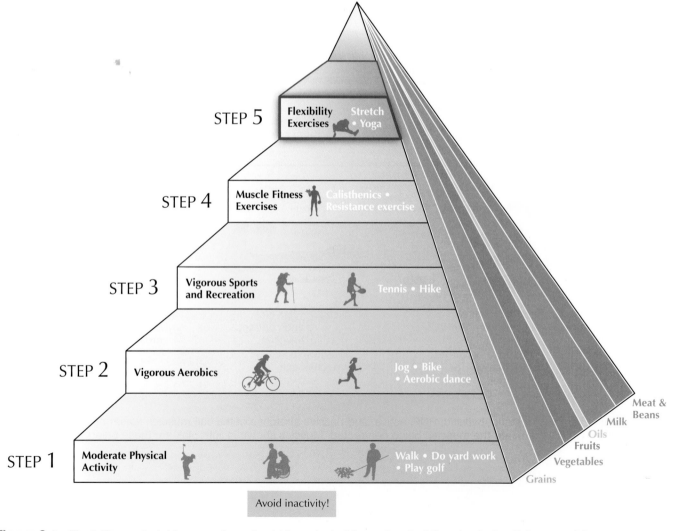

Figure 3 ▶ Flexibility or stretching exercises should be selected from step 5 of the physical activity pyramid.

stretching are to stretch just to the point of tension or just before discomfort. Exercises that do not cause an overload will not increase flexibility. Once adequate flexibility has been achieved, **range of motion (ROM) exercises** that do not require stretch greater than normal can be performed to maintain flexibility and joint range of motion.

For flexibility to be increased, you must stretch and hold muscles beyond normal length for an adequate amount of time. When a muscle is stretched (lengthened), the stretch reflex acts to resist the stretch (see Figure 4). Sensory receptors (A) in the muscle-tendon unit send a signal to the sensory neurons (B), and these neurons signal the motor neurons (C) to contract (shorten) the muscles (D). This reflex restricts initial efforts at stretching; however, if the stretch is held and maintained over time, the stretch reflex subsides and allows the muscle to lengthen (this phase is called the development phase because this is when improvements occur). We emphasize this reflex because it explains why it is important to hold a stretch for an extended period of time. Attempts to stretch for shorter durations are limited by the opposing action of the stretch reflex (see Figure 4). Recent studies suggest that to get the most benefit for the least effort stretching for at least 15 seconds and up to 30 to 60 seconds for each repetition is recommended (see Figure 5). The ACSM suggests that 10 seconds may be an adequate threshold when performing PNF (stretch after muscle contraction).

For flexibility to be increased, you must repeat stretching exercises an adequate number of times. Figure 5 shows the typical responses to a stretched muscle during a series of stretches. Tension in a muscle decreases as the stretch is held. Most of the decrease occurs in the first 15 seconds. The tension curves are lower with each successive repetition of stretching, which is why multiple sets of stretching are recommended. The ACSM recommends a minimum of 4 repetitions because this number seems to give the most benefits for the amount of time spent in exercise. While 3 to 5 reps are recommended (see Table 1), even 1 or 2 repetitions can benefit healthy people not interested in high-level performance.

Principles of overload and progression can be applied to a regular stretching program to both improve and maintain flexibility. Threshold of training refers to the minimum amount of stretching required to make gains and/or maintain a level of flexibility. Target zone refers to the overload needed to make significant gains in flexibility or to progress one's level of flexibility following a plateau. Principles of threshold and target zones are presented in Table 1 for each type of stretching. Stretching should be done at least 3 days a week (preferably daily), but 1 day a week is still better than none. The ACSM recommends stretching for a minimum of 10 minutes 2 to 3 days a week (preferably daily), but 1 day a week is still better than none. Multiple

Agonist Muscles Muscle group being stretched.

Range of Motion (ROM) Exercises Exercises used to maintain existing joint mobility (to prevent loss of ROM).

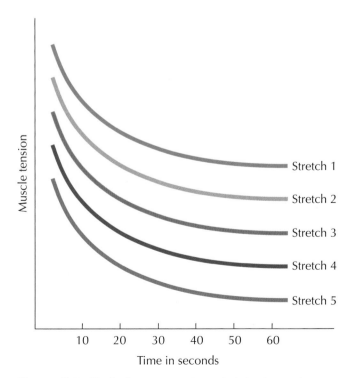

Figure 4 ▶ The stretch reflex.
Source: Shier, Butler, and Lewis.

Figure 5 ▶ Typical responses to a stretched muscle during a series of stretches.

Table 1 ▶ Flexibility Threshold of Training and Target Zones

	Static		Ballistic		PNF (CRAC)	
	Threshold	Target	Threshold	Target	Threshold	Target
Frequency	At least 2 to 3 days a week (threshold)	2–7 days a week	At least 2 to 3 days a week (threshold)	2–7 days a week	At least 2 to 3 days a week (threshold)	2–7 days a week
Intensity	Stretch as far as possible without pain. Slowly move to hold at end of range of motion.	Add passive assistance. Avoid overstretching or pain.	Stretch beyond normal length with gentle bounce or swing. Do not exceed 10% of static range of motion.	Same as ballistic threshold	Same as static threshold, except use a maximum isometric contraction of muscle prior to stretch.	Perform 4–5 reps with 6-second contractions, each followed by a 10–30-second assisted stretch. Thirty seconds between reps.
Duration	Perform 4 reps. Hold each for 15 seconds. Rest 30 seconds between reps.	Perform 4–5 reps. Hold each for 15–60 seconds. Rest 30 seconds between reps.	Perform 1 set involving 30 continuous seconds.	Perform 1–3 sets of 30 consecutive seconds of motion. Rest 1 minute between sets.	Perform 4 reps with a 6-second contraction followed by 10–30-second assisted stretch. Thirty seconds between reps.	Perform 1–3 sets of 3–5 reps of 3-second contraction and 15-second to 60-second hold. Rest 30 seconds between reps. Rest 1 minute between sets.

Table 2 ▶ Do and Don't List for Stretching

Do	Don't
Do warm muscles before you attempt to stretch them.	Don't stretch to the point of pain. Remember, you want to stretch muscles, not joints.
Do stretch with care if you have osteoporosis or arthritis.	Don't use ballistic stretches if you have osteoporosis or arthritis.
Do use static or PNF stretching rather than ballistic stretching if you are a beginner.	Don't perform ballistic stretches with passive assistance unless you are under the supervision of an expert.
Do stretch weak or recently injured muscles with care.	Don't ballistically stretch weak or recently injured muscles.
Do use great care in applying passive assistance to a partner; go slowly and ask for feedback.	Don't overstretch a muscle after it has been immobilized (such as in a sling or cast) for a long period.
Do perform stretching exercises for each muscle group and at each joint where flexibility is desired.	Don't bounce muscles through excessive range of motion. Begin ballistic stretching with gentle movements and gradually increase intensity.
Do make certain the body is in good alignment when stretching.	Don't stretch swollen joints without professional supervision.
Do stretch muscles of small joints in the extremities first; then progress toward the trunk with muscles of larger joints.	Don't stretch several muscles at one time until you have stretched individual muscles. For example, stretch muscles at the ankle, then the knee, then the ankle and knee simultaneously.

stretches of major muscle groups are recommended. For optimal results, stretching sessions of greater length are recommended.

The FIT formula varies for each of the three different methods of stretching. As described in the previous pages and illustrated in Figure 2, there are three principal types of stretching for use in building flexibility: static stretch, PNF, and ballistic stretch. The recommended frequency and duration of the exercise session is similar for all forms of stretching. However, as noted in Table 1, the duration of the stretch is slightly different for ballistic stretch than for static stretch and PNF.

The best time for stretching is following a general cardiovascular warm-up. The ACSM recommends a general aerobic warm-up of at least 10 minutes before beginning your stretching session. Studies have shown that performing warm-up activity prior to stretching can increase internal muscle temperature and the extensibility of soft tissues, allowing for a more effective stretch.

Other studies have failed to find a difference between the flexibility of subjects who warmed up and those who did not warm up. Some experts believe that cooling the muscle with ice packs in the final phases of stretching aids in lengthening the muscle, but one study failed to confirm this. Until scientists reach a consensus, it seems wise to perform the stretching phase of your workout when the muscles are warm. This means that stretching can be done in the middle or near the end of the workout. Since some people do not want to interrupt their workout in the middle, they prefer to stretch at the end. Stretching at the end of the workout serves a dual purpose—building flexibility and cooling down. It is, however, appropriate to stretch at any time in the workout after the muscles have been active and are warm.

Some experts worry that the requirement of a 10-minute warm-up before a stretching workout will be an obstacle for those who have limited time to exercise. As with almost all forms of exercise, something is better than nothing. So it would be better to do static stretching or PNF without a warm-up than to do no stretching at all, especially for people who are not interested in participating in ballistic activities. Some general suggestions for safe and effective stretching are provided in Table 2.

Flexibility-Based Activities

(i) **The popularity of flexibility-based activity has increased in recent years.** In recent FEATURE 3 years, there has been increasing interest in movement disciplines related to flexibility and stretching. Data from the recent Superstudy of Sports Participation conducted by the Sporting Goods Manufacturers Association (SGMA) indicated that yoga and tai chi were among the fastest growing activities. Increases in Pilates classes have been even more pronounced, with rates of irregular participants doubling in the past years. The popularity of these activities suggests that people may be more interested in flexibility-related activity when it is presented in an engaging and interactive format. Some of the growth may also be attributed to increased acceptance of these activities by medical professionals. Distinctions between these activities are provided below.

Tai chi is one of the safest and more established movement disciplines. Tai chi (often translated as Chinese shadow boxing) is considered a martial art but involves the execution of slow, flowing movements called "forms." Numerous studies have supported the benefits of tai chi on a variety of health-related parameters, including flexibility, muscular strength, balance, posture, pain relief, stress, weight reduction, and cardiovascular

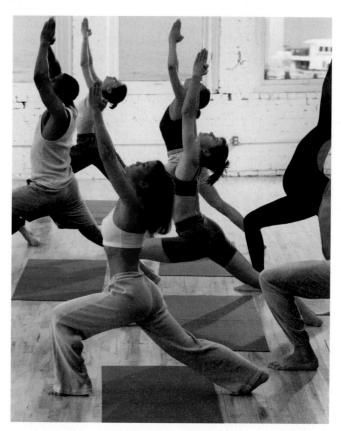

Yoga and other movement classes involving stretching are increasingly popular.

fitness. Recent studies have shown that tai chi can be particularly useful in helping people with arthritis. A unique advantage for arthritic patients is that it effectively strengthens muscles by using both isometric (holding) and isotonic (moving) muscle contractions. Studies have shown strength gains of 15 to 20 percent in elderly tai chi participants. This improved strength translates into joint protection and stability, as well as increased strength for daily living tasks. The highly cited FICSIT study demonstrated significant benefits of tai chi on balance and risk of falls in the elderly. Young participants can benefit as well.

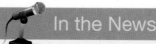

In the News

Flexibility and Stretching Trends

(i) A 2010 survey of Worldwide Fitness Trends NEWS indicates that stretching and flexibility are very much in the forefront. Of the 20 top trends, 6 relate to flexibility. Included are yoga, functional fitness training, special training for older adults, core training, Pilates, and sport-specific training. More information on these trends can be found at the associated Web link.

Technology Update
High-Tech, Low-Tech Stretching

TECH

One advantage of stretching exercises for flexibility is that they typically do not need much equipment to perform. Much of the equipment for use in stretching to improve flexibility is considered to be low tech. A recent high-tech option for those interested in flexibility is Wii Fit Plus, which includes a yoga program. More information about these low- and high-tech options is available at the associated Web link.

Yoga is a diverse and controversial movement discipline. *Yoga* is an umbrella term that refers to a number of yoga traditions. The foundation for most yoga traditions is hatha yoga, which incorporates a variety of asanas (postures). Iyengar yoga is another popular variation. It uses similar asanas as hatha yoga but uses props and cushions to enhance the movements. Emphasis is placed on balance through coordinated breathing and precise body alignment. Most forms of yoga are considered to be safe, but positions in some of the extreme yoga disciplines have been criticized by movement specialists and physical therapists as causing more harm than good, so care should be used when performing some movements. Evidence for health benefits of yoga are not as established as those for tai chi.

Pilates classes are a popular offering at many fitness centers and health clubs. Pilates is a therapeutic exercise regimen that combines strength and flexibility movements. It was originally developed as more of a therapeutic form of exercise, but it is increasingly being promoted as an overall form of conditioning. Emphasis in Pilates exercise is on core stabilization movements and enhanced body awareness, but classes typically include some stretching activities as well.

Check the qualifications of instructors conducting flexibility-related classes. The popularity of flexibility exercise has led to an increasing array of classes, videos, and resources available for tai chi, yoga, and Pilates. When reviewing these programs and materials, keep in mind that presently there is not a strong scientific basis for yoga and Pilates programming. When performed safely with a qualified instructor, they probably can be beneficial. However, many of the positions and movements may be contraindicated exercises that could increase risk for injuries. If you choose to participate in these activities, seek qualified instructors and progress gradually. See Concept 11 for more information about safe and contraindicated exercises.

Guidelines for Safe and Effective Stretching Exercise

There is a correct way to perform flexibility exercises. Remember that stretching can *cause* muscle soreness, so "easy does it." Start at your threshold if you are unaccustomed to stretching a given muscle group; then increase within the target zone. The list in Table 2 will help you gain the most benefit from your exercises.

Stretching is specific to each muscle or muscle group. No single exercise can produce total flexibility. For example, stretching tight hamstrings can increase the length of these muscles but will not lengthen the muscles in other areas of the body. For total flexibility, it is important to stretch each of the major muscle groups and to use the major joints of the body through full range of normal motion.

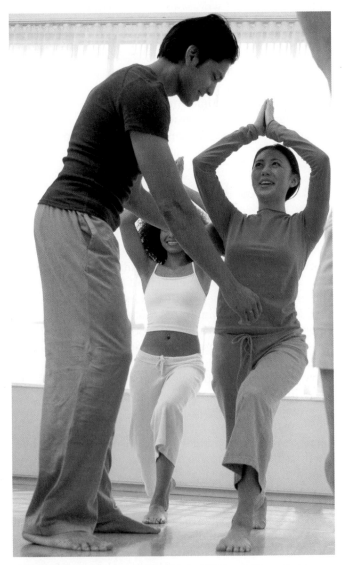

To get the most out of yoga, tai chi, and Pilates classes, find a qualified instructor.

Specialized equipment may help improve the effectiveness and ease of stretching exercise. One advance in equipment technology for flexibility training is the development of "stretching ropes." These ropes have multiple loops, which enable individuals to change the length of the rope and perform a variety of different exercises. This feature provides an easy way to put muscles on stretch and to vary the degree of stretch. Because you can apply resistance through the elastic straps, it is even possible to perform PNF stretching without the assistance of a partner. A variety of stretching ropes are available on the market, and they all provide similar functionality.

Strategies for Action

An important step for developing and maintaining flexibility is assessing your current status. An important early step in taking action to improve fitness is self-assessment. There are dozens of tests of flexibility. Four tests that assess range of motion in the major joints of the body, that require little equipment, and that can be easily administered are presented in the *Lab Resources Materials* at the end of this concept. In Lab 10A, you will get an opportunity to try these self-assessments. It is recommended that you perform these assessments before you begin your regular stretching program and use these assessments to reevaluate your flexibility periodically.

Scores on flexibility tests may be influenced by several factors. Your range of motion at any one time may be influenced by your motivation to exert maximum effort, warm-up preparation, muscular soreness, tolerance for pain, room temperature, and ability to relax. Recent studies have found a relationship between leg or trunk length and the scores made on the sit-and-reach test. The sit-and-reach test used in this book is adapted to allow for differences in body build.

Select exercises that promote flexibility in all areas of the body. For total body flexibility, 8 to 10 stretching exercises for the major muscle groups of the body are recommended. Table 3 describes some of the most effective exercises for a basic flexibility routine. Individual stretching needs may vary, but the most common areas to target are the trunk, the legs, and the arms. A variety of stretches for these areas are described in Tables 3, 4, and 5. Most are designed for static stretching, but the pectoral stretch and back-saver hamstring stretch use PNF techniques. Ballistic stretching exercises are discussed in more detail in Concept 12.

Keeping records of progress will help you adhere to a stretching program. An activity logging sheet is provided in Lab 10B to help you keep records of your progress as you regularly perform stretching exercises to build and maintain good flexibility.

Web Resources

Additional websites with information related to Concept 10 are available at the associated Web link.

CDC Physical Activity for Everyone **www.cdc.gov/ physicalactivity/everyone/guidelines/adults.html**

National Center for Complementary and Alternative Medicine—NCCAM **http://nccam.nih.gov/about/ plans/2005/page2.htm**

National Institute for Aging—Stretching Guidelines **www.nia.nih.gov/HealthInformation/Publications/**

Orthopedic Physical Therapy Products (source for stretching ropes) **www.optp.com**

Suggested Readings

Selected readings and references are listed below. A more comprehensive list is available at the associated Web link.

ACSM. 2010. *ACSM's Guidelines for Exercise Testing and Prescription.* 8th ed. Philadelphia: Lippincott, Williams & Wilkins, Chapter 7.

Faigenbaum, A., and J. E. McFarland. 2007. Guidelines for implementing a dynamic warm-up for physical education. *Journal of Physical Education, Recreation and Dance* 78(3):25–28.

Kovacs, M. 2009. *Dynamic Stretching: The Revolutionary New Warm-up Method to Improve Power, Performance and Range of Motion.* Berkeley, CA: Ulysses Press.

McAtee, R., and J. Charland. 2007. *Facilitated Stretching.* 3rd ed. Champaign, IL: Human Kinetics.

Nelson, J. G., and J. J. Kokkonen. 2007. *Stretching Anatomy.* Champaign, IL: Human Kinetics.

Nieman, D. C. 2008. You asked for it. The merits of stretching. *ACSM's Health and Fitness Journal* 12(4):5–6.

Table 3

Table 3 The Basic Eight for Trunk Stretching Exercises

1. Upper Trapezius/Neck Stretch

This exercise stretches the muscles on the back and sides of the neck. To stretch the right trapezius, place left hand on top of your head. Gently look down toward your left underarm, tucking your chin toward your chest. Let the weight of your arm gently draw your head forward. Hold. Repeat to the opposite side.

  Scalenes: The stretch above may be modified to stretch the muscles on the front and sides of the neck. Start from the stretch position described above. Keep your left ear near your left shoulder. Turn your head slightly and look up toward the ceiling, lifting your chin 2–3″. Hold.

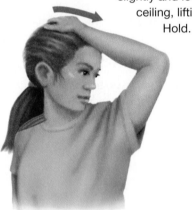

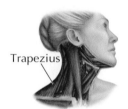

Trapezius

2. Chin Tuck

This exercise stretches the muscles at the base of the skull and reduces headache symptoms. Sit up straight, with chest lifted and shoulders back. Gently tuck in the chin by making a slight motion of nodding "yes." Imagine a string attached to the back of your head, which is pulling your head upward, like a puppet. As your chin draws inward, attempt to lengthen the back of your neck. Hold.

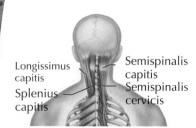

Longissimus capitis
Semispinalis capitis
Splenius capitis
Semispinalis cervicis

3. Pectoral Stretch

This exercise stretches the chest muscles (pectorals).
1. Stand erect in doorway, with arms raised 45 degrees, elbows bent, hands grasping the doorjamb, and feet in front-stride position. Press out on door frame, contracting your arms maximally for 6 seconds. Relax and shift weight forward on legs. Lean into doorway, so that the muscles on the front of your shoulder joint and chest are stretched. Hold.
2. Repeat with your arms raised 90 degrees.
3. Repeat with your arms raised 135 degrees. This exercise is useful to prevent or correct round shoulders and sunken chest.

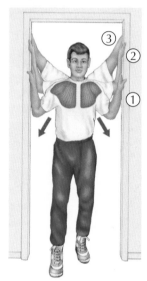

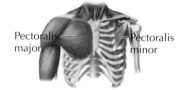

Pectoralis major
Pectoralis minor

4. Lateral Trunk Stretch

This exercise stretches the trunk muscles. Sit on the floor. Stretch the left arm over your head, to the right. Bend to the right at the waist, reaching as far to the right as possible with your left arm and as far as possible to the left with your right arm; hold. Do not let your trunk rotate. Repeat on the opposite side. For less stretch, your overhead arm may be bent at the elbow. This exercise can be done in the standing position, but is less effective.

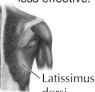

Latissimus dorsi

The Basic Eight for Trunk Stretching Exercises **Table 3**

5. Leg Hug

This exercise stretches the hip and back extensor muscles. Lie on your back. Bend one leg and grasp your thigh under the knee. Hug it to your chest. Keep the other leg straight and on the floor. Hold. Repeat with the opposite leg.

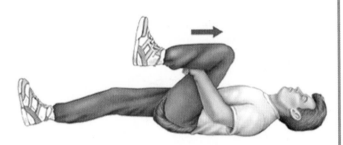

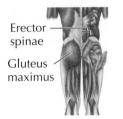

Erector spinae

Gluteus maximus

7. Trunk Twist

This exercise stretches the trunk muscles and the muscles on the outside of the hip. Sit with your right leg extended, left leg bent and crossed over the right knee. Place your right arm on the left side of the left leg and push against that leg while turning the trunk as far as possible to the left. Place the left hand on the floor behind the buttocks. Stretch and hold. Reverse position and repeat on the opposite side.

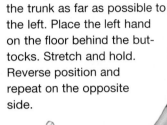

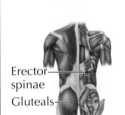

Erector spinae

Gluteals

6. Heel Sit

This exercise stretches the muscles of the lower back. Begin on hands and knees with eyes looking down toward the floor. Keep your hands on the floor directly below your shoulders. Rock backwards, bringing your buttocks toward your heels. Gently round the lower back outward. Hold.

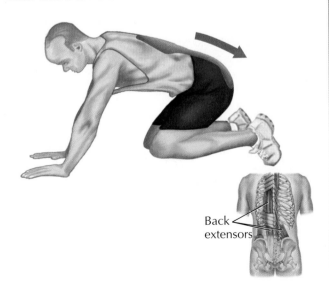

Back extensors

8. Spine Twist

This exercise stretches the trunk rotators and lateral rotators of the thighs. Start in hook-lying position, arms extended at shoulder level. Cross your left knee over the right. Push the right knee to the floor, using the pressure of the left knee and leg. Keep your arms and shoulders on the floor while touching your knees to the floor on the left. Stretch and hold. Reverse leg position and lower your knees to right.

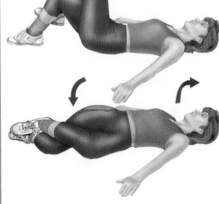

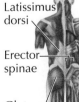

Latissimus dorsi

Erector spinae

Gluteus maximus

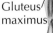

213

Table 4 The Basic Eight for Leg Stretching Exercises

Table 4

1. Calf Stretch

This exercise stretches the calf muscles and Achilles tendon. Face a wall with your feet 2′ or 3′ away. Step forward on your left foot to allow both hands to touch the wall. Keep the heel of your right foot on the ground, toe turned in slightly, knee straight, and buttocks tucked in. Lean forward by bending your front knee and arms and allowing your head to move nearer the wall. Hold. Bend your right knee, keeping your heel on floor. Stretch and hold. Repeat with the other leg.

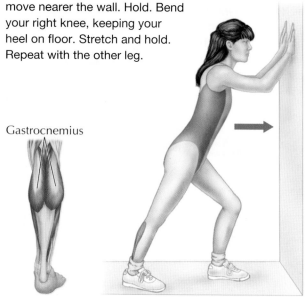

Gastrocnemius

2. Shin Stretch

This exercise relieves shin muscle soreness by stretching the muscles on the front of the shin. Kneel on both knees, turn to the right, and press down and stretch your right ankle with your right hand. Move your pelvis forward. Hold. Repeat on the opposite side. Except when they are sore, most people need to strengthen rather than stretch these muscles.

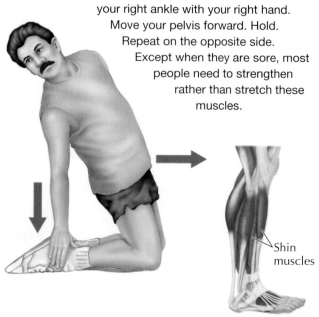

Shin muscles

3. Back-Saver Hamstring Stretch

This exercise stretches the hamstrings and calf muscles and helps prevent or correct backache caused in part by short hamstrings. Sit on the floor with the feet against the wall or an immovable object. Bend left knee and bring foot close to buttocks. Clasp hands behind back. Contract the muscles on the back of the upper leg (hamstrings) by pressing the heel downward toward the floor; hold; relax. Bend forward from hips, keeping lower back as straight as possible. Let bent knee rotate outward so trunk can move forward. Lean forward keeping back flat; hold and repeat on each leg.

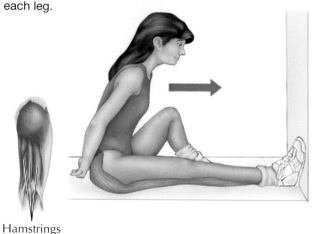

Hamstrings

4. Hip and Thigh Stretch

This exercise stretches the hip (iliopsoas) and thigh muscles (quadriceps) and is useful for people with lordosis and back problems. Place your right knee directly above your right ankle and stretch your left leg backward so your knee touches the floor. If necessary, place your hands on floor for balance.

1. Tilt the pelvis backward by tucking in the abdomen and flattening the back.
2. Then shift the weight forward until a stretch is felt on the front of the thigh; hold. Repeat on the opposite side. Caution: Do not bend your front knee more than 90 degrees.

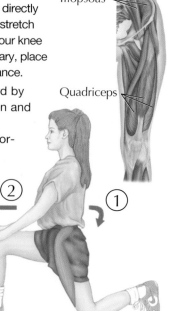

Iliopsoas

Quadriceps

5. Sitting Stretch

This exercise stretches the muscles on the inside of the thighs. Sit with the soles of your feet together; place your hands on your knees or ankles and lean your forearms against your knees; resist (contract) by attempting to raise your knees. Hold. Relax and press the knees toward the floor as far as possible; hold. This exercise is useful for pregnant women and anyone whose thighs tend to rotate inward, causing backache, knock-knees, and flat feet.

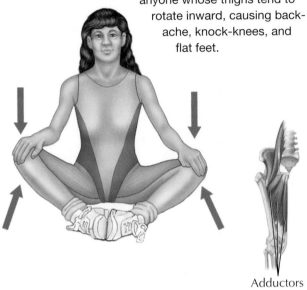

Adductors

7. Inner Thigh Stretch

This exercise stretches the muscles of the inner thigh. Stand with feet spread wider than shoulder-width apart. Shift weight onto the right foot and bend the right knee slightly. Straighten left knee and raise toes of left foot off the floor. Lean forward slightly from the waist keeping back straight/shoulders back. Shift weight back over the right foot by moving hips diagonally away from the left foot. Hold. Repeat in the opposite direction.

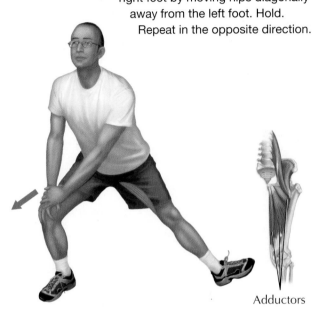

Adductors

6. Lateral Thigh and Hip Stretch

This exercise stretches the muscles and connective tissue on the outside of the legs (iliotibial band and tensor fascia lata). Stand with your left side to the wall, left arm extended and palm of your hand flat on the wall for support. Cross the left leg behind the right leg and turn the toes of both feet out slightly. Bend your left knee slightly and shift your pelvis toward the wall (left) as your trunk bends toward the right. Adjust until tension is felt down the outside of the left hip and thigh. Stretch and hold. Repeat on the other side.

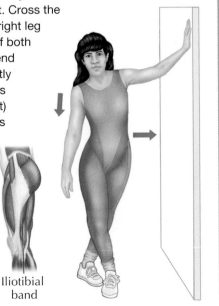

Iliotibial
band

8. Deep Buttock Stretch

This exercise stretches the deep buttock muscles, such as the piriformis. Lie on your back with knees bent and one ankle crossed over opposite knee. Hold thigh of bottom leg and pull gently toward your chest. Hold. Repeat on the other side.

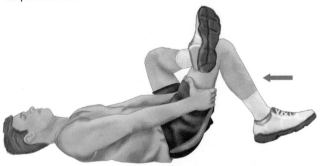

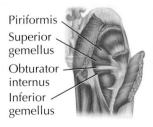

Piriformis
Superior
gemellus
Obturator
internus
Inferior
gemellus

Table 5

Table 5 The Basic Four for Arm Stretching Exercises

1. Forearm Stretch

This exercise stretches the muscles on the front and back sides of the lower arm. It is particularly useful in relieving stress from excessive keyboarding activity. Hold your right arm straight out in front, with your palm facing down. Use your left hand to gently stretch the fingertips of your right hand toward the floor. Hold. Turn your right arm over with your palm facing up. Use your left hand to gently stretch the fingertips of your right hand toward the floor. Hold. Repeat on the opposite side.

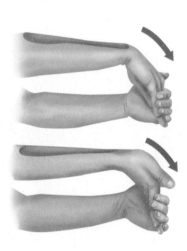

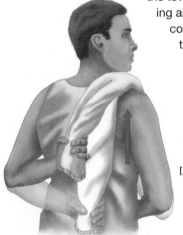

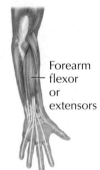

Forearm flexor or extensors

2. Back Scratcher

Stand straight with back of left hand held flat against back. With right hand, throw one end of a towel over right shoulder from front to back. Grab end of towel with left hand. Pull down gently on the towel with right hand, raising arm in back as high as is comfortable. Hold. Repeat to opposite side.

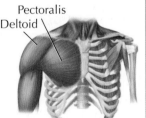

Pectoralis
Deltoid

3. Overhead Arm Stretch

This exercise stretches the triceps and latissimus dorsi muscles. Stretch your arms up overhead. Grasp your right elbow with your left hand. Pull your right elbow back behind your head. Hold. Repeat on opposite side.

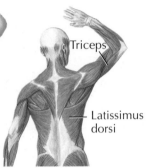

Triceps

Latissimus dorsi

4. Arm Pretzel

This exercise stretches the shoulder muscles (lateral rotators). Stand or sit with your elbows flexed at right angles, palms up. Cross your right arm over your left; grasp your right thumb with your left hand and pull gently downward, causing your right arm to rotate laterally. Stretch and hold. Reverse arm position and repeat on your left arm.

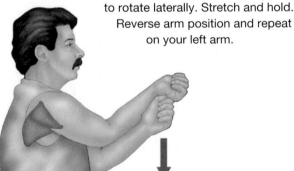

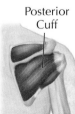

Posterior Cuff

Lab Resource Materials: Flexibility Tests

Directions: To test the flexibility of all joints is impractical. These tests are for joints used frequently. Follow the instructions carefully. Determine your flexibility using Chart 1.

Test

1. *Modified Sit-and-Reach* (Flexibility Test of Hamstrings)

   a. Remove shoes and sit on the floor. Place the sole of the foot of the extended leg flat against a box or bench. Bend opposite knee and place the head, back, and hips against a wall with a 90-degree angle at the hips.

   b. Place one hand over the other and slowly reach forward as far as you can with arms fully extended. Keep head and back in contact with the wall. A partner will slide the measuring stick on the bench until it touches the fingertips.

   c. With the measuring stick fixed in the new position, reach forward as far as possible, three times, holding the position on the third reach for at least 2 seconds while the partner records the distance on the ruler. Keep the knee of the extended leg straight (see illustration).

   d. Repeat the test a second time and average the scores of the two trials.

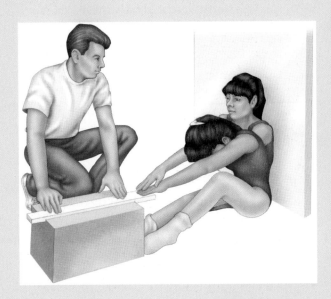

Test

2. *Shoulder Flexibility* ("Zipper" Test)

   a. Raise your arm, bend your elbow, and reach down across your back as far as possible.

   b. At the same time, extend your left arm down and behind your back, bend your elbow up across your back, and try to cross your fingers over those of your right hand as shown in the accompanying illustration.

   c. Measure the distance to the nearest half-inch. If your fingers overlap, score as a plus. If they fail to meet, score as a minus; use a zero if your fingertips just touch.

   d. Repeat with your arms crossed in the opposite direction (left arm up). Most people will find that they are more flexible on one side than the other.

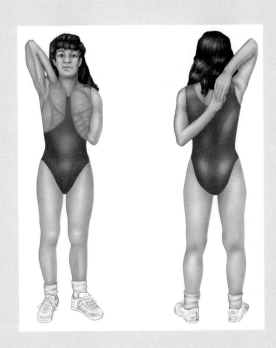

Test

3. *Hamstring and Hip Flexor Flexibility*

   a. Lie on your back on the floor beside a wall.

   b. Slowly lift one leg off the floor. Keep the other leg flat on the floor.

   c. Keep both legs straight.

   d. Continue to lift the leg until either leg begins to bend or the lower leg begins to lift off the floor.

   e. Place a yardstick against the wall and underneath the lifted leg.

   f. Hold the yardstick against the wall after the leg is lowered.

   g. Using a protractor, measure the angle created by the floor and the yardstick. The greater the angle, the better your score.

   h. Repeat with the other leg.*

*Note: For ease of testing, you may want to draw angles on a piece of posterboard, as illustrated. If you have goniometers, you may be taught to use them instead.

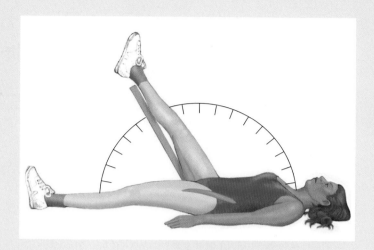

Test

4. *Trunk Rotation*

   a. Tape two yardsticks to the wall at shoulder height, one right side up and the other upside down.

   b. Stand with your left shoulder an arm's length (fist closed) from the wall. Toes should be on the line, which is perpendicular to the wall and even with the 15-inch mark on the yardstick.

   c. Drop the left arm and raise the right arm to the side, palm down, fist closed.

   d. Without moving your feet, rotate the trunk to the right as far as possible, reaching along the yardstick, and hold it 2 seconds. Do not move the feet or bend the trunk. Your knees may bend slightly.

   e. A partner will read the distance reached to the nearest half-inch. Record your score. Repeat two times and average your two scores.

   f. Next, perform the test facing the opposite direction. Rotate to the left. For this test, you will use the second yardstick (upside down) so that, the greater the rotation, the higher the score. If you have only one yardstick, turn it right side up for the first test and upside down for the second test.

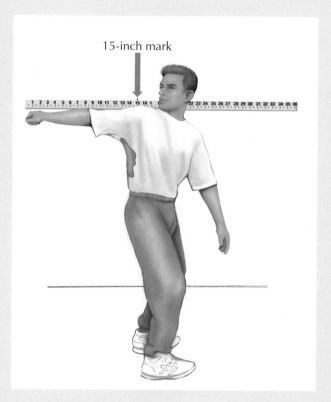

15-inch mark

Chart 1 ▶ Flexibility Rating Scale for Tests 1–4

Classification	Men					Women				
	Test 1	Test 2		Test 3	Test 4	Test 1	Test 2		Test 3	Test 4
		Right Up	Left Up				Right Up	Left Up		
High performance*	16+	5+	4+	111+	20+	17+	6+	5+	111+	20.5 or >
Good fitness zone	13–15	1–4	1–3	80–110	16–19.5	14–16	2–5	2–4	80–110	17–20
Marginal zone	10–12	0	0	60–79	13.5–15.5	11–13	1	1	60–79	14.5–16.5
Low zone	<9	<0	<0	<60	<13.5	<10	<1	<1	<60	<14.5

*Though performers need good flexibility, hypermobility may increase injury risk.

Lab 10A Evaluating Flexibility

Name   Section   Date

Purpose: To evaluate your flexibility in several joints

Procedures

1. Take the flexibility tests outlined in *Lab Resource Materials.*
2. Record your scores in the Results section.
3. Use Chart 1 in *Lab Resource Materials* to determine your ratings on the self-assessments; then place an X over the circle for the appropriate rating.

Results

Flexibility Scores and Ratings

Record Scores			Record Ratings			
			High Performance	Good Fitness	Marginal	Poor
Modified sit-and-reach						
Test 1	Left		○	○	○	○
	Right		○	○	○	○
Zipper						
Test 2	Left		○	○	○	○
	Right		○	○	○	○
Hamstring/hip flexor						
Test 3	Left		○	○	○	○
	Right		○	○	○	○
Trunk rotation						
Test 4	Left		○	○	○	○
	Right		○	○	○	○

Do any of these muscle groups need stretching? Check one circle for each muscle group.

	Yes	No
Back of the thighs and knees (hamstrings)	◯	◯
Calf muscles	◯	◯
Lower back (lumbar region)	◯	◯
Front of right shoulder	◯	◯
Back of right shoulder	◯	◯
Front of left shoulder	◯	◯
Back of left shoulder	◯	◯
Most of the body	◯	◯
Trunk muscles	◯	◯

Conclusions and Implications: In several sentences, discuss your current flexibility and your flexibility needs for the future. Include comments about your current state of flexibility, need for improvement in specific areas, and special flexibility needs for sports or other special activities.

Lab 10B Planning and Logging Stretching Exercises

Name	**Section**	**Date**

Purpose: To set 1-week lifestyle goals for stretching exercises, to prepare a stretching for flexibility plan, and to self-monitor progress in your 1-week plan

Procedures

1. Using Chart 1, provide some background information about your experience with stretching exercise, your goals, and your plans for incorporating these exercises into your normal exercise routine.
2. In Chart 2, keep a log of your actual participation in stretching exercise. You can choose from any of the stretching exercises described in Table 3, 4, or 5. Try to pick at least eight exercises and try to perform them at least 3 days in the week (ideally every day).
3. Describe your experiences with your stretching exercise program. Be sure to comment on your plans for future stretching exercise.

Chart 1 ▶ Stretching Exercise Survey

1. Determine your current stage for flexibility exercise. Check only the stage that represents your current activity level.

   ◯ Precontemplation. I do not meet flexibility exercise guidelines and have not been thinking about starting.

   ◯ Contemplation. I do not do exercise guidelines but have been thinking about starting.

   ◯ Preparation. I am planning to start doing regular flexibility exercises to meet guidelines.

   ◯ Action. I do flexibility exercises, but I am not as regular as I should be.

   ◯ Maintenance. I regularly meet guidelines for flexibility exercises.

2. What are your primary goals for flexibility exercise?

   ◯ General conditioning

   ◯ Sports improvement (specify sport:_____)

   ◯ Health benefits

3. Are you currently involved in a regular stretching program? If yes, describe your program. If no, describe barriers that have prevented you from stretching.

   ◯ Yes

   ◯ No

   _____

Results

	Yes	No
Did you do eight exercises at least 3 days in the week?	◯	◯
Did you do eight exercises more than 3 days in the week?	◯	◯

Chart 2 ▶ Stretching Exercise Log

List the stretching exercises you actually performed and the days on which you performed them.	Day 1 Date:	Day 2 Date:	Day 3 Date:	Day 4 Date:	Day 5 Date:	Day 6 Date:	Day 7 Date:
1.							
2.							
3.							
4.							
5.							
6.							
7.							
8.							

Conclusions and Interpretations

1. Do you feel that you will use stretching exercises as part of your regular lifetime physical activity plan, either now or in the future? Use several sentences to explain your answer.

2. Discuss the exercises you feel benefited you and the ones that did not. What exercises would you continue to do and which ones would you change? Use several sentences to explain your answer.

Body Mechanics: Posture, Questionable Exercises, and Care of the Back and Neck

Health Objectives for the Year 2020

- Attain high-quality, longer lives free of preventable injury.
- Reduce activity limitations due to chronic back pain.
- Reduce joint pain in adults who have doctor-diagnosed arthritis.
- Reduce proportion of adults with arthritis limitations—preserve independence/reduce job loss.
- Reduce prevalence of osteoporosis and hip fractures.
- Reduce sports and recreation injuries.
- Increase access to employee-based exercise facilities and programs.

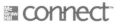 **connect** | FITNESS AND WELLNESS   **http://connect.mcgraw-hill.com**

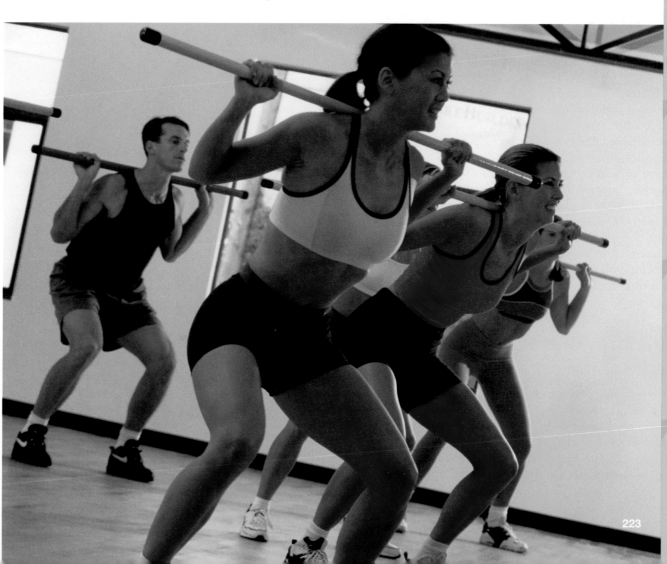

The health, integrity, and function of the neck and back are influenced by modifiable as well as nonmodifiable factors. Maintaining a healthy neck and back can be attained by using good posture, good body mechanics, and safe exercise technique.

The neck and back serve vital roles in supporting the weight of the head and body, producing movement, carrying loads, and protecting the spinal cord and nerves. These roles are facilitated by optimal alignment of the vertebrae and a balance between muscular strength and flexibility. Impairment of one or more of these functions can lead to injuries to the muscles, vertebrae, discs, ligaments, or nerves of the spine. Neck and back pain are common in today's society, with nearly 80 percent of the population experiencing an episode of low back pain sometime in their lives. Back pain is second only to headache as a common medical complaint, and an estimated 30 to 70 percent of Americans have recurring back problems. The multiple functions of the spinal column may predispose this area to injuries. The spine helps to produce an array of movements while bearing significant loads.

Chronic back and neck pain are associated with many personal health problems. Some cases of back pain are "idiopathic" (no known cause), but some are clearly preventable. This concept provides information about the interrelated function of the spine and trunk musculature to help you be more informed about back health. Specific information is provided about core training, posture, body mechanics, and safe exercise performance to help you adopt preventive measures that may reduce your risk for back and neck problems. This information is intended to provide a basic foundation of knowledge. Persons with neck or back pain should always seek direction from their own medical provider.

Anatomy and Function of the Spine

The spinal column is arranged for movement. The bones that make up the spine are called vertebrae. There are 33 vertebrae in the spine, and most are separated from one another by an **intervertebral disc** (see Figure 1). The vertebrae are divided into three main regions commonly referred to as cervical (neck), thoracic

(upper back), and lumbar (low back). The fused vertebrae that form the tailbone are called the sacrum and coccyx. The connections among the vertebrae of the cervical, thoracic, and lumbar spine allow the trunk to move in complex ways. The spine is capable of flexion (forward bending), extension (backward bending), side bending, and rotation, but functionally, these movements often

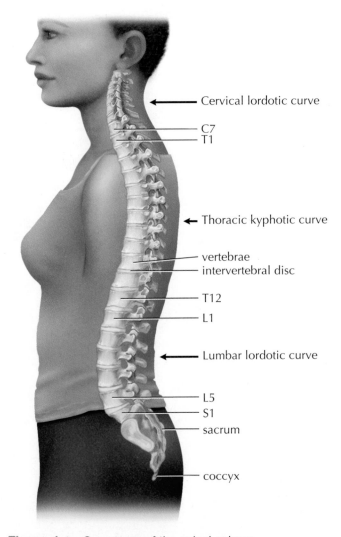

Figure 1 ▶ Curvatures of the spinal column.

Labels on figure:
- Cervical lordotic curve
- C7
- T1
- Thoracic kyphotic curve
- vertebrae
- intervertebral disc
- T12
- L1
- Lumbar lordotic curve
- L5
- S1
- sacrum
- coccyx

occur in combination. For example, in executing a tennis serve, the spine both extends and rotates. The spine is at risk for injury when movements are performed repetitively, performed beyond a joint's healthy range of motion, or performed under conditions of heavy or inefficient lifting.

The spinal column has an important role in bearing loads and protecting the neck and back from injury. The widest portion of each vertebra articulates with the intervertebral disc to form a strong pillar of support extending from the skull to the pelvis. The unique structure of the intervertebral discs is critical in distributing force and absorbing shock. The bony structure of the spine allows you to bear loads and provides protection to the spinal cord and spinal nerves. Poor posture and poor body mechanics can damage discs and vertebrae, resulting in pain and disability.

Anatomy and Function of the Core Musculature

(i) **The core is part of an integrated system that provides stability to the spine.** The
FEATURE 1 core includes musculature of the abdominals, back extensors, lateral trunk flexors, diaphragm, pelvic floor, and hips. A few of the more familiar muscles of the core include the lumbar multifidus, transversus abdominis, and internal oblique. There is no definitive list of muscles belonging to the core. Some sources may describe the core in terms of 6 or fewer key muscle groups, while other sources may include as many as 20 different muscle groups. Regardless, muscles of the core all share a common anatomical trait: their location and attachment to either the spine, pelvis or rib cage. Collectively, the core musculature form a three-dimensional cylinder that encompasses the body's center of gravity. This three-dimensional cylinder is inclusive of the lumbar spine, pelvis, and hips (see Figure 2).

Core stability refers to the body's ability to maintain the spine in a "neutral" postural zone, one in which the physiologic load on the spine is minimized. The overall function of the spinal stabilization system depends on the contribution of three components: a passive restraint system (ligaments, discs, vertebrae, and joints), active restraint system (muscle-tendon units), and neural control system (proprioception and feed-forward mechanisms of the nervous system). Core muscles incorporate functions of both the active restraint and neural control systems to maintain ideal postural alignment, thereby minimizing excessive stress and strain to the spine.

Muscles of the core are commonly classified as either mobilizers or stabilizers. In general, the mobilizers are those muscles that are more superficial and contract concentrically to produce trunk movements. The stabilizers are muscles that are more deeply located and contract isometrically or eccentrically to stabilize the trunk during arm and leg movements. The stabilizer group is further divided into two categories, local and global. These groups are distinguished by differences in anatomy and function.

The **local core stabilizers** provide stiffness and stability to the spine. They include muscles that possess a small cross-sectional area, are deeply located, and may span just one or two vertebral levels at a time. Functionally, these muscles provide local spinal support, control motion between adjacent vertebrae, increase intra-abdominal pressure, and provide proprioception input to the body to avoid injury. The most notable example of a local core stabilizer is the lumbar multifidus. Also included in the group are muscles that indirectly influence the stability of the spine due to their role in increasing intra-abdominal pressure and their supportive attachment to the fascia of the back. These muscles include the transversus abdominis, internal oblique, diaphragm, and pelvic floor muscles. The local core muscles are believed to maintain the spine in "neutral" via isometric co-contractions, thereby minimizing excessive loading of the spine.

The **global core stabilizers** function to produce trunk motion as well as trunk stability based on their attachments to the pelvis. These muscles tend to have a larger cross-sectional area, are more superficially located, often span multiple vertebral levels, and possess attachments to the pelvis, rib cage and/or thoracic spine. Examples include the rectus abdominis, external oblique, quadratus lumborum, and erector spinae. Also included are muscles of the hip, which indirectly influence lumbar stability by altering tilt of the pelvis. Functionally the global core stabilizers generate movement of the trunk as well as provide stabilization.

Intervertebral Discs Spinal discs; cushions of cartilage between the bodies of the vertebrae. Each disc consists of a fibrous outer ring (annulus fibrosus) and a pulpy center (nucleus pulposus).

Local Core Stabilizers Deep core muscles that provide stiffness and stability to the spine.

Global Core Stabilizers Superficial core muscles that produce motion and aid in stabilization.

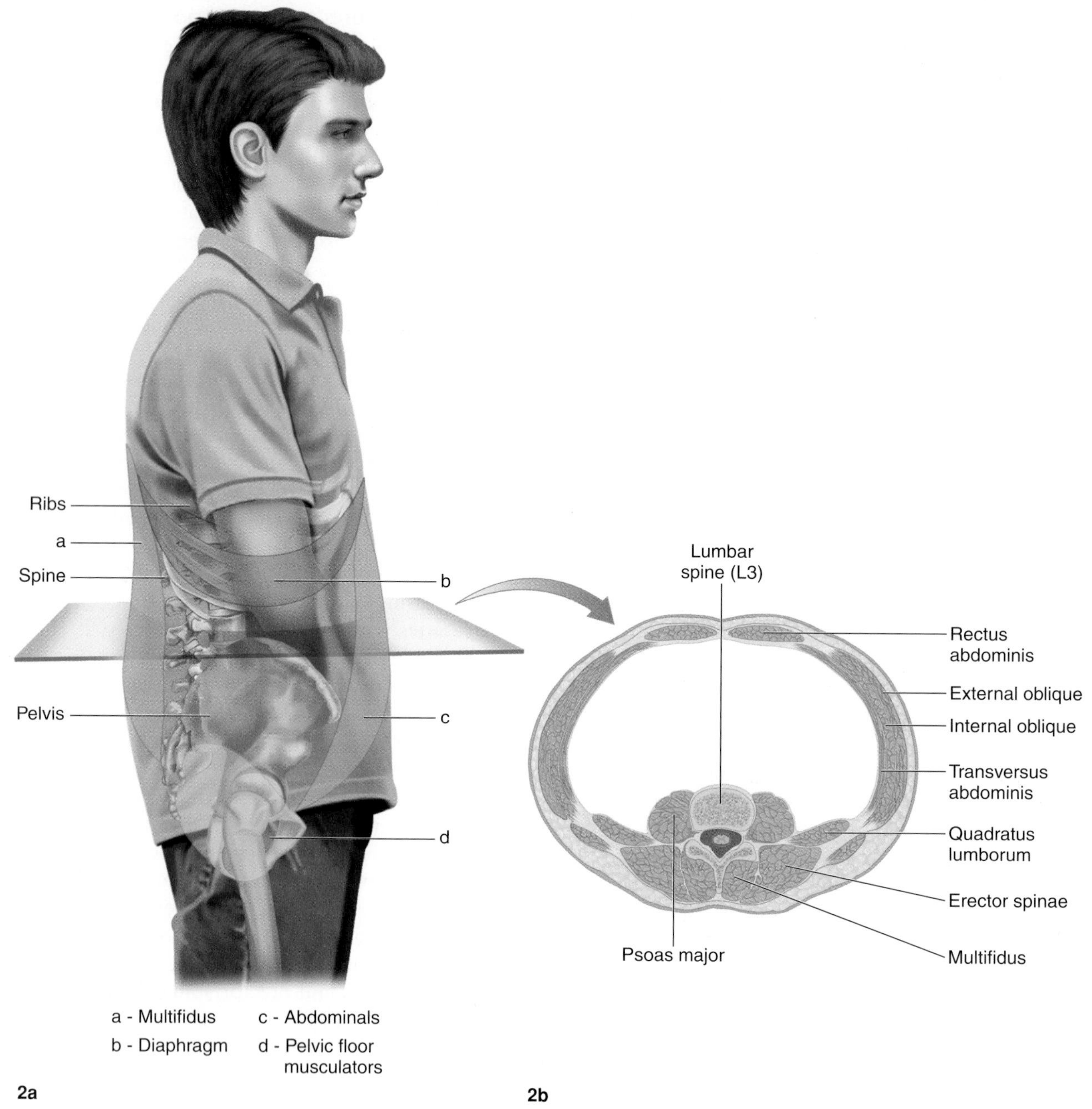

a - Multifidus   c - Abdominals
b - Diaphragm   d - Pelvic floor
                      musculators

2a   2b

Figure 2 ▶ Cross section showing layers of core musculature.

Causes and Consequences of Back and Neck Pain

Most back and neck pain stems from lifestyle choices or life experiences. The original cause (or causes) of back and neck pain are typically hard to identify. Although back and neck problems can result from an acute injury (e.g., a diving accident or car accident), most are caused by accumulated stresses over a lifetime. These factors include the avoidable effects of poor posture and body mechanics as well as performance of questionable exercises that put the back at risk (exercises to avoid are discussed later in the concept). Musculoskeletal injuries and degenerative changes to the discs, vertebrae, joint surfaces, muscles, or ligaments can predispose you to back and neck problems. Depression, cancer, infections, and some visceral diseases (kidney, pelvic organs) can also contribute to back problems. Although people have some control over these causes, some back pain stems directly from structural or functional disorders that a person is born with. Inherited causes include anomalies of the spine, such as **scoliosis.**

To reduce risk for back pain, it is important to try to reduce the risk factors that you have control over.

Modifiable risk factors (factors you can change) include regular heavy labor, use of vibrational tools, routines of prolonged sitting, smoking, a hypokinetic lifestyle, coronary artery disease, and obesity. Nonmodifiable risk factors include a family history of joint disease, age, and direct trauma (e.g., a fall or rough athletic activity when young). Lab 11A provides a questionnaire for assessing your potential risk for back and neck pain.

ⓘ **The nervous system and various pain-sensitive structures contribute to**
FEATURE 2 **back pain.** Back pain can result from direct or indirect causes. Direct causes are typically the result of tissue trauma to areas in or around the spinal column. The most common sources of pain are ligaments, intervertebral discs, nerve roots, spinal joints, and muscles. Indirect causes stem from the release of pain-causing chemicals from injured tissues. These chemicals cause nerves in the area to remain irritated and sensitive. Processes within the brainstem, spinal cord, and peripheral nerves can also modulate the sensation of pain, either increasing or decreasing it. For example, some back pain can be caused by abnormal feedback loops that enhance or maintain the perception of pain—even when the original cause or problem is corrected.

The integrity of the neck and back are jeopardized by excessive stress and strain. Forces are constantly at work to bend, twist, shear, compress, or lengthen tissues of the body. Stress on these tissues may eventually create strain, a change in the tissue's size or dimension. Healthy tissues typically return to their normal state once the force is removed. Injury occurs when excessive stress and strain prevent the tissue from returning to its normal state.

Poor posture (e.g., slouching or forward head positions) can cause body segments to experience stress and strain. When body segments are out of alignment, muscles in the back and neck must work hard to compensate. This creates excessive stress and strain in the affected area(s). Over time, tension in these muscles can lead to **myofascial trigger points,** causing headache or **referred pain** in the face, scalp, shoulder, arm, and chest. The chronic stress from poor alignment can also lead to other postural deviations and degenerative changes in the neck.

Bad body mechanics and improper lifting techniques also contribute to stress and strain on the spine. The lumbar vertebrae and the sacrum are most vulnerable to this type of injury due to the significant weight they support and the thinner ligamentous support at this level.

Some exercises and movements can produce microtrauma, which can lead to back and neck pain. Most people are familiar with acute injuries, such as ankle sprains. These injuries are associated with immediate onset of pain and swelling. **Microtrauma** is a "silent injury"—a subtle form of injury that results from accumulated damage over time. Microtrauma can result from repeatedly performing unsafe exercises or from repeatedly performing the same repetitive motion. For example, the common workplace injury of carpal tunnel syndrome is typically caused by long and extended periods of typing on a keyboard with poor hand positioning. Other terms that frequently appear in the scientific literature include *repetitive motion syndrome, repetitive strain injury (RSI), cumulative trauma disorder (CTD),* and *overuse syndrome.*

The common characteristic of microtrauma is the repeated nature of the position or the contraindicated movement. We may violate the integrity of our joints by performing, for example, 40 backward arm circles with the palms down 3 days per week for 10 or 20 years. We don't usually notice the wear and tear until the friction over time causes microscopic changes in the joint, such as fibrosis of the synovial lining, abnormal thickening of the surrounding joint capsule, thinning and roughening of the articular cartilage cushioning joint surfaces, and calcifications in the rotator cuff tendon. Because these changes are unseen and often unfelt, we view the exercise as harmless. Later in life, microtrauma becomes apparent, resulting in tendonitis, bursitis, arthritis, or nerve compression. Chances are, when the injury reaches an acute stage, the cause of the injury is not identified and is typically attributed to aging.

The lumbar intervertebral discs are particularly susceptible to injury and herniation. The intervertebral discs located between the vertebrae of the spine are composed of a tirelike outer ring (annulus fibrosus) surrounding a gel-like center (nucleus pulposus). The greatest risk for injury to the discs occurs during excessive loading and twisting motions of the spine. While most people think that disc injuries occur from an acute injury, disc herniation typically reflects a degenerative process that takes place over time. With

---

Scoliosis A lateral curvature with some rotation of the spine; the most serious and deforming of all postural deviations.

Myofascial Trigger Points Tender spots in the muscle or muscle fascia that refer pain to a location distant to the point.

Referred Pain Pain that appears to be located in one area, though it actually originates in another area.

Microtrauma Injury so small it is not detected at the time it occurs.

repeated microtrauma, small tears begin to occur in the inner fibers of the annulus. The nucleus begins to move outward (**herniated disc**), much like toothpaste moving within a squeezed tube. Disc herniation is termed *incomplete* or *contained* as long as the migrating edge of the nucleus remains within the fibers of the annulus. As damage continues (often the result of years of cumulative microtrauma), the annular fibers may reach a point of rupture at their periphery (see Figure 3). At this point (termed *disc extrusion*), the nucleus pulposus moves into the space around the spinal cord or nerve root. At this stage, herniation is termed *complete* or *noncontained.*

The risk of disc herniation is greater for younger adults. Disc herniation is frequently listed as a cause of back pain, but studies show that only 5 to 10 percent of persons with herniated discs experience pain. The reason for this is that pain is often not experienced until complete herniation occurs. The pain is experienced as the nuclear material begins to press on pain-sensitive structures in its path. Interestingly, the risk for disc herniation is greatest for individuals in their 30s and 40s. Risk decreases with increasing years as the disc degenerates and becomes less soft and pliable.

Degenerative disc disease is a common part of aging and a source of back pain. Many elderly adults get shorter as they age, often due to degenerative changes within the vertebral bodies and discs. One notable change is flattening of the discs as a result of lost water content. This reduces the space between vertebrae and increases the compressive forces on the small facet joints and the large vertebral bodies.

This results in a decrease in the size of the spinal canal, which in turn increases the likelihood of nerve impingement, bone spur development, and arthritis, all of which can contribute to back pain and disability (see Figure 4).

Injury to the spine negatively affects the function of the core musculature. One of the more important core muscles, the lumbar multifidus, is adversely affected by back pain. Studies demonstrate that with low back pain, the muscle becomes inhibited (exhibiting decreased levels of activation and increased fatigability), is subject to atrophy, and becomes infiltrated with fatty deposits. In the healthy individual, the multifidus is believed to be responsible for providing more than two-thirds of the dynamic rigidity to the lumbar spine and serves an important role in proprioception and kinesthetic awareness. Research studies have shown specific spinal stabilization exercises to be effective in reversing some of the adverse changes to the multifidus, including positive gains in cross-sectional area/muscle bulk and improved neural recruitment. More importantly, participation in a program of core training exercise has also been shown to improve pain tolerance and function. Rehabilitation of the lumbar multifidus appears critical in the recovery period following back pain.

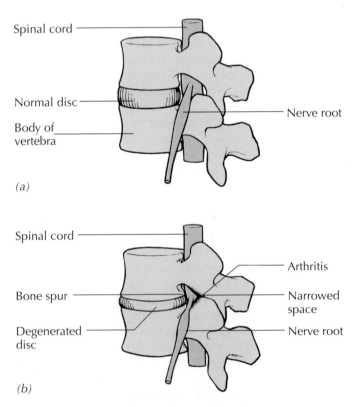

(a)

(b)

Figure 4 ▶ Normal disc (*a*) and degenerated disc with nerve impingement and arthritic changes (*b*).

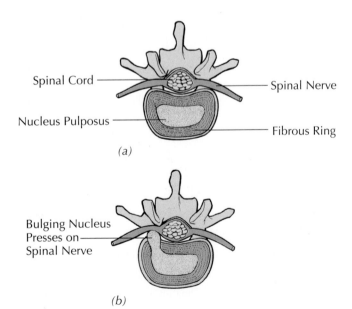

(a)

(b)

Figure 3 ▶ Normal disc (*a*) and herniated disc (*b*).

Medical intervention is sometimes needed for neck or back pain. Most cases of back pain resolve spontaneously, with 70 percent having no symptoms at the end of 3 weeks and 90 percent recovered after 2 months. However, medical approaches have been shown to speed up recovery from acute back/neck pain and to improve pain tolerance and function in chronic cases. Conservative treatment typically involves the use of anti-inflammatory medications, muscle relaxants, heat, cryotherapy, traction, or electrical stimulation. It can also include therapeutic exercise, massage and joint mobilization. When conservative care is unsuccessful, referral may occur to an alternative therapy, such as acupuncture, or to a pain clinic for steroidal anti-inflammatory injections. As a last measure, surgery may be needed for removal of a herniated portion of a disc.

Prevention of and Rehabilitation from Back and Neck Problems

Exercise is a frequently prescribed treatment for back or neck pain. Exercise has been found to be helpful in treating many types of chronic pain. (Resistance exercises and aerobic exercise are frequently used in pain clinics.) Exercises that are selected specifically to help correct pain-related problems are classified as therapeutic. These exercises are aimed at correcting the underlying cause of neck or back pain by strengthening weak muscles, stretching short ones, and improving circulation to and nourishment of tissues of the body. Both therapeutic and health-related fitness exercises may be considered preventive. Done faithfully, and with the appropriate FIT formula, they improve the health of the musculoskeletal system, allowing greater efficiency of function and reduced incidence of injury.

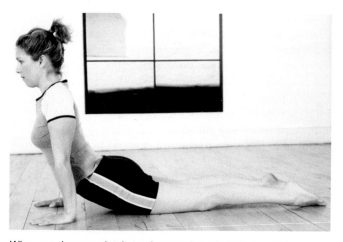

When used appropriately track extension can help maintain a healthy back.

Use of specific core stabilization exercises may reduce low back pain and functional disability. The integrity of individual vertebral segments of the spine is often compromised with injury to the neck or back. One or more components of the passive restraint system (ligaments, discs, vertebrae, or joints) may be damaged, creating a weak link in the stabilization system. In addition, optimal function of the dynamic and neural control systems is often adversely affected by injury. This may make a specific segment of the spine more vulnerable to delayed healing or further injury. Core training may enhance stability to the injured area by improving the function of the dynamic and neural control systems. Historically, core training programs for treating low back pain became widely used after several studies in the mid-1990s demonstrated significant long-term improvements in both pain level and functional status following participation in a program of spinal stabilization exercise. Studies also demonstrated reduced recurrence rates for back pain following participation in a core training program. Subsequent research has not been able to replicate these findings. In fact, more recent research has demonstrated similar levels of improvement in pain and disability with use of a general exercise program. Further research may help elucidate subsets of people who may benefit from one type of exercise program over another.

ⓘ **Core stability training and core strengthening training can promote good**
FEATURE 3 **back health.** As described in Concept 9, building **core strength** is important for overall muscular fitness. However, to reduce the risks for back and neck problems, it is also important to train the muscles involved in core stabilization. There are two main types of core training programs, and they each require somewhat different methods.

Core stability training refers to the training of the deeper ("local") core musculature. Physiologically, the

Herniated Disc The soft nucleus of the spinal disc that protrudes through a small tear in the surrounding tissue; also called prolapse.

Core Strength Strength of muscles that demonstrate optimal firing patterns and tension-generating capabilities to create movement of the trunk.

Core Stability Strength of muscles that demonstrate optimal firing patterns and tension-generating capabilities to "brace" the trunk in anticipation of, and during, movement of the head, arms, or legs.

Technology Update
New Training Aids for Core Training

TECH   Core training is an immensely popular concept across the fields of sport, fitness, and rehabilitation. The popularity of core training programs and classes has led to an expanding array of core-training devices. One category of devices includes those that provide an unstable surface for challenging balance and stability. Rocker boards, air-filled domes, therapy balls, foam rollers, and sliding disks are a few examples. Participants creatively position themselves on these devices in various postures—standing,

lunging, kneeling, or on hands and knees. A second category of devices includes equipment that provides a dynamic challenge to the arms or legs. Elastic tubing, stretch cords, vibrating wands, kettle bells and medicine balls are used to overload the extremities and elicit a corresponding and supportive contraction of the core stabilizers. The devices mentioned here are only a few of the many core-training devices currently available to fitness participants. Creative new devices enter the fitness market on a monthly basis, giving exercise participants fresh new ideas for their workout regimen. Additional detail and examples are available at the associated Web link.

local core stabilizers are slow-twitch endurance muscles that are poorly recruited, demonstrate low force production, and often sag/lengthen due to weakness. Training principles for the local core stabilizers are based on the respective physiology of the muscles. In general, exercises should involve slow and controlled movements and be held for long durations. The focus should be on improving trunk muscle endurance, since endurance of the trunk musculature appears to be more important than strength for reducing the risk of low back pain. Therefore, exercises should emphasize lower resistance and involve more repetitions. Exercises for improving local core stability are described and illustrated in the exercise section at the end of the concept.

Core strength training refers to the training of the more superficial "global" core musculature. Physiologically, these muscles are fast-twitch in nature, contract at higher resistance levels, possess greater potential for force production, work in a noncontinuous fashion, and are preferentially recruited over the local stabilizers. They are often in a shortened (tight) position. Based on the physiologic function of the global core muscles, recommended training principles include shorter duration holds, faster speeds of concentric contractions, greater resistance, and fewer numbers of repetitions. Core training of the global core stabilizers improves core strength. Traditional abdominal and trunk extensor strengthening exercises are included in the exercise section at the end of the concept.

Resistance exercise can often correct muscle imbalance, the underlying cause of many
TECH **postural and back problems.** If the muscles on one side of a joint are stronger than the muscles on the opposite side, the body part is pulled in the direction of the stronger muscles. Corrective exercises are usually designed to strengthen the long, weak muscles and to stretch the short, strong ones in order to have equal pull in both directions. For example, people with lumbar lordosis may need to strengthen the abdominals and gluteal muscles and also stretch the lower back and hip flexor muscles.

Although general resistance training may help improve the strength and endurance of the back muscles, the exercises may not be specific enough to target the areas that contribute to risk for low back pain. Because of this, increased attention has been given to the development of back exercise machines that can more effectively rehabilitate and/or strengthen back musculature. The machines help isolate the muscles by restraining or preventing other muscles from assisting. For example, pelvic muscles are restrained in a back extension machine to help isolate the lumbar muscles. This isolation helps strengthen the lumbar muscles, an important target for reducing risks for back problems.

Good Posture Is Important for Neck and Back Health

Good posture has aesthetic benefits. Posture is an important part of nonverbal communication. The first impression a person makes is usually a visual one, and good posture can help convey an impression of alertness, confidence, and attractiveness.

Proper posture allows the body segments to be balanced. Segments of the human body (i.e., the head, shoulder girdle, pelvic girdle, rib cage, and spine) are balanced in a vertical column by muscles and ligaments. Proper posture helps maintain an even distribution of force across the body, helps improve shock absorption, and helps minimize the degree of active muscle tension required to maintain upright posture. When viewed from the side, three normal curvatures of the spine are present, causing the vertebral column to appear S-shaped. These curvatures are created by the **lordotic** (inward) **curve** of the cervical and lumbar spines and the **kyphotic** (outward) **curve** of the thoracic spine (see Figure 1). The curves help balance forces on the body and minimize muscle tension. They are also responsible for humans' unique ability to walk upright on two legs while maintaining a forward gaze.

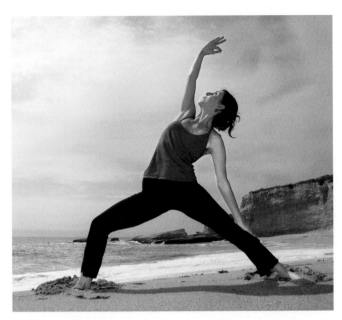

Movement disciplines like yoga and tai chi can promote body awareness and contribute to back health.

The degree of curvature is influenced by the tilt of the pelvis. A forward pelvic tilt increases curvature in the neck and lower back, whereas a backward pelvic tilt flattens the lower back. The most desirable position is a **neutral spine** in which the spine has neither too much nor too little lordotic curvature. The forces across the spine are balanced and muscular tension is at a minimum.

Awareness of good standing posture is important to a healthy spine. In the standing position, the head should be centered over the trunk; the shoulders should be down and back but relaxed, with the chest high and the abdomen flat. The spine should have gentle curves when viewed from the side but should be straight when seen from the back. When the pelvis is tilted properly, the pubis falls directly underneath the lower tip of the sternum. The knees should be relaxed, with the kneecaps pointed straight ahead. The feet should point straight ahead, and the weight should be borne over the heel, on the outside border of the sole, and across the ball of the foot and toes (see Figure 5).

Awareness of good seated posture is important to a healthy spine. A large percentage of our days are spent sitting as we attend class, commute to work, sit at a computer, dine out, or relax in front of the television. Good seated posture decreases pressure within the discs of the lower back and reduces fatigue of lower back muscles. In sitting, the head should be centered over the trunk, the shoulders down and back. If one is using a computer, the monitor should be at eye level with the screen 18–24 inches from the eyes. The seat of the chair should be at an angle that allows the knees to be positioned slightly lower than the hips. The back should firmly rest against the chair, with support to the lumbar spine. Feet should

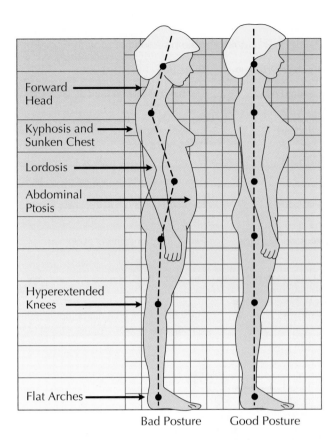

Forward Head

Kyphosis and Sunken Chest

Lordosis

Abdominal Ptosis

Hyperextended Knees

Flat Arches

Bad Posture   Good Posture

Figure 5 ▶ Comparison of bad and good posture.

be supported on the floor and arms supported on armrests for ideal unloading of the spine (see Figure 6).

Poor posture contributes to a variety of health problems. When posture deviates from neutral, weight distribution becomes uneven and tissues are at risk for injury. Examples of common postural deviations are described in Table 1, along with associated health problems. Two of those highlighted are that of lumbar lordosis (excessive curvature of the lower back) and flat back (reduced curvature of the lower back).

Posture The relationship among body parts, whether standing, lying, sitting, or moving. Good posture is the relationship among body parts that allows you to function most effectively, with the least expenditure of energy and with a minimal amount of stress and strain on the body.

Lordotic Curve The normal inward curvature of the cervical and lumbar spine that is necessary for good posture and body mechanics.

Kyphotic Curve The normal outward curvature of the thoracic spine that is necessary for good posture and body mechanics.

Neutral Spine Proper position of the spine to maintain a normal lordotic curve. The spine has neither too much nor too little lordotic curve.

Table 1 ▶ Health Problems Associated with Poor Posture

Posture Problem	Definition	Health Problem
Forward head	The head aligned in front of the center of gravity	Headache, dizziness, and pain in the neck, shoulders, or arms
Kyphosis	Excessive curvature (flexion) in the upper back; also called humpback	Impaired respiration as a result of sunken chest and pain in the neck, shoulders, and arms
Lumbar lordosis	Excessive curvature (hyperextension) in the lower back (sway back), with a forward pelvic tilt	Back pain and/or injury, protruding abdomen, low back syndrome, and painful menstruation
Flat back	Reduced curvature in the lower back	Back pain, increased risk for injury due to reduced shock absorption
Abdominal ptosis	Excessive protrusion of abdomen	Back pain and/or injury, lordosis, low back syndrome, and painful menstruation
Hyperextended knees	The knees bent backward excessively	Greater risk for knee injury and excessive pelvic tilt (lordosis)
Pronated feet	The longitudinal arch of the foot flattened with increased pressure on inner aspect of foot	Decreased shock absorption, leading to foot, knee, and lower back pain

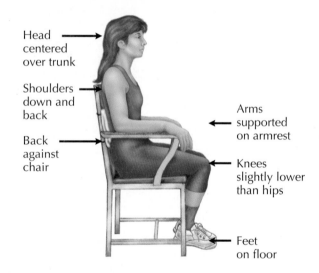

Head centered over trunk

Shoulders down and back

Back against chair

Arms supported on armrest

Knees slightly lower than hips

Feet on floor

Figure 6 ▶ Good sitting posture.

Lumbar lordosis posture occurs when the pelvis is tipped forward from a position of neutral tilt. With this posture, the hip flexor muscles become shortened and tight, while the abdominal muscles become weak and long (with a reduced ability to "hold" within inner range). This muscle imbalance shifts body segment alignment toward a position of uneven loading, increasing pressure on the facet joints of the vertebrae. Over time, degenerative changes may occur, including a narrowing of the openings where spinal nerves exit, thus increasing risk for pain.

Flat back posture, on the other hand, occurs when the pelvis is tipped backward from a position of neutral tilt. With this posture, the lumbar spine is flexed, the lower back muscles are in a lengthened (weak) position, and the hamstring muscles are shortened and tight. A reduced lumbar curvature increases pressure on the intervertebral bodies and decreases shock absorption capabilities.

Relative differences in flexibility between tight hamstring and long trunk muscles may also increase risk for injury. Laws of physics demonstrate that the body takes the path of least resistance during a chain of movement (e.g., forward bending), with the most flexible segment (i.e., the back) providing a greater contribution to the total range of movement. It follows that regions of greater movement will experience greater tissue strain. In the case of flat back posture, tight hamstrings may limit the contribution of hip motion during forward bending tasks, thus predisposing the lower back to become the fulcrum for movement and the site of injury.

Correcting postural deviations begins with restoring adequate muscle fitness and muscle length. Many postural problems are caused by a combination of weak and inflexible muscles. It is important to strengthen weak muscles in a shortened position and stretch tight muscles to help correct postural imbalance. For example, lumbar lordosis posture may be corrected by strengthening the abdominal muscles that pull the bottom of the pelvis upward and the hamstring muscles that keep the top of the pelvis tipped backward (see Figure 7). Postural correction is further enhanced by stretching tight hip flexor muscles.

In addition to body alignment problems, hereditary, congenital, and disease conditions, as well as certain environmental factors, can cause poor posture. Some environmental factors that contribute to poor posture include ill-fitting clothing and shoes, chronic fatigue, improperly fitting furniture (including poor chairs, beds, and mattresses), emotional and personality problems, poor work habits, poor physical fitness due to inactivity, and lack of knowledge relating to good posture. Some posture problems, such as scoliosis, may be congenital, hereditary, or acquired but can be improved

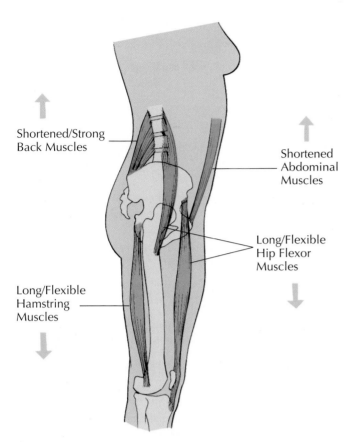

Shortened/Strong Back Muscles

Shortened Abdominal Muscles

Long/Flexible Hip Flexor Muscles

Long/Flexible Hamstring Muscles

Figure 7 ▶ Balanced muscle strength and length permit good postural alignment.

with exercise, braces, and/or other medical procedures. Early detection is critical in treating scoliosis.

Good Body Mechanics Is Important for Neck and Back Health

Proper body mechanics can help prevent back and neck injury. Biomechanics is a discipline that applies mechanical laws and principles to study how the body performs more efficiently and with less energy. Good body mechanics, as applied to back care, implies maintaining a neutral spine during activities of daily living. A neutral spine maintains the normal curvature of the spine, thus allowing an optimal balance of forces across the spine, reducing compressive forces, and minimizing muscle tension. Table 2 (page 234) provides specific recommendations for (and examples of) good body mechanics in a variety of settings and positions.

(i) **Ergonomics is a discipline that uses biomechanical principles to develop tools FEATURE 4 and workplace settings that put the least amount of strain on the body.** The modification of tools and occupational workstations can improve body

mechanics and improve job efficiency. Many employers take an active interest in ergonomic principles, since repetitive motion injuries and other musculoskeletal conditions are the leading cause of work-related ill health. One application of ergonomics is the design of effective workstations for computer users. Properly fitting desks and chairs and the effective positioning of computer screens and keyboards have been shown to minimize problems such as carpal tunnel syndrome (CTS), a painful and debilitating injury of the median nerve at the wrist. More information on ergonomics, also known as human factors engineering, can be found at the associated Web link.

Good lifting technique focuses on using the legs. Keep in mind that the muscles of the legs are relatively large and strong, compared with the back muscles. Likewise, the hip joint is well designed for motion. It is less likely to suffer the same amount of wear and tear as the smaller joints of the spine. When lifting an object from the floor, an individual should do the following: straddle the object with a wide stance; squat down by hinging through the hips and bending the knees; maintain a slight arch to the lower back by sticking out the buttocks; test the load and get help if it is too heavy or awkward; rise by tightening the leg muscles, not the back; keep the load close to the waist; don't pivot or twist (see Figure 8 on page 235).

Poor body mechanics can increase risks for back pain. A common cause of backache is muscle strain, frequently precipitated by poor body mechanics in daily activities, such as lifting or exercising. If lifting is done improperly, great pressure is exerted on the lumbar discs, and excessive stress and strain are placed on the lumbar muscles and ligaments. Many popular exercises involve the use of poor body mechanics and should be viewed with caution. Poor postures (e.g., sleeping on a soft mattress or slouching in a chair) can also cause back strain. Descriptions and examples of unsafe exercises and postures are provided later in the concept. By avoiding bad body mechanics, you can reduce your risk for back pain.

Exercise Guidelines for Back Health

Some exercises and movements may put the back and neck at risk. The human body is designed for motion. Nevertheless, certain movements can put the joints and musculoskeletal system at risk and should therefore be avoided. With respect to care of the spine, many **contraindicated** movements involve the extremes

Contraindicated Not recommended because of the potential for harm.

Table 2 ▶ Body Mechanics Guidelines for Posture and Back/Neck Care	
Sitting	• Use a hard chair with a straight back and armrests, placing the spine against the back of the chair. A footrest reduces fatigue (see Figure 6). • Keep one or both knees lower than the hips and feet supported on the floor. • If your back flattens when you sit, place a lumbar roll behind your lower back. • When sitting at a table, keep the back and neck in good alignment. • Do not sit in front-row theater seats, which forces you to tip your head back. • When driving a car, pull the seat forward, so the legs are bent when operating the pedals. If your back flattens when you drive, use a lumbar support pillow. • Whenever possible, sit while working, but stand occasionally.
Standing	• When standing for long periods, keep the lower back flat by propping a foot on a stool; alternate feet. • Avoid tilting the head backward (when shaving or washing your hair).
Lying	• Avoid lying on the abdomen. • When lying on the back, a pillow or lift should be placed under the knees. Do not use a thick head pillow. • When lying on your side, keep your knees and hips bent; place a pillow between the knees.
Lifting and Carrying	• When lifting, avoid bending at the waist. Keep the back straight, bend the knees, and lift with the legs. Assume a side-stride position with the object between the feet to allow you to get low and near the object. • Perform one-hand lifting the same way as two-hand lifting; use the nonlifting hand for support. • When lifting, do not twist the spine. This can be more damaging from a sitting position than from a standing position. • When lifting, keep the object close to the body; do not reach to lift. Tighten the abdominal muscles before lifting. • If possible, avoid carrying objects above waist level. • When objects must be carried above the waist, carry them in the midline of the body, preferably on the back (use a backpack). Keep backpack weight low and use both straps for support. • Push or pull heavy objects, rather than lifting them. It takes 34 times more force to lift than to slide an object across the floor. Pushing is preferred over pulling. • Do not lift or carry loads too heavy for you. The most economical load for the average adult is about 35 percent of the body weight. Obviously, with strength training, you can lift a greater load, but heavy loads are a backache risk factor. • Divide the load if possible, carrying half in each hand/arm. If the load cannot be divided, alternate it from one side of the body to the other. • When lifting and lowering an object from overhead, avoid hyperextending the neck and the back. Any lift above waist level is inefficient. • When objects must be carried in front of the body above the level of the waist, lean backward to balance the load, and avoid arching the back.
Working	• When working above head level, get on a stool or ladder to avoid tipping the head backward. • Work at eye level; for example, computer monitors should not be too high or low. • To avoid back and neck strain, climb a ladder or stand on a stool so you don't have to raise your arms over your head. • When working with the hands, the workbench or kitchen cabinet should be about 2 to 4 inches below the waist. The office desk should be about 29 to 30 inches high for the average man and about 27 to 29 inches high for the average woman. • Tools most often used should be the closest to reach. • Avoid constant arm extension, whether forward or sideward. • The arms should move either together or in opposite directions. When the conditions allow, use both hands in opposite and symmetrical motions while working. • Organize work to save energy. Vary the working position by changing from one task to another before feeling fatigued. When working at a desk, get up and stretch occasionally to relieve tension. • Use proper tools and equipment to reduce neck strain; for example, use a paint roller with an extension to reach overhead, thus reducing the need to hold the arms overhead and to hyperextend the neck. • Avoid stooping or unnatural positions that cause strain.

of hyperflexion and hyperextension. Hyperflexion causes increased pressure in the discs, potentially leading to disc herniation. Hyperextension causes compressive wear and tear on the facet joints that join vertebral segments (see Figure 9 on page 236). Hyperextension of the spine also causes narrowing of the intervertebral canal, potentially causing nerve impingement. Extremes of motion can be harfmul to other joints as well. For example, knee

hyperextension places excessive stress on structures at the back of the knee, whereas hyperflexion increases compressive forces under the kneecap (patello-femoral joint).

Following established exercise guidelines is important for safe exercise. "Safe" exercises are defined as those performed with normal body posture, mechanics, and movement in mind. They don't compromise the

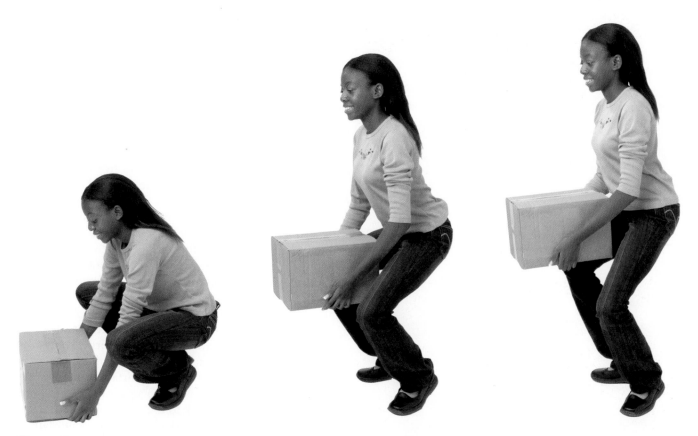

Figure 8 ▶ Proper body mechanics is important for reducing risk of back problems.

integrity or stability of one body part to the detriment of another. "Questionable" exercises, on the other hand, are exercises that may violate normal body mechanics and place the joints, ligaments, or muscles at risk for injury. No harm may occur from doing the exercise once, but repeated use over time can lead to injury. A number of commonly used exercises are regarded as poor choices (contraindicated) for nearly everyone in the general population due to the reasonable risk for injury over time. A separate category of questionable exercises are regarded as poor choices for only certain segments of the population because of a specific health issue or known physical problem.

Differentiating exercises as "safe" or "questionable" can be difficult—even experts in the field have different opinions on the subject. These views are known to change over time as new knowledge and research findings reshape our understanding of the effect of exercise on the human body.

When considering the merits and risks of different exercises, it may be necessary to consult an expert. Professionals such as athletic trainers, biomechanists, physical educators, physical therapists, and certified strength and conditioning specialists are appropriate people to consult. These individuals typically have

college degrees and 4 to 8 years of study in such courses as anatomy, physiology, kinesiology, preventive and therapeutic exercise, and physiology of exercise. On-the-job training, a good physique or figure, and good athletic or dancing ability are not sufficient qualifications for teaching or advising about exercise. Most fitness centers prefer to hire instructors and personal trainers with appropriate certifications. Unfortunately, certification is not a requirement. When searching for advice on training or exercise, it is certainly appropriate to inquire about an individual's qualifications.

Exercises prescribed for a particular individual differ from those that are good for everyone (mass prescription). In a clinical setting, a therapist works with one patient. A case history is taken and tests made to determine which muscles are weak or strong, short or long. Exercises are then prescribed for that person. For example, a wrestler with a recent history of shoulder dislocation would probably be prescribed specific shoulder-strengthening exercises to regain stability in the joint. Common shoulder stretching exercises would likely be contraindicated for this individual. In this case, the muscles and joint capsule on the front of the shoulder are already quite lax to have allowed dislocation to occur in the first place.

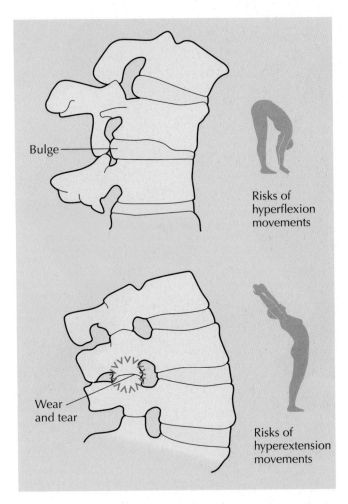

Figure 9 ▶ Risks of hyperflexion and hyperextension.

Exercises prescribed or performed as a group cannot typically take individual needs into account. For example, when a physical educator, an aerobics instructor, or a coach leads a group of people in exercise, there is little (if any) consideration for individual differences, except for some allowance made in the number of repetitions or in the amount of weight or resistance used. Some of the exercises performed in this type of group setting may not be appropriate for all individuals. Similarly, an exercise that is appropriate for a certain individual may not be appropriate for all members of a group. Since it is not always practical to prescribe individual exercise routines for everyone, it is often necessary to provide general recommendations that are appropriate for most individuals. The classification of exercises in this concept should be viewed in this context.

The risks associated with physical activity can be reduced by modifying the variables or conditions under which the activity is performed. While some exercises are contraindicated, it is almost always possible to find safer alternatives. Modifications in the way the exercise is performed can also reduce risks. The variables that are typically under the direct control of the participant include exercise frequency (the number of repetitions performed in a given time span), duration (the length of time activity is sustained), intensity (the amount of resistance), speed (the velocity of activity, or rate, at which resistance is applied), and quality (the posture and mechanics of the body parts involved in the movement). Table 3 highlights these five activity variables, illustrates how each might be involved in potential injury, and provides suggestions for modifying the variable to reduce the risk for injury. In some cases, changing a single variable may significantly reduce risk, but in other cases, multiple factors may need to be changed. In many cases, the best strategy is to look for a safer exercise. A variety of contraindicated exercises and safer alternatives are presented in Table 4 (pages 240–246) at the end of the concept.

Risks from exercise can't be completely avoided. Variables that are not always under the direct control of the participant include environmental conditions, such as temperature, humidity, or exercise surface. Likewise, the demands of sport and certain occupations may require individuals to train or work to the maximal limit of these variables (up to or just short of injury). Circumstances may not always permit every variable to be modified to suit an individual. However, making an active effort to adjust variables that are modifiable will make a difference in reducing injury risk.

Some additional general guidelines will help prevent postural, back, and neck problems. In addition to the suggestions for improving body mechanics noted in the previous sections, the following guidelines should be helpful:

- Do exercises to strengthen abdominal and hip extensors and to stretch the hip flexors and lumbar muscles if they are tight (see Tables 4–11).

 Health is available to Everyone for a **LIFETIME**, and it's Personal

According to the National Institutes of Health, the most common medical problem in the United States is back pain, which is very often caused by degeneration of the disks in the spine. Preventative measures include maintaining a healthy weight over the life span, using proper lifting techniques, and engaging in regular exercise, particularly strength training and flexibility exercises.

What steps are you taking today to help prevent back problems later in life?

Table 3 ▶ Controllable Variables in Reducing Risk for Injury

Variables	Activity Examples	Potential Injury	Modifications to Reduce Risk
Frequency	• Repeated back hyperextension in a gymnast • Repeated wrist movement in an assembly-line worker	Microtrauma to the joints undergoing repeated motions	• Maintain a balance of flexibility and strength in the vulnerable regions of the body. • Provide rest/rotate workstations within the shift. • Use ergonomic modifications to the worksite.
Duration	• Sustained position of a deep squat in a baseball catcher • Forward head posture of an office worker	Stress and strain to the muscles and ligaments used to hold the posture	• Strengthen the muscles of the knees and maintain leg muscle flexibility in the catcher. • Take regular posture breaks in the office worker and modify computer station for good seated posture.
Intensity	Excessive loads and reaction forces experienced by a • Power lifter • Runner • Construction worker	Stress and strain to the musculoskeletal system, especially the weaker portions of the back and shoulders	• Do a proper warm-up and correct training progression. • Wear supportive shoes and clothing. • Be aware of personal limits, seeking help or a spot when needed.
Speed	High-velocity movement of • A 50-yd sprinter • The rapid fingering of a concert pianist	• Motions applied over a short time under conditions of high tension predispose the muscles and tendons to injury. • With fast-paced motions, precision is often sacrificed (particularly with fatigue), possibly leading to faulty movement patterns.	• Follow activity-specific training protocols to optimize recruitment of appropriate muscle fiber types. • Maintain balance of flexibility and strength. • Use deep muscles for stability and superficial muscles for mobility.
Movement quality	• Extended range of motion during ballistic shoulder stretching of swimmers • Poor body mechanics when shoveling snow	• Movement through extreme ranges or at the limit of normal motion can lead to instability or wear/tear of joints. • Poor balance of forces throughout the body increases risk for stress and strain.	• Balance flexibility with strength and respect pain, the body's signal of injury. • Use good posture and body mechanics in recreational and lifestyle activities to balance forces.

- Avoid hazardous exercises.
- Do regular physical activity for the entire body, such as walking, jogging, swimming, and bicycling.
- Warm up before engaging in strenuous activity.
- Sleep on a moderately firm mattress or place a 3/4-inch-thick plywood board under the mattress.
- Avoid sudden, jerky back movements, especially twisting.
- Avoid obesity. The smaller the waistline, the less the strain on the lower back.
- Use appropriate back and seat supports when sitting for long periods.
- Maintain good posture when carrying heavy loads; do not lean forward, sideways, or backward.
- Adjust sports equipment to permit good posture; for example, adjust a bicycle seat and handle bars to permit good body alignment.
- Avoid long periods of sitting at a desk or driving; take frequent breaks and adjust the car seat and headrest for maximum support.

In the News

Clinical Applications (and Implications) of New Gaming Technology

 The Wii (and other interactive game platforms such as Nintendo and Sony Playstation) have ushered in a new era of video game technology. Participants actively participate in the game experience by moving a controller as part of the game. The technology has spawned a variety of sport and clinical applications since it creates an engaging and motivational climate for medical rehabilitation. Many physical therapy clinics now use the Wii to promote interest and motivation in patients. The games can be set up to require similar postures and body movements needed for traditional therapy exercises. Patients may tire of repetitive exercise but become engrossed in the task of the game and forget that they are exercising. The potential of the tools for rehabilitation is clearly a positive application but new studies report some clinical problems associated with excessive gaming—prompting some to characterize new conditions of Wii-itis and Nintendin-itis. Additional information on applications and implications of active gaming are at the associated Web link.

▶▶ Strategies for Action

An important step in taking action is assessing your current status. The Healthy Back Tests consist of eight pass or fail items that will give you an idea of the areas in which you might need improvement. The Healthy Back Tests are described in Lab Resource Materials. You will take these tests in Lab 11A. Experts have identified behaviors associated with potential future back and neck problems. A questionnaire is also provided for assessing these risk factors.

Learning to adopt and maintain good posture is an effective way to promote good back health. Lab 11B includes a posture test to help you evaluate your posture. Identifying possible postural problems can help you take appropriate corrective action that can reduce stress and strain on your back and neck.

Specific exercises are sometimes needed to prevent or help rehabilitate postural, neck, and back problems. Exercises included in previous concepts were presented with health-related fitness in mind. The exercises included in this concept are not so different. They are either flexibility or strength/muscle endurance exercises for specific muscle groups; however, each is selected specifically to help correct a postural problem or to remove the cause of neck and back pain. To that extent, these exercises may be classified as therapeutic. The same exercises may be called preventive because they can be used to prevent postural or spine problems. People who have back and neck pain should seek the advice of a physician to make certain that it is safe for them to perform the exercises.

The exercises in Tables 5–11 are not necessarily intended for all people. Rather, you should choose exercises based on your own individual needs. Use your results on the Healthy Back Tests and the posture test to determine the exercises that are most appropriate for you. Table 4 (pages 240–246) provides information on "Questionable Exercises and Safe Alternatives."

To facilitate the use of these exercises for back or postural problems, the most effective exercises for various maladies are organized in Tables 5–11. Lab 11C is designed to help you choose specific exercises related to test items in Lab 11A.

Keeping records of progress is important to adhering to a back care program. Lab 11C provides an activity logging sheet to help you keep records of your progress as you regularly perform exercises to build and maintain good back and neck fitness.

Web Resources

Additional websites with information related to Concept 11 are available at the associated Web link.

American Back Care Company **www.americanback.com**

Back and Body Care **www.backandbodycare.com**

Back Pain (Medline Plus-NIH) **www.nlm.nih.gov/medlineplus/backpain.html**

Guide to Clinical Preventive Services
http://odphp.osophs.dhhs.gov/pubs/guidecps

Low Back Pain (American Academy of Orthopaedic Surgeons)
http://orthoinfo.aaos.org/topic.cfm?topic=A00311

Low Back Pain Fact Sheet (NIH) **www.ninds.nih.gov/disorders/backpain/detail_backpain.htm**

MedX **www.medxonline.com**

National Osteoporosis Foundation **www.nof.org**

National Safety Council **www.nsc.org**

Suggested Readings

Selected readings and references are listed below. A more comprehensive list is available at the associated Web link.

Bergman, S. 2007. Public health perspective—How to improve the musculoskeletal health of the population. *Best Practice & Research in Clinical Rheumatology* 21(1):191–204.

Bonis, J. 2007. Acute Wiiitis. *New England Journal of Medicine* 356(23):2431–2432.

Brumitt, J. 2010. *Core Assessment and Training*. Champaign, IL: Human Kinetics.

Christensen. 2007. Active lifestyle protects against incident low back pain in seniors. *Spine* 32(1): 76–81.

Eley, K. 2010. A Wii fracture. *New England Journal of Medicine* 362(5):473–474.

Freburger J.K., et al. 2009. The rising prevalence of chronic low back pain. *Archives of Internal Medicine* 169(3): 251–258.

Hooper, M. M., et al., 2007. Musculoskeletal findings in obese subjects before and after weight loss following bariatric surgery. *International Journal of Obesity* 31(1):114–120.

Martin, R. A., et al. 2008. Expenditures and health status among adults with back and neck problems. *Journal of the American Medical Association* 299(6):656–664.

Nelson, A. and J. Kokkonen. 2007. *Stretching Anatomy*. Champaign, IL: Human Kinetics.

Oleske, D. M., et al. 2007. Are back supports plus education more effective than education alone in promoting recovery from low back pain? Results from a randomized clinical trial. *Spine* 32(19):2050–2057.

Rahman, S., et al. 2010. The association between obesity and low back pain: A meta-analysis. *American Journal of Epidemiology* 171(2):135–154.

Ratliff, J., A. Hilibrand, and A. R. Vaccaro. 2008. Spine-related expenditures and self-reported health status. *Journal of the American Medical Association* 299(22):2627.

Sanders, M. E. 2009. Off the floor exercises for back health. *ACSM's Health and Fitness Journal* 13(6):33–35.

Takeshima, N., et al. 2007. Functional fitness gain varies in older adults depending on exercise mode. *Medicine and Science in Sports and Exercise* 39(11):2036–2043.

Zhu, K., et al. 2007. Association of back pain frequency with mortality, coronary heart events, mobility, and quality of life in elderly women. *Spine* 32(18):2012–2018.

Table 4 Questionable Exercises and Safer Alternatives

1. Questionable Exercise: The Swan

This exercise hyperextends the lower back and stretches the abdominals. The abdominals are too long and weak in most people and should not be lengthened further. Extension can be harmful to the back, potentially causing nerve impingement and facet joint compression. Other exercises in which this occurs include: cobras, backbends, straight-leg lifts, straight-leg sit-ups, prone-back lifts, donkey kicks, fire hydrants, backward trunk circling, weight lifting with the back arched, and landing from a jump with the back arched.

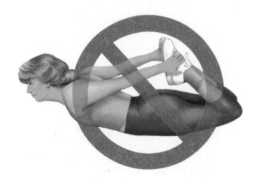

Safer Alternative Exercise: Back Extension

Lie prone over a roll of blankets or pillows and extend the back to a neutral or horizontal position.

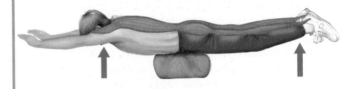

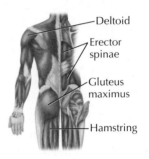

- Deltoid
- Erector spinae
- Gluteus maximus
- Hamstring

2. Questionable Exercise: Back-Arching Abdominal Stretch

This exercise can stretch the hip flexors, quadriceps, and shoulder flexors (such as the pectorals), but it also stretches the abdominals, which is not desired. Because of the armpull, it can potentially hyperflex the knee joint and strain neck musculature.

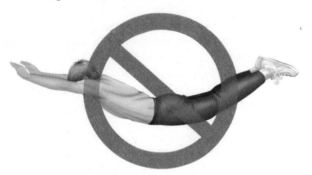

> Note: All safer alternative exercises should be held 15 to 30 seconds unless otherwise indicated.

Safer Alternative Exercise: Wand Exercise

This exercise stretches the front of the shoulders and chest. Sit with wand grasped at ends. Raise wand overhead. Be certain that the head does not slide forward. Keep the chin tucked and neck straight. Bring wand down behind shoulder blades. Keep spine erect. Hold. Press forward on the wand simultaneously by pushing with the hands. Relax; then try to move the hands lower, sliding the wand down the back. Hold again. Hands may be moved closer together to increase stretch

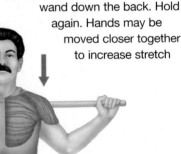

on chest muscles. If this is an easy exercise for you, try straightening the elbows and bringing the wand to waist level in back of you.

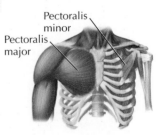

- Pectoralis minor
- Pectoralis major

Table 4

3. Questionable Exercise: Seated Forward Arm Circles with Palms Down

This exercise (arms straight out to the sides) may cause pinching of the rotator cuff and biceps tendons between the bony structures of the shoulder joint and/or irritate the bursa in the shoulder. The tendency is to emphasize the use of the stronger chest muscles (pectorals) to perform the motion rather than emphasizing the weaker upper back muscles.

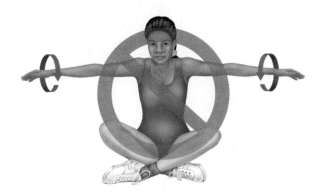

Safer Alternative Exercise: Seated Backward Arm Circles with Palms Up

Sit, turn palms up, pull in chin, and contract abdominals. Circle arms backward.

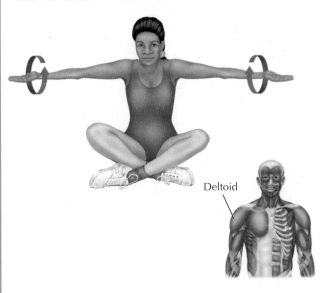

Deltoid

4. Questionable Exercise: Double-Leg Lift

This exercise is usually used with the intent of strengthening the abdominals, when in fact it is primarily a hip flexor (iliopsoas) strengthening exercise. Most people have overdeveloped the hip flexors and do not need to further strengthen those muscles because this may cause forward pelvic tilt. Even if the abdominals are strong enough to contract isometrically to prevent hyperextension of the lower back, the exercise produces excess stress on the discs.

Safer Alternative Exercise: Reverse Curl

This exercise strengthens the lower abdominals. Lie on your back on the floor and bring your knees in toward the chest. Place the arms at the sides for support. For movement, pull the knees toward the head, raising the hips off the floor. Do not let knees go past the shoulders. Return to starting position and repeat.

Rectus abdominis

Table 4 Questionable Exercises and Safer Alternatives

Table 4

5. Questionable Exercise: The Windmill

This exercise involves simultaneous rotation and flexion (or extension) of the lower back, which is contraindicated. Because of the orientation of the facet joints in the lumbar spine, these movements violate normal joint mechanics, placing tremendous torsional stress on the joint capsule and discs.

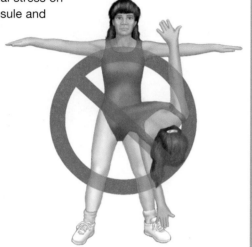

Safer Alternative Exercise: Back-Saver Toe Touch

Sit on the floor. Extend leg and bend the other knee, placing the foot flat on the floor. Bend at the hips and reach forward with both hands. Grasp one foot, ankle, or calf depending upon the distance you can reach. Pull forward with your arms and bend forward. Slight bend in the knee is acceptable. Hold. Repeat with the opposite leg.

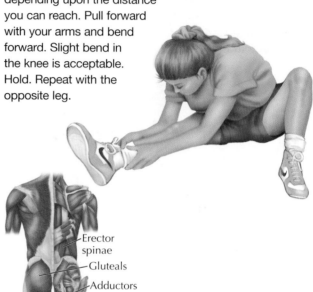

Erector spinae
Gluteals
Adductors

6. Questionable Exercise: Neck Circling

This exercise and other exercises that require neck hyperextension (e.g., neck bridging) can pinch arteries and nerves in the neck and at the base of the skull, cause wear and tear to small joints of the spine, and produce dizziness or myofascial trigger points. In people with degenerated discs, it can cause dizziness, numbness, or even precipitate strokes. It also aggravates arthritis and degenerated discs.

Safer Alternative Exercise: Head Clock

This exercise relaxes the muscle of the neck. Assume a good posture (seated with legs crossed or in a chair), and imagine that your neck is a clock face with the chin at the center. Flex the neck and point the chin at 6:00, hold, lift the chin; repeat pointing chin to 4:00, to 8:00, to 3:00 and finally to 9:00. Return to center position with chin up after each movement.

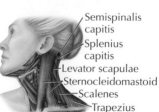

Semispinalis capitis
Splenius capitis
Levator scapulae
Sternocleidomastoid
Scalenes
Trapezius

7. Questionable Exercise: Shoulder Stand Bicycle

This exercise and the yoga positions called the plough and the plough shear (not shown) force the neck and upper back to hyperflex. It has been estimated that 80 percent of the population has forward head and kyphosis (humpback) with accompanying weak muscles. This exercise is especially dangerous for these people. Neck hyperflexion results in excessive stretch on the ligaments and nerves. It can also aggravate preexisting arthritic conditions. If the purpose for these exercises is to reduce gravitational effects on the circulatory system or internal organs, lie on a tilt board with the feet elevated. If the purpose is to warm up the muscles in the legs, slow jog in place. If the purpose is to stretch the lower back, try the leg hug exercise.

Safer Alternative Exercise: Leg Hug

Lie on your back with the knees bent at about 90 degrees. Bring your knees to the chest and wrap the arms around the back of the thighs. Pull knees to chest and hold.

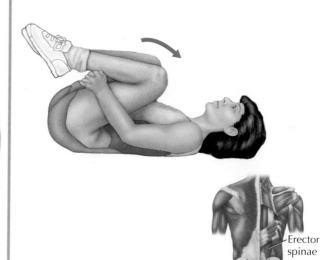

Erector spinae

Gluteals

8. Questionable Exercise: Straight-Leg and Bent-Knee Sit-Ups

There are several valid criticisms of the sit-up exercise. Straight-leg sit-ups can displace the fifth lumbar vertebra, causing back problems. A bent-knee sit-up creates less shearing force on the spine, but some recent studies have shown it produces greater compression on the lumbar discs than the straight-leg sit-up. Placing the hands behind the neck or head during the sit-up or during a crunch results in hyperflexion of the neck.

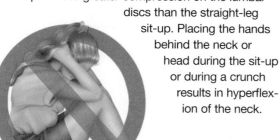

Safer Alternative Exercise: Crunch

Lie on your back with the knees bent more than 90 degrees. Curl up until the shoulder blades lift off the floor, then roll down to starting position and repeat. There are several safe arm positions. The easiest is with the arms extended straight in front of the body. Alternatives are with the arms crossed over the chest or the palms or fist held beside the ears.

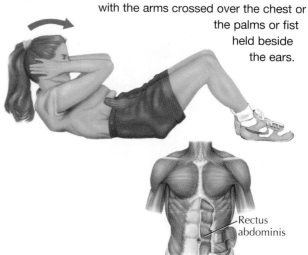

Rectus abdominis

Table 4 Questionable Exercises and Safer Alternatives

Table 4

9. Questionable Exercise: Standing Toe Touches or Double-Leg Toe Touches

These exercises—especially when done ballistically—can produce degenerative changes at the vertebrae of the lower back. They also stretch the ligaments and joint capsule of the knee. Bending the back while the legs are straight may cause back strain, particularly if the movement is done ballistically. If performed only on rare occasions as a test, the chance of injury is less than if incorporated into a regular exercise program. Safer stretches of the lower back include the leg hug, the single knee-to-chest, the hamstring stretcher, and the back-saver toe touch.

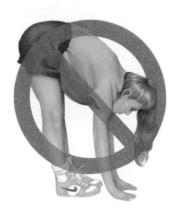

Safer Alternative Exercise:
Back-Saver Hamstring Stretch

This exercise stretches the hamstring and lower back muscles. Sit with one leg extended and one knee bent, foot turned outward and close to the buttocks. Clasp hands behind back. Bend forward from the hips, keeping the low back as straight as possible. Allow bent knee to move laterally so trunk can move forward. Stretch and hold. Repeat with the other leg.

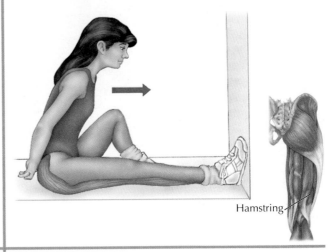

Hamstring

10. Questionable Exercise: Bar Stretch

This type of stretch may be harmful. Some experts have found that when the extended leg is raised 90 degrees or more and the trunk is bent over the leg, it may lead to **sciatica** and **piriformis syndrome,** especially in the person who has limited flexibility.

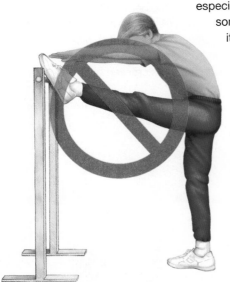

Safer Alternative Exercise:
One-Leg Stretch

This exercise stretches the hamstring muscles. Stand with one foot on a bench, keeping both legs straight. Hinge forward from the hips keeping shoulders back and chest up. Bend forward until a pull is felt on the back side of the thigh. Hold. Repeat.

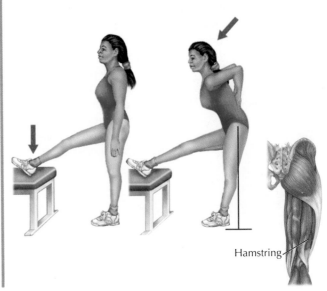

Hamstring

11. Questionable Exercise: Shin and Quadriceps Stretch

This exercise causes hyperflexion of the knee. When the knee is hyperflexed more than 120 degrees and/or rotated outward by an external **torque,** the ligaments and joint capsule are stretched, and damage to the cartilage may occur. Note: one of the quadriceps, the rectus femoris, is not stretched if the trunk is allowed to bend forward because it crosses the hip as well as the knee joint. If the exercise is used to stretch the quadriceps, substitute the hip and thigh stretch. For most people it is not necessary to stretch the shin muscles, since they are often elongated and weak; however, if you need to stretch the shin muscles to relieve muscle soreness, try the shin stretch.

Safer Alternative Exercise: Hip and Thigh Stretch

Kneel so that the front leg is bent at 90 degrees (front knee directly above the front ankle). The knee of the back leg should touch the floor well behind the front foot. Press the pelvis forward and downward. Hold. Repeat with the opposite leg forward. Do not bend the front knee more than 90 degrees.

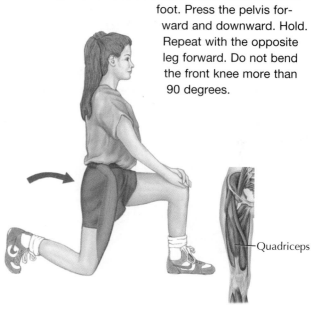

Quadriceps

12. Questionable Exercise: The Hero

Like the shin and quadriceps stretch, this exercise causes hyperflexion of the knee. It also causes torque on the hyperflexed knee. For these reasons the ligaments and joint capsule are stretched and the cartilage may be damaged. For most people it is not necessary to stretch the shin muscles since they are often elongated and weak; however, if you need to stretch the shin muscles, use the shin stretch. If this exercise is used to stretch the quadriceps, substitute the hip and thigh stretch.

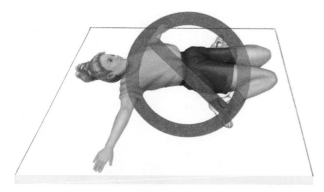

Safer Alternative Exercise: Shin Stretch

Kneel on your knees, turn to right and press down on right ankle with right hand. Hold. Keep hips thrust forward to avoid hyperflexing the knees. Do not sit on the heels. Repeat on the left side.

Tibialis anterior

Extensor digitorum longus

Extensor hallucis longus

Sciatica Pain along the sciatic nerve in the buttock and leg.

Piriformis Syndrome Muscle spasm and nerve entrapment in the pyriformis muscle of the buttocks region, causing pain in the buttock and referred pain down the leg (sciatica).

Torque A twisting or rotating force.

Table 4

Table 4 Questionable Exercises and Safer Alternatives

13. Questionable Exercise: Deep Squatting Exercises

This exercise, with or without weights, places the knee joint in hyperflexion, tends to "wedge it open," stretching the ligaments, irritating the synovial membrane, and possibly damaging the cartilage. The joint has even greater stress when the lower leg and foot are not in straight alignment with the knee. If you are performing squats to strengthen the knee and hip extensors, try substituting the alternate leg kneel or half-squat with free weight or leg presses on a resistance machine.

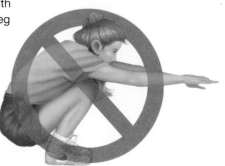

Safer Alternative Exercise: Half Squat

This exercise develops the muscles of the thighs and buttocks. Stand upright with feet shoulder width apart. Squat slowly by moving hips backwards, then bending knees. Keep shins vertical. Bend knees 45–90 degrees. Repeat.

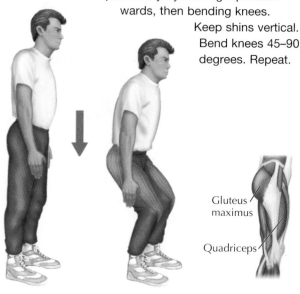

Gluteus maximus

Quadriceps

14. Questionable Exercise: Knee Pull-Down

This exercise can result in hyperflexion of the knee. The arms or hands placed on top of the shin places undue stress on the knee joint.

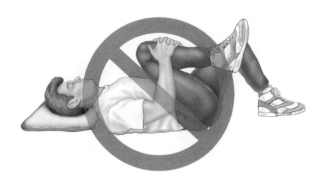

Safer Alternative Exercise: Single Knee-to-Chest

Lie down with both knees bent, draw one knee to the chest by pulling on the thigh with the hands, then extend the knee and point the foot toward the ceiling. Hold. Pull to chest again and return to starting position. Repeat with other leg.

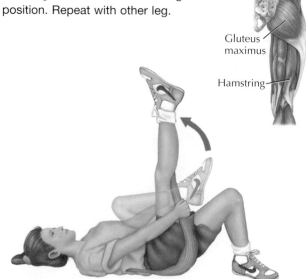

Gluteus maximus

Hamstring

Stretching Exercises for the Hip Flexors and Hamstrings Table 5

When performed on a regular basis, these exercises will help maintain neutral spine posture and improve the flexibility of the hip flexor and hip extensor musculature. (Tightness of these muscles can, respectively, contribute to a forward or backward pelvic tilt due to their attachments to the pelvis.) Hold stretches for 15 to 30 seconds.

Table 5

1. Back-Saver Hamstring Stretch

This exercise stretches the hamstrings and calf muscles. Sit on the floor with the feet against the wall or an immovable object. Bend left knee and bring foot close to buttocks. Clasp hands behind back. Bend forward from hips, keeping lower back as straight as possible. Let bent knee rotate outward so trunk can move forward keeping back flat. Hold and repeat on each leg.

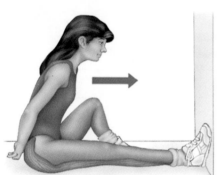

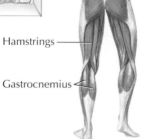

Hamstrings

Gastrocnemius

2. Single Knee-to-Chest

This exercise stretches the lower back, gluteals, and hamstring muscles. Lie on your back with knees bent. Use hands on back of thigh to draw one knee to the chest. Hold. Then extend the knee and point the foot toward the ceiling. Hold. Return to the starting position without arching your back. Repeat with other leg.

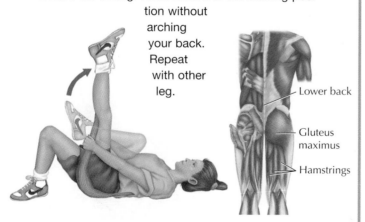

Lower back

Gluteus maximus

Hamstrings

3. Hip and Low Back Stretch

This exercise stretches the hip flexors of one leg and the gluteals and lumbar muscles of the opposite leg. Lie on your back. Draw one knee up to the chest and pull thigh toward chest with the hands; then slowly return to the original position. Repeat with other knee. Do not grasp knee—grasp thigh. If a partner or a weight stabilizes the extended leg, the hip flexor muscles on that leg will be stretched.

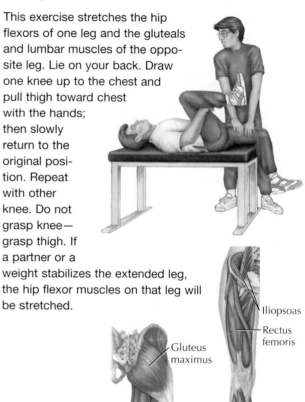

Iliopsoas

Rectus femoris

Gluteus maximus

4. Hip and Thigh Stretch

This exercise stretches the hip flexor muscles and helps prevent or correct forward pelvic tilt, lumbar lordosis, and backache. Place right knee directly above right ankle and stretch left leg backward so knee touches floor. If necessary, place hands on floor for balance. Press pelvis forward and downward. Hold. Repeat on opposite side. Caution: Do not bend front knee more than 90 degrees.

Iliopsoas

Rectus femoris

Table 6

Table 6 Core Stabilization Exercises

These exercises help train the abdominal and buttock muscles to provide postural stability by maintaining the pelvis in a neutral position during activity. They help prevent or correct lumbar lordosis, abdominal ptosis (see Table 1), and backache. Hold exercises for 15 to 30 seconds.

1. Abdominal Hollowing on Hands and Knees

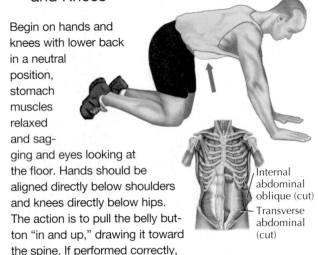

Begin on hands and knees with lower back in a neutral position, stomach muscles relaxed and sagging and eyes looking at the floor. Hands should be aligned directly below shoulders and knees directly below hips. The action is to pull the belly button "in and up," drawing it toward the spine. If performed correctly, the muscles below the umbilicus will flatten, rather than bulge. Recruitment of the transverse abdominus may be facilitated by coughing and then holding the muscle contraction. The exercise is held for 10–30 seconds. Breathe normally throughout the contraction. Repeat 10 times.

Internal abdominal oblique (cut)
Transverse abdominal (cut)

2. Abdominal Hollowing in Wall Support

Begin standing with feet 6 inches from the wall and back gently resting against the surface. Maintain a neutral spine. Contract the muscles below the belly button by pulling the abdominal wall "in and up." The pelvic floor may be contracted at the same time by pulling it "up and in" in a gripping motion. Breathe throughout the contraction. Hold 10–30 seconds. Repeat 10 times.

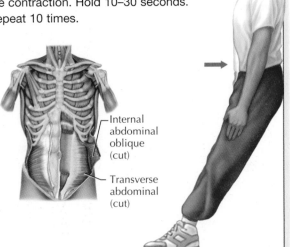

Internal abdominal oblique (cut)

Transverse abdominal (cut)

3. Horizontal Side Support

Begin in side lying position with the body resting on the forearm. Slowly lift the pelvis until the body forms a straight line from foot to shoulder. Hold 10 - 30 seconds. Repeat 8–12 times.

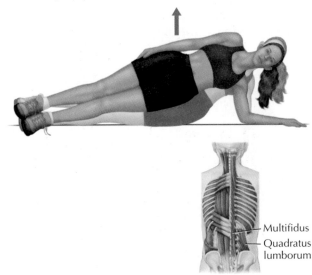

Multifidus
Quadratus lumborum

4. Head Nod

Lie flat on the back without a pillow. Gently nod the head in a "yes" motion. Motion should result in the tightening of muscles deep in the front of the neck. Place two fingers over the sides of the neck to monitor for the undesirable substitution of stronger muscles in this region. Hold 10–30 seconds (or as long as can be maintained without substitution). Repeat 10 times. Progress this exercise by first nodding "yes" and then lifting the head ¼ inch to ½ inch off the surface.

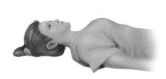

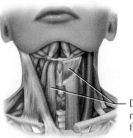

Deep neck flexors

Exercises for Muscle Fitness of the Abdominals Table 7

Table 7

These exercises are designed to increase the strength of the abdominal muscles. Strong abdominal muscles are important for maintaining a neutral pelvis, maintaining good posture, and preventing backache associated with lordosis.

1. Reverse Curl

Lie on your back. Bend the knees and bring knees in toward the chest. Place arms at sides for balance and support. Pull the knees toward the chest, raising the hips off the floor. Do not let the knees go past the shoulders. Return to the starting position. Repeat.

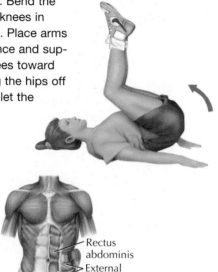

Rectus abdominis

External obliques

2. Crunch (Curl-Up)

Lie on your back with your knees bent and palms on ears. If desired, legs may rest on bench to increase difficulty. For less resistance, place hands at side of body. For more resistance, move hands higher. Curl up until shoulder blades leave floor, then roll down to the starting position. Repeat. Variation: extend the arms or cross the arms over your chest.

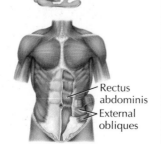

Rectus abdominis

External obliques

3. Crunch with Twist (on Bench)

Lie on your back with your feet on a bench, knees bent at 90 degrees. Arms may be extended or on shoulders or hands on ears (the most difficult). Same as crunch except twist the upper trunk so the right shoulder is higher than the left.

Reach toward the left knee with the right elbow. Hold. Return and repeat to the opposite side. (This exercise is not recommended for people with lower back pain due to the combined motions of flexion and rotation.)

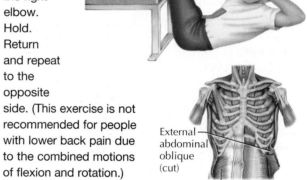

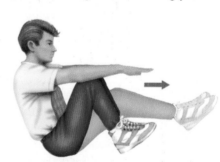

External abdominal oblique (cut)

Internal abdominal oblique

4. Sitting Tucks

Sit on floor with feet raised, arms extended for balance. Alternately bend and extend legs without letting your back or feet touch floor. (This is an advanced exercise and is not recommended for people who have back pain.)

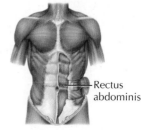

Rectus abdominis

Table 8

Table 8 Stretching and Strengthening Exercises for the Muscles of the Neck

These exercises are designed to increase strength in the neck muscles and to improve neck range of motion. They are helpful in preventing and resolving symptoms of neck pain and for relieving trigger points. Hold stretches for 15 to 30 seconds.

1. Neck Rotation Exercise

This PNF exercise strengthens and stretches the neck rotators. It should always be done with the head and neck in axial extension (good alignment). It is particularly useful for relieving trigger point pain and stiffness. Place palm of left hand against left cheek. Point fingers toward ear and point elbow forward. Turn head and neck to the left; contract while gently resisting with left hand. Contract neck muscle for 6 seconds. Relax and turn head to right as far as possible; hold stretch. Repeat four times; repeat on opposite side.

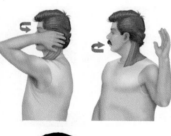

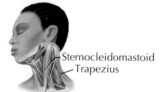

Sternocleidomastoid
Trapezius

2. Isometric Neck Exercises

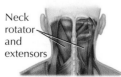

This exercise strengthens the neck muscles. Sit and place one or both hands on the head as shown. Assume good head and neck posture by tucking the chin, flattening the neck, and pushing the crown of the head up (axial extension). Apply resistance (a) sideward, (b) backward, and (c) forward. Contract the neck muscles to prevent the head and neck from moving. Hold contraction for 6 seconds. Repeat each exercise up to six times. Note: for neck muscles, it is probably best to use a little less than a maximal contraction, especially in the presence of arthritis, degenerated discs, or injury.

Neck flexors

Neck rotator and extensors

3. Chin Tuck

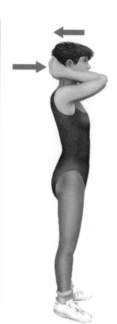

This exercise stretches the muscles at the base of the skull and reduces headache symptoms. Place hands together at the base of the head. Tuck in the chin and gently press head backward into your hands, while looking straight ahead. Hold.

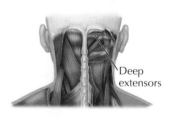

Deep extensors

4. Upper Trapezius Stretch

This exercise stretches the upper trapezius muscle and relieves neck pain and headache. To stretch the right upper trapezius, place left hand on top of head, right hand behind back. Gently turn head toward left underarm and tilt chin toward chest. Increase stretch by gently drawing head forward with left hand. Hold. Repeat to opposite side.

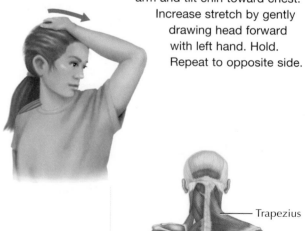

Trapezius

Table 9

Exercises for the Trunk Mobility **Table 9**

These exercises are designed to increase the strength and mobility of the muscles that move the trunk. They are especially helpful for people with chronic back pain. Hold stretches for 15 to 30 seconds.

1. Upper Trunk Lift

Lie on a table, bench, or special-purpose bench designed for trunk lifts with the upper half of the body hanging over the edge. Have a partner stabilize the feet and legs while the trunk is raised parallel to the floor; then lower the trunk to the starting position. Lift smoothly, one segment of the back at a time. Place hands behind neck or on ears. Do not raise past the horizontal or arch the back or neck.

Back extensors

3. Side Bend

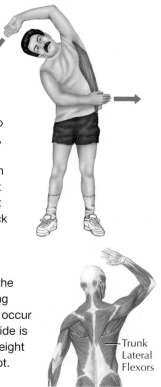

This exercise stretches the trunk lateral flexors. Stand with feet shoulder-width apart. Stretch left arm overhead to right. Bend to right at waist, reaching as far to right as possible with left arm; reach as far as possible to the left with right arm. Hold. Do not let trunk rotate or lower back arch. Repeat on opposite side. Note: this exercise is more effective if a weight is held down at the side in the hand opposite the side being stretched. More stretch will occur if the hip on the stretched side is dropped and most of the weight is borne by the opposite foot.

Trunk Lateral Flexors

2. Trunk Lift

This exercise develops the muscles of the upper back and corrects round shoulders. Lie face down with hands clasped behind the neck. Pull the shoulder blades together, raising the elbows off the floor. Slowly raise the head and chest off the floor by arching the upper back. Return to the starting position. Repeat. For less resistance, hands may be placed under thighs. Caution: Do not arch the lower back or neck. Lift only until the sternum (breastbone) clears the floor.

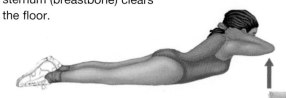

Variations: arms down at sides (easiest), hands by head, hands extended (hardest).

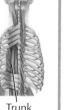

Trunk extensors

4. Supine Trunk Twist

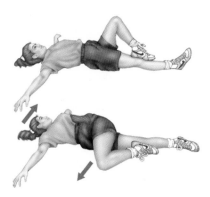

This exercise increases the flexibility of the spine and stretches the rotator muscles. Lie on your back with your arms extended at shoulder level. Place left foot on right knee cap. Twist the lower body by lowering left knee to touch floor on right. Turn head to left. Keep shoulders and arms on floor. Hold.

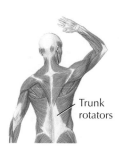

Trunk rotators

Table 9 Exercises for the Trunk and Mobility

Table 9

5. Lower Trunk Lift

This exercise develops low back and hip strength. Lie on your stomach on a bench or table with legs hanging over the edge. Have a partner stabilize the upper back or grasp the edges of the table with hands. Raise the legs parallel to the floor and lower them. Do not raise past the horizontal or arch the back. Suggested progression: (1) Begin by alternating legs; (2) when you can do 25 reps, add ankle weights; (3) when you can do 25 reps, lift both legs simultaneously (no weights).

Erector spinae

Gluteus maximus

6. Press-Up (McKenzie Extension Exercise)

This exercise increases flexibility of the lumbar spine and restores normal lordotic curve, especially for people with a flat lumbar spine. Lie on your stomach with hands under the face. Slowly press up to a rest position on forearms. Keep pelvis on floor. Relax and hold 10 seconds. Perform 5-10 repetitions. Do several times a day. Progress to gradually straightening the elbows while keeping the pubic bone on the floor. Caution: do not perform if you have lordosis or if you feel any pain or discomfort in the back or legs. Note: a prone press-up will feel good as a stretch after doing abdominal strength or endurance exercises. This relaxed lordotic position can be performed while standing. Place the hands in the small of the back and gently arch the back and hold. This should feel good after sitting for a long period with the back flat.

These exercises are designed to stretch the muscles of the chest and strengthen the muscles that keep the shoulders pulled back in good alignment (scapular adduction).

1. Arm Lift

This exercise strengthens the scapular adductors. Lie on stomach with arms in reverse-T. Rest forehead on floor. Maintain the arm position and contract the muscles between the shoulder blades, lifting the arms as high as possible without raising head and trunk. Hold. Relax and repeat. Note: if the arms are first pressed against the floor before lifting, this becomes a PNF exercise and range of motion may be greater. Variation: this more advanced exercise is performed in the same way except the arms are extended overhead.

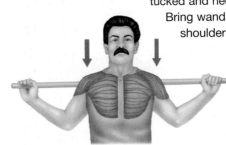

Rhomboids
Trapezius

2. Seated Rowing

This exercise strengthens the scapular adductors (rhomboid and trapezius). Sit facing pulley, feet braced and knees slightly bent. Grasp bar, palms down with hands shoulder-width apart. Pull bar to chest, keeping elbows high, and return.

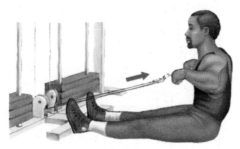

Rhomboids
Trapezius

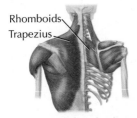

3. Wand Exercise

This exercise stretches the muscles on the front of the shoulder joint. Sit with wand grasped at ends. Raise wand overhead. Be certain that the head does not slide forward into a "poke neck" position. Keep the chin tucked and neck straight. Bring wand down behind shoulder blades. Keep spine erect; hold. Hands may be moved closer together to increase stretch on chest muscles.

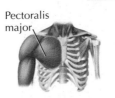

Pectoralis major

4. Pectoral Stretch

This exercise stretches the chest muscle (pectorals).
1. Stand erect in doorway with arms raised 45 degrees, elbows bent, and hands grasping door jambs, feet in front stride position. Press out on door frame, contracting the arms maximally for 3 seconds. Relax and shift weight forward on legs. Lean into doorway, so muscles on front of shoulder joint and chest are stretched. Hold.
2. Repeat with arms raised 90 degrees.
3. Repeat with arms raised 135 degrees.
(This exercise is not recommended for people with shoulder instability. Discontinue if it causes numbness in the arms or hands.)

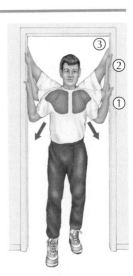

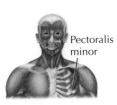

Pectoralis minor

Table 11

Table 11 Lumbar Stabilization Exercises with Stability Balls

These exercises are designed to help improve the ability of the back to stabilize and support the trunk. The physioballs provide a useful way to learn to balance the body in these positions.

1. Balancing

Contract abdominal muscles. Straighten one knee and raise opposite arm over head. Alternate sides. To increase difficulty, position ball farther from your body. Variation: slowly walk ball forward or backward with legs. Be careful not to arch back.

3. Wall Support

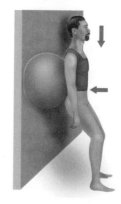

Stand against a wall with ball supporting low back. Contract abdominal muscles. Slowly bend knees 45 to 90 degrees and hold 5 seconds. Straighten knees and repeat. Raise both arms over head to increase difficulty.

2. Marching

Sit up straight with hips and knees bent 90 degrees. Contract abdominal muscles. Slowly raise one heel off the ground and opposite arm over head. Alternate sides. To increase difficulty, slowly raise one foot 2 inches from floor, alternating sides.

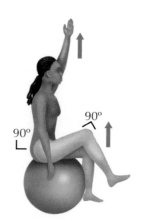

4. Stomach Roll

Lie prone over ball with abdominal region supported. Lower back and neck should be in neutral position with hands supported on floor directly under shoulders. Raise one leg off the floor while maintaining balance and a neutral spine. Alternate sides. To increase difficulty, raise one leg and opposite arm.

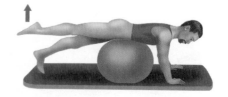

Lab Resource Materials: Healthy Back Tests

Chart 1 ▶ Healthy Back Tests

Physicians and therapists use these tests, among others, to make differential diagnoses of back problems. You and your partner can use them to determine if you have muscle tightness that may put you at risk for back problems. Discontinue any of these tests if they produce pain, numbness, or tingling sensations in the back, hips, or legs. Experiencing any of these sensations may be an indication that you have a low back problem that requires diagnosis by your physician. Partners should use *great caution* in applying force. Be gentle and listen to your partner's feedback.

FLEXIBILITY

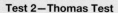

Test 1—Straight-Leg Lift

Lie on your back with hands behind your neck. The partner on your left should stabilize your right leg by placing his or her right hand on your knee. With the left hand, your partner should grasp your left ankle and raise your left leg as near to a right angle as possible. In this position (as shown in the diagram), your lower back should be in contact with the floor. Your right leg should remain straight and on the floor throughout the test.

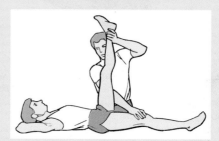

If your left leg bends at the knee, this indicates short hamstring muscles. If your back arches and/or your right leg does not remain flat on the floor this indicates short lumbar muscles or hip flexor muscles. To pass the test each leg should be able to reach approximately 90 degress without the knee or back bending (Both sides must pass in order to pass the test.)

Test 2—Thomas Test

Lie on your back on a table or bench with your right leg extended beyond the edge of the table (approximately one-third of your thigh off the table). Bring your left knee to your chest and pull your thigh down tightly with your hands. Lower your right leg. Your lower back should remain flat against the table, as shown in the diagram. To pass the test, your right thigh should be at table level or lower.

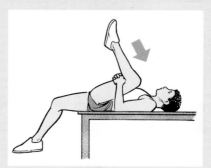

Test 3—Ober Test

Lie on your left side with your left leg flexed 90 degrees at the hip and 90 degrees at the knee. A partner should place your right hip in slight extension and right knee with just a slight bend (~20 degrees flexion). Your partner stabilizes your pelvis with the left hand to prevent movement. Your partner then allows the weight of the top leg to lower the leg to the floor. To pass the test your knee or upper leg should be able to touch the table.

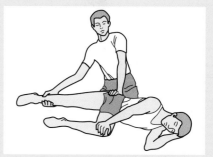

CORE TRUNK ENDURANCE TESTS

Test 4—Leg Drop Test*

Lie on your back on a table or on the floor with both legs extended overhead. Flatten your low back against the table or floor by tightening your abdominals. Slowly lower your legs while keeping your back flat.

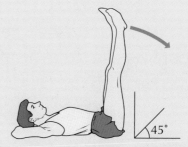

If your back arches before you reach a 45-degree angle, your abdominal muscles are too weak and you fail the test. A partner should be ready to support your legs if needed to prevent your lower back from arching or strain to the back muscles.

*The double leg drop is suitable as a diagnostic test when performed one time. It is not a good exercise to be performed regularly by most people. If it causes pain, stop the test.

Chart 1 ► **Healthy Back Tests** *(Continued)*

Test 5—Isometric Abdominal Test Lie supine with hips bent 45 degrees, feet flat on the floor and arms by the side. Draw a line 4 1/2 inches beyond fingertips. Tuck chin and curl trunk forward, touching line with fingers. To pass, hold for 30 seconds.

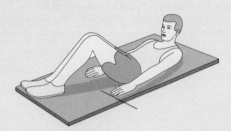

Test 6—Isometric Extensor Test Lie on a table with upper half of the body hanging over the edge and arms crossed in front of chest. Have a partner stabilize your feet and legs. Raise your trunk smoothly until your back is in a horizontal position parallel to the floor. Do not arch the back. To pass the test hold this position for 30 seconds.

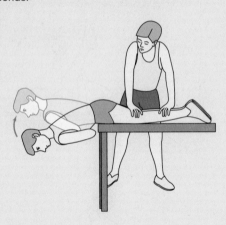

Test 7—Prone Bridge Support yourself on the floor by resting on forearms and balls of feet, body extended and back straight. Elbows are placed directly underneath shoulders. Look straight down toward hands. Do not arch the back. To pass the test hold this position for 30 seconds.

Test 8— Quadruped Stabilization Begin on hands and knees. Place hands directly below shoulders and knees directly below hips. Draw abdominals in. Extend one arm and opposite leg to a horizontal position. Do not allow back to arch or body to sway. To pass, hold position for 30 seconds.

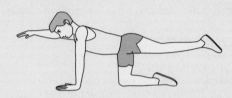

Test 9—Right Lateral Bridge Lie on your right side with legs extended. Raise pelvis off the floor until trunk is straight and body weight is supported on arm and feet. Do not roll forward or backward. Do not arch back. Hold this position for 30 seconds.

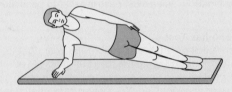

Test 10— Left Lateral Bridge Lie on your left side with legs extended. Raise pelvis off the floor until trunk is straight and body weight is supported on arm and feet. Do not roll forward or backward or arch back. To pass the test hold this position for 30 seconds.

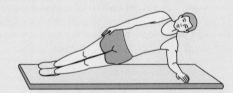

Chart 2 ► **Healthy Back Test Ratings**

Classification	Number of Tests Passed
Excellent	8–10
Very good	7
Good	6
Fair	5
Poor	1–4

Lab 11A The Healthy Back Tests and Back/Neck Questionnaire

Name	**Section**	**Date**

Purpose: To self-assess your potential for back problems using the Healthy Back Tests and the back/neck questionnaire

Procedures

1. Answer the questions in the following back/neck questionnaire. Count your points for nonmodifiable factors, modifiable factors, and total score, and record these scores in the Results section. Use Chart 1 to determine your rating for all three scores and record them in the Results section.
2. With a partner, administer the Healthy Back Tests to each other (see *Lab Resource Materials*). Determine your rating using Chart 2. Record your score and rating in the Results section. If you did not pass a test, list the muscles you should develop to improve on that test.
3. Complete the Conclusions and Implications section.

Risk Factor Questionnaire for Back and Neck Problems

Directions: Place an X in the appropriate circle after each question. Add the scores for each of the circles you checked to determine your modifiable risk, nonmodifiable risk, and total risk scores.

Nonmodifiable

1. Do you have a family history of osteoporosis, arthritis, rheumatism, or other joint disease? (0) No ⊗   (1) Yes

2. What is your age? (0) <40 ⊗   (1) 40–50   (2) 51–60   (3) 61+

3. Did you participate extensively in these sports when you were young: gymnastics, football, weight lifting, skiing, ballet, javelin, or shot put? (0) No   (1) Some ⊗   (3) Extensive

4. How many previous back or neck problems have you had? (0) None ⊗   (1) 1   (2) 2   (5) 3+

Modifiable

5. Does your daily routine involve heavy lifting? (0) No ⊗   (1) Some ⊗   (3) A lot

6. Does your daily routine require you to stand for long periods? (0) No ⊗   (1) Some   (3) A lot

7. Do you have a high level of job-related stress? (0) No ⊗   (1) Some   (3) A lot

8. Do you sit for long periods of time (computer operator, typist, or similar job)? (0) No   (1) Some   (3) A lot ⊗

9. Does your daily routine require doing repetitive movements or holding objects (e.g., baby, briefcase, sales suitcase) for long periods of time? (0) No ⊗   (1) Some   (3) A lot

10. Does your daily routine require you to stand or sit with poor posture (e.g., sitting in a low car seat, reaching overhead with head tilted back)? (0) No ⊗   (1) Some   (3) A lot

11. What is your score on the Healthy Back Tests? (0) 6–7   (1) 5   (3) 4   (5) 0–3

12. What is your score on the posture test in Lab 11B? (0) 0–2   (1) 3–4   (3) 5–7   (5) 8+

257

Results

Tests	Pass	Fail	If you failed, what exercise should you do?
1. Straight-leg lift	◯	◯	
2. Thomas test	◯	◯	
3. Ober's test	◯	◯	
4. Leg drop test	◯	◯	
5. Isometric abdominal test	◯	◯	
6. Isometric extensor test	◯	◯	
7. Prone bridge	◯	◯	
8. Right lateral bridge	◯	◯	
9. Left lateral bridge	◯	◯	
10. Quadruped stabilization	◯	◯	

Total ▢

Chart 1 ▶ Back/Neck Questionnaire Ratings

Rating	Modifiable Score	Nonmodifiable Score	Total Score
Very high risk	7+	12+	19+
High risk	5–6	8–11	13–17
Average risk	3–4	4–7	7–11
Low risk	0–2	0–3	0–5

Chart 2 ▶ Healthy Back Tests Ratings

Classification	Number of Tests Passed
Excellent	8–10
Very good	7
Good	6
Fair	5
Poor	1–4

Back/Neck Questionnaire

Score ▢   Rating ▢

Back Tests

Score ▢   Rating ▢

Conclusions and Implications: In several sentences, discuss your need to do exercises for care of the back and neck. Include in your discussion whether you think your muscles are fit enough to prevent problems, the areas in which you are most likely to experience problems, and steps you might take to prevent future problems. Use your test results to answer.

Lab 11B Evaluating Posture

Name	Section	Date

Purpose: To learn to recognize postural deviations and thus become more posture conscious and to determine your postural limitations in order to institute a preventive or corrective program

Procedures

1. Wear as little clothing as possible (bathing suits are recommended) and remove shoes and socks.
2. Work in groups of two or three, with one person acting as the subject while partners serve as examiners; then alternate roles.
   a. Stand by a vertical plumb line.
   b. Using Chart 1 and Figure 1, check any deviations and indicate their severity using the following point scale (0 = none, 1 = slight, 2 = moderate, and 3 = severe).
   c. Total the score and determine your posture rating from the Posture Rating Scale (Chart 2).
3. If time permits, perform back and posture exercises (see Lab 11C).
4. Complete the Conclusions and Implications section.

Results

Record your posture score:

Record your posture rating from the Posture Rating Scale in Chart 2:

Chart 1 ▶ Posture Evaluation

Side View	Points
Forward head	
Rounded shoulders	
Excessive lordosis (lumbar)	
Abdominal ptosis	
Hyperextended knees	
Total scores	

Chart 2 ▶ Posture Rating Scale

Classification	Total Score
Excellent	0–3
Very good	4–6
Good	7–9
Fair	10–12
Poor	12 or more

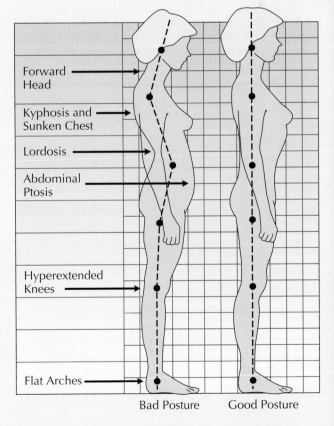

Bad Posture   Good Posture

Figure 1 ▶ Comparison of bad and good posture.

Conclusions and Implications

Were you aware of the deviations that were found?   Yes ◯   No ◯

1. List the deviations that were moderate or severe (use several complete sentences).

2. In several sentences, describe your current posture status. Include in this discussion your overall assessment of your current posture, whether you think you will need special exercises in the future, and the reasons your posture rating is good or not so good.

Lab 11C Planning and Logging Exercises: Care of the Back and Neck

Name		Section	Date

Purpose: To select several exercises for the back and neck that meet your personal needs and to self-monitor progress for one of these

Procedures

1. On Chart 1, check the tests from the Healthy Back Tests that you did *not* pass. Select at least one exercise from the group associated with those items. In addition, select several more exercises (a total of 8 to 10) that you think will best meet your personal needs. If you passed all of the items, select 8 to 10 exercises that you think will best prevent future back and neck problems. Check the exercises you plan to perform in Chart 1.
2. Perform each of the exercises you select 3 days in 1 week.
3. Keep a 1-week log of your actual participation using the last three columns in Chart 1. If possible, keep the log with you during the day. Place a check by each of the exercises you perform for each day, including ones that you didn't originally plan. If you cannot keep the log with you, fill in the log at the end of the day. If you choose to keep a log for more than 1 week, make extra copies of the log before you begin.
4. Answer the question in the Results section.

Chart 1 ▶ Back and Neck Exercise Plan

Check the tests you failed.	✓	Write in a selected exercises for each test that you can plan to perform this week [The core tests (5-10) may be used as strengthening exercies]. Check the dates you performed the exercises.	Day 1 Date:	Day 2 Date:	Day 3 Date:
1. Straight-leg lift					
2. Thomas test					
3. Ober test					
4. Leg drop test					
5. Isometric abdominal test					
6. Isometric extensor test					
7. Prone bridge					
8. Right lateral bridge					
9. Left lateral bridge					
10. Quadruped stabilization					

Results

Did you do 8 to 10 exercises at least 3 days in the week?　　Yes ◯　No ◯

Conclusions and Interpretations

1. Do you feel that you will use back and neck exercises as part of your regular lifetime physical activity plan, either now or in the future? Use several sentences to explain your answer.

2. Discuss the exercises you did. What exercises would you continue to do, and which ones would you change? Use several sentences to explain your answer.

Performance Benefits
of Physical Activity

Health Objectives for the Year 2020

- Reduce sports and recreation injuries.
- Reduce injuries from overexertion.
- Increase the proportion of adults who meet guidelines for aerobic and muscle fitness activity.
- Reduce steroid use by adolescents.
- Reduce percentage of adults who do no leisure-time activity.
- Increase access to employee-based exercise facilities and programs.
- Reduce adverse events from medical products.

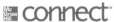

|FITNESS AND WELLNESS   http://connect.mcgraw-hill.com

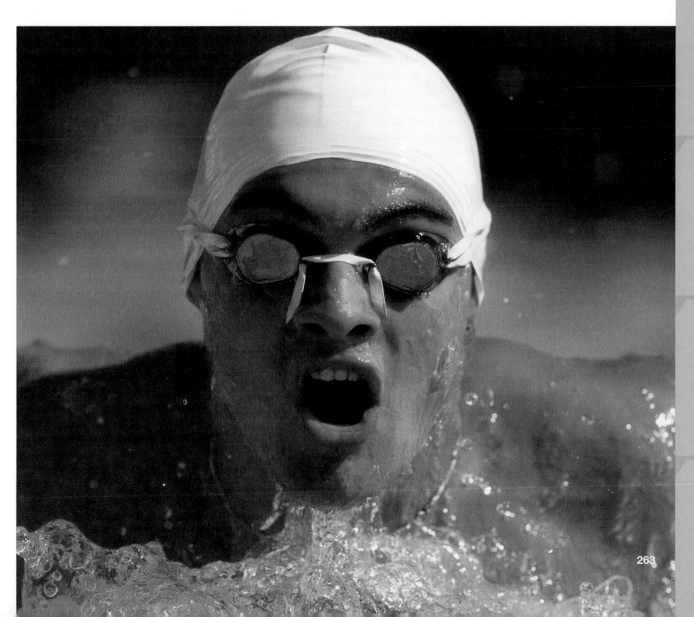

Specialized forms of training are needed to optimize adaptations to exercise and performance in sports.

Sports and competitive athletics provide opportunities for individuals to explore the limits of their ability and to challenge themselves in competition. Some individuals enjoy challenges associated with competitive aerobic activities, such as running, cycling, swimming, and triathlons. Others enjoy the challenges associated with competitive resistance training activities, such as powerlifting and bodybuilding. High-level performance is also a requirement for some types of work, such as fire safety, military service, and police work.

In this concept, specific attention is devoted to the methods used to train for high-level performance. Several types of training are discussed in detail, including endurance and speed training, specialized forms of resistance training, and other advanced training techniques, such as plyometrics, ballistic stretching, and functional balance training. Strategies for maximizing skill-related fitness and planning effective programs are also presented.

A full understanding of performance training requires a working knowledge of exercise physiology, an area of exercise science devoted to understanding how the body responds and adapts to exercise. The content provided in this concept provides a basic introduction to these principles and some practical guidelines for individuals interested in athletic performance.

High-Level Performance and Training Characteristics

Improving performance requires more specific training than the type needed to improve health. High levels of performance require good genetics, high levels of motivation, and a commitment to regular training. The amount of effort and training required to excel in sports, competitive athletics, or work requiring high-level performance is greater than the amount required for good health and wellness. Because adaptations to exercise are specific to the type of activity that is performed, training should be matched to the specific needs of a given activity.

High-level performance requires health-related, skill-related fitness and the specific motor skills necessary for the performance. To succeed in sports and certain jobs, high-performance levels of health-related physical fitness are necessary, over and above what the normal person needs to enhance health. This is illustrated in Figure 1. **Training** (regular physical activity)

builds health-related fitness to enhance health and high-level performance. This is why arrows in Figure 1 extend from health-related fitness to both health and high-level performance. High-performance levels are not necessary for all people, only those who need exceptional performances. A distance runner needs exceptional cardiovascular fitness and muscular endurance, a lineman in football needs exceptional strength, and a gymnast needs exceptional flexibility.

Exceptional performance also requires high-level skill-related physical fitness and good physical and motor skills. It is important to understand that skill-related fitness and skills are not the same thing. Skill-related fitness components are abilities that help you learn skills faster and better, thus the arrow in Figure 1 from skill-related fitness to skills. Skills, on the other hand, are things such as throwing, kicking, catching, and hitting a ball. Practice enhances skills. Practicing the specific skills of a sport or a job is more productive to performance enhancement than more general drills associated with changing skill-related fitness.

Success in endurance sports requires a high aerobic capacity. Distance runners, cyclists, and swimmers must be able to perform activity for long periods of time without stopping. are good examples. These types of performers are in special need of high levels of cardiovascular fitness, defined as aerobic capacity. In aerobic exercise, adequate oxygen is available to allow the body to rebuild the high-energy fuel the muscles need to sustain performance. Aerobic exercise increases aerobic capacity (cardiovascular fitness) by enhancing the body's ability to supply oxygen to the muscles as well as their ability to use it. Slow-twitch muscle fibers are most suited for aerobic exercise, and these fibers adapt most to aerobic training. Any performance that involves sustained performance places

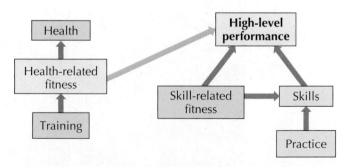

Figure 1 ▶ Factors influencing high-level performance.

special demands on the slow-twitch fibers and requires a high level of aerobic capacity (see Concept 7).

(i) FEATURE 1 **Many types of high-level performance require anaerobic capacity.** While all athletes benefit from a good level of aerobic fitness, success in many sports is determined more by speed, strength, and power. The sprinting, jumping, and powerful movements needed in most competitive sports are good examples. Strength competitions and sprint events in running, bicycling, and swimming also require short bursts of high-intensity activity. These activities use more energy than can be provided with aerobic metabolism. Anaerobic processes (i.e., processes that do not require oxygen) provide the additional energy needs, but a by-product of these processes (**lactic acid**) eventually causes the muscles to fatigue.

When you do anaerobic exercise the body cannot supply enough oxygen to sustain performance. So the body uses a high-energy fuel that the body has stored. When the high-energy fuel is used up, you cannot continue to perform. After the exercise you keep breathing fast and the heart continues to beat fast for a while, because the body needs to take in extra oxygen to rebuild the stores of the high-energy fuel used in anaerobic exercise. This is sometimes called **oxygen debt.** The body "borrows" oxygen that it cannot provide when it is using high-energy fuel during anaerobic exercise and then "pays back the debt" by supplying extra oxygen after the anaerobic

exercise. Your body also breaks down lactic acid during the recovery period after anaerobic exercise. In some ways "borrowing" oxygen during anaerobic exercise, and paying back the oxygen debt later, is like using a credit card to borrow money that is paid back later.

Athletes involved in anaerobic activities typically perform specialized forms of **anaerobic exercise** to help improve their bodies' ability to produce energy anaerobically and to tolerate higher levels of lactic acid. Using the credit card analogy, this is equivalent to the increases in available credit that are provided to customers who demonstrate that they can pay their credit card bills. Fast-twitch muscle fibers are used primarily during intense anaerobic activity, and these fibers are more likely to adapt and respond to anaerobic exercise. Most sports require a combination of aerobic and anaerobic capacity, so it is important to conduct training that is most specific to the needs of a given activity.

Genetics can influence a person's potential for high-level performance. Each person inherits a unique genetic profile, which may predispose him or her to success in different sports and activities. A higher percentage of slow-twitch muscle fibers allow a person to adapt most effectively to aerobic exercise, while a higher percentage of fast-twitch muscle fibers enhance adaptations from and performance in anaerobic exercise. Heredity also influences the dimensions of skill-related fitness, such as balance, coordination, and reaction time, that enhance development of motor skills. The most successful performers are those who inherit good potential for health- and skill-related fitness, who train to improve their health-related fitness, and who do extensive practice to improve the skills associated with the specific activity in which they hope to excel.

Performance in most sports requires good levels of fitness (health-related and skill-related) as well as practice to improve skills.

Training The type of physical activity performed by people interested in high-level performance—e.g., athletes, people in specialized jobs.

Lactic Acid Substance that results from the process of supplying energy during anaerobic exercise; a cause of muscle fatigue.

Oxygen Debt A term used to describe the body's ability to use high-energy fuel in anaerobic exercise without the presence of oxygen, and its ability to supply oxygen after the exercise to rebuild the supply of high-energy fuel.

Anaerobic Exercise *Anaerobic* means "in the absence of oxygen." Anaerobic exercise is performed at an intensity so great that the body's demand for oxygen exceeds its ability to supply it.

Training for Endurance and Speed

Specific forms of training are needed to optimize endurance performance and speed. Speed and endurance are at opposite ends of the performance continuum. Speed events in running are as short as 100 meters, while endurance events, such as a marathon, last 26 miles. Middle-distance events, such as the mile run, fall between these extremes and present unique challenges, since it is important for athletes to have both speed and endurance. While these examples all involve running, the types of training needed for these events are very different.

One feature that is common in advanced training programs is the need to continually challenge the body. Involvement in regular physical activity will lead to increases in cardiovascular fitness in most people, but improvements are harder to achieve once a good level of fitness has been attained (the principle of diminishing returns). To maximize performance, it is necessary to perform more specific types of workouts that provide a greater challenge (overload) to the cardiovascular system. Serious athletes may exercise 6 or 7 days a week, but easier workouts are generally done after harder and more intense workouts. The hard workouts are generally very specific and are designed to challenge the body in different ways. Supplemental training to improve technique and efficiency are also used to enhance performance.

Long-slow distance training is important for endurance performance. Extended periods of aerobic exercise are needed to achieve high-level endurance performance. Athletes generally refer to this type of training as **long-slow distance (LSD) training.** Emphasis is placed on the overall duration or length of the exercise session rather than on speed. The reason for this is that specific adaptations take place within the muscles when used for long periods of time. These adaptations improve the muscles' ability to take up and use the oxygen in the bloodstream. Adaptations within the muscle cell also improve the body's ability to produce energy from fat stores. Long-slow distance training involves performances longer than the event for which you are performing but at a slower pace. For example, a mile runner will regularly perform 6- to 7-mile runs (at 50 to 60 percent of racing pace) to improve aerobic conditioning, even though the event is much shorter. A marathoner may perform runs of 20 miles or more to achieve even higher levels of endurance. Although this 20-mile distance is shorter than the marathon race distance, research suggests that ample adaptations occur from this volume of exercise. Excess mileage in this case may just wear the body down. Long-slow distance training should be performed once every 1 to 2 weeks, and a

rest day is recommended on the subsequent day to allow the body to recover fully.

Improved anaerobic capacity can contribute to performance in activities considered to be aerobic. Many physical activities commonly considered to be aerobic—such as tennis, basketball, and racquetball—have an anaerobic component. These activities require periodic vigorous bursts of exercise. Regular anaerobic training will help you resist fatigue in these activities. Even participants in activities such as long-distance running can benefit from anaerobic training, especially if performance times or winning races is important. A fast start may be anaerobic, a sprint past an opponent may be anaerobic, and a kick at the end is certainly anaerobic. Anaerobic training can help prepare a person for these circumstances.

(*i*) **Interval training can be effective in building both aerobic and anaerobic capacity.** FEATURE 2 High-level performance requires high-level training. **Interval training** is commonly used by many competitive athletes. The premise behind interval training is that by providing periodic rest you can increase the overall intensity of the exercise session and provide a

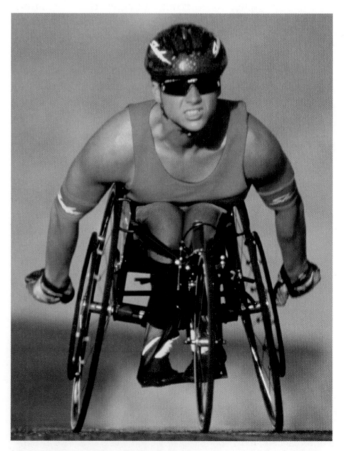

Interval training can be adapted for performers in a variety of activities.

Table 1 ▶ Aerobic Interval Training Schedules for a 10-Kilometer Runner

Best 10-km Times (Min:Sec)	Reps	Distance (Meters)	Rest (Sec)	Pace (Min:Sec)
46:00	20	400	10–15	2:00
43:00	20	400	10–15	1:52
40:00	20	400	10–15	1:45
37:00	20	400	10–15	1:37
34:00	20	400	10–15	1:30

Source: Wilmore and Costill.

Table 2 ▶ Sample Anaerobic Interval Training Program (Moderate Intensity)

Short Intervals	Long Intervals
1. Do a flexibility and cardio-vascular warm-up.	1. Do a flexibility and cardio-vascular warm-up.
2. Run at 100% speed for 10 seconds (approximately 70–100 yards).	2. Run at 90% speed for 1 minute (approximately 300–500 yards).
3. Rest for 10 seconds by walking slowly.	3. Rest for 4 minutes by walking slowly.
4. Alternately repeat steps 2 and 3 until 20 runs have been completed.	4. Alternately repeat steps 2 and 3 until 5 runs have been completed.

greater stimulus to the body. Interval training can be performed in different ways to achieve different training goals.

In aerobic interval training, the goal is to challenge the aerobic system to work near maximal levels for extended periods of time. Research suggests that a period of 4 to 6 minutes of activity is needed to cause the aerobic system to elicit maximal adaptations that will improve aerobic capacity (VO_2 max). The use of repeated mile runs at a faster than normal training pace would provide this type of challenge to the aerobic system. Alternately, shorter exercise bouts can be performed with brief rest periods to achieve the same goal. For example, a series of quarter-mile repeats with short rests is suitable as long as the total time at a high intensity is similar. In this case, the rest intervals must be short enough to allow only partial recovery between intervals.

Aerobic intervals are typically conducted at paces slower than the pace an individual would use in a race. An example of a schedule of aerobic interval training for a 10-km runner is illustrated in Table 1. To use the schedule, locate your typical 10-km time in the left-hand column. Perform 400-meter runs at the time specified in the "Pace" column. Repeat 20 times with intervals of 10 to 15 seconds between runs. Similar schedules can be developed with other activities, such as swimming and cycling.

In anaerobic interval training, the goal is to challenge the anaerobic energy systems. This is typically accomplished with repeated high-intensity bouts of activity. In response to this training, the body improves its ability to produce energy anaerobically and improves its ability to tolerate and remove lactic acid from the blood.

Anaerobic interval training can be performed with either short or long intervals. Short-interval workouts should use maximum speed with rest intervals lasting from 10 seconds to 2 minutes. These should be repeated 8 to 30 times. Long-interval training should use 90 to 100 percent speed, with rest intervals lasting from 3 to 15 minutes.

These should be repeated 4 to 15 times. A sample short anaerobic interval program and a sample long-interval running program are presented in Table 2. These plans can be modified for use with other types of activities.

Principles of interval training can be adapted for different activities. The principles of interval training can be integrated into workouts in less structured ways. Runners sometimes use *fartlek* training to break up their workouts. A fartlek training run incorporates bursts of higher-intensity running followed by recovery periods of lower intensity. The difference from interval training is that the intermittent bursts in fartlek training are dictated by the nature of the terrain or the feelings of the moment. The term is from a Swedish word meaning "speed play," because the unstructured nature is more relaxed than structured interval training.

Many competitive sports involve alternating bursts of high-intensity activity followed by periods of recovery. Basketball, for example, involves intermittent sprints and jumps interspersed with periods of short recovery. Similarly, tennis involves bursts of activity separated by short recovery periods between points. To prepare for success in sports, it is important for athletes to incorporate intermittent interval-type training into their conditioning. Simulated games that require repeated sprints up and down the basketball court are a form of interval training specific to basketball players. Tennis players can

Long-Slow Distance (LSD) Training Training technique used by marathon runners and other endurance performers that emphasizes long, slow distance, rather than speed.

Interval Training A training technique often used for high-level aerobic and anaerobic training; uses repeated bouts of activity followed by rest to maximize the quality of the workout.

incorporate a variety of forward and lateral movements into a high-intensity agility drill to improve conditioning for tennis.

Too much strength and flexibility training may impair endurance performance. The principle of specificity dictates that adaptations are specific to the type of training that is performed. While athletes should strive for a good balance of strength and flexibility, studies show that too much training in these areas can actually cause decreases in performance. Additional muscle mass from resistance training can reduce efficiency and impair performance. The use of weighted wristlets, ankles, or belts is also not recommended, as they may alter running mechanics and stride efficiency.

Flexibility has always been thought to be important for minimizing risks for injury, but recent studies have shown that running economy (the energy cost required to run a specific speed) is not as good in people with high flexibility as in those who have poorer flexibility. Because running economy is an advantage for distance running performance, this suggests that extra flexibility may actually reduce performance. The theory behind these findings is that stiffer muscle-tendon structures may help facilitate elastic energy return during running movements. This result shouldn't discourage you from stretching, but it does illustrate the complexities of high-level training. Regular stretching is still of value for most runners and endurance athletes.

Training for Strength and Muscular Endurance

ⓘ **Specific progressive resistance training programs are needed to achieve** FEATURE 3 **high-level muscular performance.** A basic progressive resistance program for overall good health might involve performing a single exercise for each major muscle group two or three times a week. This level of training provides a regular stimulus to maintain healthy levels of muscular strength and endurance. However, many people enjoy challenging themselves to achieve higher levels of muscular performance. Olympic weight-lifting competitors use free weights and compete in two exercises: the snatch and the clean and jerk. Powerlifting competitors use free weights and compete in three lifts: the bench press, squat, and dead lift. Bodybuilding competitors use several forms of resistance training and are judged on muscular hypertrophy (large muscles) and **definition of muscle.** Performers in these activities and athletes in strength-related sports need to use more advanced training methods to reach their full potential. The essential goal in high-level training is to provide the optimal stimulus, so that the muscles adapt in the desired way. Because the goals are clearly different for athletes interested in strength/power, muscular hypertrophy, or muscular endurance, it is important to follow appropriate programs. The essential aspects of these different training programs are described in the sections that follow. The basic concepts are summarized in Figure 2.

Performers training for high-level strength should use multiple sets with heavier weights. The best stimulus for strength gains is repeated lifts with very heavy loads. Guidelines for intermediate lifters call for multiple sets of 6 to 12 reps performed using 70 to 80 percent of 1RM values. The load and intensity guidelines are higher for advanced lifters (1 to 12 reps performed using 70 to 100 percent 1RM) because they may need to use a higher overload to get continued improvements. Rest intervals must be long (2 to 3 minutes) for high-intensity strength training to allow full recovery of the muscles between sets.

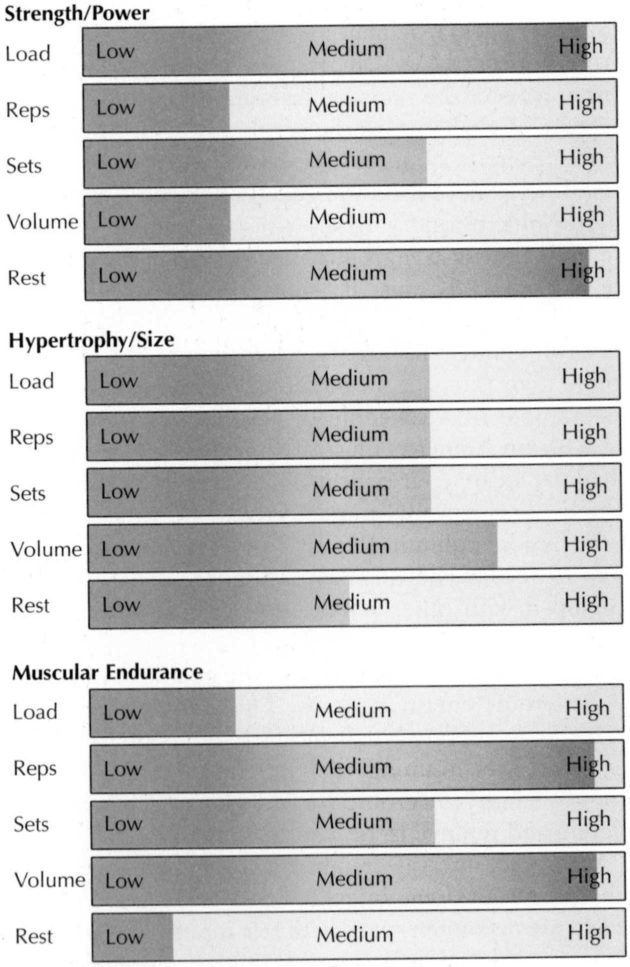

Figure 2 ▶ Differences in training stimulus for different resistance training programs.

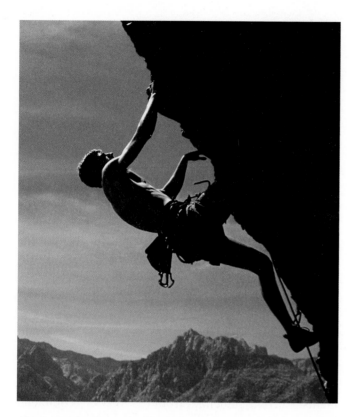

Good muscular endurance (and strength) are needed for performance in rock climbing.

Multiple joint exercises, such as the bench press, have been found to be more effective in strength enhancement, since they allow a greater load to be lifted. The sequencing of exercises within a workout is also an important consideration for strength development. When training all major muscle groups in a workout, large muscle groups should be done before small muscle groups, and multiple-joint exercises should be done before single-joint ones.

Performers training for muscular endurance should emphasize many repetitions with lighter weights. Completing multiple sets of 10 to 25 repetitions is required to build endurance. Short rest periods of 1 to 2 minutes are recommended for high-repetition sets, and periods of less than 1 minute should be used for lower-repetition sets. This challenges the muscles to perform repeatedly and with little or no rest. Variation in the order in which exercises are performed is also recommended to vary the stimulus. Intermediate lifters should aim for two to four times per week, but advanced lifters may perform up to six sessions per week if appropriate variation in muscle groups is used between workouts.

Performers training for bulk and definition often use extra reps and/or sets. Bodybuilders are more interested in definition and hypertrophy than in absolute strength. Gaining both size and definition requires a

balance between strength and muscle endurance training. Most bodybuilders use 3 to 7 sets of 10 to 15 repetitions, rather than the 3 sets of 3 to 8 repetitions recommended for most weight lifters. Sometimes definition is difficult to obtain because it is obscured by fat. It should be noted that people with the largest-looking muscles are not always the strongest.

Training for cardiovascular fitness along with strength training can limit adaptations. The body adapts to the type of training that is performed. If too much endurance training is performed, the body tries to adapt to the needs of aerobic activity, and this makes it more difficult to gain muscle mass or achieve maximal increases in strength. The effect would only be an issue for competitive strength or power athletes and should not deter people from getting the important health benefits associated with moderate amounts of aerobic activity. Regular aerobic activity is considered essential for bodybuilders to help them reduce unwanted body fat.

Training for Power

Power is a combination of strength and speed, and it is both health-related and skill-related. Most experts classify power as a skill-related component of fitness because it depends partially on speed. On the other hand, power also depends on strength and can be classified as a health-related component to the extent that strength is involved. Thus, power falls somewhere between the two distinct groups of fitness attributes.

Some experts consider power to be the most functional mode in which all human motion occurs. Power is exceptionally important in sport activities such as hitting a baseball, blocking in football, putting the shot, and throwing the discus. Power is also essential for good vertical jumping—a movement critical for basketball and many other sports. A typical progressive resistance exercise program will build sufficient power for normal activities of daily living; however, people interested in high-level performance should consider using additional exercises that specifically develop power.

The stronger person is not necessarily the more powerful. Power is the amount of work per unit of time. To increase power, you must do more work in the same time or the same work in less time. If you extend your knee and move a 100-pound weight through a 90-degree arc in 1 second, you have twice as much power as a person

Definition of Muscle The detailed external appearance of a muscle.

Performers who need explosive power to perform their events should use training that closely resembles those events. Jumpers, for example, should jump as a part of their training programs in order to learn correct timing and mechanics. If they use machines, it is better to use the leg press than a knee extension machine because the press more nearly resembles the leg action of the jump.

The performer's program should use similar speed, force, angle, and range of motion as the activity. However, if a performer is unable to do the specific skill because of weather or injury or is seeking variety, then plyometrics, isokinetics, and weight training (especially with free weights or pulleys if simulating a sport skill) are effective means of developing power.

Power training can be done with weight equipment, but care is needed to ensure safety and efficacy. Resistance training can be performed to optimize power development, but these movements are not recommended for beginning lifters. Studies have shown that heavy resistance training can actually decrease power unless training also includes some explosive movements. Current guidelines from the ACSM recommend heavy loading (85 to 100 percent of 1RM) to increase the force component of the power equation and light to moderate loading (30 to 60 percent of 1RM) performed at an explosive velocity to enhance the speed component of power. The guidelines recommend that a multiple-set power program (3–6 sets) be integrated within an overall strength training program. Exercises for power are most effectively done with free weights or pulleys to simulate sport-related movements more effectively. Isokinetic devices, such as isokinetic swim benches, may also be useful for enhancing sport-specific power.

Plyometrics may be useful in training for tasks or events requiring power. **Plyometrics** is an advanced training technique used by many athletes. It takes advantage of a quick prestretch prior to a movement to increase power. By repeatedly doing these movements in training, athletes can provide a greater stimulus to their muscles and improve their body's ability to perform power movements. Track and field athletes may do a hopping drill for 30 to 100 meters or alternate jumping from a box to the floor and back to the box (called depth jumping, drop jumping, or bounce loading). As the body lands, some of the major leg muscles lengthen in an eccentric contraction, then follow immediately with a strong concentric contraction as the legs push off for the next jump or stride. The prestretch of the muscle during landing adds an elastic recoil that provides extra force to the push-off (see Table 3).

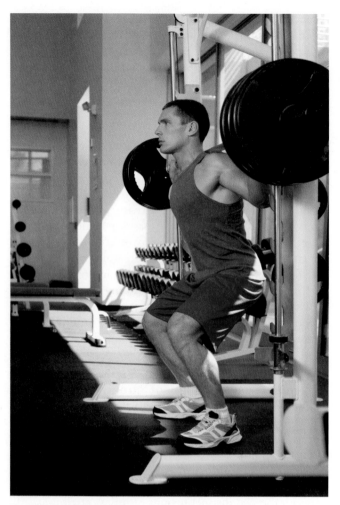

Training for high-level performance requires focus and determination.

who needs 2 seconds to complete the same movement. Power requires both strength and speed. Increasing one without the other limits power. Some power athletes (for example, football players) might benefit more by achieving less strength and more speed.

The principle of specificity applies to power development. If you need power for an activity in which you are required to move heavy weights, then you need to develop *strength-related power* by working against heavy resistance at slower speeds. If you need to move light objects at great speed, such as in throwing a ball, you need to develop *speed-related power* by training at high speeds with relatively low resistance. There must be trade-offs between speed and power because the heavier the resistance, the slower the movement. Training adaptations are also specific to the type of training performed. Power exercises done at high speeds will help enhance muscular endurance, whereas power exercises that use heavy resistance at lower speeds will increase strength.

Table 3 ▶ Plyometric Exercise—a Technique for Developing Power

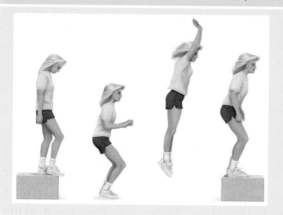

In this plyometric exercise, called the "depth jump," the athlete jumps off a box and then quickly bounds upward to land on another box. The first phase of the exercise involves an eccentric contraction (shortening of muscle fibers to slow the body during the landing phase). This is followed immediately by a concentric lengthening of muscle fibers to leap onto the next box. The recoiling of the fibers increases the force that can be applied to the muscles. Several repetitions of this type of exercise should be performed, followed by brief rests. Because of the eccentric contractions, plyometric exercises can promote greater amounts of muscle soreness, so it is important to work up to this gradually.

Table 4 ▶ Safety Guidelines for Plyometrics

- Plyometrics for growing teens should begin moderately and progress slowly, compared with plyometrics for adults.

- Progression should be gradual to avoid extreme muscle soreness.

- Adequate strength should be developed prior to plyometric training. (As a general rule, you should be able to do a half-squat with one-and-a-half times your body weight.)

- Get a physician's approval prior to doing plyometrics if you have a history of injuries or if you are recovering from injury to the body part being trained.

- The landing surface should be semiresilient, dry, and unobstructed.

- Shoes should have good lateral stability, be cushioned with an arch support, and have a nonslip sole.

- Obstacles used for jumping-over should be padded.

- The training should be preceded by a general and specific warm-up.

- The training sequence should…
  - precede all other workouts (while you are fresh);
  - include at least one spotter;
  - be done no more than twice per week, with 48 hours' rest between bouts;
  - last no more than 30 minutes;
  - include 3 or 4 drills (for beginners), with 2 or 3 sets per drill, 10–15 reps per set, and 1–2 minutes' rest between sets.

Source: Adapted from Brittenham.

Plyometrics are used to apply the specificity principle to training for certain skills. Because eccentric exercise tends to result in more muscular soreness, it would be wise to proceed slowly with this type of training. It would also be important to have good flexibility before beginning a plyometrics program. Table 4 lists safety guidelines for plyometrics.

Training for Balance and Flexibility

Functional balance training is used by some athletes to improve performance. Functional balance training involves the execution of skilled movements that improve **proprioception** and promote balance. The unique aspect of the movements is that they typically require movement and stabilization force production at the same time. In other words, one part of the body is in motion while another is stabilized. These actions essentially train the body's many somatic sensory organs to respond and adjust to different postures and positions—thereby improving balance. Functional balance training is frequently performed with exercise balls, balance boards, or BOSU trainers (see Concept 9). It is important to start slowly with easy movements and work up to more challenging positions and movements. This type of training is not recommended for people who have had recent orthopedic injuries, who have degenerative joint disease, or individuals with knee instability.

(i) **Stretching techniques for performance are very different from those recommended** FEATURE 4 **for general health.** Static stretching is generally recommended for people interested in improving flexibility because it is both safe and effective. More

Plyometrics A training technique used to develop explosive power. It involves the use of concentric-isotonic contractions performed after a prestretch or an eccentric contraction of a muscle.

Proprioception Awareness of body movements and orientation of the body in space; often used synonymously with *kinesthesis*.

Risk of Injuries in Sports

Ankle Sprains. Recent research indicates that nearly 1.5 million ankle sprains occur annually, and 49 percent of these injuries are related to athletic performance. Injuries occur most frequently in the teen years but are very prevalent among college-age adults. This may be because of the higher athletic and sports participation of younger people. Men have more sprains than women before age 30, and women have more sprains after 30. African Americans are at greater risk of ankle injuries than other populations. The sports with the greatest risk for ankle sprains are basketball (41%), football (9%), soccer (8%), running (7%), volleyball (4%), softball (4%), and baseball (3%). Running was the only non-team sport in the top five. More information on ankle sprains is available at the associated Web link.

mode. To use this indicator, you should regularly monitor your resting heart rate before getting out of bed in the morning. Another indicator that is increasingly used by elite endurance athletes is compressed or reduced "heart rate variability." A lower beat-to-beat variability indicates fatigue or overtraining, since it reflects sympathetic dominance over the normally dominant parasympathetic system that exists during more rested states. Newer heart rate monitors provide an indicator of heart rate variability.

Rest and a history of regular exercise are important for reducing the risks for overuse injuries. Rest is a critical part of training programs for serious athletes. Adequate rest helps the body recover from the stress of vigorous training—it promotes the physiological adaptations that improve performance and reduces the likelihood of developing overuse injuries.

A history of regular exercise is also important for reducing risks for injury. Research conducted by the military has determined that recruits with a history of regular exercise were less likely to get injured during basic training than recruits without this experience. This suggests that regular exercise can build up the strength and integrity of bones and joints and reduce the risk for injury. In other words, experienced athletes can perform higher levels of training without injury because they have built up a greater tolerance.

Periodization of training may help prevent overtraining. When a person trains for a single performance or perhaps several competitive events, such as games or matches during a sport season, he or she must plan carefully to reach peak performance at the right time and to avoid overtraining and injuries. *Periodization* is a modern concept of manipulating repetition, resistance, and exercise selection so there are periodic peaks and valleys during the training program. The peaks are needed to challenge the body, and the valleys are needed to allow the body to recover and adapt fully. Over the course of the season, there should be a gradual progression that allows the person to peak at just the right time. To accomplish this, training begins with an emphasis on base training, in which the volume of training is gradually increased (increasing reps or performing large numbers of sets). As the season progresses, the emphasis shifts to the intensity of training (going faster or lifting heavier weights). Because higher-intensity exercise requires more time for recovery, the volume of training should be reduced at these times. A key concept in periodization is to provide opportunities for the body to adapt and recover fully prior to competition. Thus, the phase immediately prior to competition (**tapering**) is characterized by a reduced volume and intensity of training. By applying periodization to their training, athletes optimize performance and minimize the risks of overtraining (see Figure 3).

Athletes should be aware of various psychological disorders related to overtraining. Compulsive physical activity, often referred to as activity neurosis or exercise addiction, can be considered a hyperkinetic condition. People with activity neurosis become irrationally concerned about their exercise regimen. They

HEALTH is available to Everyone for a Lifetime, and it's Personal

Improved athletic performance, better attention span, and staying awake to study are just a few of the reasons given for using "energy drinks" that contain high amounts of caffeine. But most are not aware of how much caffeine they are truly consuming. An article in the *Journal of American College Health* suggests that high consumption of energy drinks is a risky behavior and is associated with other risky health behaviors. While not all students consume energy drinks, limiting their use to specific situations, others find themselves reaching for energy drinks many times a day.

Do you or your friends drink energy drinks? What do you think are the benefits and drawbacks of energy drinks?

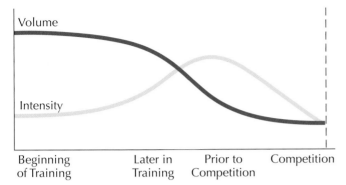

Figure 3 ▶ Volume and intensity of training during periodization.

may exercise more than once a day, rarely take a day off, or feel the need to exercise even when ill or injured. One condition related to body neurosis is an obsessive concern for having an attractive body. Among females, it is usually associated with an extreme desire to be thin, whereas among males it is more often associated with an extreme desire to be muscular. The excessive desire to be fit or thin can negatively affect other aspects of life, threaten personal relationships, and contribute high amounts of stress. Anorexia nervosa, an eating disorder associated with an excessive drive to be thin, has frequently been associated with compulsive exercise.

Performance Trends and Ergogenic Aids

Many athletes look to ergogenic aids as an additional way to improve performance. Athletes are always looking for a competitive edge. In addition to pursuing rigorous training programs, many athletes look for alternative ways to improve their performance. Substances, strategies, and treatments designed to improve physical performance beyond the effects of normal training are collectively referred to as **ergogenic aids.** People interested in improving their appearance (including those with body neurosis) also abuse products they think will enhance their appearance. Ergogenic aids can be classified as mechanical, psychological, and physiological. Each category will be discussed in the subsequent sections.

Tapering A reduction in training volume and intensity prior to competition to elicit peak performance.

Ergogenic Aids Substances, strategies, and treatments intended to improve performance in sports or competitive athletics.

Technology Update
Performance Technology

TECH

New technological developments have helped numerous athletes improve their performance. Some innovations have contributed to Olympic records and helped athletes achieve medal-winning performances. Two of these innovations are nanotechnology and friction-reducing fibers for athletic wear.

Nanotechnology: Nanoscience is the study of materials engineered at the level of the atom. *Nano* refers to nanometer, which is equal to one-billionth of a meter. The width of one nanometer is three to five atoms. Nanoscience has led to nanotechnology using very small particles to make new materials or improve existing materials. It has also resulted in the development of equipment that is lighter, yet stronger than older equipment. Examples of products made using nanotechnology include lighter golf clubs for faster swing speed; golf balls produced with high precision, for more even spin and truer flight path; lighter and stronger tennis rackets for higher serve speed; tennis balls that keep bounce longer because of a nano-composite barrier that prevents leaks; high-tech ski wax that allows faster skiing; and lighter bicycles for greater speed and more efficient performance. More information is available at the associated Web link.

Clothing Technology: The development of various types of performance-based clothing has had major impacts on a number of sports. A number of years ago, track athletes and swimmers began using whole body suits as a way to reduce drag and improve performance. The new high-tech swimsuits used by top swimmers reduce drag and improve speed. The suit uses a customized, water-repellent fabric (a combination of spandex and nylon yarn) that makes it feel almost slippery to the touch. It weighs 70 percent less than other swimsuits and retains almost no water. Additional details are provided on the associated Web link along with other examples.

Mechanical ergogenics may improve efficiency and performance. Mechanical ergogenic aids consist of equipment or devices that aid performance. Examples include oversized tennis racquets, more flexible poles for pole vaulting, spring-loaded ice skates (klap skates) for skating, lycra body suits for reducing drag in swimming and running, and carbon fiber bike frames to increase stiffness and force transmission. Consumers are presented with many options in the sport and fitness industry, and it is difficult to keep up with all the innovations.

While mechanical ergogenic aids may help maximize performance, the advantages provided by the latest high-tech innovations are probably noticeable only for highly elite athletes. For example, a recreational athlete may not play any better with an expensive tennis racquet or new golf clubs. Expert players, on the other hand, can appreciate subtle differences in equipment and may benefit. New developments in nanotechnology will likely usher in a new era of technological advances (see Tech Update). Athletes, however, should continue to focus on improving fitness and practicing skills, since these will have bigger impacts on performance.

Psychological ergogenics can improve concentration, improve motivation, and reduce anxiety during competitive activities. Many competitive activities require extreme levels of concentration, motivation, and focus. Athletes who maintain a mental edge during an event are at a clear advantage over athletes who cannot. Competitive anxiety can impair performance, and psychological ergogenics can help competitors reduce anxiety before and during an event. Types of psychological ergogenics include mental imagery, hypnosis, modeling performance, and establishing skill routines, to name but a few. Sources containing useful information about psychological ergogenics are provided in the Web Resources and Suggested Readings.

ⓘ **Physiological ergogenics are designed to improve performance by enhancing**
FEATURE 6 **biochemical and physiological processes in the body.** Physiological ergogenics are primarily nutritional supplements thought to have a positive effect on various metabolic processes. Because the supplement industry is largely unregulated, many products are developed and marketed with little or no research to document their effects. Producers of these products prey on an athlete's lack of knowledge and concern

over performance. Products with little or no evidence of benefits also have questionable safety, so consumers should be cautious.

For example, protein supplements are unregulated products for which evidence of effectiveness is lacking. Many strength athletes continue to believe that extra protein in the diet can contribute to strength and muscle mass gains, despite the fact that this has been clearly refuted in the scientific literature. The aggressive marketing and propaganda in many muscle-related fitness publications convince many people to buy and try unproven supplements. Consumers are encouraged not to be swayed by ads and unsubstantiated claims.

Physiological ergogenics with established performance benefits are described below. Additional information about ergogenic aids and links to performance are provided at the associated Web link. Concept 23 presents strategies for detecting quackery.

- *Fluid replacement beverages and energy bars.* Fluid replacement beverages, such as Gatorade, Exceed, and Power Aide, contain carbohydrates needed for endurance exercise. People exercising for more than an hour can benefit from these supplements, and research shows that they can replace fluid lost in sweat at the same or a faster rate than water. Energy bars (e.g., Power Bars and Clif Bars), energy gels (e.g., GU), or energy chews (e.g., Clif Shot Blocks) also provide valuable energy for extended endurance exercise. Consumers should be wary of other "energy" products that tout energy without calories. These are simply stimulants or caffeine products.

- *Creatine.* As described in Concept 9, creatine is a nutrient involved in the production of energy during intense exercise. The body produces it naturally from foods containing protein, but some athletes take creatine supplements (usually a powder dissolved in a liquid) to increase the amounts available in the muscle. The idea behind supplementation is that additional creatine intake enhances energy production and therefore increases the body's ability to maintain force and delay fatigue. Some studies have shown improvements in performance and anaerobic capacity, but recent reviews indicate that the supplement may be effective only for athletes who are already well trained. Products containing creatine do not work by themselves; instead, they only help athletes maximize their training or performance during an event. Effects are not evident unless training is performed while taking the supplements.

Strategies for Action

Select activities that match your abilities. People differ in many factors, including skills and abilities that influence sports and athletic performance. You may be well suited to some sports but not to others. Behavioral scientists have also determined that perceptions of competence are important predictors of long-term exercise adherence. To give yourself the best chance of being successful in sports (and exercise involvement), choose activities that are well matched to your abilities. Lab 12A provides an assessment that will allow you to evaluate your levels of skill-related physical fitness. By referring to Table 5, you can determine the sports and activities that best match your individual abilities.

The assessments provided in Lab 12A are but a few of the many tests that can be done for each of the skill-related fitness parts. You may want to try other tests if you want more information about your abilities. If you have a personal desire to train for a specific sport or activity, but do not have a fitness profile that predicts success, you should not be deterred. Lab 12A will help you find an activity that you will enjoy and in which you have a good chance of success. People with good motivation, who persist in training, can often excel over others with greater ability.

Take time to plan and record your training sessions. Success in sports and competitive athletics requires careful planning and a lot of effort. To maximize your potential, take time to plan your training program. Coaches handle these tasks for many competitive athletes, but recreational athletes typically have to plan their own program. Although you can contract with personal trainers to help with this task, adequate planning can be done by applying the principles described in this book. The key is to write a workout plan and keep careful records of your progress. This will allow you to monitor how your training program is progressing.

Get adequate rest and listen to your body. Because high-performance training can be quite intense, it is important to get adequate rest. Many athletes make the mistake of training too hard. An essential part of a good training program is rest. Without rest, the body does not have sufficient time to make the needed adaptations, and overtraining syndrome can result. Lab 12B provides an assessment to help you learn how to monitor for signs of overtraining.

Web Resources

Additional websites with information related to Concept 12 are available at the associated Web link.

Gatorade Sports Science Institute **www.gssiweb.com**

National Athletic Trainers Association **www.nata.org**

National Collegiate Athletic Association **www.ncaa.org**

National Strength and Conditioning Association **www.nsca-cc.org**

Promote Performance Newsletter (free) **www.performancemattersinc.com/newsletters**

Special Olympics International **www.specialolympics.org**

Sports Injuries (Medline Plus-NIH) **www.nlm.nih.gov/medlineplus/sportsinjuries.html**

Sports Injuries (NIAMSD) **www.niams.nih.gov/Health_Info/sports_injuries/**

United States Olympic Committee **www.usoc.org**

Women's Sports Foundation **www.womenssportsfoundation.org**

Suggested Readings

Selected readings and references are listed below. A more comprehensive list is available at the associated Web link.

Bahr, R., et al. 2003. Risk factors for sports injuries— A methodological approach. *British Journal of Sports Medicine* 37:384–392.

Bompa, T. and G. G. Haff. 2009. *Periodization*. 5th ed. Champaign, IL: Human Kinetics.

Borchers, J. R., et al. 2009. Metabolic syndrome and insulin resistance in Division 1 collegiate football players. *Medicine and Science in Sports and Exercise* 41(12):2105–2110.

Brotherhood, J. R. 2008. Heat stress and strain in exercise and sport. *Journal of Science and Medicine in Sport* 11(1):3–5.

Faigenbaum, A. D. 2009. Overtraining in young athletes: How much is too much? *ACSM's Health and Fitness Journal* 13(4):8–13.

Gibala, M. J. 2010. A practical model of low-volume high-intensity interval training induces mitochondrial biogenesis in human skeletal muscle: potential mechanisms. *Journal of Physiology* 588:1011–1022.

Hibbs, A. E., et al. (2008). Optimizing performance by improving core stability and core strength. *Sports Medicine* 38(12):995–1008.

Kovacs, M. 2009. *Dynamic Stretching: The Revolutionary New Warm-up Method to Improve Power, Performance and Range of Motion*. Berkeley, CA: Ulysses Press.

Kruscall, L. J., et al. 2009. Caffeine and exercise performance: What's all the buzz about? *ACSM's Health and Fitness Journal* 13(6):1723.

Lederman E. 2010. The myth of core stability. *Journal of Bodywork and Movement Therapies* 14(1):84–98.

Murray, B. 2007. Hydration and physical performance. *Journal of the American College of Nutrition* 26(5):542s–548s.

Nemet, D., and A. Eliakim. 2007. Protein and amino acid supplementation in sport. *International Sports Medicine Journal* 8(1):11–23.

Noakes, T. D. 2008. Heat stress in sport—Fact or fiction. *Journal of Science and Medicine in Sport* 11(1):3–5.

Orlick, T. 2008. *In Pursuit of Excellence*. 4th ed. Champaign, IL: Human Kinetics.

Stewart, M., et al. 2007. Warm-up or stretch as preparation for sprint performance? *Journal of Science and Medicine in Sport* 10(6):403–410.

Lab Resource Materials: Skill-Related Physical Fitness

Important Note: Because skill-related physical fitness does not relate to good health, the rating charts used in this section differ from those used for health-related fitness. The rating charts that follow can be used to compare your scores with those of other people. You *do not* need exceptional scores on skill-related fitness to be able to enjoy sports and other types of physical activity; however, it is necessary for high-level performance. After the age of 30, you should adjust ratings by 1 percent per year.

Evaluating Skill-Related Physical Fitness

I. Evaluating Agility: The Illinois Agility Run

An agility course using four chairs 10 feet apart and a 30-foot running area will be set up as depicted in this illustration. The test is performed as follows:

1. Lie prone with your hands by your shoulders and your head at the starting line. On the signal to begin, get on your feet and run the course as fast as possible.

2. Your score is the time required to complete the course.

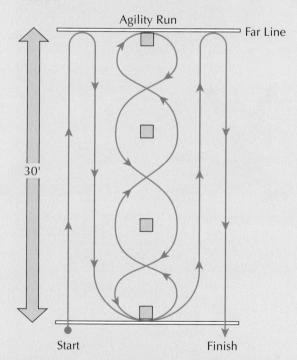

II. Evaluating Balance: The Bass Test of Dynamic Balance

Eleven circles (9½ inches) are drawn on the floor as shown in the illustration. The test is performed as follows:

1. Stand on the right foot in circle X. *Leap* forward to circle 1, then circle 2 through 10, alternating feet with each leap.

2. The feet must leave the floor on each leap and the heel may not touch. Only the ball of the foot and toes may land on the floor.

3. Remain in each circle for 5 seconds before leaping to the next circle. (A count of 5 will be made for you aloud.)

4. Practice trials are allowed.

5. The score is 50, plus the number of seconds taken to complete the test, minus the number of errors.

6. For every error, deduct 3 points each. Errors include touching the heel, moving the supporting foot, touching outside a circle, and touching any body part other than the supporting foot to the floor.

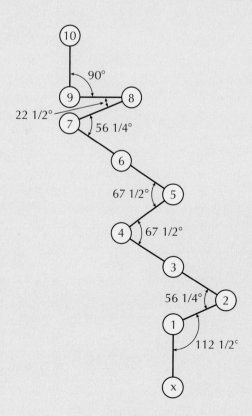

Chart 1 ▶ Agility Rating Scale

Classification	Men	Women
Excellent	15.8 or faster	17.4 or faster
Very good	16.7–15.9	18.6–17.5
Good	18.6–16.8	22.3–18.7
Fair	18.8–18.7	23.4–22.4
Poor	18.9 or slower	23.5 or slower

Source: Adams et al.

Chart 2 ▶ Balance Test Rating Scale

Rating	Score
Excellent	90–100
Very good	80–89
Good	80–89
Fair	80–89
Poor	80–89

III. Evaluating Coordination: The Stick Test of Coordination

The stick test of coordination requires you to juggle three wooden sticks. The sticks are used to perform a one-half flip and a full flip, as shown in the illustrations.

1. *One-half flip.* Hold two 24-inch (½ inch in diameter) dowel rods, one in each hand. Support a third rod of the same size across the other two. Toss the supported rod in the air, so that it makes a half turn. Catch the thrown rod with the two held rods.
2. *Full flip.* Perform the preceding task, letting the supported rod turn a full flip.

The test is performed as follows:

1. Practice the half-flip and full flip several times before taking the test.
2. When you are ready, attempt a half-flip five times. Score 1 point for each successful attempt.
3. When you are ready, attempt the full flip five times. Score 2 points for each successful attempt.

Chart 3 ▶ Coordination Rating Scale

Classification	Men	Women
Excellent	14–15	13–15
Very good	11–13	10–12
Good	5–10	4–9
Fair	3–4	2–3
Poor	0–2	0–1

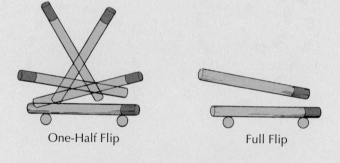

One-Half Flip   Full Flip

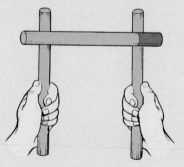

Hand Position

IV. Evaluating Power: The Vertical Jump Test

The test is performed as follows:

1. Hold a piece of chalk so its end is even with your fingertips.
2. Stand with both feet on the floor and your side to the wall and reach and mark as high as possible.
3. Jump upward with both feet as high as possible. Swing arms upward and make a chalk mark on a 5′ × 1′ wall chart marked off in half-inch horizontal lines placed 6 feet from the floor.
4. Measure the distance between the reaching height and the jumping height.
5. Your score is the best of three jumps.

Chart 4 ▶ Power Rating Scale

Classification	Men	Women
Excellent	25½″ or more	23½″ or more
Very good	21″–25″	19″–23″
Good	16 ½″–20½″	14½″–18½″
Fair	12½″–16″	10½″–14″
Poor	12″ or less	10″ or less

Metric conversions for this chart appear in Appendix A.

V. Evaluating Reaction Time: The Stick Drop Test

To perform the stick drop test of reaction time, you will need a yardstick, a table, a chair, and a partner to help with the test. To perform the test, follow this procedure:

1. Sit in the chair next to the table so that your elbow and lower arm rest on the table comfortably. The heel of your hand should rest on the table so that only your fingers and thumb extend beyond the edge of the table.
2. Your partner holds a yardstick at the top, allowing it to dangle between your thumb and fingers.
3. The yardstick should be held so that the 24-inch mark is even with your thumb and index finger. No part of your hand should touch the yardstick.
4. Without warning, your partner will drop the stick, and you will catch it with your thumb and index finger.
5. Your score is the number of inches read on the yardstick just above the thumb and index finger after you catch the yardstick.
6. Try the test three times. Your partner should be careful not to drop the stick at predictable time intervals, so that you cannot guess when it will be dropped. It is important that you react only to the dropping of the stick.
7. Use the middle of your three scores (for example: if your scores are 21, 18, and 19, your middle score is 19). The higher your score, the faster your reaction time.

Chart 5 ▶ Reaction Time Rating Scale

Classification	Score
Excellent	More than 21″
Very good	19″–21″
Good	16″–18¾″
Fair	13″–15¾″
Poor	Below 13″

Metric conversions for this chart appear in Appendix A.

VI. Evaluating Speed: 3-Second Run

To perform the running test of speed, it will be necessary to have a specially marked running course, a stopwatch, a whistle, and a partner to help you with the test. To perform the test, follow this procedure:

1. Mark a running course on a hard surface so that there is a starting line and a series of nine additional lines, each 2 yards apart, the first marked at a distance 10 yards from the starting line.

2. From a distance 1 or 2 yards behind the starting line, begin to run as fast as you can. As you cross the starting line, your partner starts a stopwatch.

3. Run as fast as you can until you hear the whistle, which your partner will blow exactly 3 seconds after the stopwatch is started. Your partner marks your location at the time the whistle was blown.

4. Your score is the distance you covered in 3 seconds. You may practice the test and take more than one trial if time allows. Use the better of your distances on the last two trials as your score.

Chart 6 ▶ Speed Rating Scale

Classification	Men	Women
Excellent	24–26 yards	22–26 yards
Very good	22–23 yards	20–21 yards
Good	18–21 yards	16–19 yards
Fair	16–17 yards	14–15 yards
Poor	Less than 16 yards	Less than 14 yards

Metric conversions for this chart appear in Appendix A.

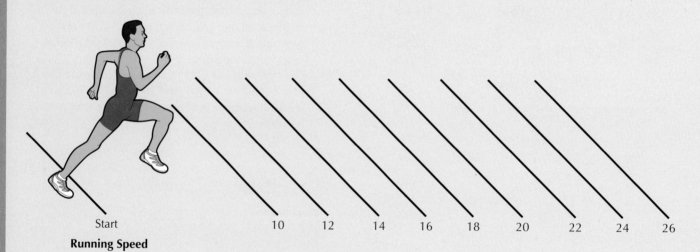

Start   10 12 14 16 18 20 22 24 26

Running Speed

Lab 12A Evaluating Skill-Related Physical Fitness

Name	Section	Date

Purpose: To help you evaluate your own skill-related fitness, including agility, balance, coordination, power, speed, and reaction time; this information may be of value in helping you decide which sports match your skill-related fitness abilities

Procedures

1. Read the direction for each of the skill-related fitness tests presented in *Lab Resource Materials.*
2. Take as many of the tests as possible, given the time and equipment available.
3. Be sure to warm up before and to cool down after the tests.
4. It is all right to practice the tests before trying them. However, you should decide ahead of time which trial you will use to test your skill-related fitness.
5. After completing the tests, write your scores in the appropriate places in the Results section.
6. Determine your rating for each of the tests from the rating charts in Lab Resource Materials.

Results

Place a check in the circle for each of the tests you completed.

Agility (Illinois run) ◯

Balance (Bass test) ◯

Coordination (stick test) ◯

Power (vertical jump) ◯

Reaction time (stick drop test) ◯

Speed (3-second run) ◯

Record your score and rating in the following spaces.

	Score	Rating	
Agility			(Chart 1)
Balance			(Chart 2)
Coordination			(Chart 3)
Power			(Chart 4)
Reaction time			(Chart 5)
Speed			(Chart 6)

Conclusions and Implications: In two or three paragraphs, discuss the results of your skill-related fitness tests. Comment on the areas in which you did well or did not do well, the meaning of these findings, and the implications of the results, with specific reference to the activities you will perform in the future.

Lab 12B Identifying Symptoms of Overtraining

Name	Section	Date

Purpose: To help you identify the symptoms of overtraining

Procedures

1. Answer the questions concerning overtraining syndrome in the Results section. If you are in training, rate yourself; if not, evaluate a person you know who is in training. As an alternative, you may evaluate a person you know who was formerly in training (and who experienced symptoms) or evaluate yourself when you were in training (if you trained for performance in the past).
2. Use Chart 1 (below) to rate the person (yourself or another person) who is (or was) in training.
3. Use Chart 2 (page 286) to identify some steps that you might take to treat or prevent overtraining syndrome.
4. Answer the questions in the Conclusions and Implications section.

Results

Answer "Yes" (place a check in the circle) to any of the questions relating to overtraining symptoms you (or the person you are evaluating) experienced.

 1. Has performance decreased dramatically in the last week or two?

 2. Is there evidence of depression?

 3. Is there evidence of atypical anger?

 4. Is there evidence of atypical anxiety?

 5. Is there evidence of general fatigue that is not typical?

 6. Is there general lack of vigor or loss of energy?

 7. Have sleeping patterns changed (inability to sleep well)?

 8. Is there evidence of heaviness of the arms and/or legs?

 9. Is there evidence of loss of appetite?

10. Is there a lack of interest in training?

Chart 1 ▶ Ratings for Overtraining Syndrome

Number of "Yes" Answers	Rating
9–10	Overtraining syndrome is very likely present. Seek help.
6–8	Person is at risk for overtraining syndrome if it is not already present. Seek help to prevent additional symptoms.
3–5	Some signs of overtraining syndrome are present. Consider methods of preventing further symptoms.
0–2	Overtraining syndrome is not present, but attention should be paid to the few symptoms that do exist.

Conclusions and Implications

Chart 2 lists some of the steps that may be taken to help eliminate or prevent overtraining syndrome. Check the steps that you think would be (or would have been) most useful to the person you evaluated.

Chart 2 ▶ Steps for Treating or Preventing Overtraining Syndrome
◯ 1. Consider a break from training.
◯ 2. Taper the program to help reduce symptoms.
◯ 3. Seek help to redesign the training program.
◯ 4. Alter your diet.
◯ 5. Evaluate other stressors that may be producing symptoms.
◯ 6. Reset performance goals.
◯ 7. Talk to someone about problems.
◯ 8. Have a medical checkup to be sure there is no medical problem.
◯ 9. If you have a coach, consider a talk with him or her.
◯ 10. Add fluids to help prevent performance problems from dehydration.

Discuss overtraining syndrome in general. Elaborate on one or two of the steps in Chart 2 that you think would be (or would have been) most effective in treating or preventing overtraining syndrome for the person you evaluated.

Body Composition

Health Objectives for the Year 2020

- Increase proportion of adults with healthy weight.
- Reduce childhood overweight and obesity.
- Reduce disorder eating among adolescents.
- Increase proportion of adults with high LDL who control weight and get activity.
- Increase proportion of people who regularly perform aerobic and muscle fitness exercises.
- Reduce percentage of adults who do no leisure-time activity.
- Increase diabetes education, screening, and care.
- Increase overall cardiovascular health in U.S. population.

- Increase work sites that offer nutrition and weight management classes and counseling.
- Increase participation in employee programs.
- Increase physician counseling on nutrition and weight management.
- Increase BMI measurement by primary doctors.
- Reduce joint pain in adults who have doctor-diagnosed arthritis.
- Increase policies that give retail food outlets incentives for foods that meet dietary guidelines.

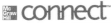

McGraw Hill **connect** | FITNESS AND WELLNESS   http://connect.mcgraw-hill.com

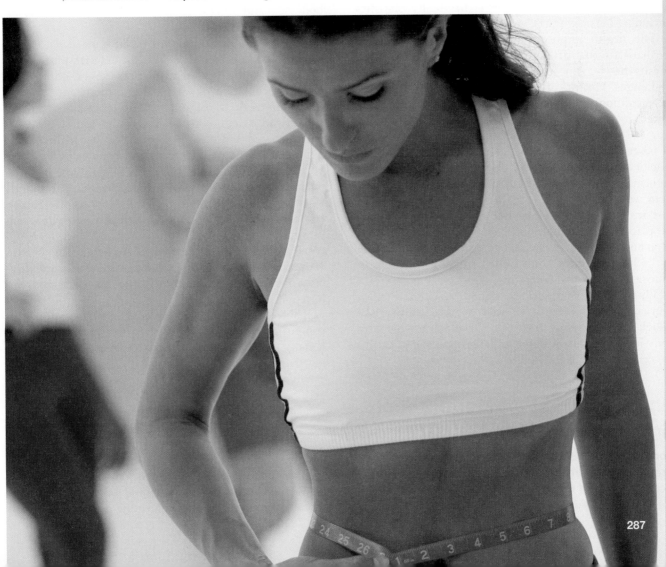

Possessing an optimal amount of body fat contributes to health and wellness.

(i)

FEATURE 1

The topic of overweight and obesity is in the news almost on a daily basis. Reports describe the health effects of obesity, the social and environmental factors that contribute to obesity, and the overall impact that it has on society. Ironically, in a society in which being thin or lean is almost obsessively valued, the incidence of overweight and obesity continues to increase. The most recent statistics indicate that approximately 17 percent of youth and 66 percent of adults are overweight or obese in the United States. Surveys indicate that only 52 percent believe they are overweight. About one-third of American adults are classified as obese, but only 12 percent classify themselves in this category. Over the past year, obesity rates have increased in 23 states, with Mississippi having the highest rate and Colorado the lowest. The Department of Defense indicates that incidence of overweight and obesity has doubled among active military personnel in the last 10 years. For more overweight/obesity statistics (including ranks by state), visit the associated Web link.

The health implications of this obesity epidemic are hard to quantify and predict, but it is clear that obesity has become one of our greatest public health challenges. Health-care dollars spent annually on medical conditions associated with obesity have been estimated at over $147 billion. It is estimated that by the year 2018 the cost will be $334 billion, accounting for 21 percent of health-care spending. Currently the yearly cost of medical care for the obese exceeds the cost for a normal-weight person by $2,460. When absenteeism from work is considered, the differences in health-care cost are even greater. Collectively, the obesity epidemic has placed a tremendous burden on our economy as well as on our health-care system. The problem is not unique to the United States, since similar trends are evident in almost all developed countries.

This concept describes issues associated with overweight and obesity as well as the health risks associated with being too lean. Developing a healthy body image and avoiding disordered patterns of eating are critical for optimal health and wellness.

Understanding and Interpreting Body Composition Measures

Body composition is considered a component of health-related fitness but can also be considered a component of metabolic fitness. Body composition is generally considered to be a health-related component of physical fitness. However, body composition is unlike the other parts of health-related physical fitness in that it is not a performance measure. Cardiovascular fitness, strength, muscular endurance, and flexibility can be assessed using movement or performance, such as running, lifting, or stretching. Body composition requires no movement or performance. This is one reason some experts prefer to consider body composition as a component of metabolic fitness. Whether you consider body composition to be a part of health-related or metabolic fitness, it is an important health-related factor.

Standards have been established for healthy levels of body fatness. Fat has important functions in the body, and it is distributed naturally into different tissues and storage depots. The indicator of **percent body fat** is typically used to reflect the overall fat content of the body. This indicator takes into account differences in body size and allows recommendations to be made for healthy levels of body fatness.

A certain minimal amount of fat is needed to allow the body to function. This level of **essential fat** is necessary for temperature regulation, shock absorption, and the regulation of essential body nutrients, including vitamins A, D, E, and K. The exact amount of fat considered essential to normal body functioning has been debated, but most experts agree that males should possess no less than 5 percent and females no less than 10 percent. For females, an exceptionally low body fat percentage (**underfat**) is of special concern, particularly when associated with overtraining, low calorie intake, competitive stress, and poor diet. **Amenorrhea** may occur, placing the woman at risk for bone loss (osteoporosis) and other health problems. A body fat level below 10 percent is one of the criteria often used by clinicians for diagnosing eating disorders, such as anorexia nervosa.

Table 1 shows the health-related standards for body composition (percent body fat) for both males and females. Because individuals differ in their response to low fatness, a borderline range is provided above the essential fat (too low) zone. Values in this zone are not necessarily considered to be healthy, but some individuals may seek to have lower body fat levels to enhance performance in certain sports. These levels can be acceptable for nonperformers if they can be maintained on a healthy diet and without overtraining. If symptoms such as amenorrhea, bone loss, and frequent injury occur, then levels of body fatness should be reconsidered, as should training techniques and eating patterns. For many

Table 1 ▶ Health-Related Standards for Body Fatness (Percent Body Fat) and Body Mass Index

	Too low	Borderline	Good fitness	Marginal	At risk	
Male	5 or less	6–9	10–20	21–25	26+	Body fatness (percent body fat)
Female	10 or less	11–16	17–28	29–35	36+	

	Too low	Borderline	Good fitness	Overweight*	Obesity*	
Male	12 or less	13–16	17–25	26–30	30+	Body mass Index (kg/m²)
Female	12 or less	13–16	17–25	26–30	30+	

*Note: Based on international standards used for BMI classification.

people in training, maintaining performance levels of body fatness is temporary; thus, the risk for long-term health problems is diminished.

Fat that is stored above essential fat levels is classified as **nonessential fat.** Just as percent body fat should not drop too low, it should not get too high. The healthy range for body fatness in males is between 10 and 20 percent, while the healthy range for women is between 17 and 28 percent. These levels are associated with good metabolic fitness, good health, and wellness. The marginal zone includes levels that are above the healthy fitness zone but not quite into the range used to reflect **obesity.** The term *obesity* often carries negative connotations and stereotypes, but it is important to understand that it is a clinical term that simply means excessively high body fat. Lab 13A provides opportunities for you to assess your level of body fatness.

(i) FEATURE 2 **Health standards have been established for the Body Mass Index.** The **Body Mass Index (BMI)** is a commonly used indicator of overweight and obesity in our society but is often misunderstood. The measure of BMI is basically an indicator of your weight relative to your height. It does not provide an indicator of body fatness, although BMI values tend to correlate with body fatness in most people. Because of this association, it is widely used in clinical settings and as a general indicator of body composition.

Because BMI is a frequently used measure, you should know how to calculate and interpret your BMI and your "healthy weight range." Mathematically, BMI is calculated with the following formula: BMI = weight (kg)/(height [m] × height [m]). Instructions and charts are provided in the *Lab Resource Materials* to simplify the calculation. There are also many BMI calculators n the Internet that make it easy to calculate (see Web link).

The accepted international standards for defining overweight and obesity are the same for both men and women. BMI values over 25 are used to define **overweight,** and values over 30 are used to define obesity. Table 1 provides additional information concerning BMI standards.

While the use of BMI is widely accepted, it does have limitations. Individuals who do regular physical activity and who possess considerable muscle mass may show up as overweight using the BMI. This is because muscle weighs more than fat, but height and weight measurements do not detect differences in muscle and fat in the body.

Percent Body Fat The percentage of total body weight that is composed of fat.

Essential Fat The minimum amount of fat in the body necessary to maintain healthful living.

Underfat Too little of the body weight composed of fat (see Table 1).

Amenorrhea Absent or infrequent menstruation.

Nonessential Fat Extra fat or fat reserves stored in the body.

Obesity A clinical term for a condition characterized by an excessive amount of body fat (or extremely high BMI).

Body Mass Index (BMI) A measure of body composition using a height-weight formula. High BMI values have been related to increased disease risk.

Overweight A clinical term that implies higher than normal levels of body fat and potential risk for development of obesity.

Assessing body weight too frequently can result in making false assumptions about body composition changes. The most common way that people gauge their body composition is by periodic assessments of body weight. While occasional checks of weight (and BMI) can be helpful, frequent body weight measurements can provide incorrect information and lead to false assumptions. For example, people vary in body weight from day to day and even hour to hour, based solely on their level of hydration. Short-term changes in weight are often due to water loss or gain, yet many people erroneously attribute the weight changes to their diet, a pill they have taken, or the exercise they recently performed. There is some evidence that monitoring weight daily can help normal-weight people from gaining weight. For people trying to lose weight, monitoring weight less frequently—once a week, for example—is more useful than taking daily or multiple daily measures. When you do weigh yourself, it is best to weigh at the same time of day, preferably early in the morning, because it reduces the chances that your weight variation will be a result of body water changes. Of course, it is best to use body composition assessments in addition to those based on body weight if accurate evaluations are expected. These are described in the next section.

Methods Used to Assess Body Composition

 Methods of body composition vary in accuracy and practicality. A number of FEATURE 3 techniques have been developed to assess body composition. The procedures vary in terms of practicality and accuracy, so it is important to understand the limitations of each method. It should be noted that even established techniques have potential for error. The most common methods are summarized below, with additional details available at the associated Web link.

Dual-energy absorptiometry (DXA) has emerged as the accepted "gold standard" measure of body composition. The DXA technique uses the attenuation of two energy sources to estimate the density of the body. A specific advantage of DXA is that it can provide whole-body measurements of body fatness as well as amounts stored in different parts of the body. For the procedure, the person lies on a table and the machine scans up along the body. While some radiation exposure is necessary with the procedure, it is quite minimal compared with X-ray and other diagnostic scans. Because the machine is quite expensive, this procedure is only found in medical centers and well-equipped research laboratories. The

 Technology Update
WiFi Scale

Most people have a scale in their house, and some have a device for assessing body fatness, such as those described in this section of the text. A new high-tech scale gives your body weight, your body fatness, and sends your daily measurement by WiFi to a source of your choice (computer or iPhone). It has the capacity to "tweet" your information to others if you choose.
A tweet is a text message of 140 characters or less using a social networking system known as Twitter. More information is available at the Web link.

DXA (also called DEXA) procedure provides scientists with a highly accurate measure of body composition for research and a criterion measure that has been used to validate other, more practical measures of body composition.

Underwater weighing and Bod Pod are two highly accurate methods. Underwater weighing is another excellent method of assessing body fatness. Before the development of DXA it was considered to be the "gold standard" method of assessment. In this technique, a person is weighed in air and underwater, and the difference in weight is used to assess the levels of body fatness. People with a lot of muscle, bone, and other lean tissue sink like a rock in water because muscle and other lean tissue are dense. Fat is less dense, so people with more fat tend to float in a water environment.

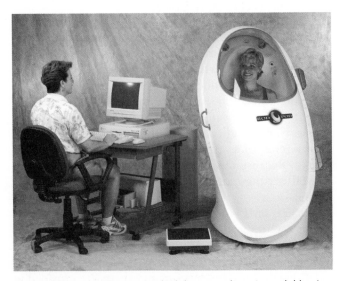

The Bod Pod uses the same principles as underwater weighing to estimate body fatness.

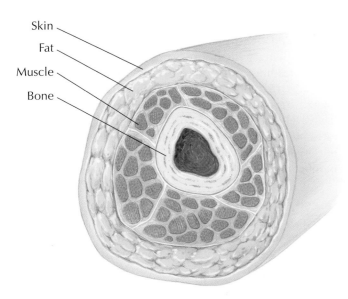

Figure 1 ▶ Location of body fat.

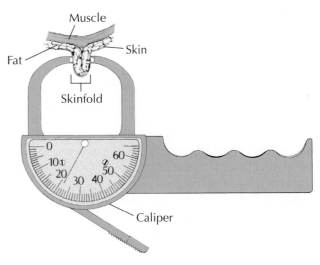

Figure 2 ▶ Measuring skinfold thickness with calipers.

People who weigh more underwater are more dense than those who weigh less in water. A limitation of this method is that participants must exhale all their air while submerged in order to obtain an accurate reading. Additional error from the estimations of residual lung volumes also tends to reduce the accuracy of this approach.

A relatively new device, called the Bod Pod, uses the same principles as underwater weighing, but relies on air displacement to assess body composition. Evidence suggests that it provides an acceptable alternative to underwater weighing and is particularly useful for special populations (obese older people and the physically challenged).

Skinfold measurements are a practical method of assessing body fatness. About one-half of the body's fat is located around the various body organs and in the muscles. The other half of the body's fat is located just under the skin, or in skinfolds. A skinfold (Figure 1) is two thicknesses of skin and the amount of fat that lies just under the skin. By measuring skinfold thicknesses of various sites around the body, it is possible to estimate total body fatness (Figure 2). Skinfold measurements are often used because they are relatively easy to do. They are not nearly as costly as underwater weighing and other methods that require expensive equipment. Research-quality skinfold calipers cost more than $100, but consumer models are available for $10–20.

In general, the more skinfolds measured, the more accurate the fatness estimate. However, measurements with two or three skinfolds have been shown to be reasonably accurate and can be done in a relatively short period. Two skinfold techniques are used in Lab 13A. You are encouraged to try both. With adequate training,

most people can learn to use calipers to get a good estimate of fatness.

Bioelectric impedance analysis has become a practical alternative for body fatness assessment. Bioelectric impedance analysis (BIA) ranks quite favorably for accuracy and has overall rankings similar to those of skinfold measurement techniques. The test can be performed quickly and is more effective for people high in body fatness (a limitation of skinfolds). The technique is based on measuring resistance to current flow. Electrodes are placed on the body and low doses of current are passed through the skin. Because muscle has greater water content than fat, it is a better conductor and has less resistance to current. The overall amount of resistance and body size are used to predict body fatness. The results depend heavily on hydration status, so it is important not to conduct testing after exercising or immediately after eating or drinking. Accuracy is also affected by the quality of the equipment. Portable BIA scales are available that allow you to simply stand on metal plates to get an estimate of body fatness. These devices are easier to use but are less accurate than those that use electrodes for both upper and lower body.

Infrared sensors are sometimes used to assess body fatness. Near-infrared interactance machines use the absorption of light to estimate body fatness. The technique was originally developed to measure the fat content of meats. Commercially available units for humans have not been shown to be effective for estimating body fat, and at least one company has faced sanctions from the government for selling an unapproved product. For this reason, this type of device is not recommended.

Health Risks Associated with Overfatness

Obesity contributes directly and indirectly to a number of major health problems. The presence of excess body fat impairs the function of most systems of the body (e.g., the cardiovascular system, the pulmonary system, the skeletal system, the reproductive system, and the metabolic system). It also increases risks for a variety of diseases, including a variety of cancers. The American Heart Association classifies obesity as a primary risk factor, along with high blood pressure and high blood lipids (both associated with overweight and obesity). When all the evidence is considered, it is clear that overweight is associated with many health problems and obesity places a person at special risk (see Figure 3).

Studies in previous years have indicated that overweight and obesity and associated unhealthy lifestyles (e.g., sedentary living and unhealthy eating) are the second leading actual cause of death. One current study indicates that obesity and smoking are equal in their overall burden on the health-care system. Smoking has decreased 18.5 percent from 1993 to 2008, while obesity rates increased by 85 percent. If current trends continue, obesity and overweight will soon surpass smoking as the number 1 cause of early death.

Obesity contributes to early death. In addition to the higher incidence of certain diseases and health problems, evidence shows that people who are moderately overfat have a 40 percent higher than normal risk of shortening their life span. More severe obesity results in a 70 percent

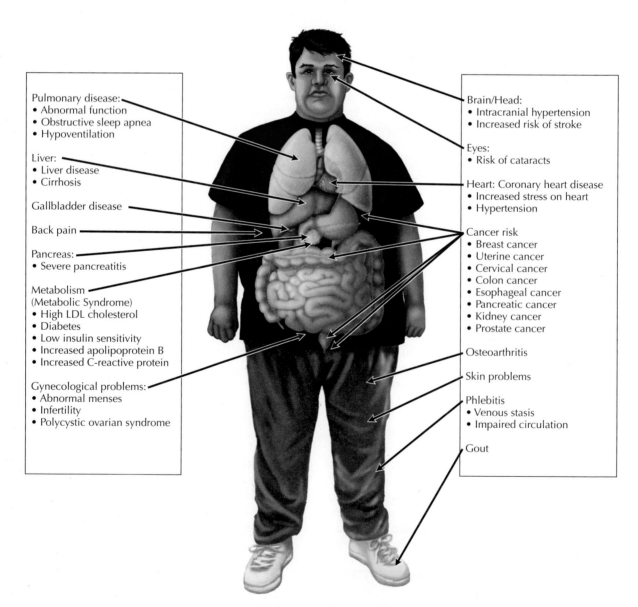

Figure 3 ▶ Diseases and medical complications associated with obesity.

higher than normal death rate. A study of nearly one million adults suggests that obesity can cut 8 to 10 years from life expectancy. Another recent study indicates that extreme obesity shortens life by 12 years.

Statistics indicate that underweight people also have a higher than normal risk for premature death. Though adequate evidence shows extreme leanness (e.g., anorexia nervosa) can be life threatening, underweight people may have lost weight because of a medical condition such as cancer. It appears that the medical problems are often the reason for low body weight rather than low body weight being the source of the medical problem. Most experts agree that people who are free from disease and who have lower than average amounts of body fat have a lower than average risk for premature death.

(i) **Physical fitness provides protection from the health risks of obesity.** A general
FEATURE 4 assumption in our society is that if you are thin, you are probably fit and healthy and that if you are overweight, you are unfit and unhealthy. A series of studies from the Aerobic Center Longitudinal Study (a large cohort study of patients from the Cooper Clinic in Dallas, Texas) has demonstrated that the health risks associated with overweight are greatly reduced by regular physical activity and reasonable levels of cardiovascular fitness (see Figure 4). In fact, the findings consistently show that active people who have a high BMI are at less risk than inactive people with normal BMI levels. Even high levels of body fatness may not be especially likely to increase disease risk if a person has good metabolic fitness as indicated by healthy blood fat levels, normal blood pressure, and normal blood sugar levels. It is when several of these factors are present at the same time that risk levels increase dramatically. For this reason, it is important to consider your cardiovascular and metabolic fitness levels before drawing conclusions about the effects of high body weight or high body fat levels on health and wellness. This information also points out the importance of periodically assessing your cardiovascular and metabolic fitness levels.

Excessive abdominal fat and excessive fatness of the upper body can increase the risk for various diseases. The location of body fat can influence the health risks associated with obesity. Fat in the upper part of the body is sometimes referred to as "Northern Hemisphere" fat, and a body type high in this type of fat is sometimes called the "apple" shape (see Figure 5). Upper-body fat is also referred to as android fat because it is more characteristic of men than women. Postmenopausal women typically have a higher amount of upper body fat than premenopausal women. Lower body fat, such as in the hips and upper legs, is sometimes referred to as "Southern Hemisphere" fat. This body type is sometimes called the "pear" shape. Lower-body fat is also referred to as gynoid fat because it is more characteristic of women than men.

Body fat located in the core of the body is referred to as central fat or visceral fat. Visceral fat is located in the abdominal cavity (see Figure 5), as opposed to subcutaneous fat, which is located just under the skin. Though subcutaneous fat (skinfold measures) can be used to estimate body fatness, it is not a good indicator of central fatness. A useful indicator of fat distribution is the waist-to-hip circumference ratio (see *Lab Resource Materials*). A high waist

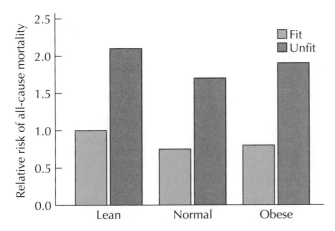

Figure 4 ▶ Risks of fatness vs. fitness.
Source: Lee, C. D., et al.

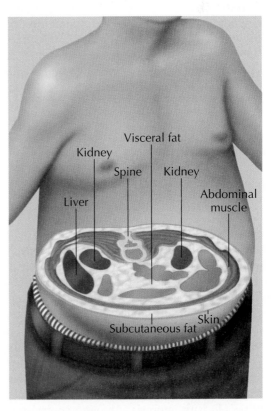

Figure 5 ▶ Visceral, or abdominal, fat is associated with increased disease risk.

circumference relative to hip circumference yields a high ratio indicative of high visceral fat. Visceral fat is associated with high blood fat levels as well as other metabolic problems. It is also associated with high incidence of heart attack, stroke, chest pain, breast cancer, and early death.

Part of the benefit of aerobic activity for health appears to be its ability to promote the preferential loss of abdominal body fat. Several recent studies have demonstrated that higher levels of activity and/or higher cardiorespiratory fitness are associated with lower levels of abdominal body fatness independent of body mass index. In other words, if one person who is fit and active has the same height and weight as a less active person, he or she will likely have a lower amount of abdominal fat. Abdominal body fat is considered to be more harmful than other forms. These studies provide a clear understanding of how fitness may protect against the health risks of obesity and improve overall health.

Health Risks Associated with Excessively Low Body Fatness

ⓘ **Excessive desire to be thin or low in body weight can result in health problems.** In
FEATURE 5 Western society, the near obsession with thinness has been, at least in part, responsible for eating disorders. Eating disorders, or altered eating habits, involve extreme restriction of food intake and/or regurgitation of food to avoid digestion. The most common disorders are anorexia nervosa, bulimia, and anorexia athletica. All of these disorders are most common among highly achievement-oriented girls and young women, although they affect virtually all segments of the population. Patterns of "disordered eating" are not the same as clinically diagnosed eating disorders. People who adopt disordered eating, however, tend to have a greater chance of developing an eating disorder. It is interesting to note that in 1974 the percentage of underweight Americans was 3.6. Today half that percentage (1.8) of Americans is classified as underweight.

Anorexia nervosa is the most severe eating disorder. If untreated, it is life threatening. Anorexics restrict food intake so severely that their bodies become emaciated. Among the many characteristics of anorexia nervosa are fear of maturity and inaccurate body image. The anorexic starves himself or herself and may exercise compulsively or use laxatives to prevent the digestion of food in an attempt to attain excessive leanness. The anorexic's self-image is one of being too fat, even when the person is too lean for good health. Assessing body fatness using procedures such as skinfolds and observation of the eating habits may help identify people with anorexia. Among anorexic girls and women, development of an adult figure is often feared. People with this disorder must obtain medical and psychological help immediately, as the consequences are severe. About 25 percent of those with anorexia do compulsive exercise in an attempt to stay lean. Anorexia is a very serious medical condition that deserves more discussion than can be provided in this book.

Binge-eating is a disorder that can be treated. Binge-eating is the most common eating disorder in the United States. According the American Psychiatric Association, you are a binge-eater if you meet these three criteria: (1) eat larger amounts of food than most people eat in a short time; (2) feel out of control while bingeing at least once a week for three months; and (3) do three or more behaviors such as feeling depressed about your binges, eating alone to avoid embarrassment about amounts eaten, eating large amounts when not hungry, eating more rapidly than normal, or continuing to eat when you feel full. While binge-eating can be a serious disorder, it can be treated effectively. One recent study showed that 64 percent of binge-eaters who received therapy and reading material were binge free after only one year.

Bulimia is a common eating disorder characterized by bingeing and purging. Disordered eating patterns become habitual for many people with bulimia. They alternate between bingeing and purging. Bingeing means periodically eating large amounts of food at one time. A binge might occur after a relatively long period of dieting and often consists of junk foods containing empty calories. After a binge, the bulimic purges the body of the food by forced regurgitation or the use of laxatives. Another form of bulimia is bingeing on one day and starving on the next. The consequences of bulimia include serious mental, gastrointestinal, and dental problems. Bulimics may or may not be anorexic. It may not be possible to use measures of body fatness to identify bulimia, as the bulimic may be lean, normal, or excessively fat.

Anorexia athletica is a more recently identified eating disorder that appears to be related to participation in sports and activities emphasizing body leanness. Studies show that participants in sports such as gymnastics, wrestling, and bodybuilding and activities such as ballet and cheerleading are most likely to develop anorexia athletica. This disorder has many of the symptoms of anorexia nervosa, but not of the same severity. In some cases, anorexia athletica leads to anorexia nervosa.

Female athlete triad is an increasingly common condition among female athletes. The triad refers to the relationship among energy availability, menstrual function, and bone mineral density. *Energy availability* refers to the amount and quality of food taken in, minus exercise energy expenditure. Low energy intake, especially in the presence of high energy expenditure, can have clinical manifestations, including eating disorders, amenorrhea and/or irregular menstrual cycles, and osteoporosis.

The female athlete triad is one of the more challenging conditions to treat because it often goes undetected. Once identified or diagnosed, it is hard to change because the three components of the triad are thought to be linked pathophysiologically. The athlete is very serious about performance and has likely developed altered eating patterns to control body weight. Efforts to bring about change often result in resistance, since the compulsion to be thin and perform well overrides other concerns, such as eating well, moderating exercise, and having a normal menstrual cycle. A position statement by the ACSM recommends regular screening exams to identify those with the triad and rule changes in women's sports to "discourage unhealthy weight loss practices." Nutrition counseling is recommended for those with the triad, and psychotherapy is recommended for athletes with eating disorders.

Many female athletes train extensively and have relatively low body fat levels but experience none of the symptoms of the triad. Eating well, training properly, using stress-management techniques, and monitoring health symptoms are the keys to their success.

Muscle dysmorphia is an emerging problem among male athletes. Muscle dysmorphia is characterized as a body dysmorphic disorder in which a male becomes preoccupied with the idea that his body is not sufficiently lean and/or muscular. Athletes with this condition may be more inclined to use performance-enhancing drugs, to exercise while sick, or to have an eating disorder. Additional risks include depression and social isolation.

Fear of obesity and purging disorder are other identified conditions. Fear of obesity is most common among achievement-oriented teenagers who impose a self-restriction on caloric intake because they fear obesity. Consequences include stunting of growth, delayed puberty, delayed sexual development, and decreased physical attractiveness. Purging disorder, a condition that results in purging similar to bulimia, but without the bingeing, has recently been identified. People with these conditions should seek assistance.

The Origin of Fatness

Obesity is a multifactorial disease that is influenced by both genetics and the environment. The evidence documenting a genetic component to human obesity is quite compelling. There is clear clustering of obesity within families, and studies have documented high concordance of body composition in identical twins. Studies of adopted children have also demonstrated that there is an association between the BMI of adoptees and the biologic parents but not between adoptees and adoptee parents. Despite the clear evidence, the role of genetic factors is still not well understood. Genetic mapping studies suggest that a number of genes may work in combination to influence susceptibility to obesity. These *susceptibility genes* may not lead directly to obesity but may predispose a person to overweight or obesity if exposed to certain environmental conditions. Two recent studies suggest that regular physical activity can overcome some genetic predispositions to fatness. The first study showed that teens with a variant gene referred to as the "fatso" gene can maintain normal body weight with 60 minutes of activity per day. The second study of Amish people who had a genetic variation (common to 30 percent of Caucasians) found that the risk of obesity could be blunted by regular physical activity.

Thus, the prevailing model guiding obesity research is that complex genetic and environmental variables interact to increase potential risks for obesity. Genetic factors, by themselves, cannot account for the rapid changes in the prevalence of obesity because the gene pool does not change that rapidly. Recent research has demonstrated that lack of sleep can increase risk for overweight (particularly in youth). Research has also demonstrated that excessive screen time (TV and computer use) and sitting time increase risk of obesity. Future research will allow genetic factors to be integrated with behavioral and environmental data so that the combined effects can be better understood.

Body weight is regulated and maintained through complex regulatory processes. Some scholars have suggested that the human body type, or **somatotype**, is inherited. Clearly, some people have more difficulty than others controlling fatness, and this may be because of their somatotype and genetic predisposition. Regulatory processes appear to balance energy intake and energy expenditure so that body weight stays near a biologically determined **set-point**. The regulation is helpful for maintaining body weight but can be frustrating for people trying to lose weight. If a person slowly tries to cut calories, the body perceives an energy imbalance and initiates processes

Somatotype A term that refers to a person's body type. One researcher (Sheldon) suggested that there are three basic body types: ectomorph (linear), mesomorph (muscular), and endomorph (round).

Set-point A theoretical concept that describes the way the body protects current weight and resists change.

In the News

Creating Social Change to Reverse Obesity

The childhood obesity epidemic represents one of the biggest public health challenges facing our country. A number of national campaigns have been created to mobilize action and create change. These initiatives use a variety of social media to generate interest and momentum. Three prominent examples are highlighted below.

- We Can! or "Ways to Enhance Children's Activity & Nutrition" is a national education program developed by the National Institutes of Health (NIH) to help prevent childhood obesity. The We Can program focuses on programs and activities for parents and families because they have a primary influence over shaping the home environment.

- Let's Move! is a program established by First Lady Michelle Obama to help address childhood obesity. The program adopts a broad community approach to enlist a variety of partners (community leaders, physicians, teachers, and parents) to help create healthier environments. The goal is to solve the epidemic of childhood obesity within a generation.
- The ActiveLifeMovement is an innovative social movement aimed at mobilizing individuals, groups, and communities to create change in society. They have developed a growing network of change agents and have made it possible for them to connect with others to create and advocate for change.

Learn more about these campaigns (and see how you can help) at the associated Web link.

---

to protect the current body weight. The body can accommodate to a new, higher set-point if weight gain takes place over time, but there is greater resistance to adopting a lower set-point. Many people lose weight, only to see the weight come back months later. One of the reasons exercise is so critical for weight maintenance is that it may help in resetting this set-point.

In recent years, the mechanisms involved in the regulation of the biological set-point have become better understood. The current view is that there are complex feedback loops among fatty tissues, the brain, and endocrine glands, such as the pancreas and the thyroid. A compound known as leptin plays a crucial role in altering appetite and in speeding up or slowing down the metabolism. Leptin levels rise during times of energy excess in order to suppress appetite and fall when energy levels are low to stimulate appetite. Resistance to leptin has been hypothesized as a possible contributor to obesity. A number of other compounds also appear to be involved in the complex processes regulating energy balance. Problems with the thyroid gland can lead to impairments in metabolic regulation, but these do not contribute to overfatness in most people.

Fatness early in life leads to adult fatness. Research has documented that body composition levels tend to track through the life span. Although there are exceptions, individuals who are overweight or obese as children are more likely to be overweight or obese as adults. One explanation for this is that overfatness in children causes the body to produce more fat cells. Research has even suggested that the neonatal environment that the child is exposed to during development may also influence future risks for obesity.

It appears that hormones and lipids circulating in the maternal blood can interact with genetic factors to establish metabolic conditions that contribute to overfatness. While these factors influence body composition, it is still possible to improve body composition by adopting healthy lifestyles.

Maintaining healthy levels of body fat is an important objective for children and adults. It was previously thought that only adult obesity was related to health problems, but it is now apparent that teens who are overfat are at a greater risk for heart problems and cancer than leaner peers. Obese children have been found to have symptoms of "adult-onset diabetes," and obese children have a higher than normal risk of premature death, indicating that the effects of obesity can impair health, even for young people. Concerns about the current and future implications of childhood obesity have made it one of the greatest public health concerns facing our country. A variety of national organizations have targeted obesity prevention as a top priority. The Let's Move campaign recently put forth by Michelle Obama has set out the ambitious goal of reversing the epidemic of childhood obesity within a generation. The momentum generated from these campaigns is encouraging, but it must translate into progressive policies and programming to create such a change. See the In the News content for more information.

Changes in basal metabolic rate can be the cause of obesity. The amount of energy you expend each day must be balanced by your energy intake if you are to maintain your body fat and body weight over time. Your energy intake is determined solely by the **calories** you eat, while your energy expenditure is determined by a number of related factors. The **basal metabolic rate (BMR)** is the largest component of total daily energy expenditure. BMR is the amount of calories needed to maintain your body function under resting conditions. Other contributions to energy expenditure come from processing the food you eat and from the physical activity performed during the day.

BMR is highest during the growing years. The amount of food eaten increases to support this increased energy expenditure. When growing ceases, if eating does not decrease or activity level increase, fatness can result. Basal metabolism also decreases gradually as you grow older. One major reason for this is the loss of muscle mass associated with inactivity. Regular physical activity throughout life helps keep the muscle mass higher, resulting in a higher BMR. Evidence suggests that regular exercise can contribute in other ways to increased BMR. The higher BMR of active people helps them prevent overfatness, particularly in later life.

"Creeping obesity" is a problem as you grow older. People become less active and their BMR gradually decreases with age. Caloric intake does seem to decrease somewhat with age, but the decrease does not adequately compensate for the decreases in BMR and activity levels. For this reason, body fat increases gradually with age for the typical person (see Figure 6). This increase in fatness over time is commonly referred to as "creeping obesity" because the increase in fatness is gradual. For a typical person, creeping obesity can result in a gain of 1/2 to 1 pound per year. People who stay active can keep muscle mass high and delay changes in BMR. For those who are not active, it is suggested that caloric intake decrease by 3 percent each decade after 25 so that by age 65 caloric intake is at least 10 percent less than it was at age 25. The decrease in caloric intake for active people need not be as great.

College students are susceptible to creeping obesity. College is a time when activity and eating patterns can change dramatically, often resulting in weight gain. Some have referred to extra weight gained in the first year of college as "the freshman 15," suggesting that

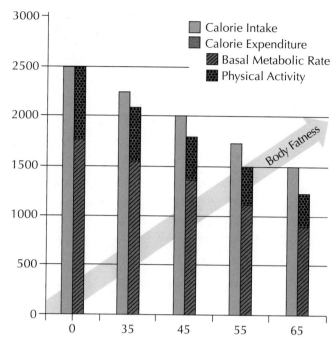

Figure 6 ▶ Creeping obesity.

the typical student gains 15 pounds in the first year of college. Recent studies show that the average gain is less than 15 pounds (5–9 pounds), but still quite significant. Sixty percent of freshmen gained weight, citing such factors as being less active, eating when stressed, and drinking more. Another study found that weight gained in college resulted in long-term weight gain. Students in this study gained 10 pounds over 4 years of college.

The Relationship between Physical Activity and Body Composition

A combination of regular physical activity and dietary restriction is the most effective means of losing body fat. Studies indicate that regular physical activity combined with dietary restriction is the most effective method of losing fat. **Diet** alone can contribute to weight loss, but much of this loss is actually lean tissue.

Calories Units of energy supplied by food; the quantity of heat necessary to raise the temperature of a kilogram of water 1°C (actually, a kilocalorie, but usually called a calorie for weight control purposes).

Basal Metabolic Rate (BMR) Energy expenditure in a basic, or rested, state.

Diet The usual food and drink for a person or an animal.

Table 2 ▶ Threshold of Training and Target Zones for Body Fat Reduction

	Threshold of Training*		Target Zones*	
	Physical Activity	**Diet**	**Physical Activity**	**Diet**
Frequency	• To be effective, activity must be regular, preferably daily, though fat can be lost over the long term with almost any frequency that results in increased caloric expenditure.	• Reduce caloric intake consistently and daily. To restrict calories only on certain days is not best, though fat can be lost over a period of time by reducing caloric intake at any time.	• Daily moderate activity is recommended. For people who do regular vigorous activity, 3 to 6 days per week may be best.	• It is best to diet consistently and daily.
Intensity	• To lose 1 pound of fat, you must expend 3,500 calories more than you normally expend.	• To lose 1 pound of fat, you must eat 3,500 calories fewer than you normally eat.	• Slow, low-intensity aerobic exercise that results in no more than 1 to 2 pounds of fat loss per week is best.	• Modest caloric restriction resulting in no more than 1 to 2 pounds of fat loss per week is best.
Time	• To be effective, exercise must be sustained long enough to expend a considerable number of calories. At least 15 minutes per exercise bout are necessary to result in consistent fat loss.	• Eating moderate meals is best. Do not skip meals.	• Exercise durations similar to those for achieving aerobic cardiovascular fitness seem best. Exercise of 30 to 60 minutes in duration is recommended.	• Eating moderate meals is best. Skipping meals or fasting is not most effective.

*It is best to combine exercise and diet to achieve the 3,500-calorie imbalance necessary to lose a pound of fat. Using both exercise and diet in the target zone is most effective.

When physical activity and diet are both used in a weight loss program, the same amount of weight may be lost but more of it is from fat. This is obviously beneficial for appearance and for participation in physical activity, but it can also help maintain resting metabolic rate at a higher level. This can contribute to further weight loss or facilitate weight maintenance. For optimal results, all weight loss programs should combine a lower caloric intake with a good physical exercise program. Table 2 presents thresholds of training and target zones for body fat reduction, including information for both physical activity and diet. A general guideline is to try to lose no more than 1–2 pounds a week. Because a pound of fat contains 3,500 calories, this requires a caloric deficit of approximately 500 calories per day. Individuals interested in maintaining body composition should aim for **caloric balance.** Individuals who want to increase lean body mass need to increase caloric intake while carefully increasing the intensity and duration of their physical activity (mainly muscular activity).

Physical activity can help expend extra energy needed to promote weight loss. The ACSM and national activity guidelines recommend a minimum of 30 minutes of moderate to vigorous activity a day or 150 minutes per week (see Table 2) but acknowledge that this may not be enough for some people. Both sources suggest that more is often needed either to maintain weight over time, or to lose weight. The new ACSM guidelines suggest that it may be necessary to work progressively up to 200 to 300 minutes a week. One recent study showed

that daily walks of 60 minutes resulted in fat loss among female cancer patients, and another found that women who maintained weight across the life span average approximately 60 minutes of activity per day.

Energy balance principles apply for weight maintenance and weight gain. Table 2 focuses on weight loss because overweight and obesity are prevalent in our society and because so many adults are currently dieting (approximately 33 percent) and another one-third are taking other steps to lose weight. For normal-weight people, maintenance is important, and balancing energy intake with energy expenditure is the key. There is little doubt that preventing overweight will help people avoid the more difficult task of losing weight. For those interested in weight gain, extra calorie intake is required, following the sound eating practices described in Concepts 14 and 15. Resistance training is also recommended because it builds muscle mass.

Whether you are trying to maintain, gain, or lose weight, you will need to know the number of calories you consume in food and the number of calories expended in the activities you perform. Table 3 lists calories expended in various activities.

Caloric Balance Consuming calories in amounts equal to the number of calories expended.

Table 3 ► Calories Expended per Hour in Various Physical Activities (Performed at a Recreational Level)*

| Activity | Calories Used per Hour | | | | |
	100 lb. (46 kg)	120 lb. (55 kg)	150 lb. (68 kg)	180 lb. (82 kg)	200 lb. (91 kg)
Archery	180	204	240	276	300
Backpacking (40-lb. pack)	307	348	410	472	513
Badminton	255	289	340	391	425
Baseball	210	238	280	322	350
Basketball (half-court)	225	255	300	345	375
Bicycling (normal speed)	157	178	210	242	263
Bowling	136	164	205	245	273
Canoeing (4 mph)	276	344	414	504	558
Circuit training	247	280	330	380	413
Dance, aerobics	315	357	420	483	525
Dance, ballet (choreographed)	240	300	360	432	480
Dance, modern (choreographed)	240	300	360	432	480
Dance, social	174	222	264	318	348
Fencing	225	255	300	345	375
Fitness calisthenics	232	263	310	357	388
Football	225	255	300	345	375
Golf (walking)	187	212	250	288	313
Gymnastics	232	263	310	357	388
Handball	450	510	600	690	750
Hiking	225	255	300	345	375
Horseback riding	180	204	240	276	300
Interval training	487	552	650	748	833
Jogging (5 1/2 mph)	487	552	650	748	833
Judo/karate	232	263	310	357	388
Mountain climbing	450	510	600	690	750
Pool/billiards	97	110	130	150	163
Racquetball/paddleball	450	510	600	690	750
Rope jumping (continuous)	525	595	700	805	875
Rowing, crew	615	697	820	943	1025
Running (10 mph)	625	765	900	1035	1125
Sailing (pleasure)	135	153	180	207	225
Skating, ice	262	297	350	403	438
Skating, roller/inline	262	297	350	403	438
Skiing, cross-country	525	595	700	805	875
Skiing, downhill	450	510	600	690	750
Soccer	405	459	540	621	775
Softball (fast-pitch)	210	238	280	322	350
Softball (slow-pitch)	217	246	290	334	363
Surfing	416	467	550	633	684
Swimming (fast laps)	420	530	630	768	846
Swimming (slow laps)	240	272	320	368	400
Table tennis	180	204	240	276	300
Tennis	315	357	420	483	525
Volleyball	262	297	350	403	483
Walking	204	258	318	372	426
Waterskiing	306	390	468	564	636
Weight training	352	399	470	541	558

Source: Corbin and Lindsey.

*Locate your weight to determine the calories expended per hour in each of the activities shown in the table based on recreational involvement. More vigorous activity, as occurs in competitive athletics, may result in greater caloric expenditures.

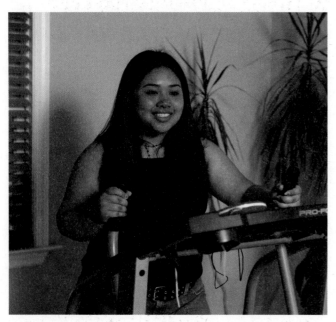

Physical activity can help in regulating body fatness.

Appendices B and C give calories in some common foods. Web links to calories in foods are also provided in Concepts 14 and 15.

Strength training can be effective in maintaining a desirable body composition. Performing exercises from the strength and muscular endurance level of the physical activity pyramid can be effective in maintaining desirable body fat levels. People who do strength training increase their muscle mass (lean body mass). This extra muscle mass expends extra calories at rest, resulting in a higher metabolic rate. Also, people with more muscle mass expend more calories when doing physical activity.

 ## Strategies for Action

Doing a variety of self-assessments can help you make informed decisions about body composition. In Labs 13A and 13B, you will take various body composition self-assessments. It is important that you take all of the measurements and consider all of the information before making final decisions about your body composition. Each of the self-assessment techniques has its strengths and weaknesses, and you should be aware of these when making personal decisions. The importance you place on one particular measure may be different from the importance another person places on that measure because you are a unique individual and should use information that is more relevant for you personally.

Self-assessment information—especially body composition information—is personal and confidential. Body composition self-assessment information is personal and should be confidential. There are steps that can be taken to assure confidentiality. When performing the self-assessments, be aware of the following:

1. If doing a self-assessment around other people makes you self-conscious, do the measurement in private. If the measurement requires the assistance of another person, choose a person you trust and feel comfortable with.
2. Estimates of body composition from even the best techniques may be off by as much as 2 to 3 percent. The values should be interpreted only as estimates.
3. The formulas used to determine body fatness from skinfolds and other procedures are based on typical body types. Measurement will be larger for the very lean and for people with higher than normal levels of fat.
4. Some measurements, such as the thigh skinfold, are hard to take on some people. This is one reason two different skinfold procedures are presented.
5. Self-assessments require skill. With practice, you can become skillful in making measurements. Your first few attempts will, no doubt, lack accuracy.
6. Use the same measuring device each time you measure (scale, calipers, measuring tape, etc.). This will assure that any measurement error is constant and will allow you to track your progress over time.
7. Once you have tried all of the self-assessments in Lab 13A, choose the ones you want to continue to do and use the same measurement techniques each time you do the measurements. Consider having your body composition assessed with some of the other techniques described in the concept.

Estimating your BMR can help you determine the number of calories you expend each day. In Lab 13C, you can estimate your BMR. This will give you an idea of how much energy you expend when you are resting. You can use this information together with the information about the energy you expend in activities to help you balance the calories you consume with the calories you expend each day.

Logging your daily activities can help you determine the number of calories you expend each day in these activities. In Lab 13C, you will also log the activities you perform in a day. You can then determine your energy expenditure in these activities. You can combine this information with the information about your basal metabolism to determine your total daily energy expenditure.

Take steps to balance calories during the college years. As noted earlier in this concept, the average student gains weight in the first year of college and over the college years. Many students think they do more activity than they actually do. Many are less active than in high school. Selecting and preparing

foods may be new to some. Finding ways to stay active and eat well to balance intake and expenditure are the keys to maintaining a healthy weight while in college.

Accumulation of low-intensity activity during the day can be important. Most people spend the majority of their day sitting, but simple changes in lifestyle, such as standing instead of sitting, can have a big impact on energy expenditure. Researchers at the Mayo Clinic (led by Dr. Jim Levine) have coined the term *NEAT (non-exercise activity thermogenesis)* to refer to calories that can be expended from light-intensity activities. His team has been working on ways to reengineer activity into typical activities of daily living. To test these ideas, Dr. Levine developed a mobile workstation that allows him to walk on a treadmill at very slow speeds (~.5–1.0 mph) while working on a computer and answering his phone. The adaptation allows him to expend far more calories per day than if he were sitting at his desk.

Web Resources

Additional websites with information related to Concept 13 are available at the associated Web link.

American Anorexia/Bulimia Association **www.aabainc.org**

Centers for Disease Control and Prevention BMI Information **www.cdc.gov/nccdphp/dnpa/bmi/adult_BMI/about _adult_BMI.htm**

Centers for Disease Control and Prevention Growth Chart Information **www.cdc.gov/growthcharts**

FDA Consumer **www.fda.gov/fdac**

Let's Move Campaign **www.letsmove.gov**

National Heart Lung and Blood Institute (BMI Calculator) **www.nhlbisupport.com/bmi**

Nutriwatch (nutrition facts and fallacies) **www.nutriwatch.org**

Partnership for Healthy Weight Management **www.consumer.gov/weightloss/bmi.htm**

Shape Up America **www.shapeup.org**

STOP Obesity Alliance **www.stopobesityalliance.org**

Surgeon General's Call to Reduce Overweight and Obesity **www.surgeongeneral.gov/topics/obesity**

"We Can" Program **www.nhlbi.nih.gov/health/public/heart/ obesity/wecan/index.htm**

Suggested Readings

Selected readings and references are listed below. A more comprehensive list is available at the associated Web link.

ACSM. 2010. *ACSM's Resource Manual for Guidelines for Exercise Testing and Prescription.* 6th ed. Philadelphia: Lippincott, Williams & Wilkins, Chapter 10.

Chan, R. S., and J. Woo. 2010. Prevention of overweight and obesity: How effective is the current public health approach. *International Journal of Environmental Research on Public Health* 7(3):765–783.

Christakis, N. A., and J. H. Fowler. 2007. The spread of obesity in a large social network over 32 years. *New England Journal of Medicine* 375(4):370–379.

Christian, J. G., et al. 2008. Clinic-based support to help overweight patients with type 2 diabetes increase physical activity and lose weight. *Archives of Internal Medicine* 168(2):141–146.

Cohen, D. A., et al. 2010. Not enough fruit and vegetables or too many cookies, candies, salty snacks, and soft drinks? *Public Health Reports* 125(1):88–95.

Eisenmann, et al. 2008. Combined influence of physical activity and television viewing on the risk of overweight in US youth. *International Journal of Obesity* 32(4):613–618.

Fairburn, C. G. 2008. *Cognitive Behavior Therapy and Eating Disorders.* New York: Guilford Press.

Finkelstein, E., et al. 2007. A pilot study testing the effect of different levels of financial incentives on weight loss among overweight employees. *Journal of Occupational and Environmental Medicine* 49(9):981–989.

Finkelstein, E. A. 2010. Individual and aggregate years of life lost associated with overweight and obesity. *Obesity* 18(2):333–339.

Flegal, K. M., and B. I. Graubard. 2009. Estimates of excess deaths associated with body mass index and other anthropometric variables. *American Journal of Clinical Nutrition* 89(4):1213–1219.

Flegal, K. M., et al. 2010. Prevalence and trends in obesity among U.S. adults, 1999–2008. *Journal of the American Medical Association* 303(3):235–241.

Flegal, K. M., et al. 2007. Cause-specific excess deaths associated with underweight, overweight, and obesity. *Journal of the American Medical Association* 298(17): 2028–2037.

Hardy, L. L., et al. 2010. Screen time and metabolic risk factors among adolescents. *Archives of Pediatric and Adolescent Medicine* 164(7):643–649.

Haskell, W. L., et al. 2007. Physical activity and public health: Updated recommendations for adults from the American College of Sports Medicine. *Medicine and Science in Sports and Exercise* 39(8):1424–1434.

Herman, K. M., et al. 2009. Tracking of obesity and physical activity from childhood to adulthood: The Physical Activity Longitudinal Study. *International Journal of Pediatric Obesity* 4(4):281–288.

Hickey, M. S., and R. G. Israel. 2007. Obesity drugs and drugs in the pipeline. *ACSM's Health and Fitness Journal* 11(4):20–25.

Institute of Medicine. 2004. *Preventing Childhood Obesity: Health in the Balance.* Washington, DC: Institute of Medicine.

John, J., et al. 2010. Recent economic findings on childhood obesity: Cost-of-illness and cost-effectiveness of interventions. *Current Opinions in Clinical Nutrition and Metabolic Care* 13(3):305–313.

Keel, P. K., et al., 2007. Clinical features and psychological response to a test meal in purging disorder and bulimia nervosa. *Archives of General Psychiatry* 64:1058–1066.

Kuk, J. L., et al. 2006. Visceral fat is an independent predictor of all-cause mortality in men. *Obesity Research* 14:336–341.

Lee. I., et al. 2010. Physical activity and weight gain prevention. *Journal of the American Medical Association* 303(12):1173–1179.

Levine, J. A., and J. M. Miller. 2007. The energy expenditure of using a "walk-and-work" desk for office workers with obesity. *British Journal of Sports Medicine* 41:558–561.

Li, S., and R. J. Loos. 2008. Progress in the genetics of common obesity: Size matters. *Current Opinions in Lipidology* 19(2):113–121.

Liou, Y. M., et al. 2010. Obesity among adolescents: Sedentary leisure time and sleeping as determinants. *Journal of Advances in Nursing* 66(6):1246–1256.

Lynch, F. L., et al. 2010. Cognitive behavioral guided self-help for the treatment of recurrent binge eating. *Journal of Consulting and Clinical Psychology* 78(3):312–321.

Lynch, F. L., et al. 2010. Cost-effectiveness of guided self-help treatment for recurrent binge eating. *Journal of Consulting and Clinical Psychology* 78(3):322–333.

Nelson, T. F., et al. 2007. Vigorous physical activity among college students in the U.S. *Journal of Physical Activity and Health* 4(4):495–508.

Ogden, C. L., et al. 2010. Prevalence of high body mass index in US children and adolescents. *Journal of the American Medical Association* 303(3):242–249.

Perusse, L., et al. 2005. The human obesity gene map: The 2004 update. *Obesity Research* 13(3):381–490.

Phillips, K. A., et al. 2010. Body dysmorphic disorder: Some key issues for DSM-V. *Depression and Anxiety* 27(6):573–591.

Prospective Studies Collaboration. 2009. Body-mass index and cause-specific mortality in 900,000 adults: Collaborative analyses of 57 prospective studies. *Lancet* 373(9669):1083–1096.

Puhl, R. M., and C. M. Wharton. 2007. Weight bias: A primer for the fitness industry. *ACSM's Health and Fitness Journal* 11(3):7–11.

Ruiz, J. R., et al. 2010. Attenuation of the effect of the FTO rs9939609 polymorphism on total and central body fat by physical activity in adolescents: The HELENA Study. *Archives of Pediatric and Adolescent Medicine* 164(4):328–333.

Stewart, S. 2009. Forecasting the effects of obesity and smoking on U.S. life expectancy. *New England Journal of Medicine* 361(23):2252–2260.

Sui, M. J., et al. 2007. Cardiorespiratory fitness and adiposity as mortality predictors in older adults. *Journal of the American Medical Association* 298(21):2507–2516.

Surgeon General's Vision for a Healthy and Fit Nation. 2010 (fact sheet). Available at **www.surgeongeneral.gov.**

Vella-Zarb, R. A., and F. J. Elgar. 2009. The 'freshman 5': A meta-analysis of weight gain in the freshman year of college. *Journal of American College Health* 58(2): 161–166.

Wang, Y., et al. 2008. Will all Americans become overweight or obese? Estimating the progression and cost of the U.S. obesity epidemic. *Obesity* 16(10):2323–2330.

Westcott, W. 2009. ACSM strength training guidelines: Role in body composition and health enhancement. *ACSM's Health and Fitness Journal* 13(4):14–22.

Lab Resource Materials: Evaluating Body Fat

General Information about Skinfold Measurements

It is important to use a consistent procedure for "drawing up" or "pinching up" a skinfold and making the measurement with the calipers. The following procedures should be used for each skinfold site.

1. Lay the calipers down on a nearby table. Use the thumbs and index fingers of both hands to draw up a skinfold, or layer of skin and fat. The fingers and thumbs of the two hands should be about 1 inch apart, or 1/2 inch on each side of the location where the measurement is to be made.

2. The skinfolds are normally drawn up in a vertical line rather than a horizontal line. However, if the skin naturally aligns itself less than vertical, the measurement should be done on the natural line of the skinfold, rather than on the vertical.

3. Do not pinch the skinfold too hard. Draw it up so that your thumbs and fingers are not compressing the skinfold.

4. Once the skinfold is drawn up, let go with your right hand and pick up the calipers. Open the jaws of the calipers and place them over the location of the skinfold to be measured and 1/2 inch from your left index finger and thumb. Allow the tips, or jaw faces, of the calipers to close on the skinfold at a level about where the skin would be normally.

5. Let the reading on the calipers settle for 2 or 3 seconds; then note the thickness of the skinfold in millimeters.

6. Three measurements should be taken at each location. Use the middle of the three values to determine your measurement. For example, if you had values of 10, 11, and 9, your measurement for that location would be 10. If the three measures vary by more than 3 millimeters from the lowest to the highest, you may want to take additional measurements.

Skinfold Measurement Methods

You will be exposed to two methods of using skinfolds. The first method (Fitnessgram) uses the same sites for men and women. It was originally developed for use with schoolchildren but has since been modified for adults. The second method (Jackson-Pollock) is the most widely used method. It uses different sites for men and women and considers your age in estimating your body fat percentage. You are encouraged to try both methods.

Calculating Fatness from Skinfolds (FITNESSGRAM Method)

1. Sum the three skinfolds (triceps, abdominal, and calf) for men and women. Use horizontal abdominal measure.

2. Use the skinfold sum and the appropriate column (men or women) to determine your percent fat using Chart 1. Locate your sum of skinfold in the left column at the top of the chart. Your estimated body fat percentage is located where the values intersect.

3. Use the Standards for Body Fatness (Chart 2) to determine your fatness rating.

FITNESSGRAM Locations (Men and Women)

Triceps

Make a mark on the back of the right arm, one-half the distance between the tip of the shoulder and the tip of the elbow. Make the measurement at this location.

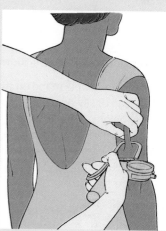

Abdominal

Make a mark on the skin approximately 1 inch to the right of the navel. Make a horizontal measurement.

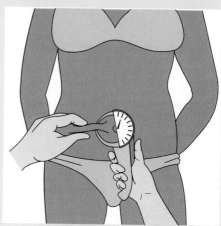

303

FITNESSGRAM Locations (continued)

Calf skinfold

Make a mark on the inside of the calf of the right leg at the level of the largest calf size (girth). Place the foot on a chair or other elevation so that the knee is kept at approximately 90 degrees. Make a vertical measurement at the mark.

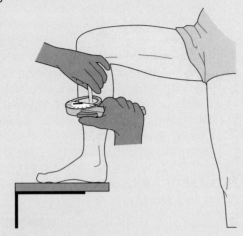

Self-Measured Triceps Skinfold

This measurement is made on the left arm so that the calipers can easily be read. Hold the arm straight at shoulder height. Make a fist with the thumb faced upward. Place the fist against a wall. With the right hand, place the calipers over the skinfold as it "hangs freely" on the back of the tricep (halfway from the tip of the shoulder to the elbow).

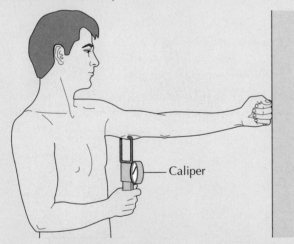

Caliper

Chart 1 ▶ Percent Fat for Sum of Triceps, Abdominal, and Calf Skinfolds (Fitnessgram)

Men		Women	
Sum of Skinfolds	Percent Fat	Sum of Skinfolds	Percent Fat
8–10	3.2	23–25	16.8
11–13	4.1	26–28	17.7
14–46	5.0	29–31	18.5
17–19	6.0	32–34	19.4
20–22	6.0	35–37	20.2
23–25	7.8	38–40	21.0
26–28	8.7	41–43	21.9
29–31	9.7	44–46	22.7
32–34	10.6	47–49	23.5
35–37	11.5	50–52	24.4
38–40	12.5	53–55	25.2
41–43	13.4	56–58	26.1
44–46	14.3	59–61	26.9
47–49	15.2	62–64	27.7
50–52	16.2	65–67	28.6
53–55	17.1	68–70	29.4
56–58	18.0	71–73	30.2
59–61	18.9	74–76	31.1
62–64	19.9	77–79	31.9
65–67	20.8	80–82	32.7
68–70	21.7	83–85	33.6
71–73	22.6	86–88	34.4
74–76	23.6	89–91	35.5
77–79	24.5	92–94	36.1
80–82	25.4	95–97	36.9
83–85	26.4	98–100	37.8
86–88	27.3	101–103	38.6
89–91	28.2	104–106	39.4
92–94	29.1	107–109	40.3
95–97	30.1	110–112	41.1
98–100	31.0	113–115	42.0
101–103	31.9	116–118	42.8
104–106	32.8	119–121	43.6
107–109	33.8	122–124	44.5
110–112	34.7	125–127	45.3
113–115	35.6	128–130	46.1
116–118	36.6	131–133	47.0
119–121	37.5	134–136	47.8
122–124	38.4	137–139	48.7
125–127	39.3	140–142	49.5

Chart 2 ▶ Standards for Body Fatness (Percent Body Fat)

	Too Low	Borderline	Good Fitness (Healthy)	Marginal	Overfat
	Below Essential Fat Levels	Unhealthy for Many People	Optimal for Good Health	Associated with Some Health Problems	Unhealthy
Males	No less than 5%	6–9%	10–20%	21–25%	>25%
Females	No less than 10%	11–16%	17–28%	29–35%	>35%

Calculating Fatness from Skinfolds (Jackson-Pollock Method)

1. Sum three skinfolds (tricep, iliac crest, and thigh for women; chest, abdominal [vertical], and thigh for men).
2. Use the skinfold sum and your age to determine your percent fat using Chart 3 for women and Chart 4 for men. Locate your sum of skinfold in the left column and your age at the top of the chart. Your estimated body fat percentage is located where the values intersect.
3. Use the Standards for Body Fatness (Chart 2) to determine your fatness rating.

Jackson-Pollock Locations (Women)

Triceps

Same as Fitnessgram (see page 303).

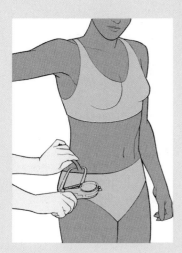

Iliac crest

Make a mark at the top front of the iliac crest. This skinfold is taken diagonally because of the natural line of the skin.

Thigh

Make a mark on the front of the thigh midway between the hip and the knee. Make the measurement vertically at this location.

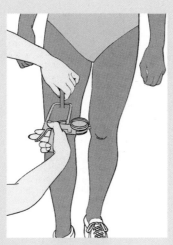

Jackson-Pollock Locations (Men)

Chest

Make a mark above and to the right of the right nipple (one-half the distance from the midline of the side and the nipple). The measurement at this location is often done on the diagonal because of the natural line of the skin.

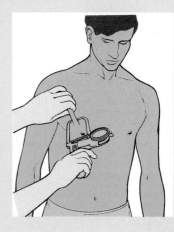

Abdominal

Make a mark on the skin approximately 1 inch to the right of the navel. Make a vertical measure for the Jackson-Pollock method and horizontally for the Fitnessgram method.

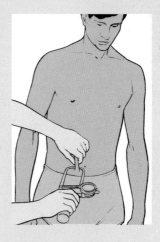

Thigh

Same as for women.

Chart 3 ▶ Percent Fat for Women (Jackson-Pollock: Sum of Triceps, Iliac Crest, and Thigh Skinfolds)

Sum of Skinfolds (mm)	Age to the Last Year								
	22 and Under	23 to 27	28 to 32	33 to 37	38 to 42	43 to 47	48 to 52	53 to 57	Over 57
23–25	9.7	9.9	10.2	10.4	10.7	10.9	11.2	11.4	11.7
26–28	11.0	11.2	11.5	11.7	12.0	12.3	12.5	12.7	13.0
29–31	12.3	12.5	12.8	13.0	13.3	13.5	13.8	14.0	14.3
32–34	13.6	13.8	14.0	14.3	14.5	14.8	15.0	15.3	15.5
35–37	14.8	15.0	15.3	15.5	15.8	16.0	16.3	16.5	16.8
38–40	16.0	16.3	16.5	16.7	17.0	17.2	17.5	17.7	18.0
41–43	17.2	17.4	17.7	17.9	18.2	18.4	18.7	18.9	19.2
44–46	18.3	18.6	18.8	19.1	19.3	19.6	19.8	20.1	20.3
47–49	19.5	19.7	20.0	20.2	20.5	20.7	21.0	21.2	21.5
50–52	20.6	20.8	21.1	21.3	21.6	21.8	22.1	22.3	22.6
53–55	21.7	21.9	22.1	22.4	22.6	22.9	23.1	23.4	23.6
56–58	22.7	23.0	23.2	23.4	23.7	23.9	24.2	24.4	24.7
59–61	23.7	24.0	24.2	24.5	24.7	25.0	25.2	25.5	25.7
62–64	24.7	25.0	25.2	25.5	25.7	26.0	26.2	26.4	26.7
65–67	25.7	25.9	26.2	26.4	26.7	26.9	27.2	27.4	27.7
68–70	26.6	26.9	27.1	27.4	27.6	27.9	28.1	28.4	28.6
71–73	27.5	27.8	28.0	28.3	28.5	28.8	28.0	29.3	29.5
74–76	28.4	28.7	28.9	29.2	29.4	29.7	29.9	30.2	30.4
77–79	29.3	29.5	29.8	30.0	30.3	30.5	30.8	31.0	31.3
80–82	30.1	30.4	30.6	30.9	31.1	31.4	31.6	31.9	32.1
83–85	30.9	31.2	31.4	31.7	31.9	32.2	32.4	32.7	32.9
86–88	31.7	32.0	32.2	32.5	32.7	32.9	33.2	33.4	33.7
89–91	32.5	32.7	33.0	33.2	33.5	33.7	33.9	34.2	34.4
92–94	33.2	33.4	33.7	33.9	34.2	34.4	34.7	34.9	35.2
95–97	33.9	34.1	34.4	34.6	34.9	35.1	35.4	35.6	35.9
98–100	34.6	34.8	35.21	35.3	35.5	35.8	36.0	36.3	36.5
101–103	35.3	35.4	35.7	35.9	36.2	36.4	36.7	36.9	37.2
104–106	35.8	36.1	36.3	36.6	36.8	37.1	37.3	37.5	37.8
107–109	36.4	36.7	36.9	37.1	37.4	37.6	37.9	38.1	38.4
110–112	37.0	37.2	37.5	37.7	38.0	38.2	38.5	38.7	38.9
113–115	37.5	37.8	38.0	38.2	38.5	38.7	39.0	39.2	39.5
116–118	38.0	38.3	38.5	38.8	39.0	39.3	39.5	39.7	40.0
119–121	38.5	38.7	39.0	39.2	39.5	39.7	40.0	40.2	40.5
122–124	39.0	39.2	39.4	39.7	39.9	40.2	40.4	40.7	40.9
125–127	39.4	39.6	39.9	40.1	40.4	40.6	40.9	41.1	41.4
128–130	39.8	40.0	40.3	40.5	40.8	41.0	41.3	41.5	41.8

Source: Baumgartner and Jackson.

Note: Percent fat calculated by the formula by Siri. Percent fat = $[(4.95/BD) - 4.5] \times 100$, where BD = body density.

Chart 4 ▶ Percent Fat for Men (Jackson-Pollock: Sum of Thigh, Chest, and Abdominal Skinfolds)

Sum of Skinfolds (mm)	Age to the Last Year								
	22 and Under	23 to 27	28 to 32	33 to 37	38 to 42	43 to 47	48 to 52	53 to 57	Over 57
8–10	1.3	1.8	2.3	2.9	3.4	3.9	4.5	5.0	5.5
11–13	2.2	2.8	3.3	3.9	4.4	4.9	5.5	6.0	6.5
14–16	3.2	3.8	4.3	4.8	5.4	5.9	6.4	7.0	7.5
17–19	4.2	4.7	5.3	5.8	6.3	6.9	7.4	8.0	8.5
20–22	5.1	5.7	6.2	6.8	7.3	7.9	8.4	8.9	9.5
23–25	6.1	6.6	7.2	7.7	8.3	8.8	9.4	9.9	10.5
26–28	7.0	7.6	8.1	8.7	9.2	9.8	10.3	10.9	11.4
29–31	8.0	8.5	9.1	9.6	10.2	10.7	11.3	11.8	12.4
32–34	8.9	9.4	10.0	10.5	11.1	11.6	12.2	12.8	13.3
35–37	9.8	10.4	10.9	11.5	12.0	12.6	13.1	13.7	14.3
38–40	10.7	11.3	11.8	12.4	12.9	13.5	14.1	14.6	15.2
41–43	11.6	12.2	12.7	13.3	13.8	14.4	15.0	15.5	16.1
44–46	12.5	13.1	13.6	14.2	14.7	15.3	15.9	16.4	17.0
47–49	13.4	13.9	14.5	15.1	15.6	16.2	16.8	17.3	17.9
50–52	14.3	14.8	15.4	15.9	16.5	17.1	17.6	18.1	18.8
53–55	15.1	15.7	16.2	16.8	17.4	17.9	18.5	18.2	19.7
56–58	16.0	16.5	17.1	17.7	18.2	18.8	19.4	20.0	20.5
59–61	16.9	17.4	17.9	18.5	19.1	19.7	20.2	20.8	21.4
62–64	17.6	18.2	18.8	19.4	19.9	20.5	21.1	21.7	22.2
65–67	18.5	19.0	19.6	20.2	20.8	21.3	21.9	22.5	23.1
68–70	19.3	19.9	20.4	21.0	21.6	22.2	22.7	23.3	23.9
71–73	20.1	20.7	21.2	21.8	22.4	23.0	23.6	24.1	24.7
74–76	20.9	21.5	22.0	22.6	23.2	23.8	24.4	25.0	25.5
77–79	21.7	22.2	22.8	23.4	24.0	24.6	25.2	25.8	26.3
80–82	22.4	23.0	23.6	24.2	24.8	25.4	25.9	26.5	27.1
83–85	23.2	23.8	24.4	25.0	25.5	26.1	26.7	27.3	27.9
86–88	24.0	24.5	25.1	25.5	26.3	26.9	27.5	28.1	28.7
89–91	24.7	25.3	25.9	25.7	27.1	27.6	28.2	28.8	29.4
92–94	25.4	26.0	26.6	27.2	27.8	28.4	29.0	29.6	30.2
95–97	26.1	26.7	27.3	27.9	28.5	29.1	29.7	30.3	30.9
98–100	26.9	27.4	28.0	28.6	29.2	29.8	30.4	31.0	31.6
101–103	27.5	28.1	28.7	29.3	29.9	30.5	31.1	31.7	32.3
104–106	28.2	28.8	29.4	30.0	30.6	31.2	31.8	32.4	33.0
107–109	28.9	29.5	30.1	30.7	31.3	31.9	32.5	33.1	33.7
110–112	29.6	30.2	30.8	31.4	32.0	32.6	33.2	33.8	34.4
113–115	30.2	30.8	31.4	32.0	32.6	33.2	33.8	34.5	35.1
116–118	30.9	31.5	32.1	32.7	33.3	33.9	34.5	35.1	35.7
119–121	31.5	32.1	32.7	33.3	33.9	34.5	35.1	35.7	36.4
122–124	32.1	32.7	33.3	33.9	34.5	35.1	35.8	36.4	37.0
125–127	32.7	33.3	33.9	34.5	35.1	35.8	36.4	37.0	37.6

Source: Baumgartner and Jackson.

Note: Percent fat calculated by the formula by Siri. Percent fat = $[(4.95/BD) - 4.5] \times 100$, where BD = body density.

Calculating Fatness from Self-Measured Skinfolds

1. Use either the Jackson-Pollock or Fitnessgram method, but make the measures on yourself rather than have a partner do the measures. When doing the triceps measure, use the self-measurement technique for men and women. (See page 304.)

2. Calculate fatness using the methods described previously.

Height-Weight Measurements

1. *Height*—Measure your height in inches or centimeters. Take the measurement without shoes, but add 2.5 centimeters or 1 inch to measurements, as the charts include heel height.

2. *Weight*—Measure your weight in pounds or kilograms without clothes. Add 3 pounds or 1.4 kilograms because the charts include the weight of clothes. If weight must be taken with clothes on, wear indoor clothing that weighs 3 pounds, or 1.4 kilograms.

3. Determine your frame size using the elbow breadth. The measurement is most accurate when done with a broad-based sliding caliper. However, it can be done using skinfold calipers or can be estimated with a metric ruler. The right arm is measured when it is elevated with the elbow bent at 90 degrees and the upper arm horizontal. The back of the hand should face the person making the measurement. Using the calipers, measure the distance between the epicondyles of the humerus (inside and outside bony points of the elbow). Measure to the nearest millimeter (1/10 centimeter). If a caliper is not available, place the thumb and the index finger of the left hand on the epicondyles of the humerus and measure the distance between the fingers with a metric ruler. Use your height and elbow breadth in centimeters to determine your frame size (Chart 5); you need not repeat this procedure each time you use a height and weight chart.

4. Use Chart 6 to determine your healthy weight range. The new healthy weight range charts do not account for frame size. However, you may want to consider frame size when determining a personal weight within the healthy weight range. People with a larger frame size typically can carry more weight within the range than can those with a smaller frame size.

Chart 5 ▶ Frame Size Determined from Elbow Breadth (mm)

Height	Elbow Breadth (mm)		
	Small Frame	Medium Frame	Large Frame
Males			
5′2″ or less	<64	64–72	>72
5′3″–5′6 ½″	<67	67–74	>74
5′7″–5′10 ½″	<69	69–76	>76
5′11″–6′2 ½″	<71	71–78	>78
6′3″ or more	<74	74–81	>81
Females			
4′10 ½″ or less	<56	56–64	>64
4′11″–5′2 ½″	<58	58–65	>65
5′3″–5′6 ½″	<59	59–66	>66
5′7″–5′10 ½″	<61	61–68	>69
5′11″ or more	<62	62–69	>69

Source: Metropolitan Life Insurance Company.

Height is given including 1-inch heels.

Chart 6 ▶ Healthy Weight Ranges for Adult Women and Men

Women			Men		
Height			Height		
Feet	Inches	Pounds	Feet	Inches	Pounds
4	10	91–119	5	9	129–169
4	11	94–124	5	10	132–174
5	0	97–128	5	11	136–179
5	1	101–132	6	0	140–184
5	2	104–137	6	1	144–189
5	3	107–141	6	2	148–195
5	4	111–146	6	3	152–200
5	5	114–150	6	4	156–205
5	6	118–155	6	5	160–211
5	7	121–160	6	6	164–216
5	8	125–164			

Source: U.S. Department of Agriculture and Department of Health and Human Services.

Chart 7 ▶ Body Mass Index (BMI)

Height	100	105	110	115	120	125	130	135	140	145	150	155	160	165	170	175	180	185	190	195	200	205	210	215	220	225	230	235	240	245	250
5'0"	20	21	21	22	23	24	25	26	27	28	29	30	31	32	33	34	35	36	37	38	39	40	41	42	43	44	45	46	47	48	49
5'1"	19	20	21	22	23	24	25	26	26	27	28	29	30	31	32	33	34	35	36	37	38	39	40	41	42	43	43	44	45	46	47
5'2"	18	19	20	21	22	23	24	25	26	27	27	28	29	30	31	32	33	34	35	36	37	37	38	39	40	41	42	43	44	45	46
5'3"	18	19	19	20	21	22	23	24	25	26	27	27	28	29	30	31	32	33	34	35	35	36	37	38	39	40	41	42	43	43	44
5'4"	17	18	19	20	21	21	22	23	24	25	26	27	27	28	29	30	31	32	33	33	34	35	36	37	38	39	39	40	41	42	43
5'5"	17	17	18	19	20	21	22	22	23	24	25	26	27	27	28	29	30	31	32	32	33	34	35	36	37	37	38	39	40	41	42
5'6"	16	17	18	19	19	20	21	22	23	23	24	25	26	27	27	28	29	30	31	31	32	33	34	35	36	36	37	38	39	40	40
5'7"	16	16	17	18	19	20	20	21	22	23	23	24	25	26	27	27	28	29	30	31	31	32	33	34	34	35	36	37	38	38	39
5'8"	15	16	17	17	18	19	20	21	21	22	23	24	24	25	26	27	27	28	29	30	30	31	32	33	33	34	35	36	36	37	38
5'9"	15	16	16	17	18	18	19	20	21	21	22	23	24	24	25	26	27	27	28	29	30	30	31	32	32	33	34	35	35	36	37
5'10"	14	15	16	17	17	18	19	19	20	21	22	22	23	24	24	25	26	27	27	28	29	29	30	31	32	32	33	34	34	35	36
5'11"	14	15	15	16	17	17	18	19	20	20	21	22	22	23	24	24	25	26	26	27	28	29	29	30	31	31	32	33	33	34	35
6'0"	14	14	15	16	16	17	18	18	19	20	20	21	22	22	23	24	24	25	26	26	27	28	28	29	30	31	31	32	33	33	34
6'1"	13	14	15	15	16	16	17	18	18	19	20	20	21	22	22	23	24	24	25	26	26	27	28	28	29	30	30	31	32	32	33
6'2"	13	13	14	15	15	16	17	17	18	19	19	20	21	21	22	22	23	24	24	25	26	26	27	28	28	29	30	30	31	31	32
6'3"	12	13	14	14	15	16	16	17	17	18	19	19	20	21	21	22	22	23	24	24	25	26	26	27	27	28	29	29	30	31	31
6'4"	12	13	13	14	15	15	16	16	17	18	18	19	19	20	21	21	22	23	23	24	25	26	26	27	27	28	29	29	30	30	30

Weight

◼ Low   ◼ Normal (good fitness zone)   ◻ Overweight   ◻ Obese

Body Mass Index (BMI)

Use the steps listed below or use Chart 7 to calculate your BMI.

1. Divide your weight in pounds by 2.2 to determine your weight in kilograms.
2. Multiply your height in inches by 0.0254 to determine your height in meters.
3. Square your height in meters (multiply your height in meters by your height in meters).
4. Divide your weight in kilograms from step 1 by your height in meters squared from step 3.
5. If you use these steps to determine your BMI, use the Rating Scale for Body Mass Index (Chart 8) to obtain a rating for your BMI.

Formula

$$\text{BMI} = \frac{\text{weight in kilograms (kg)}}{(\text{height in meters}) \times (\text{height in meters})}$$

$$\text{BMI} = \frac{(\text{weight in pounds})}{(\text{height in inches}) \times (\text{height in inches})} \times 703$$

Chart 8 ▶ Rating Scale for Body Mass Index (BMI)

Classification	BMI
Obese (high risk)	Over 30
Overweight	25–30
Normal (good fitness zone)	17–24.9
Low	Less than 17

Note: An excessively low BMI is not desirable. Low BMI values can indicate eating disorders and other health problems.

Determining the Waist-to-Hip Circumference Ratio

The waist-to-hip circumference ratio is recommended as the best available index for determining risk for disease associated with fat and weight distribution. Disease and death risk are associated with abdominal and upper body fatness. When a person has high fatness and a high waist-to-hip ratio, additional risks exist. The following steps should be taken in making measurements and calculating the waist-to-hip ratio.

1. Both measurements should be done with a nonelastic tape. Make the measurements while standing with the feet together and the arms at the sides, elevated only high enough to allow the measurements. Be sure the tape is horizontal and around the entire circumference. Record scores to the nearest millimeter or 1/16th of an inch. Use the same units of measure for both circumferences (millimeters or 1/16th of an inch). The tape should be pulled snugly but not to the point of causing an indentation in the skin.

2. *Waist measurement*—Measure at the natural waist (smallest waist circumference). If no natural waist exists, the measurement should be made at the level of the umbilicus. Measure at the end of a normal inspiration.

3. *Hip measurement*—Measure at the maximum circumference of the buttocks. It is recommended that you wear thin-layered clothing (such as a swimming suit or underwear) that will not add significantly to the measurement.

4. Divide the hip measurement into the waist measurement or use the waist-to-hip nomogram (Chart 9) to determine your waist-to-hip ratio.

5. Use the Waist-to-Hip Ratio Rating Scale (Chart 10) to determine your rating for the waist-to-hip ratio.

Chart 9 ▶ Waist-to-Hip Ratio Nomogram

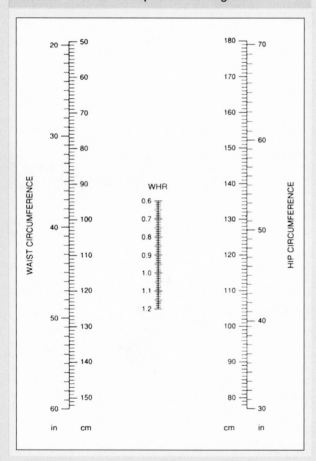

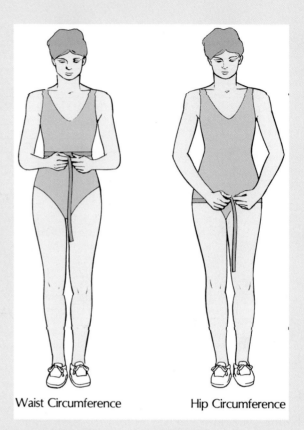

Waist Circumference   Hip Circumference

Note: Using a partner or mirror will aid you in keeping the tape horizontal.

Determining Disease Risk Based on BMI and Waist Circumference

Use Chart 11 to determine a BMI and Waist Circumference Rating. In the first column of Chart 11, locate your BMI. Locate your Waist Circumference in either column 2 or 3 depending on your age. Your rating is located at the point where the appropriate rows and columns intersect.

Chart 11 ▶ BMI and Waist Circumference Rating Scale

	Waist Circumference (in.)	
BMI	Men 40 or less Women 34.5 or less	Men above 40 Women above 34.5
Less than 18.5	Normal	Normal
18.5–24.9	Normal	Normal
25.0–29.9	Increased risk	High risk
30.0–34.9	High risk	Very high risk
35.0–39.9	Very high risk	Very high risk
40 or more	Extremely high risk	Extremely high risk

Source: Adapted from ACSM.

Chart 10 ▶ Waist-to-Hip Ratio Rating Scale

Classification	Men	Women
High risk	>1.0	>0.85
Moderately high risk	0.90–1.0	0.80–0.85
Lower risk	<0.90	<0.80

Lab 13A Evaluating Body Composition: Skinfold Measures

Name	Section	Date

Purpose: To estimate body fatness using two skinfold procedures; to compare measures made by an expert, by a partner, and by self-measurements; to learn the strengths and weaknesses of each technique; and to use the results to establish personal standards for evaluating body composition.

General Procedures: Follow the specific procedures for the two self-assessment techniques. If possible, have one set of measurements made by an expert (instructor) for each of the two techniques. Next, work with a partner you trust. Have the partner make measurements at each site for both techniques. Finally, make self-measurements for each of the sites. If you are just learning a measurement technique, it is important to practice the skills of making the measurement. If you do measurements over time, use the same instrument (if possible) each time you measure. If your measurements vary widely, take more than one set until you get more consistent results.

If you have had an underwater weighing, a bioelectric impedance measurement, a near-infrared interactance measure, or some other body fatness measurement done recently, record your results below.

Measurement Technique	% Body Fat	Rating
1.		
2.		

Skinfold Measurements (Jackson-Pollock Method)

Procedures for Jackson-Pollock Method

1. Read the directions for the Jackson-Pollock method measurements in *Lab Resource Materials.*
2. If possible, observe a demonstration of the proper procedures for measuring skinfolds at each of the different locations before doing partner or self-measurements.
3. Make expert, partner, and self-measurements (see *Lab Resource Materials*). When doing the self-measure of the triceps, use the self-measurement technique described in *Lab Resource Materials* (women only).
4. Record each of the measurements in the Results section.
5. Calculate your body fatness from skinfolds by summing the appropriate skinfold values (chest, thigh, and abdominal for men; triceps, iliac crest, and thigh for women). Using your age and the sum of the appropriate skinfolds, determine your body fatness using Charts 3 and 4 in *Lab Resource Materials.*
6. Rate your fatness using Chart 2 in *Lab Resource Materials.*

Results for Jackson-Pollock Method

Skinfolds by an Expert (If Possible)	Skinfolds by Partner	Self-Measurements
Male	**Male**	**Male**
Chest	Chest	Chest
Thigh	Thigh	Thigh
Abdominal	Abdominal	Abdominal
Sum	Sum	Sum
% body fat	% body fat	% body fat
Rating	Rating	Rating
Female	**Female**	**Female**
Triceps	Triceps	Triceps
Iliac crest	Iliac crest	Iliac crest
Thigh	Thigh	Thigh
Sum	Sum	Sum
% body fat	% body fat	% body fat
Rating	Rating	Rating

Make a check by the statements that are true about your measurements.

☐ The person doing measurements has experience with these three skinfold measurements.

☐ Self-measurements were practiced until measurements became consistent.

☐ Results of several trials for each measure are consistent (do not vary more than 2–3 mm).

☐ You are not exceptionally low or exceptionally high in body fat.

The more checks you have, the more likely your measurements are accurate.

Skinfold Measurements (Fitnessgram Method)

Procedures for Fitnessgram Method

1. Read the directions for the Fitnessgram measurements in *Lab Resource Materials.*
2. Use the procedures as for the Fitnessgram method using the triceps, abdominal, and calf sites described in *Lab Resource Materials.* When doing the self-measure of the triceps, use the self-measurement technique shown earlier.
3. Calculate your body fatness from skinfolds by summing the appropriate skinfold values (same for both men and women). Using the sum of the appropriate skinfolds, determine your body fatness using Chart 1 in *Lab Resource Materials.*
4. Rate your fatness using Chart 2 in *Lab Resource Materials.*

Results for Fitnessgram Method

**Skinfolds by
an Expert (If Possible)**

Triceps [ ]

Abdominal [ ]

Calf [ ]

Sum [ ]

% body fat [ ]

Rating [ ]

Skinfolds by Partner

Triceps [ ]

Abdominal [ ]

Calf [ ]

Sum [ ]

% body fat [ ]

Rating [ ]

Self-Measurements

Triceps [ ]

Abdominal [ ]

Calf [ ]

Sum [ ]

% body fat [ ]

Rating [ ]

Make a check by the statements that are true about your measurements.

[ ] The person doing measurements has experience with these three skinfold measurements.

[ ] Self-measurements were practiced until measurements became consistent.

[ ] Results of several trials for each measure are consistent (do not vary more than 2–3 mm).

[ ] You are not exceptionally low or exceptionally high in body fat.

The more checks you have, the more likely your measurements are accurate.

Conclusions and Implications

In the space provided below, discuss your current body composition based on the two skinfold procedures and any other measures of body fatness you did. Note any discrepancies in the measurements and discuss which of the measurements you think provide the most useful information. To what extent do you think you need to alter your level of body fatness?

Lab 13B Evaluating Body Composition: Height, Weight, and Circumference Measures

Name		Section	Date

Purpose: To assess body composition using a variety of procedures, to learn the strengths and weaknesses of each technique, and to use the results to establish personal standards for evaluating body composition

General Procedures: Follow the specific procedures for the three self-assessment techniques. If possible, work with a partner you trust to help with measurements that you have difficulty making yourself. If you are just learning a measurement technique, it is important to practice the skills of making the measurement. If you do measurements over time, use the same instrument (if possible) each time you measure. If your measurements vary widely, take more than one set until you get more consistent results. If possible, have an expert make measurements on you using these procedures.

Height and Weight Measurements

Procedures

1. Read the directions for height and weight measurements in *Lab Resource Materials*.
2. Determine your healthy weight range using Chart 6 in *Lab Resource Materials*. You may want to use your elbow breadth (Chart 5). People with a smaller frame size should typically weigh less than those with a larger frame size within the healthy weight range. You may need the assistance of a partner to make the elbow breadth measurement.
3. Record your scores in the Results section.

Results

Weight  6'0"

Height 195

Healthy weight range 140-184

Make a check by the statements that are true about your measurements.

☑ You are confident in the accuracy of the scale you used.

☑ You are confident that the height technique is accurate.

The more checks you have, the more likely your measurements are accurate.
If you are a very active person with a high amount of muscle, use this method with caution.

Body Mass Index

Procedures

1. Use the height and weight measures from above.
2. Determine your BMI score by using Chart 7 or the directions in *Lab Resource Materials*. Determine your rating using Chart 8.
3. Record your score and rating in the Results section.

Results

Body mass index 26   Rating Overweight

If you are a very active person with a high amount of muscle, use this method with caution.

Waist-to-Hip Ratio

Procedures

1. Measure your waist and hip circumferences using the procedures in *Lab Resource Materials*.
2. Divide your hip circumference into your waist circumference, or use Chart 9 in *Lab Resource Materials* to calculate your waist-to-hip ratio.
3. Determine your rating using Chart 10 in *Lab Resource Materials*.
4. Record your scores in the Results section.

Results

Waist circumference 35   Hip circumference 39   Waist-to-hip ratio 0.9

Rating Mod High

Make a check by the statements that are true about you.

- [ ] I am a male 5′9″ or less and have a waist girth of 34 inches or more.
- [ ] I am a male 5′10″ to 6′4″ and have a waist girth of 36 inches or more.
- [ ] I am a male 6′5″ or more and have a waist girth of 38 inches or more.
- [ ] I am a female 5′2″ or less and have a waist girth of 29 inches or more.
- [ ] I am a female 5′3″ to 5′10″ and have a waist girth of 31 inches or more.
- [ ] I am a female 5′11″ or more and have a waist girth of 33 inches or more.

If you checked one of the boxes above, the waist-to-hip ratio is especially relevant for you.

BMI and Waist Circumference Rating

Procedures

1. Locate your BMI and Waist Circumference from previous Results sections in this Lab.
2. Use these values to calculate your BMI and Waist Circumference Rating using Chart 11. Record the rating in the Results section.

Results

BMI and Waist Circumference Rating Increased Risk

Conclusions and Implications

In the space below, discuss your results for the height, weight, and circumference procedures. Note any discrepancies in the measurements. Indicate the strengths and weaknesses of the various methods. Which of the measures do you think provided you with the most useful information? If you also did the skinfold measures (Lab 13A), discuss your body composition based on all the information you have collected (skinfolds and height, weight, and circumference measures).

Lab 13C Determining Your Daily Energy Expenditure

Name		Section	Date

Purpose: To learn how many calories you expend in a day

Procedures

1. Estimate your basal metabolism using step 1 in the Results section in this Lab. First determine the number of minutes you sleep.
2. Monitor your activity expenditure for 1 day using Chart 1 (page 000). Record the number of 5-, 15-, and 30-minute blocks of time you perform each of the different types of physical activities (e.g., if an activity lasted 20 minutes, you would use one 15-minute block and one 5-minute block). Be sure to distinguish between moderate (Mod) and vigorous (Vig) intensity in your logging. If you perform an activity that is not listed, specify the activity on the line labeled "Other" and estimate if it is moderate or vigorous. You may want to keep copies of Chart 1 for future use. One extra copy is provided.
3. Sum the total number of minutes of moderate and vigorous activity. Determine your calories expended during moderate and vigorous activity using steps 2 and 3.
4. Determine your nonactive minutes using step 4. This is all time that is not spent sleeping or being active.
5. Determine your calories expended in nonactive minutes using step 5.
6. Determine your calories expended in a day using step 6.

Results

Daily Caloric Expenditure Estimates

Step 1:

Basal calories $= .0076 \times$ [Body wt. (lbs.)] $\times$ [Minutes of sleep] $=$ [Basal calories] (A)

Step 2:

Calories (moderate activity) $= .036 \times$ [Body wt. (lbs.)] $\times$ [Minutes of moderate activity] $=$ [Calories in moderate activity] (B)

Step 3:

Calories (vigorous activity) $= .053 \times$ [Body wt. (lbs.)] $\times$ [Minutes of vigorous activity] $=$ [Calories in vigorous activity] (C)

Step 4:

Minutes (nonactive) $= 1,440 \text{ min} -$ [Minutes of sleep] $-$ [Minutes of moderate activity] $-$ [Minutes of vigorous activity] $=$ [Nonactive minutes]

Step 5:

Calories (rest and light activity) $= .011 \times$ [Body wt. (lbs.)] $\times$ [Nonactive minutes] $=$ [Calories in other activities] (D)

Step 6:

Calories expended (per day) $=$ [(A)] $+$ [(B)] $+$ [(C)] $+$ [(D)] $=$ [**Daily calories**]

Answer the following questions about your daily caloric expenditure estimate.

Yes   **No**

☐   ☐   Were the activities you performed similar to what you normally perform each day?

☐   ☐   Do you think your daily estimated caloric expenditure is an accurate estimate?

☐   ☐   Do you think you expend the correct number of calories in a typical day to maintain the body composition (body fat level) that is desirable for you?

Conclusions and Interpretations: In several paragraphs, discuss your daily caloric expenditure. Comment on your answers to the preceding questions. In addition, comment on whether you think you should modify your daily caloric expenditure for any reason.

Chart 1 ▶ Daily Activity Log

Day of Monitoring:				
Physical Activity Category	**5 Minutes**	**15 Minutes**	**30 Minutes**	**Minutes**
Lifestyle Activity	1 2 3 4 5 6	1 2 3 4 5 6	1 2 3	
Dancing (general) — Mod				
Gardening — Mod				
Home repair/maintenance — Mod				
Occupation — Mod				
Walking/hiking — Mod				
Other: — Mod				
Aerobic Activity	1 2 3 4 5 6	1 2 3 4 5 6	1 2 3	
Aerobic dance (low-impact) — Mod / Vig				
Aerobic machines (rowing, stair, ski) — Mod / Vig				
Bicycling — Mod / Vig				
Running — Mod / Vig				
Skating (roller/ice) — Mod / Vig				
Swimming (laps) — Mod / Vig				
Other: — Mod / Vig				
Sport/Recreation Activity	1 2 3 4 5 6	1 2 3 4 5 6	1 2 3	
Basketball — Mod / Vig				
Bowling/billiards — Mod				
Golf — Mod				
Martial arts (judo, karate) — Mod / Vig				
Racquetball/tennis — Mod / Vig				
Soccer/hockey — Mod / Vig				
Softball/baseball — Mod				
Volleyball — Mod / Vig				
Other: — Mod				
Flexibility Activity	1 2 3 4 5 6	1 2 3 4 5 6	1 2 3	
Stretching — Mod				
Other: — Mod				
Strengthening Activity	1 2 3 4 5 6	1 2 3 4 5 6	1 2 3	
Calisthenics (push-ups/sit-ups) — Mod				
Resistance exercise — Mod				
Other: — Mod				

Minutes of moderate activity _____

Minutes of vigorous activity _____

Total minutes of activity _____

Chart 2 ▶ Daily Activity Log

Day of Monitoring:					
Physical Activity Category		**5 Minutes**	**15 Minutes**	**30 Minutes**	**Minutes**
Lifestyle Activity		1 2 3 4 5 6	1 2 3 4 5 6	1 2 3	
Dancing (general)	Mod				
Gardening	Mod				
Home repair/maintenance	Mod				
Occupation	Mod				
Walking/hiking	Mod				
Other:	Mod				
Aerobic Activity		1 2 3 4 5 6	1 2 3 4 5 6	1 2 3	
Aerobic dance (low-impact)	Mod				
	Vig				
Aerobic machines (rowing, stair, ski)	Mod				
	Vig				
Bicycling	Mod				
	Vig				
Running	Mod				
	Vig				
Skating (roller/ice)	Mod				
	Vig				
Swimming (laps)	Mod				
	Vig				
Other:	Mod				
	Vig				
Sport/Recreation Activity		1 2 3 4 5 6	1 2 3 4 5 6	1 2 3	
Basketball	Mod				
	Vig				
Bowling/billiards	Mod				
Golf	Mod				
Martial arts (judo, karate)	Mod				
	Vig				
Racquetball/tennis	Mod				
	Vig				
Soccer/hockey	Mod				
	Vig				
Softball/baseball	Mod				
Volleyball	Mod				
	Vig				
Other:	Mod				
Flexibility Activity		1 2 3 4 5 6	1 2 3 4 5 6	1 2 3	
Stretching	Mod				
Other:	Mod				
Strengthening Activity		1 2 3 4 5 6	1 2 3 4 5 6	1 2 3	
Calisthenics (push-ups/sit-ups)	Mod				
Resistance exercise	Mod				
Other:	Mod				

Minutes of moderate activity

Minutes of vigorous activity

Total minutes of activity

Nutrition

Health Objectives for the Year 2020

- Increase the contribution of fruits in the diet.
- Increase the variety and contribution of vegetables in the diet.
- Increase the contribution of whole grains in the diet.
- Reduce consumption of saturated fat in the diet.
- Reduce consumption of sodium.
- Increase consumption of calcium.
- Reduce iron deficiency.

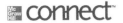 connect™
|FITNESS AND WELLNESS   http://connect.mcgraw-hill.com

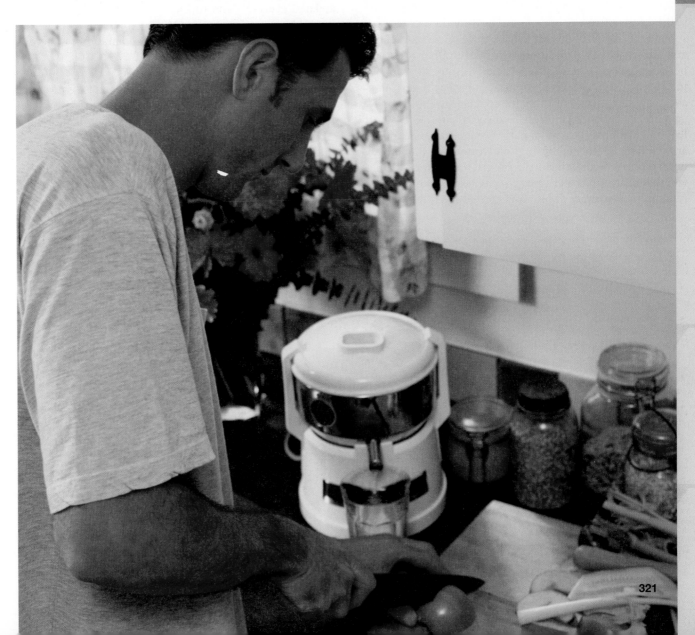

The amount and kinds of food you eat affect your health and wellness.

The importance of good nutrition for optimal health is well established. Eating patterns have been related to four of the seven leading causes of death, and poor nutrition increases the risks for numerous diseases, including heart disease, obesity, stroke, diabetes, hypertension, osteoporosis, and many cancers (e.g., colon, prostate, mouth, throat, lung, and stomach). The links to cancer are probably not fully appreciated in today's society, but the American Cancer Society estimates that 35 percent of cancer risks are related to nutritional factors. In addition to helping avoid these health risks, proper nutrition can enhance the quality of life by improving appearance and increasing the ability to carry out work and leisure-time activity without fatigue.

Most people believe that nutrition is important but still find it difficult to maintain a healthy diet. One reason for this is that foods are usually developed, marketed, and advertised for convenience and taste rather than for health or nutritional quality. Another reason is that many individuals have misconceptions about what constitutes a healthy diet. Some of these misconceptions are propagated by commercial interests and so-called experts with less than impressive credentials. Other misconceptions are created by the confusing, and often contradictory, news reports about new nutrition research. In spite of the fact that nutrition is an advanced science, many questions remain unanswered. This concept reviews important national guidelines and recommendations for healthy eating. The significance of essential dietary nutrients is also described along with strategies for adopting and maintaining a healthy diet.

Guidelines for Healthy Eating

National dietary guidelines provide a sound plan for good nutrition. The U.S. Department of Agriculture (USDA) and the Department of Health and Human Services (DHHS) recently published new dietary guidelines intended to help consumers make healthier food choices. Federal law requires that these guidelines be updated every 5 years to incorporate new research findings. The most recent USDA nutrition guidelines were published in 2010 and are summarized in the In the News feature.

(i) **The MyPyramid model conveys a variety of key nutrition principles.** MyPyramid was created as part of the USDA's nutrition guidelines program to promote education about healthy eating. The colored bars on the model represent the different food groups (grains, vegetables, fruits, oils, milk, and meat/beans) and the importance of eating a variety of foods. The width of the bars in this figure is proportional to the

KEY PRINCIPLES

- **Physical Activity** represented by steps
- **Moderation** represented by narrowing of each food group from bottom to top
- **Personalization** represented by person
- **Proportionality** represented by different widths—the widths suggest how much a person should choose from each group
- **Variety** symbolized by the different colors, which represent the five food groups

MUSCLE FITNESS EXERCISES | FLEXIBILITY EXERCISES

MyPyramid
STEPS TO A HEALTHIER YOU

SPORTS & RECREATION
VIGOROUS AEROBICS
MODERATE

GRAINS | VEGETABLES | FRUITS | MILK | MEAT & BEANS

MAIN MESSAGES

- Make 1/2 your grains "whole"
- Vary your veggies
- Focus on fruits
- Know your fats
- Eat calcium-rich foods
- Go lean on protein

Figure 1 ▶ MyPyramid presents a combination of nutrition guidelines and emphasis on daily physical activity.

Source: Adapted from the USDA 2005 MyPyramid (www.mypyramid.com) by Corbin, Welk, and LeMasurier.

In the News

New Dietary Guidelines

(i) NEWS Every 5 years the U.S. Department of Agriculture (USDA) releases new dietary guidelines. MyPyramid is one of the outcomes from the dietary guidelines issued by the USDA in 2005. The latest guidelines were issued in 2010. The guidelines are prepared by a panel of experts who report on key topical areas such as (in alphabetical order): alcoholic beverages, carbohydrates and proteins, eating patterns, energy balance and physical activity, fats, food groups, food safety, minerals, nutrient density, sodium, potassium, water, and vitamins. A summary of the 2010 guidelines is provided at the associated Web link.

amount of each food group that should be consumed. This principle of proportionality is conceptually similar to the presentation in the old food guide pyramid, which depicted grains on the bottom level, fruits and vegetables on the second layer, protein sources on the third layer, and fats on the top layer. The tapering of the bars from bottom to top is intended to illustrate the principle of moderation in food choices. The wider base stands for the healthier options that should be the base of the diet, while the narrower area at the top stands for the foods (those with more added fat and sugar) that should be consumed less often. This helps people learn to balance sweet treats with other healthier food choices. A Web-based assessment tool called MyPyramid Tracker is also available to help consumers monitor their diet and activity behaviors (see Web Resources).

The USDA nutrition guidelines also emphasize the importance of daily physical activity (60 minutes a day). The steps and the person climbing them on the left of MyPyramid serve as a specific reminder of the importance of physical activity in energy balance. People who are more active (higher up on the stairway) can typically get away with eating more of the high-calorie foods near the top of the pyramid because they burn off the excess calories. As described in previous concepts, each component in the physical activity pyramid provides important health benefits. To illustrate this, the labels from the activity pyramid are superimposed on the steps of the MyPyramid image in Figure 1.

(i) FEATURE 1 **Nutrition guidelines provide specific suggestions for healthy eating.** Unlike previous versions, the 2010 dietary guidelines have recommended a "total diet" approach rather than targets for certain nutrients. The preliminary report defined a total diet as the "combination of foods and

beverages that provide energy and nutrients and constitute an individual's complete dietary intake, on average, over time." The report further described four key components of a nutrient-dense total diet:

- *Moderate energy intake.* Effective weight control requires balancing energy intake with energy expenditure. The new guidelines encourage Americans to achieve their recommended nutrient intakes by consuming foods within a total diet that meets, but does not exceed, energy needs.
- *Reduce solid fats and added sugars (SoFAS).* Evidence indicates that solid fats and added sugars (SoFAS) contribute about 35 percent of total calories, and this leads to excessive intake of saturated fat and cholesterol and insufficient intake of dietary fiber and other nutrients. The guidelines recommend reducing consumption of SoFAS as an important diet strategy.
- *Consume nutrient-dense foods.* Reports suggest that Americans consume less than 20 percent of the recommended intakes for whole grains, less than 60 percent for vegetables, less than 50 percent for fruits, and less than 60 percent for milk and milk products. Consuming nutrient-dense foods improves the overall quality of the diet. Examples of nutrient-dense foods include vegetables, fruits, high-fiber whole grains, fat-free or low-fat fluid milk and milk products, seafood, lean meat and poultry, eggs, soy products, nuts, seeds, and oils.
- *Reduce sodium intake.* Excessive sodium in the diet can increase blood pressure and lead to health problems. The guidelines recommend reducing sodium intake.

A unique aspect of the 2010 guidelines is that they highlight a variety of dietary patterns that would achieve these overall goals. The established DASH-style dietary pattern and the Mediterranean-style dietary pattern were cited as examples of a healthy diet because they have been well supported in the scientific literature. The guidelines also referenced traditional Asian dietary patterns and vegetarian diets as examples of ways to achieve dietary goals. The new guidelines emphasize that a healthful total diet is not a rigid prescription, but rather a flexible approach to eating that can be adjusted for a variety of individual tastes and preferences.

(i) FEATURE 2 **National dietary recommendations provide a target zone for healthy eating.** About 45 to 50 nutrients in food are believed to be essential for the body's growth, maintenance, and repair. These are classified into six categories: carbohydrates (and fiber), fats, proteins, vitamins, minerals, and water. The first three provide energy, which is measured in calories. Specific dietary recommendations for each of the six nutrients are presented later in this concept.

National guidelines specifying the nutrient requirements for good health are developed by the Food and Nutrition Board of the National Academy of

Table 1 ▶ Dietary Reference Intake (DRI), Recommended Dietary Allowance (RDA), and Tolerable Upper Intake Level (UL) for Major Nutrients

B-Complex Vitamins	DRI/RDA Males	DRI/RDA Females	UL	Function
Thiamin (mg/day)	1.2	1.1	ND	Co-enzyme for carbohydrates and amino acid metabolism
Riboflavin (mg/day)	1.3	1.1	ND	Co-enzyme for metabolic reactions
Niacin (mg/day)	16	14	35	Co-enzyme for metabolic reactions
Vitamin B-6 (mg/day)	1.3	1.3	100	Co-enzyme for amino acid and glycogen reactions
Folate (µg/day)	400	400	1,000	Metabolism of amino acids
Vitamin B-12 (µg/day)	2.4	2.4	ND	Co-enzyme for nucleic acid metabolism
Pantothenic acid (mg/day)	5*	5*	ND	Co-enzyme for fat metabolism
Biotin (µg/day)	30*	30*	ND	Synthesis of fat, glycogen, and amino acids
Choline (mg/day)	550*	425*	3,500	Precursor to acetylcholine
Antioxidants and Related Nutrients				
Vitamin C (mg/day)	90	75	2,000	Co-factor for reactions, antioxidant
Vitamin E (mg/day)	15	15	1,000	Undetermined, mainly antioxidant
Selenium (µg/day)	55	55	400	Defense against oxidative stress
Bone-Building Nutrients				
Calcium (mg/day)	1,000*	1,000*	2,500	Muscle contraction, nerve transmission
Phosphorus (mg/day)	700	700	3,000	Maintenance of pH, storage of energy
Magnesium (mg/day)	400–420	310–320	350	Co-factor for enzyme reactions
Vitamin D (µg/day)	5*	5*	50	Maintenance of calcium and phosphorus levels
Fluoride (mg/day)	4*	3*	10	Stimulation of new bone formation
Micronutrients and Other Trace Elements				
Vitamin K (µg/day)	120*	90*	ND	Blood clotting and bone metabolism
Vitamin A (µg/day)	900	700	3,000	Vision, immune function
Iron (mg/day)	8	18	45	Component of hemoglobin
Zinc (mg/day)	11	8	40	Component of enzymes and proteins
Energy and Macronutrients				
Carbohydrates (45–65%)	130 g	130 g	ND	Energy (only source of energy for the brain)
Fat (20–35%)	ND	ND	ND	Energy, vitamin carrier
Protein (10–35%)	.8 g/kg	.8 g/kg	ND	Growth and maturation, tissue formation
Fiber (g/day)	38 g/day*	25 g/day*	ND	Digestion, blood profiles

Note: These values reflect the dietary needs generally for adults aged 19–50 years. Specific guidelines for other age groups are available from the Food and Nutrition Board of the National Academy of Sciences (www.iom.edu). Values labeled with an asterisk (*) are based on Adequate Intake (AI) values rather than the RDA values; ND = not determined.

Science's Institute of Medicine. **Recommended Dietary Allowance (RDA)** historically was used to set recommendations for nutrients, but the complexity of dietary interactions prompted the board to develop a more comprehensive and functional set of dietary intake recommendations. These broader guidelines, referred to as **Dietary Reference Intake (DRI),** include RDA values when adequate scientific information is available and estimated **Adequate Intake (AI)** values when sufficient data aren't available to establish a firm RDA. The DRI values also include **Tolerable Upper Intake Level (UL),** which reflects the highest level of daily intake a person can consume without adverse effects on health (see Table 1). The guidelines make it clear that although too little of a nutrient can be harmful to health, so can too much. The distinctions are similar to the concept of the target zone used to prescribe exercise levels. The Recommended Dietary Allowance (RDA) or Adequate Intake (AI) values are analogous to the threshold levels (minimal amount needed to meet guidelines), while the Upper Limit values represent amounts that should not be exceeded.

A unique aspect of the DRI values is that they are categorized by function and classification in order to facilitate awareness of the different roles that nutrients play in the diet. Specific guidelines have been developed for B-complex vitamins; vitamins C and E; bone-building nutrients, such as calcium and vitamin D; micronutrients, such as iron and zinc; and the class of macronutrients that includes carbohydrates, fats, proteins, and fiber. Table 1 includes the DRI values (including the UL values) for most of these nutrients.

Another unique aspect of the DRI values is that they were designed to accommodate individualized eating patterns. The recommended DRI values for carbohydrates range from 45 to 65 percent. The DRI values for protein range from 10 to 35 percent, while the DRI values for fat range from 20 to 35 percent. These ranges are much broader than recommendations from the USDA in previous versions of the dietary guidelines. According to the Institute of Medicine (IOM), this broader range was established to "help people make healthy and more realistic choices based on their own food preferences." Figure 2 illustrates the recommended DRI distributions for carbohydrates, fats, and proteins.

The quantity of nutrients recommended varies with age and other considerations; for example, young children need more calcium than adults and pregnant women, and postmenopausal women need more calcium than other women. Accordingly, DRIs, including RDAs, have been established for several age/gender groups. In this book, the values are appropriate for most adult men and women. The USDA has a website that calculates personally determined DRI values. You can enter data such as your gender, age, height, weight, and activity level, and the calculator determines your DRI values (**http://fnic.nal.usda .gov/interactiveDRI**). See associated Web link for details.

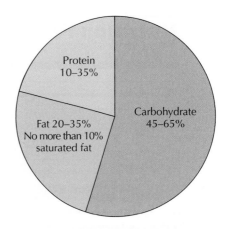

Figure 2 ▶ Dietary Reference Intake values.

Food Labels

Well-informed consumers eat better. Research indicates that most people underestimate the number of calories they consume daily and underestimate the caloric content of specific foods. Research also indicates that people who have better information about the content of their food are more likely to make wise food choices. Examples of methods to get better food choice information include accurate food labels on packages and information about food content on menus or signs in restaurants.

The content of food labels changes from time to time depending on federal guidelines and policies. The most recent change is the requirement to post trans fat content on labels (see Figure 3). This action was prompted by the clear scientific evidence that trans fats are more likely to cause atherosclerosis and heart disease than are other types of fat. Trans fats are discussed in a later section.

Reading food labels can help you be more aware of what you are eating and can help you make healthier choices in your daily eating. In particular, paying attention

Recommended Dietary Allowance (RDA) Dietary guideline that specifies the amount of a nutrient needed for almost all of the healthy individuals in a specific age and gender group.

Dietary Reference Intake (DRI) Appropriate amounts of nutrients in the diet (AI, RDA, and UL).

Adequate Intake (AI) Dietary guideline established experimentally to estimate nutrient needs when sufficient data are not available to establish an RDA value.

Tolerable Upper Intake Level (UL) Maximum level of a daily nutrient that will not pose a risk of adverse health effects for most people.

Start here

Nutrition Facts

Serving Size 1 cup (228g)
Servings Per Container 2

Amount Per Serving

Calories 250	Calories from Fat 110

	% Daily Value*
Total Fat 12g	**18%**
Saturated Fat 3g	**15%**
Trans Fat 1.5g	
Cholesterol 30mg	**10%**
Sodium 470mg	**20%**
Total Carbohydrate 31g	**10%**
Dietary Fiber 0g	**0%**
Sugars 5g	
Protein 5g	
Vitamin A	**4%**
Vitamin C	**2%**
Calcium	**20%**
Iron	**4%**

Limit these nutrients

Get enough of these nutrients

* Percent Daily Values are based on a 2,000 calorie diet. Your Daily Values may be higher or lower depending on your calorie needs.

	Calories:	2,000	2,500
Total Fat	Less than	65g	80g
Sat Fat	Less than	20g	25g
Cholesterol	Less than	300mg	300mg
Sodium	Less than	2,400mg	2400mg
Total Carbohydrate		300g	375g
Dietary Fiber		25g	30g

Footnote

Figure 3 ▶ Sample food label for macaroni and cheese.
Source: U.S. Food and Drug Administration.

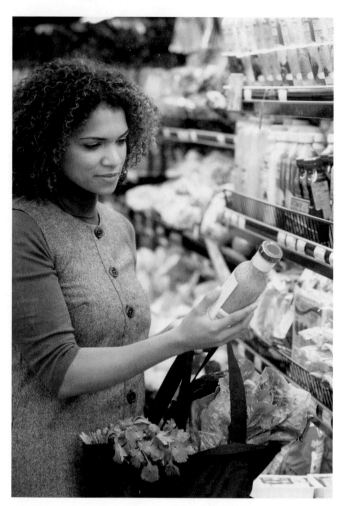

Learning to read food labels is an important skill for establishing good nutrition habits.

to the amounts of saturated fat, trans fat, and cholesterol posted on food labels will help you make heart-healthy food choices. When comparing similar food products, combine the grams (g) of saturated fat and trans fat and look for the lowest combined amount. The listing of % Daily Value (% DV) can also provide useful information. Foods low in saturated fat and cholesterol generally have % DV values less than 5 percent, while foods high in saturated fat and cholesterol have values greater than 20 percent (% DV values are not yet available for trans fat).

Supplemental food labels may not provide accurate information. Some manufacturers have used supplemental labels on foods to advertise healthy aspects of their products. An example is the "Smart Choice" designation created by a consortium of food manufacturers. The labels were placed prominently on the front of selected food packages to promote them as a healthy choice for good nutrition. While perhaps well-intentioned, the claims and designations were not approved by the FDA and could have swayed consumers to select the product. National nutrition groups criticized the name (Smart Choice) as well as the location and content of the labels. This action prompted the FDA to require manufacturers to cease using the potentially confusing labels.

The FDA has also become more strict in enforcing other claims placed on packages. The FDA warned General Mills to stop making inappropriate claims about cholesterol and heart disease risk reduction on Cheerios boxes and warned Kellogg about claims related to increased disease immunity. Specific requirements must be satisfied to warrant health claims, and food companies may not post claims to sway consumers before the claims are formally approved. Care should be taken when considering claims on food packages.

Guides to food contents in restaurants can help consumers eat better. A provision of the health-care bill passed in 2010 requires that restaurant chains with 20 or more locations post the calorie counts in each menu item. Daily special items are exempt. The calorie counts must be posted on signboards both inside the restaurant and near the drive-through window as well as on vending machines. In addition, information about specific nutrients must be provided (e.g., protein, carbohydrate, salt, fiber). The FDA is charged with regulating the program designed to make the public more aware of what they eat. For example, many people are not aware that coffee drinks may contain as many as 1,000 calories, and a single sandwich (e.g., loaded hamburger) may contain more than half of the day's allotted calories.

Dietary Recommendations for Carbohydrates

FEATURE 4

Complex carbohydrates should be the principal source of calories in the diet. Carbohydrates have gotten a bad rap in recent years due to the hype associated with low-carbohydrate diets. Carbohydrates have been unfairly implicated as a cause of obesity. The suggestion that they cause insulin to be released and that insulin, in turn, causes the body to take up and store excess energy as fat is overly simplistic and doesn't take into account differences in types of carbohydrates. Simple sugars (such as sucrose, glucose, and fructose) found in candy and soda lead to quick increases in blood sugar and tend to promote fat deposition. Complex carbohydrates (e.g., bread, pasta, rice), on the other hand, are broken down more slowly and do not cause the same effect on blood sugar. They contribute valuable nutrients and fiber in the diet and should constitute the bulk of a person's diet. Lumping simple and complex carbohydrates together is not appropriate, since they are processed differently and have different nutrient values.

A number of low-carb diet books have used an index known as the glycemic index (GI) as the basis for determining if foods are appropriate in the diet. Foods with a high GI value produce rapid increases in blood sugar, while foods with a low GI value produce slower increases. While this seems to be a logical way to categorize carbohydrates, it is misleading, since it doesn't account for the amount of carbohydrates in different servings of a food. A more appropriate indicator of the effect of foods on blood sugar levels is called the glycemic load. Carrots, for example, are known to have a very high GI value, but the overall glycemic load is quite low. The carbohydrates from most fruits and vegetables exhibit similar properties.

Despite the intuitive and logical appeal of this classification system, neither the glycemic index nor glycemic load have been consistently associated with body weight. Evidence also indicates no difference on weight loss between high glycemic index and low glycemic index diets. There is some evidence linking glycemic load to a higher risk for diabetes but no associations with cancer risk.

Additional research is needed, but excess sugar consumption appears to be problematic only if caloric intake is larger than caloric expenditure. Carbohydrates are the body's preferred form of energy for physical activity, and the body is well equipped for processing extra carbohydrates. Athletes and other active individuals typically have no difficulty burning off extra energy from carbohydrates. Sugar consumption, among people with an adequate diet, is also not associated with major chronic diseases.

Reducing dietary sugar can help reduce risk of obesity and heart disease. Although sugar consumption has not been viewed as harmful, people who consume high amounts of sugar also tend to consume excess calories. The new dietary guidelines clearly recommend decreasing consumption of added sugars to reduce risk of excess calorie consumption and weight gain. The American Heart Association also endorsed this position in a scientific statement entitled "Dietary Sugars Intake and Cardiovascular Health."

The document notes that excessive consumption of sugars (sugars added to foods and drinks) contributes to overconsumption of discretionary calories. Among Americans, the current average daily sugars consumption is 355 calories per day (22.2 teaspoons) as opposed to 279 calories in 1970. Soft drinks and sugar-sweetened beverages are the primary sources of added sugars in the American diet. The AHA's scientific statement recommends no more than 100 calories of added sugars for most women and not more than 150 calories for most men. A typical 12-ounce sweetened soft drink contains 150 calories, mostly sugar. Reducing consumption of sugar-sweetened beverages is a simple (but important) diet modification.

Increasing consumption of dietary fiber is important for overall good nutrition and health. Studies clearly demonstrate that diets high in complex carbohydrates and **fiber** are associated with a low incidence of coronary

Fiber Indigestible bulk in foods that can be either soluble or insoluble in body fluids.

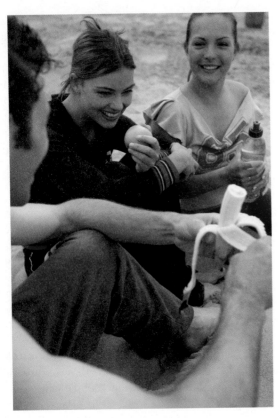

Plan ahead for healthy, low-fat snacks when on the run.

heart disease, stroke, and some forms of cancer. Long-term studies indicate that high-fiber diets may also be associated with a lower risk for diabetes mellitus, diverticulosis, hypertension, and gallstone formation. It is not known whether these health benefits are directly attributable to high dietary fiber or other effects associated with the ingestion of vegetables, fruits, and cereals.

The American Dietetics Association has released a position statement on dietary fiber that summarizes the health benefits and importance of fiber in a healthy diet. It indicates that high-fiber diets provide bulk, are more satiating, and have been linked to lower body weights. It also points out that a fiber-rich diet often has a lower fat content, is larger in volume, and is richer in micronutrients, all of which have beneficial health effects. Evidence for health benefits has become strong enough that the FDA has stated that specific beneficial health claims can be made for specific dietary fibers. The National Cholesterol Education Program has also recommended dietary fiber as part of overall strategies for treating high cholesterol in adults.

In the past, clear distinctions were made between soluble fiber and insoluble fiber because they appeared to provide separate effects. Soluble fiber (typically found in fruits and oat bran) was more frequently associated with improving blood lipid profiles, while insoluble fiber (typically found in grains) was mainly thought to help speed up digestion and reduce risks for colon and rectal cancer. Difficulties in measuring these compounds in typical mixed diets led a National Academy of Sciences panel to recommend eliminating distinctions between soluble and insoluble fibers and instead to use a broader definition of fiber.

Currently, few Americans consume the recommended amounts of dietary fiber. The average intake of dietary fiber is about 15 g/day, which is much lower than the recommended 25–35 g/day. Foods in the typical American diet contain little, if any, dietary fiber, and servings of commonly consumed grains, fruits, and vegetables contain only 1–3 g of dietary fiber. Therefore, individuals have to look for ways to ensure that they get sufficient fiber in their diet. Manufacturers are allowed to declare a food as a "good source of fiber" if it contains 10 percent of the recommended amount (2.5 g/serving) and an "excellent source of fiber" if it contains 20 percent of the recommended amount (5 g/serving). Because fiber has known health benefits, the new dietary guidelines encourage consumers to select foods high in dietary fiber, such as whole-grain breads and cereals, legumes, vegetables, and fruit, whenever possible.

Fruits and vegetables are essential for good health. Fruits and vegetables are a valuable source of dietary fiber, are packed with vitamins and minerals, and contain many additional phytochemicals, which may have beneficial effects on health. The International Agency of Research on Cancer (IARC), an affiliate of the World Health Organization, did a comprehensive review on the links between dietary intake of fruits and vegetables and cancer. It concluded that both human studies and animal experimental studies "indicate that a higher intake of fruits and vegetables is associated with a lower risk of various types of cancer." The clearest evidence of a cancer-protective effect from eating more fruits is for stomach, lung, and esophageal cancers. A higher intake of vegetables is also associated with reduced risks for cancers of the esophagus and colon-rectum. This evidence—plus the evidence of the beneficial effects of fruits and vegetables on other major diseases, such as heart disease—indicates that individuals should strive to increase their intake of these foods. Reports from the 2010 Dietary Guidelines Advisory Committee indicate that beneficial effects on health appear to be linked to a minimum of five servings of fruits and vegetables per day. Additional benefits were noted at even higher consumption levels. These findings contributed to the increased emphasis being placed on a plant-based diet in the new dietary guidelines.

Some recommendations can be followed to assure healthy amounts of carbohydrates in the diet. The following list summarizes key strategies to achieve dietary guidelines for carbohydrate content in the diet:

- Consume a variety of fiber-rich fruits and vegetables.
- Select whole-grain foods when possible.
- Choose and prepare foods and beverages with little added sugars or caloric sweeteners.

Dietary Recommendations for Fat

(i) FEATURE 5 **Fat is an essential nutrient and an important energy source.** Humans need some fat in their diet because fats are carriers of vitamins A, D, E, and K. They are a source of essential linoleic acid, they make food taste better, and they provide a concentrated form of calories, which serve as a vital source of energy during moderate to vigorous exercise. Fats have more than twice the calories per gram as carbohydrates.

There are several types of dietary fat. **Saturated fats** come primarily from animal sources, such as red meat, dairy products, and eggs, but they are also found in some vegetable sources, such as coconut and palm oils. **Unsaturated fats** are of two basic types: polyunsaturated and monounsaturated. Polyunsaturated fats are derived principally from vegetable sources, such as safflower, cottonseed, soybean, sunflower, and corn oils (omega-6 fats), and cold-water fish sources, such as salmon and mackerel (omega-3 fats). Monounsaturated fats are derived primarily from vegetable sources, including olive, peanut, and canola oil.

Saturated fat is associated with an increased risk for disease, but polyunsaturated and monounsaturated fats can be beneficial. Excessive total fat in the diet (particularly saturated fat) is associated with atherosclerotic cardiovascular diseases and breast, prostate, and colon cancer, as well as obesity. Excess saturated fat in the diet contributes to increased cholesterol and increased low-density lipoprotein (LDL) cholesterol in the blood. For this reason, no more than 10 percent of your total calories should come from saturated fats.

Unsaturated fats are generally considered to be less likely to contribute to cardiovascular disease, cancer, and obesity than saturated fats. Polyunsaturated fats can reduce total cholesterol and LDL cholesterol, but they also decrease levels of high-density lipoprotein (HDL) cholesterol. Omega-3 fatty acids (a special type of polyunsaturated fat found in cold-water fish) have received a lot of attention due to their potential benefits in reducing the risk of cardiovascular disease. A plant source of omega-3 fatty acids (alpha-linolenic acid) found in walnuts, flaxseed, and canola oil may have similar benefits.

Monounsaturated fats have been shown to decrease total cholesterol and LDL cholesterol without an accompanying decrease in the desirable HDL cholesterol. Past dietary guidelines recommended a diet low in saturated fat and cholesterol but moderate in total fat. This distinction made it clear that excess saturated fat is the main concern and acknowledges that some fat is necessary in the diet. Guidelines suggest that fat should account for 20 to 35 percent of calories in the diet, with no more than 10 percent of total calories from saturated fat. The remaining fat should come from plant-based sources, especially monounsaturated fats.

Trans fats and hydrogenated vegetable oils should be minimized in the diet. For decades, the public has been cautioned to avoid saturated fats and foods with excessive cholesterol. Many people switched from using butter to margarine because margarine is made from vegetable oils that are unsaturated and contain no cholesterol. The hydrogenation process used to convert oils into solids, however, is known to produce **trans fats**, which are just as harmful as saturated fats, if not more so. Trans fats are known to cause increases in LDL cholesterol and have been shown to contribute to the buildup of atherosclerotic plaque. Because of these effects, it is important to try to minimize consumption of trans fats in your diet.

The requirement to post trans fat content on food labels has prompted companies to look for ways to remove excess trans fats from products. New types of oils are showing promise because they require little or no hydrogenation. Lay's now uses cottonseed oil instead of sunflower oil to help eliminate trans fats from Fritos, Tostitos, and Cheetos. A number of margarines are also available with little or no trans fat (e.g., Smart Balance). It is important to note that foods containing less than .5 g of trans fat per serving may still be listed as having no trans fat. Therefore, you should also look for foods that contain little or no hydrogenated vegetable oil.

Saturated Fats Dietary fats that are usually solid at room temperature and come primarily from animal sources.

Unsaturated Fats Monounsaturated or polyunsaturated fats that are usually liquid at room temperature and come primarily from vegetable sources.

Trans Fats Fats that result when hydrogen is added to liquid oil to make it more solid. Hydrogenation transforms unsaturated fats so that they take on the characteristics of saturated fats, as is the case for margarine and shortening.

Fat substitutes and neutraceuticals in food products may reduce fat consumption and lower cholesterol. Olestra is a synthetic fat substitute that passes through the gastrointestinal system without being digested. Thus, foods prepared with Olestra have fewer calories. For example, a chocolate chip cookie prepared in a normal way would have 138 calories, but an Olestra cookie would have 63. To date, studies examining the effects of Olestra have not noted any harmful effects. Still, some consumer groups warn that the promotion of Olestra-containing products may make individuals more likely to snack on less energy-dense snack foods. They also express concern that Olestra inhibits absorption of many naturally occurring antioxidants that have been shown to have many beneficial effects on health.

Several other new products offer potential to modify the amount and effect of dietary fat in our diets. The first is a naturally occurring compound included in several margarines (Benecol and Take Control). The active ingredient in this compound (sitostanol ester) comes from pine trees and has been shown to reduce total and LDL cholesterol in the blood. Several clinical trials have confirmed that these margarines are both safe and effective in lowering cholesterol levels. The products must be used regularly to be effective and may be useful only in individuals who have high levels of cholesterol. Food products that contain these medically beneficial compounds are often referred to as *neutraceuticals*, or *functional foods*, because they are a combination of pharmaceuticals and food.

Some recommendations can be followed to assure healthy amounts of fat in the diet. The 2010 Dietary Guidelines Advisory Committee emphasized that significant health benefits can be achieved by making several changes in consumption of dietary fats and cholesterol.

- Limit saturated fatty acid intake to less than 10 percent of total calories, with continued reductions down to 7 percent. Individuals should gradually reduce saturated fats and try to substitute food sources of mono- or polyunsaturated fatty acids.
- Limit dietary cholesterol to less than 300 mg per day (200 mg per day for persons with or at high risk for cardiovascular disease or Type II diabetes).
- Avoid trans fatty acids from processed foods (except the small amounts that occur naturally from ruminant sources in animals).
- Limit cholesterol-raising fats (saturated fats exclusive of stearic acid and trans fatty acids) to less than 5 to 7 percent of energy.
- Consume two servings of seafood per week to provide healthy amounts of omega-3 fatty acids from marine sources (e.g., docosahexaenoic acid [DHA] and eicosapentaenoic acid [EPA].

Dietary Recommendations for Proteins

Protein is the basic building block for the body, but dietary protein constitutes a relatively small amount of daily caloric intake. Proteins are often referred to as the building blocks of the body because all body cells are made of protein. More than 100 proteins are formed from 20 different **amino acids.** Eleven of these amino acids can be synthesized from other nutrients, but 9 **essential amino acids** must be obtained directly from the diet. One way to identify amino acids is the -*ine* at the end of their name. For example, arginine and lysine are two of the amino acids. Only 3 of the 20 amino acids do not have the -*ine* suffix. They are aspartic acid, glutamic acid, and tryptophan.

Certain foods, called complete proteins, contain all of the essential amino acids, along with most of the others. Examples of complete proteins are meat, dairy products, and fish. Incomplete proteins contain some, but not all, of the essential amino acids. Examples of incomplete proteins are beans, nuts, and rice.

Protein should account for at least 10 percent of daily calorie consumption, and this need can be met easily with complete (animal) or incomplete (vegetable) sources of protein. A person consuming a typical 2,000-calorie diet would need to consume approximately 200 calories from protein. Protein provides 4 calories per gram, so minimum daily protein needs are as low as 50 grams per day. Figure 4 shows the relative protein content of various foods.

To provide more flexibility, dietary guidelines indicate that protein can account for as much as 35 percent of calorie intake. Experts, however, agree that there are no known benefits and some possible risks associated with consuming excess protein, particularly animal protein.

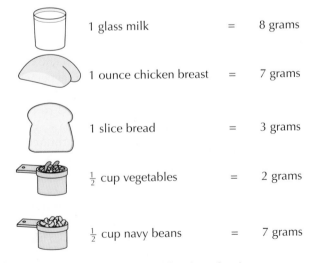

1 glass milk	=	8 grams
1 ounce chicken breast	=	7 grams
1 slice bread	=	3 grams
$\frac{1}{2}$ cup vegetables	=	2 grams
$\frac{1}{2}$ cup navy beans	=	7 grams

Figure 4 ▶ Protein content of various foods.

Source: Williams, M.

High-protein diets are damaging to the kidneys, as the body must process a lot of extra nitrogen. Excessive protein intake can also lead to urinary calcium loss, which can weaken bones and lead to osteoporosis.

People who eat a variety of foods, including meat, dairy, eggs, and plants rich in protein, virtually always consume more protein than the body needs. Because of the negative consequences associated with excess intake, dietary supplements containing extra protein are not recommended for the general population.

(i) **Vegetarian diets provide sufficient protein and may offer health benefits.**
FEATURE 6 Vegetarian diets provide ample sources of protein as long as a variety of protein-rich food sources are included in the diet. According to the American Dietetics Association, well-planned vegetarian diets "are appropriate for all stages of the life cycle, including during pregnancy, and lactation," and can "satisfy the nutrient needs of infants, children, and adolescents." You can get enough protein as long as the variety and amounts of foods consumed are adequate. **Vegans** must supplement the diet with vitamin B-12 because this vitamin's only source is animal foods. **Lacto-ovo vegetarians** do not have the same concerns. The guidelines also emphasize the need for vegans to take care that, especially for children, the diet contains adequate vitamin D and calcium, because most people get these nutrients from milk products.

An increasing array of soy foods are available to provide alternative sources of protein. Soybeans and soy-based foods are a high-quality source of protein. Evidence suggests that soy foods may have beneficial effects on blood pressure and cholesterol levels, possibly contributing to reductions in risk for coronary heart disease. Soy-based foods also contain compounds called isoflavones, a phytoestrogen that contributes to bone health, immune function, and maintenance of menopausal health in women. A variety of soy-based food products are commercially available as alternatives to traditional meat foods. Some common options include tofu, tempeh, soy milk, or textured vegetable (soy) protein. Grocery stores carry a variety of other meatless products based on soy (e.g., veggie burgers). Soy foods that contain at least 6.25 grams per serving can be labeled with FDA-approved health claims.

Some recommendations can be followed to assure healthy amounts of protein in the diet. The following list summarizes some key dietary recommendations for protein:

- Of the three major nutrients that provide energy, protein should account for the smallest percentage of total calories consumed (10–35 percent).

- Protein in the diet should meet the RDA of 0.8 gram per kilogram (2.2 pounds) of a person's weight (about 54 grams for a 150-pound person).
- People on low-calorie diets need to consume a higher percentage of protein in the diet. In contrast, people consuming a lot of calories need a lower percentage.
- Vegetarians must eat a combination of foods to assure an adequate intake of essential amino acids. Vegans should supplement their diet with vitamin B-12.
- Excess protein can be harmful to the kidneys. Protein in the diet should not exceed twice the RDA (1.6 grams per kilogram of body weight).
- Dietary supplements of protein, such as tablets and powders, are not recommended.

Dietary Recommendations for Vitamins

Adequate vitamin intake is necessary for good health and wellness, but excessive vitamin intake is not necessary and can be harmful. Consuming foods containing the minimum RDA of each of the vitamins is essential to the prevention of disease and maintenance of good health. Vitamins serve a variety of functions within the body. For example, they serve as co-enzymes for metabolism of different nutrients, contribute to the regulation of energy stores, and assist in immune function. Some vitamins (e.g., B-complex vitamins and vitamin C) are water soluble and are excreted in urine. These vitamins must be consumed on a daily basis. Other vitamins, such as A, D, E, and K, are fat soluble. These vitamins are stored over time, so daily doses of these vitamins are not necessary. Excess consumption of fat-soluble vitamins can actually build to toxic levels and harm cell function and health. The specific DRI values (minimal amounts) for some of the more important vitamins are shown in Table 1, along with the Tolerable Upper Intake Levels (maximum amounts).

Amino Acids The 20 basic building blocks of the body that make up proteins.

Essential Amino Acids The nine basic amino acids that the human body cannot produce and that must be obtained from food sources.

Vegans Strict vegetarians, who exclude not only all forms of meat from the diet but also dairy products and eggs.

Lacto-Ovo Vegetarians Vegetarians who include dairy and eggs in the diet.

Some vitamins act as antioxidants, but health benefits may depend on other compounds in foods. Carotenoid-rich foods, such as carrots and sweet potatoes, contain high amounts of vitamin A and high amounts of beta-carotene. Diets high in vitamin C (e.g., citrus fruits) and vitamin E (e.g., green leafy vegetables) are also associated with reduced risk of cancer. Vitamin E has also been associated with reduced risk of heart disease.

Vitamins A, C, and E (as well as beta-carotene) act as **antioxidants** within the body, so the health benefits of many vitamin-rich foods have been attributed to antioxidant properties. However, several large-scale studies have shown no benefit (and possible risks) from taking beta-carotene supplements. Another study of over 20,000 people failed to find health benefits associated with consumption of a daily mixture of vitamin E, vitamin C, and beta-carotene. These results were difficult for scientists to interpret, but it is now known that there may be other beneficial substances in foods that contribute health benefits.

As mentioned earlier, the designation of *"functional foods"* has been coined to refer to foods or dietary components that may provide a health benefit beyond basic nutrition. Fruits and vegetables, for example, are loaded with a variety of powerful phytochemicals that have been shown to have potential health benefits (see Table 2).

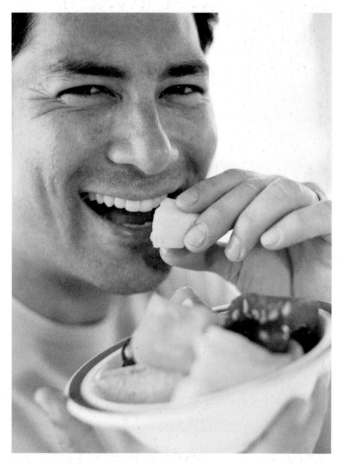

Fruits and vegetables contain vitamins as well as health-promoting phytochemicals.

The relative importance to health of each compound is difficult to determine because the compounds may act synergistically with each other (and with antioxidant vitamins) to promote positive outcomes.

Other examples of functional foods include the beneficial types of fiber and beta glucan in whole grains, the isoflavones in soy products, the omega-3 fatty acids in cold-water fish, and the probiotic yeasts and bacteria in yogurts and other cultured dairy products. Most vitamins and minerals are also classified as functional foods, since they have functions beyond their primary role in basic nutrition. The examples listed here and in Table 2 should not be viewed as "magic bullets," since research is still accumulating on these compounds. In general, diets containing a lot of fruits and vegetables and whole grains

Table 2 ▶ Examples of Functional Foods and Potential Benefits

Carotenoids	Potential Benefits
Beta-carotene: found in carrots, pumpkin, sweet potato, cantaloupe	May bolster cellular antioxidant defenses
Lutein, zeaxanthin: found in kale, collards, spinach, corn, eggs, citrus	May contribute to healthy vision
Lycopene: Found in tomatoes, watermelon, red/pink grapefruit	May contribute to prostate health
Flavonoids	**Potential Benefits**
Anthocyanins: found in berries, cherries, red grapes *Flavanones:* found in citrus foods *Flavonols:* found in onions, apples, tea, broccoli	May bolster antioxidant defenses; maintain brain function and heart health
Isothiocyanates	**Potential Benefits**
Proanthocyanidins: found in cranberries, cocoa, apples, strawberries, grapes, peanuts	May contribute to maintenance of urinary tract health and heart health
Sulforaphane: found in cauliflower, broccoli, brussels sprouts, cabbage, kale, horseradish	May enhance detoxification of undesirable compounds; bolsters cellular antioxidant defenses
Phenolic Acids	**Potential Benefits**
Caffeic/ferulic acids: found in apples, pears, citrus fruits, some vegetables, coffee	May bolster cellular antioxidant defenses; may contribute to maintenance of healthy vision
Sulfides/Thioles	**Potential Benefits**
Sulfides: found in garlic, onions, leeks, scallions *Dithiolthiones:* found in cruciferous vegetables	May enhance detoxification of undesirable compounds; may contribute to maintenance of heart health and healthy immune function

(as recommended in MyPyramid) will provide adequate intake of vitamins and other healthy food components.

Fortification of foods has been used to ensure adequate vitamin intake in the population. National policy requires many foods to be fortified—milk is fortified with vitamin D, low-fat milk with vitamins A and D, and margarine with vitamin A. These foods were selected because they are common food sources for growing children. Many common grain products are fortified with folic acid because low folic acid levels increase the risk for birth defects in babies. Fortification is considered essential, since more than half of all women do not consume adequate amounts of folic acid in the diet during the first months of gestation (before most women even realize they are pregnant). Research has clearly demonstrated the value of fortification. One study showed that neural tube defects are 19 percent less likely today than in 1996 (prior to fortification). Though factors other than fortification may have contributed to this decline, the study supports the benefits of fortification for improving nutritional intakes.

Taking a daily multiple vitamin supplement may be a good idea. Sometimes supplements are needed to meet specific nutrient requirements for specific groups. For example, older people may need a vitamin D supplement if they get little exposure to sunlight, and iron supplements are often recommended for pregnant women. Vitamin supplements at or below the RDA are considered safe; however, excess doses of vitamins can cause health problems. For example, excessively high amounts of vitamin C are dangerous for the 10 percent of the population who inherit a gene related to health problems. Excessively high amounts of vitamin D are toxic, and mothers who take too much vitamin A risk birth defects in unborn children.

In the past some medical groups recommended a daily multivitamin to insure adequate daily intake. However, the 2010 Dietary Guidelines specifically note that "For the general, healthy population, there is no evidence to support a recommendation for the use of multivitamin/mineral supplements in the primary prevention of chronic disease." In spite of this recommendation, some people will choose to take a multivitamin/mineral supplement. Guidelines for those who make this choice are presented in Table 3.

Some recommendations can be followed to assure healthy amounts of vitamins in the diet. Vitamins in the amounts equal to the RDAs should be included in the diet each day. The following guidelines will help you implement this recommendation:

- Eat a diet containing the recommended servings for carbohydrates, proteins, and fats.
- Consume extra servings of green and yellow vegetables, citrus and other fruits, and other nonanimal food sources high in fiber, vitamins, and minerals.

Table 3 ▶ Issues to Consider Regarding the Use of Vitamin and Mineral Supplements

- Limit the use of supplements unless warranted because of a health problem or a specific lack of nutrients in the diet.

- If you decide that supplementation is necessary, select a multivitamin/mineral supplement that contains micronutrients in amounts close to the recommended levels (e.g., "one-a-day"-type supplements).

- If your diet is deficient in a particular mineral (e.g., calcium or iron), it may be necessary to incorporate dietary sources or an additional mineral supplement as well, since most multivitamins do not contain the recommended daily amount of minerals.

- Choose supplements that provide between 50 and 100 percent of the AI or RDA, and avoid those that provide many times the recommended amount. The use of supplements that hype "megadoses" of vitamins and minerals can increase the risk for some unwanted nutrient interactions and possible toxic effects.

- Buy supplements from a reputable company and look for supplements that carry the U.S. Pharmocopoeia (USP) notation (www.usp.org).

Source: Manore.

- People with special needs should seek medical advice before selecting supplements and should inform medical personnel as to the amounts and content of all supplements (vitamin and other).

Dietary Recommendations for Minerals

Adequate mineral intake is necessary for good health and wellness, but excessive mineral intake is not necessary and can be harmful. Like vitamins, minerals have no calories and provide no energy for the body. They are important in regulating various bodily functions. Two particularly important minerals are calcium and iron. Calcium is important to bone, muscle, nerve, and blood development and function and has been associated with reduced risk for heart disease. Iron is necessary for the blood to carry adequate oxygen. Other important minerals are phosphorus, which builds teeth and bones; sodium, which regulates water in the body; zinc, which aids in the healing process; and potassium, which is necessary for proper muscle function.

Antioxidants Vitamins that are thought to inactivate "activated oxygen molecules," sometimes called free radicals. Free radicals may cause cell damage that leads to diseases of various kinds. Antioxidants may inactivate the free radicals before they do their damage.

RDAs are established to determine the amounts of each mineral necessary for healthy daily functioning. A sound diet provides all of the RDA for minerals. Evidence indicating that some segments of the population may be mineral-deficient has led to the establishment of health goals identifying a need to increase mineral intake for some people.

A National Institutes of Health (NIH) consensus statement indicates that a large percentage of Americans fail to get enough calcium in their diet and emphasizes the need for increased calcium—particularly for pregnant women, postmenopausal women, and people over 65, who need 1,500 mg/day, which is higher than previous RDA amounts. The NIH has indicated that a total intake of 2,000 mg/day of calcium is safe and that adequate vitamin D in the diet is necessary for optimal calcium absorption to take place. Though getting these amounts in a calcium-rich diet is best, calcium supplementation for those not eating properly seems wise. Many multivitamins do not contain enough calcium for some classes of people, so some may want to consider additional calcium. Check with your physician or a dietitian before you consider a supplement because individual needs vary.

Another concern is iron deficiency among very young children and women of childbearing age. Low iron levels may be a special problem for women taking birth control pills because the combination of low iron levels and birth control pills has been associated with depression and generalized fatigue. Eating the appropriate number of servings from the food guide pyramid provides all the minerals necessary for meeting the RDA for minerals. Nutrition goals for the nation emphasize the importance of adequate servings of foods rich in calcium, such as green, leafy vegetables and milk products; adequate servings of foods rich in iron, such as beans, peas, spinach, and meat; and reduced salt in the diet.

Some recommendations can be followed to assure healthy amounts of minerals in the diet. The following list includes basic recommendations for mineral content in the diet:

- Minerals in amounts equal to the RDAs should be consumed in the diet each day.
- In general, a calcium dietary supplement is not recommended for the general population; however, supplements (up to 1,000 mg/day) may be appropriate for adults who do not eat well. For postmenopausal women, a calcium supplement is recommended (up to 1,500 mg/day for those who do not eat well). A supplement may also be appropriate for people who restrict calories, but RDA values should not be exceeded unless the person consults with a registered dietitian or a physician.

The following guidelines will help you implement these recommendations:

- A diet containing the food servings recommended for carbohydrates, proteins, and fats will more than meet the RDA standards.

- Extra servings of green and yellow vegetables, citrus and other fruits, and other nonanimal sources of foods high in fiber, vitamins, and minerals are recommended as a substitute for high-fat foods.

Reducing salt in the diet can reduce health risks. A high priority was placed on reducing salt in the diet in the new 2010 Dietary Guidelines. The amount of salt recommended in the diet was reduced from 2.5 grams, slightly less than one teaspoon per day, to 1.5 grams (about ½ half a teaspoon) for both adults and children. This is because of the strong link between salt intake and high blood pressure. The guidelines note that it will take time for most people to reduce salt intake so it may be done gradually. Increased potassium in the diet is recommended because it helps reduce the effects of sodium on blood pressure. New research indicates that cutting salt intake by ½ teaspoon a day could save 44,000 to 92,000 lives a year. In 2010 the Institute of Medicine issued a report entitled "Strategies to Reduce Sodium Intake in the United States." A principal recommendation is that manufacturers reduce salt content in processed foods. Of course, taking responsibility for lowering salt in the diet is the best way for an individual to make change. A study of 17 fast-food chains showed that 85 percent of meals served had more than a full day's allotment of salt.

Dietary Recommendations for Water and Other Fluids

Water is a critical component of a healthy diet. Though water is not in the food guide pyramid because it contains no calories, provides no energy, and provides no key nutrients, it is crucial to health and survival. Water is a major component of most of the foods you eat, and more than half of all body tissues are composed of it. Regular water intake maintains water balance and is critical to many bodily functions. Though a variety of fluid-replacement beverages are available for use during and following exercise, replacing water is the primary need.

Beverages other than water are a part of many diets, but some beverages can have an adverse effect on good health. Coffee, tea, soft drinks, and alcoholic beverages are often substituted for water in the diet. Too much caffeine consumption has been shown to cause symptoms such as irregular heartbeat in some people. Tea has not been shown to have similar effects, though this may be because tea drinkers typically consume less volume than coffee drinkers, and tea has less caffeine per cup than coffee. Many soft drinks also have caffeine, though drip coffee typically contains two to three times the caffeine of a typical cola drink.

Excessive consumption of alcoholic beverages can have negative health implications because the alcohol often replaces nutrients. Excessive alcohol consumption is associated with increased risk for heart disease, high blood pressure, stroke, and osteoporosis. Long-term excessive alcoholic beverage consumption leads to cirrhosis of the liver and to increased risk for hepatitis and cancer. Alcohol consumption during pregnancy can result in low birth weight, fetal alcoholism, and other damage to the fetus. The National Dietary Guidelines indicate that alcohol used in moderation can "enhance the enjoyment of meals" and is associated with a lower risk for coronary heart disease for some individuals.

Some recommendations can be followed to assure healthy amounts of water and other fluids in the diet. The following list includes basic recommendations for water and other fluids in the diet:

- In addition to foods containing water, the average adult needs about eight glasses (8 ounces each) of water every day. Active people and those who exercise in hot environments require additional water.
- Coffee, tea, and soft drinks should not be substituted for sources of key nutrients, such as low-fat milk, fruit juices, or foods rich in calcium.
- Limit daily servings of beverages containing caffeine to no more than three.
- Limit sugared soft drinks.
- If you are an adult and you choose to drink alcohol, do so in moderation. The dietary guidelines for Americans indicate that moderation means no more than one drink per day for women and no more than two drinks per day for men (one drink equals 12 ounces of regular beer, 5 ounces of wine [small glass], or one average-size cocktail [1.5 ounces of 80-proof alcohol]).

Sound Eating Practices

Consistency (with variety) is a good general rule of nutrition. Eating regular meals every day, including a good breakfast, is wise. Many studies have shown breakfast to be an important meal, in which one-fourth of the day's calories should be consumed. Skipping breakfast impairs performance because blood sugar levels drop in the long period between dinner the night before and lunch the following day. Eating every 4 to 6 hours is wise.

Moderation is a good general rule of nutrition. Just as too little food can cause problems, so can excessive intake of various nutrients. More is not always better. Moderation in food choices is advised. You do not have to permanently eliminate foods that you really enjoy, but some of your favorite foods may not be among the best choices. Enjoying special foods on occasion is part of moderation. The key is to limit food choices high in empty calories.

Considerable evidence indicates that portion sizes have increased in recent years. Large portions are featured in advertising campaigns to lure customers. Cafeteria-style restaurants (and others) sometimes offer all you can eat for a specific price, encouraging large portions. Reducing portion size is very important when eating out and at home (see Concept 15 for more information).

Minimizing your reliance on fast foods is a sound eating practice. Many Americans rely on fast foods as part of their normal diet. Recent estimates suggest that 63 percent of Americans eat fast food one to three times a week and an additional 3 percent eat fast food three to five times a week. Unfortunately, many fast foods are poor nutritional choices. Many hamburgers are high in fat. French fries are high in fat because they are usually cooked in saturated fat. Even choices deemed to be more nutritious, such as chicken or fish sandwiches, are often high in fat and calories because they are cooked in fat and covered with high-fat/high-calorie sauces. Minimizing consumption of fast food can help you avoid excess calories and fat. Nutritional analyses for various fast foods are presented in Appendix D. Fast foods are also discussed in more detail in Concept 15. Minimizing consumption of fast foods can greatly improve overall nutrition patterns.

Minimize your consumption of overly processed foods and foods high in saturated fat or hydrogenated fats. Many foods available in grocery stores have been highly processed to enhance shelf life and convenience. In many cases, the processing of

Technology Update
Web Technology

The Internet provides opportunities to promote education and awareness about nutrition. Listed below are websites that can be useful in analyzing food content and learning about healthy eating. Also listed is a nutrition application (app) for an iPod.

- *MyPyramid:* The MyPyramid Tracker program has been one of the most widely visited and used websites for people interested in nutrition. The MyPyramid program is a free computerized diet software tool that provides a detailed assessment of diet patterns. www.mypyramidtracker.gov
- *MyFoodapedia:* This website allows you to enter the name of a specific food and get immediate feedback concerning the calorie content of that food. www.myfoodapedia.gov
- *Fat Translator:* The AHA website helps you make decisions concerning healthy food intake. www.myfattranslator.com
- *Calorie Tracker:* This iPhone app helps you track your daily physical activities as well as what you eat (calories, fat, and cholesterol). http://itunes.apple.com/us/app/calorie-tracker-achieve-your/id295305241?mt=8

foods removes valuable food nutrients and includes other additives that may compromise overall nutrition. Processing of grains, for example, typically removes the bran and germ layers, which contain fiber and valuable minerals. In regard to additives, there has been considerable attention on the possible negative effects of high fructose corn syrup, as well as the pervasive use of hydrogenated vegetable oils containing trans fatty acids. One way to enhance overall nutrition is to minimize your reliance on processed foods. Table 4 compares food quality in each of the main food categories. To the extent possible, you should aim to choose foods in the "more desirable" category instead of those in the "less desirable" category.

Healthy snacks can be an important part of good nutrition. Snacking is not necessarily bad. For people interested in losing weight or maintaining their current weight, small snacks of appropriate foods can help fool the appetite. For people interested in gaining weight, snacks provide additional calories. For people trying to maintain or lose weight, the calories consumed in snacks will probably necessitate limiting the calories consumed at meals. The key is proper selection of the foods for snacking.

As with your total diet, the best snacks are nutritionally dense. Too many snacks are high in calories, fats, simple sugar, and salt. Check the content of snacks. Even foods sold as "healthy snacks," such as granola bars, are often high in fat and simple sugar. Some common snacks, such as chips, pretzels, and even popcorn, may be high in salt and may be cooked in fat. Some suggestions for healthier snacks include ice milk (instead of ice cream), fresh fruits, vegetable sticks, popcorn not cooked in fat and with little or no salt, crackers, and nuts with little or no salt.

Consider eating organic foods to reduce exposure to carcinogens. Consumers are often confused about what the designation "organic" means. Organic food differs from conventionally produced food primarily in the way it is grown, handled, and processed. Organic food is produced without conventional pesticides and using natural fertilizers. Organic meat, poultry, eggs, and dairy products come from animals that are given no antibiotics or growth hormones. An additional distinction is that organic foods are typically produced by farmers who emphasize the use of renewable resources and the conservation of soil and water.

The U.S. Department of Agriculture (USDA) has recently established a new set of standards for foods labeled as "organic." The current labeling requires that a government-approved certifier inspect the farm where the food is grown or produced to ensure that the farmer is following all the rules necessary to meet USDA organic standards. Companies that handle, process, or sell organic food must also be certified. The USDA does not imply that organically produced food is safer or more nutritious than conventionally produced food, but many health experts recommend organic foods to reduce exposure to pesticides and other chemicals and to help support more sustainable and environmentally friendly agricultural practices.

The benefits of organic farming production have led to initiatives to encourage farmers to adopt organic practices. The U.S. Farm Bill, currently in review, calls for a national plan (coordinated through state extension networks) to help introduce farmers to organic practices. The bill proposes $50 million to be allocated to an Organic Conversion Assistance Program to directly assist farmers who are transitioning into organic agriculture. On the consumer side, many farm-to-field initiatives have been launched to facilitate the consumption of locally grown produce.

Table 4 ► Comparing the Quality of Similar Food Products

Food Product	Less Desirable Option	More Desirable Option	Benefit of More Desirable Option in Nutrition Quality
Bread	White bread	Wheat bread	More fiber
Rice	White rice	Brown rice	More fiber
Juice	Sweetened juice	100% juice	More fiber and less fructose corn syrup
Fruit	Canned	Fresh	More vitamins, more fiber, less sugar
Vegetables	Canned	Fresh	More vitamins, less salt
Potatoes	French fries	Baked potato	Less saturated fat
Milk	2% milk	Skim milk	Less saturated fat
Meat	Hamburger	Lean beef	Less saturated fat
Oils	Vegetable oil	Canola oil	More monounsaturated fat
Snack food	Fried chips	Baked chips	Less fat/calorie content, less trans fat

Nutrition and Physical Performance

Some basic dietary guidelines exist for active people. In general, the nutrition rules described in this concept apply to all people, whether active or sedentary, but some additional nutrition facts are important for exercisers and athletes. Because active people often expend calories in amounts considerably above normal, they need extra calories in their diet. To avoid excess fat and protein, complex carbohydrates should constitute as much as 70 percent of total caloric intake. A higher amount of protein is generally recommended for active individuals (1.2 grams per kg of body weight) because some protein is used as an energy source during exercise. Extra protein is obtained in the additional calories consumed. While the IOM range of 10 to 35 percent allows a "broader range" of choice, intake above 15 percent is not typically necessary.

Carbohydrate loading and carbohydrate replacement during exercise can enhance sustained aerobic performances. Athletes and vigorously active people must maintain a high level of readily available fuel, especially in the muscles. Consumption of complex carbohydrates is the best way to assure this.

Prior to an activity requiring an extended duration of physical performance (more than 1 hour in length, such as a marathon), **carbohydrate loading** can be useful. Carbohydrate loading is accomplished by resting 1 or 2 days before the event and eating a higher than normal amount of complex carbohydrates. This helps build up maximum levels of stored carbohydrate (**glycogen**) in the muscles and liver so it can be used during exercise. The key in carbohydrate loading is not to eat a lot but, rather, to eat a higher percentage of carbohydrates than normal.

Ingesting carbohydrate beverages during sustained exercise can also aid performance by preventing or forestalling muscle glycogen depletion. Drinking fluids that have no more than 6 to 8 percent sugar helps prevent dehydration and replenishes energy stores. Fluid-replacement drinks containing 6 to 8 percent carbohydrates are very helpful in preventing dehydration and replacing energy stores. A number of companies also make concentrated carbohydrate gels that deliver carbohydrates (generally 80 percent complex, 20 percent simple) in a format the body can absorb quickly for energy. Examples are PowerGel and Gu. Energy bars, such as Powerbars and Clif bars, are also commonly eaten during or after exercise to enhance energy stores. The various carbohydrate supplements have been shown to be effective for exercise sessions lasting over an hour and are good for replacing glycogen stores after exercise. Studies show that consuming carbohydrates 15 to 30 minutes following exercise can aid in rapid replenishment of muscle glycogen, which may enhance future performance or training sessions.

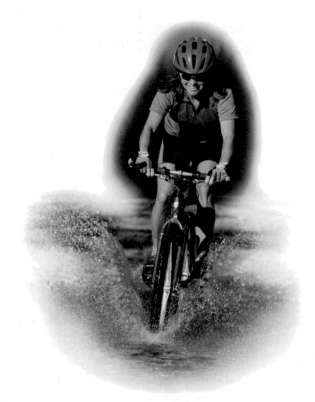

Good nutrition is essential for active people.

These supplements have little benefit for shorter bouts of exercise. Because they contain considerable calories, they are not recommended for individuals primarily interested in weight control.

The timing may be more important than the makeup of a pre-event meal. If you are racing or doing high-level exercise early in the morning, eat a small meal prior to starting. Eat about 3 hours before competition or heavy exercise to allow time for digestion. Generally, athletes can select foods on the basis of experience, but easily digested carbohydrates are best. Generally, fat intake should be minimal because fat digests more slowly; proteins and high-cellulose foods should be kept to a moderate amount prior to prolonged events to avoid urinary and bowel excretion. Drinking 2 or 3 cups of liquid will ensure adequate hydration.

Consuming simple carbohydrates (sugar, candy) within an hour or two of an event is not recommended because it may cause an insulin response, resulting in weakness and fatigue, or it may cause stomach distress, cramps, or nausea.

Carbohydrate Loading The extra consumption of complex carbohydrates in the days prior to sustained performance.

Glycogen A source of energy stored in the muscles and liver necessary for sustained physical activity.

Strategies for Action

An analysis of your current diet is a good first step in making future decisions about what you eat. Many experts recommend keeping a log of what you eat over an extended period so you can determine the overall quality of your diet. In Lab 14A, you will have an opportunity to analyze your diet over several days. In addition to computing the amount of carbohydrates, fats, and proteins, you will also be able to monitor your consumption of fruits and vegetables. A number of online tools and personal software programs can make dietary calculations for you and provide a more comprehensive report of nutrient intake. Whether you use a Web-based tool or a paper and pencil log doesn't really matter—the key is to learn how to monitor and evaluate the quality of your diet.

Making small changes in diet patterns can have a big impact. Experts in nutrition emphasize the importance of making small changes in your diet over time rather than trying to make comprehensive changes at one time. Try cutting back on sweets or soda. Simply adding a bit more fruit and vegetables to your diet can lead to major changes in overall diet quality. In Lab 14B, you will be given the opportunity to compare a "nutritious diet" to a "favorite diet." Analyzing two daily meal plans will help you get a more accurate picture as to whether foods you think are nutritious actually meet current healthy lifestyle goals.

Web Resources

Additional websites with information related to Concept 14 are available at the associated Web link.

American Dietetic Association **www.eatright.org**
Berkeley Nutrition Services **www.nutritionquest.com**
Center for Nutrition Policy and Promotion **www.usda.gov/cnpp**
Center for Science in the Public Interest **www.cspinet.org**
FDA Food Website **www.fda.gov/Food/default.htm**
Food and Drug Administration (FDA) **www.fda.gov**
Food Safety Database **www.foodsafety.gov**
Institute of Medicine **www.iom.edu**
Institute of Medicine—Food and Nutrition
    www.iom.edu/Global/Topics/Food-Nutrition.aspx
International Food Information Council **www.ific.org**
MyPyramid Website **www.mypyramid.gov**
National Nutrition Summit Database
    www.nlm.nih.gov/pubs/cbm/nutritionsummit.html
Nutrition.gov **www.nutrition.gov**
Office of Dietary Supplements **http://ods.od.nih.gov**
Rudd Center for Food Policy and Obesity
    (Yale University) **www.yaleruddcenter.org**
U.S. Department of Agriculture (USDA) **www.usda.gov**
USDA Food and Nutrition Information Center
    www.nal.usda.gov/fnic
USDA MyFoodapedia (calorie calculator)
    www.myfoodapedia.gov

Suggested Readings

Selected readings and references are listed below. A more comprehensive list is available at the associated Web link.

Clark, N. 2008. *Nancy Clark's Sports Nutrition Guidebook.* Champaign, IL: Human Kinetics.

Clark, N. 2008. "Strategies to Better Eating." ACSM's Fit Society Page. Summer, available at www.acsm.org.

Finkelstein, E. A., and L. Zuckerman. 2008. *The Fattening of America.* Hoboken, NJ: John Wiley and Sons.

Institute of Medicine, Food and Nutrition Board. 2010. *Strategies to Reduce Sodium Intake in the United States.* Washington, DC: National Academies Press.

Johnson, R. K., et al. 2009. Dietary sugars intake and cardiovascular health: A scientific statement from the American Heart Association. *Circulation* 120(11):1011–1020.

Kessler, D. 2009. *The End of Overeating: Taking Control of the Insatiable American Appetite.* New York: Rodale Press.

Otten, J. J., Helwig, J. P., and L. D. Meyers (Eds.). 2006. *Dietary Referenced Intakes: The Essential Guide to Nutrient Requirements.* Washington, DC: Institute of Medicine, National Academy of Science Press.

Roberto, C. A., et al. 2010. Evaluating the impact of menu labeling on food choices and intake. *American Journal of Public Health* 100(2):312–318.

Wardlaw, G. M. 2011. *Contemporary Nutrition.* New York: McGraw-Hill Higher Education.

Lab 14A Nutrition Analysis

Name	Section	Date

Purpose: To learn to keep a dietary log, to determine the nutritional quality of your diet, to determine your average daily caloric intake, and to determine necessary changes in eating habits

Procedures

1. Record your dietary intake for 2 days using the Daily Diet Record sheets (see pages 341–342). Record intake for 1 weekday and 1 weekend day. You may wish to make copies of the record sheet for future use.
2. Include the actual foods eaten and the amount (size of portion in teaspoons, tablespoons, cups, ounces, or other standard units of measurement). Be sure to include all drinks (coffee, tea, soft drinks, etc.). Include *all* foods eaten, including sauces, gravies, dressings, toppings, spreads, and so on. Determine your caloric consumption for each of the 2 days. Use the calorie guides at the **mypyramid.gov** website to assist in evaluating your diet.
3. List the number of servings from each food group by each food choice.
4. Estimate the proportion of complex carbohydrate, simple carbohydrate, protein, and fat in each meal and in snacks, as well as for the total day.
5. Answer the questions in Chart 1 on back of this sheet, using information for a typical day based on the Daily Diet Record sheets. Score 1 point for each "yes" answer. Then use Chart 2 to rate your dietary habits (circle rating).
6. Complete the Conclusions and Implications sections

Results

Record the number of calories consumed for each of the 2 days.

Weekday [ ] calories   Weekend [ ] calories

Conclusions and Implications: In several sentences, discuss your diet as recorded in this lab. Explain any changes in your eating habits that may be necessary. Comment on whether the days you surveyed are typical of your normal diet.

Chart 1 ▶ Dietary Habits Questionnaire

Yes No   Answer questions based on a typical day (use your Daily Diet Records to help).

Yes	No	Question
○	○	1. Do you eat three normal-sized meals?
○	○	2. Do you eat a healthy breakfast?
○	○	3. Do you eat lunch regularly?
○	○	4. Does your diet contain 45 to 65 percent carbohydrates with a high concentration of fiber?*
○	○	5. Are less than one-fourth of the carbohydrates you eat simple carbohydrates?
○	○	6. Does your diet contain 10 to 35 percent protein?*
○	○	7. Does your diet contain 20 to 35 percent fat?*
○	○	8. Do you limit the amount of saturated fat in your diet (no more than 10 percent)?
○	○	9. Do you limit salt intake to acceptable amounts?
○	○	10. Do you get adequate amounts of vitamins in your diet without a supplement?
○	○	11. Do you typically eat 6 to 11 servings from the bread, cereal, rice, and pasta group of foods?
○	○	12. Do you typically eat 3 to 5 servings of vegetables?
○	○	13. Do you typically eat 2 to 4 servings of fruits?
○	○	14. Do you typically eat 2 to 3 servings from the milk, yogurt, and cheese group of foods?
○	○	15. Do you typically eat 2 to 3 servings from the meat, poultry, fish, beans, eggs, and nuts group of foods?
○	○	16. Do you drink adequate amounts of water?
○	○	17. Do you get adequate minerals in your diet without a supplement?
○	○	18. Do you limit your caffeine and alcohol consumption to acceptable levels?
○	○	19. Is your average caloric consumption reasonable for your body size and for the amount of calories you normally expend?

	Total number of "yes" answers

*Based on USDA standards.

Chart 2 ▶ Dietary Habits Rating Scale

Score	Rating
18–19	Very good
15–17	Good
13–14	Marginal
12 or less	Poor

Daily Diet Record

Day 1

Breakfast Food	Amount (cups, tsp., etc.)	Calories	Food Servings				Estimated Meal Calorie %
			Bread/Cereal	Fruit/Veg.	Milk/Meat	Fat/Sweet	
							☐ % Protein
							☐ % Fat
							☐ % Complex carbohydrate
							☐ % Simple carbohydrate
							100% Total
Meal Total	✕						

Lunch Food	Amount (cups, tsp., etc.)	Calories	Food Servings				Estimated Meal Calorie %
			Bread/Cereal	Fruit/Veg.	Milk/Meat	Fat/Sweet	
							☐ % Protein
							☐ % Fat
							☐ % Complex carbohydrate
							☐ % Simple carbohydrate
							100% Total
Meal Total	✕						

Dinner Food	Amount (cups, tsp., etc.)	Calories	Food Servings				Estimated Meal Calorie %
			Bread/Cereal	Fruit/Veg.	Milk/Meat	Fat/Sweet	
							☐ % Protein
							☐ % Fat
							☐ % Complex carbohydrate
							☐ % Simple carbohydrate
							100% Total
Meal Total	✕						

Snack Food	Amount (cups, tsp., etc.)	Calories	Food Servings				Estimated Snack Calorie %
			Bread/Cereal	Fruit/Veg.	Milk/Meat	Fat/Sweet	
							☐ % Protein
							☐ % Fat
							☐ % Complex carbohydrate
							☐ % Simple carbohydrate
							100% Total
Meal Total							

Estimated Daily Total Calorie %

☐ % Protein
☐ % Fat
☐ % Complex carbohydrate
☐ % Simple carbohydrate
100% Total

| Daily Totals | ✕ | Calories | Servings | Servings | Servings | Servings | |

Daily Diet Record

Day 2

Breakfast Food	Amount (cups, tsp., etc.)	Calories	Food Servings				Estimated Meal Calorie %
			Bread/Cereal	Fruit/Veg.	Milk/Meat	Fat/Sweet	
							☐ % Protein
							☐ % Fat
							☐ % Complex carbohydrate
							☐ % Simple carbohydrate
							100% Total
Meal Total	✕						

Lunch Food	Amount (cups, tsp., etc.)	Calories	Food Servings				Estimated Meal Calorie %
			Bread/Cereal	Fruit/Veg.	Milk/Meat	Fat/Sweet	
							☐ % Protein
							☐ % Fat
							☐ % Complex carbohydrate
							☐ % Simple carbohydrate
							100% Total
Meal Total	✕						

Dinner Food	Amount (cups, tsp., etc.)	Calories	Food Servings				Estimated Meal Calorie %
			Bread/Cereal	Fruit/Veg.	Milk/Meat	Fat/Sweet	
							☐ % Protein
							☐ % Fat
							☐ % Complex carbohydrate
							☐ % Simple carbohydrate
							100% Total
Meal Total	✕						

Snack Food	Amount (cups, tsp., etc.)	Calories	Food Servings				Estimated Snack Calorie %
			Bread/Cereal	Fruit/Veg.	Milk/Meat	Fat/Sweet	
							☐ % Protein
							☐ % Fat
							☐ % Complex carbohydrate
							☐ % Simple carbohydrate
							100% Total
Meal Total							**Estimated Daily Total Calorie %**
Daily Totals	✕						☐ % Protein
		Calories	Servings	Servings	Servings	Servings	☐ % Fat
							☐ % Complex carbohydrate
							☐ % Simple carbohydrate
							100% Total

Lab 14B Selecting Nutritious Foods

Name		Section	Date

Purpose: To learn to select a nutritious diet, to determine the nutritive value of favorite foods, and to compare nutritious and favorite foods in terms of nutrient content

Procedures

1. Select a favorite breakfast, lunch, and dinner from the foods list in Appendix D. Include between-meal snacks with the nearest meal. If you cannot find foods you would normally choose, select those most similar to choices you might make.
2. Select a breakfast, lunch, and dinner from foods you feel would make the most nutritious meals. Include between-meal snacks with the nearest meal.
3. Record your "favorite foods" and "nutritious foods" on page 344. Record the calories for proteins, carbohydrates, and fats for each of the foods you choose.
4. Total each column for the "favorite" and the "nutritious" meals.
5. Determine the percentages of your total calories that are protein, carbohydrate, and fat by dividing each column total by the total number of calories consumed.
6. Comment on what you learned in the Conclusions and Implications section.

Results: Record your results below. Calculate percentage of calories from each source by dividing total calories into calories from each food source (protein, carbohydrates, or fat).

Food Selection Results

Source	Favorite Foods		Nutritious Foods	
	Calories	% of Total Calories	Calories	% of Total Calories
Protein				
Carbohydrates				
Fat				
Total 100%		100%		100%

Conclusions and Implications: In several sentences, discuss the differences you found between your nutritious diet and your favorite diet. Discuss the quality of your nutritious diet as well as other things you learned from doing this lab.

"Favorite" versus "Nutritious" Food Choices for Three Daily Meals

Breakfast Favorite	Food Choices				Breakfast Nutritious	Food Choices			
Food No.	Cal.	Pro. Cal.	Car. Cal.	Fat Cal.	Food No.	Cal.	Pro. Cal.	Car. Cal.	Fat Cal.
Totals					Totals				

Lunch Favorite	Food Choices				Lunch Nutritious	Food Choices			
Food No.	Cal.	Pro. Cal.	Car. Cal.	Fat Cal.	Food No.	Cal.	Pro. Cal.	Car. Cal.	Fat Cal.
Totals					Totals				

Dinner Favorite	Food Choices				Dinner Nutritious	Food Choices			
Food No.	Cal.	Pro. Cal.	Car. Cal.	Fat Cal.	Food No.	Cal.	Pro. Cal.	Car. Cal.	Fat Cal.
Totals					Totals				
Daily Totals (Calories)					Daily Totals (Calories)				
Daily % of Total Calories					Daily % of Total Calories				

Managing Diet and Activity for Healthy Body Fatness

Health Objectives for the Year 2020

- Increase policies that give retail food outlets incentives for foods that meet dietary guidelines.
- Increase work sites that offer nutrition and weight management classes and counseling.
- Increase participation in employee wellness programs.
- Increase BMI measurement by primary care physicians.

- Increase physician counseling on nutrition and weight management.
- Reduce percentage of adults who do no leisure-time activity.
- Reduce consumption of calories from solid fats and added sugars.
- Increase proportion of adults with healthy weight.
- Reduce childhood overweight and obesity.

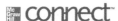 **connect**

FITNESS AND WELLNESS   http://connect.mcgraw-hill.com

Concept 15

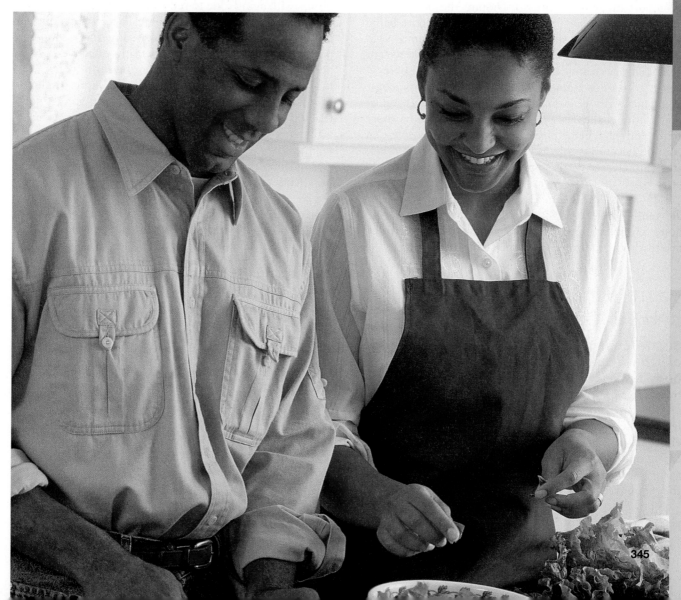

345

Various management strategies for eating and performing physical activity are useful in achieving and maintaining optimal body composition.

The fact that more than 67 percent of the American adult population is classified as overweight is clear evidence that weight control is a vexing problem for the majority of the population. Most Americans recognize the importance of the problem and want to correct it. In fact, a recent national survey by the International Food Information Council (IFIC) reported that nearly two-thirds of Americans were either very concerned or somewhat concerned about their weight.

Too often, the focus is on appearance rather than health and on weight loss rather than fat loss. In attempts to lose weight, the dietary (energy intake) side of the energy balance equation is typically emphasized. Evidence suggests that the energy expenditure side of the equation is just as important, if not more so. Despite the documented benefits, few people trying to lose weight report being physically active. A state-based survey determined that approximately one-half of individuals trying to lose weight do not engage in any physical activity, and only 15 percent report exercising regularly. The challenges many people experience with weight control may be an indirect reflection of the challenges people face in trying to be more active. Although being physically active cannot ensure that you will become as thin as you desire, it may allow you to attain a body size that is appropriate for your genetics and body type.

The focus in this concept is on lifestyle patterns (both diet and physical activity) that will assist with losing body fat rather than weight. Guidelines for maintaining healthy body fat levels over time are also presented.

Factors Influencing Weight and Fat Control

Subtle changes in diet and activity patterns can have major effects on body weight and body fatness. Experts have concluded that the recent trends in obesity are due in large part to environmental influences that make it difficult to manage body fat levels. The term *obesigenic* has been used to describe the elements of our environment that collectively promote eating and inactivity. The model in Figure 1 shows the various aspects of the obesigenic environment and how they influence the energy balance equation.

The essence of the model is that we are continually confronted with environments that make it easy to consume large quantities of energy-dense food. We also live in an environment in which most physical tasks are no longer necessary and people have less apparent time available for active recreation. Small increases in energy intake combined with small decreases in energy expenditure lead to the storage of fat. Awareness of these environmental influences is important if we desire to maintain a healthy body fat level and weight.

Physical activity contributes to energy balance in a number of ways. By maintaining an active lifestyle, you can burn off extra calories, keep your body's metabolism high, and prevent the decline in basal metabolic rate that typically occurs with aging (due to reduced muscle mass). All types of physical activity from the physical activity pyramid can be beneficial to weight control (see Figure 2). Moderate physical activity (step 1) is especially effective because people of all ages and abilities can perform it. It can be maintained for long periods of time and results in significant calorie expenditure. Long-term studies show that 60 or more minutes of moderate activity such as walking is quite effective for long-term weight loss and maintenance.

Vigorous physical activity (steps 2 and 3) can also be effective in maintaining or losing weight. For some people, especially older adults, vigorous activity may be more difficult to adhere to over a long time. However, for those who stick with it, vigorous activity expends more calories in a shorter time, and for this reason, it can be a very good way to expend calories. The evidence that muscle fitness exercise (step 4) is effective in maintaining a healthy body weight has expanded in recent years.

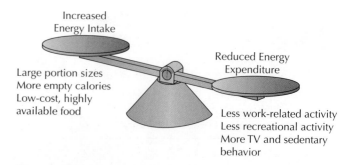

Figure 1 ▶ Factors contributing to increased energy intake and reduced energy expenditure.

Source: Model adapted from Hill, et al.

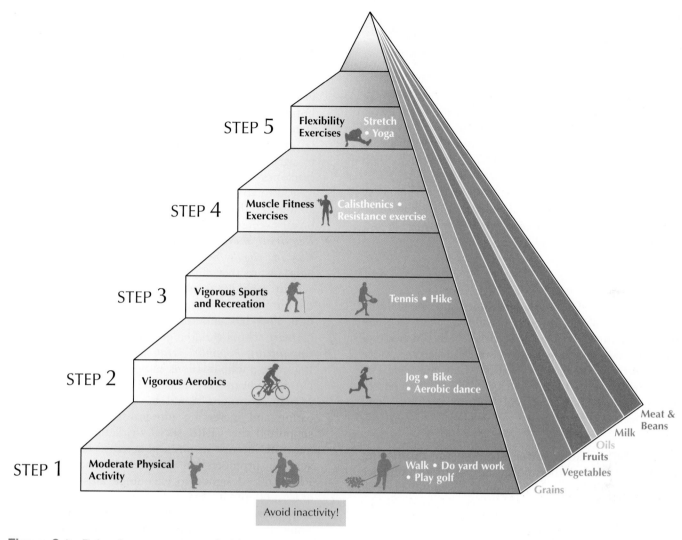

STEP 5 · **Flexibility Exercises** · Stretch • Yoga

STEP 4 · **Muscle Fitness Exercises** · Calisthenics • Resistance exercise

STEP 3 · **Vigorous Sports and Recreation** · Tennis • Hike

STEP 2 · **Vigorous Aerobics** · Jog • Bike • Aerobic dance

STEP 1 · **Moderate Physical Activity** · Walk • Do yard work • Play golf

Meat & Beans · Milk · Oils · Fruits · Vegetables · Grains

Avoid inactivity!

Figure 2 ► Balancing energy expended (steps in pyramid) with energy taken in (color bands at right) is necessary for healthy weight maintenance

Muscle fitness exercise expends calories and increases muscle mass, leading to an increase in calories expended at rest. Flexibility exercises (step 5) also expend calories, but are of lower intensity than other types of activities on the pyramid. They can still contribute to energy expenditure, however.

Although it is not included in the physical activity pyramid, light activity results in energy expenditure and can contribute to maintaining a healthy body weight over time, especially if it replaces inactivity such as watching television or working on a computer. Non-exercise activity thermogenesis (NEAT) that results from unintentional or very low intensity movement throughout the day may account for as much as 15 percent of total daily energy expenditure among sedentary people and up to 50 percent in highly active people with active jobs. The weight maintenance benefits of light or NEAT activity are greatest when the activities replace sedentary activities such as sitting (TV watching and computer use).

Avoiding inactivity is critical to weight maintenance over time. One reason why the typical college student gains 10 pounds over four years is the replacement of former moderate-to-vigorous activities with inactivity.

Awareness and dietary restraint are needed to avoid excess caloric intake. Energy expended in activities from the physical activity pyramid must be balanced by energy intake from food (see color bars at right of Figure 2). However, many forces make it difficult to keep energy intake at healthy levels. Sugar intake, especially from soft drink and beer consumption, results in increases in caloric intake for college students. Fast foods high in empty calories are easily available and are frequent selections of college students, who are often responsible for their food selection or preparation for the first time in their lives. For older college students, the demands of school and part- or full-time jobs make fast food an easy choice. Other factors, such as increasing portion size, easy

HELP

Health is available to Everyone for a Lifetime,
and it's **PERSONAL**

A recent online survey of American adults indicated that 67% of those interviewed did not know how many calories that they should consume in a day. Many did not know that recommend daily calorie intake values vary by gender, age, and activity level. Evidence suggests that most people exceed daily calorie limits because they eat more calories than they think, or they think that their calorie limits are higher than they really are.

What steps can you take to make sure that you do not exceed recommended daily calorie requirements for your age, gender, and activity level?

access to junk food in vending machines, and lack of information about calorie contents of food, contribute to excessive calorie intake. Using food labels to become aware of food content can help college students become more aware of the nutritional value of the foods they eat. The guidelines presented later in this concept are designed to provide information that will lead to healthier food selections.

New public policies offer promise for promoting weight control. Public policy has a strong influence on behavior, because it has the potential to influence all segments of the population. Examples of recent public policy changes that have potential for helping reduce overweight are described below.

- *Posting food values in restaurants.* As noted in Concept 14, chain restaurants with 20 or more outlets must post calorie and other nutrition values for the foods they serve. Posting food values has been shown to be effective in reducing calorie consumption in people eating at fast food restaurants.
- *Restricting use of non-FDA food labels.* Research shows that supplemental food labels provided by manufacturers are often deceptive. The FDA has established policies restricting this practice due to concerns that the industry labels may take attention away from the official food labels.
- *Restricting food commercials that target children.* The food industry adopted self-regulation on foods targeted for children, especially high-sugar, low-nutrient foods. Studies show that these self-regulations have made only small changes in advertising. Nutrition groups have proposed regulation requiring the food industry to advertise nutritious foods more often and to reduce advertising of non-nutritious foods during children's TV shows.

- *Restricting foods sold in vending machines in schools.* Children average 576 calories a day from snacks—more than 25 percent of daily calories. Today, 98 percent of children snack as compared to 74 percent 30 years ago. Efforts are under way to limit foods in school vending machines to healthy foods dense in nutrients and to eliminate foods with empty calories.
- *Removing sweetened soft drinks from schools.* Efforts by groups such as the Clinton Foundation have led to agreements with industry to remove soft drink machines from schools. Coca-Cola and Pepsi have agreed to voluntary removal by 2012. Coca-Cola also announced that by 2011 calorie labels will be included on all sweetened soft drinks.
- *Requiring more physical activity and physical education in schools.* Schools provide an infrastructure to help ensure that children get some regular physical activity each day. A national health goal is to increase the number of children who get daily physical education. The CDC indicates that only 3.8 percent of elementary school children get daily physical education.
- *Conducting public relations campaigns.* Various statewide public relations campaigns to reduce smoking have been very effective. Experts suggest that similar campaigns would be effective in improving eating and increasing physical activity. The CDC supported the VERB social marketing campaign to generate interest in physical activity. The NFL now actively promotes an integrated campaign called PLAY 60 designed to encourage kids to be active at least 60 minutes every day.
- *Implementing empty calorie tax (also called fat tax).* Some public health experts have proposed a tax on foods low in nutritional density, such as sweetened soft drinks, candy, and fast food. Several states are considering taxes of this kind, and one has been under consideration in the United Kingdom. Advocates of this type of tax propose that the proceeds go to campaigns to improve nutrition and increase activity levels.

Public support is strong for many of the policies listed above. However, some people argue that policy changes such as a "fat tax" infringe on personal liberties. Nevertheless, changes in public policy have resulted in major reductions in smoking and smoking-related deaths over the past 20 years, and experts feel that similar policy changes can decrease obesity in America and reduce medical costs associated with obesity.

The most effective diet for fat loss is a low-calorie diet that you can and will stick with over a long period of time. Research has consistently shown that a key to losing weight over the long haul is to modestly restrict calories using a diet that you will stick with. A recent study in the *New England Journal of Medicine* noted

Table 1 ▶ Guidelines for Weight Loss Treatment

Questions about Weight Loss	Recommendations
Who should consider weight loss?	Individuals with a BMI of >25 or in the marginal or overfat zone *should consider* reducing their body weight—especially if it is accompanied by abdominal obesity. Individuals with a BMI of >30 *are encouraged to seek* weight loss treatment.
What types of goals should be established?	Overweight and obese individuals should target reducing their body weight by a minimum of 5–10% and should aim to maintain this long-term weight loss.
What about maintenance?	Individuals should strive for long-term weight maintenance and the prevention of weight regain over the long term, especially when weight loss is not desired or when attainment of ideal body weight is not achievable.
What should be targeted in a weight loss program?	Weight loss programs should target both eating and exercise behaviors, as sustained changes in both behaviors have been associated with significant long-term weight loss.
How should diet be changed?	Overweight and obese individuals should reduce their current intake by 500–1,000 kcal/day to achieve weight loss (<30% of calories from fat). Individualized level of caloric intake should be established to prevent weight regain after initial loss.
How should activity be changed?	Overweight and obese individuals should progressively increase to a minimum of 150 minutes of moderate-intensity physical activity per week for health benefits. However, for long-term weight loss, the program should progress to higher amounts of activity (e.g., 200–300 minutes per week or >2,000 kcal/week).
What about resistance exercise?	Resistance exercise should supplement the endurance exercise program for individuals undertaking modest reductions in energy intake to lose weight.
What about using drugs for weight loss?	Pharmocotherapy (medicine/drugs) for weight loss should be used only by individuals with a BMI >30 or those with excessive body fatness. Weight loss medications should be used only in combination with a strong behavioral intervention that focuses on modifying eating and exercise behaviors.

Source: American College of Sports Medicine.

that reduced-calorie diets result in clinically meaningful weight loss regardless of which micronutrients they emphasize, as long as they are not high in saturated fat. The report notes that regular exercise is crucial to long-term fat loss and that diets high in grains, fruits, and vegetables are typically low in calories and easy to adhere to. This and other studies refute the notion that specific nutrients are the key to success.

Guidelines for Losing Body Fat

Following appropriate weight loss guidelines is important for the best long-term results. There is considerable misinformation about diet and weight loss strategies. The information leads many people to use unsafe or ineffective weight loss supplements or to follow inappropriate exercise programs. Fat, weight, and body proportions are all factors that can be changed, but people often set goals that are impossible to achieve. Starting with small goals and aiming for reasonable rates of weight loss (1–2 pounds a week) are recommended. Setting unrealistic goals may result in eating disorders, failure to meet goals, or failure to maintain weight loss over time. Table 1

provides a summary of weight loss guidelines from the American College of Sports Medicine (ACSM).

Behavioral goals are more effective than outcome goals. Researchers have shown that setting **outcome goals,** or goals that set a specific amount of weight or fat loss (or gain), can be discouraging. If a **behavioral goal** of eating a reasonable number of calories per day and expending a reasonable number of calories in exercise is met, outcome goals will be achieved. Most experts believe that behavioral goals work better than weight or fat loss goals, especially in the short term.

Outcome Goal Statement of intent to achieve a specific test score or a specific standard associated with good health or wellness—for example, "I will lower my body fat level by 3 percent."

Behavioral Goal Statement of intent to perform a specific behavior (changing a lifestyle) for a specific period of time—for example, "I will reduce the calories in my diet by 200 a day for the next 4 weeks."

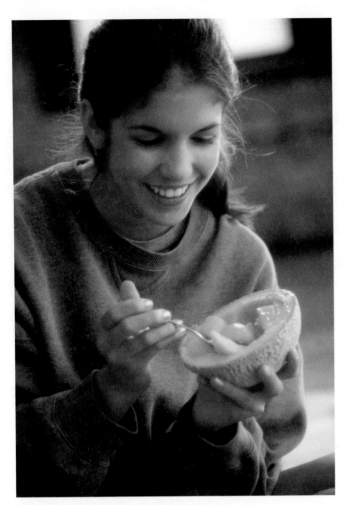

Fruits and vegetables are good snack choices to help reduce total calorie consumption and improve health.

Fad diets and extreme diets are not likely to be effective. Consumers are barraged with products and advertisements that claim easy weight loss solutions. Various fad diets capitalize on the consumer's concern about weight as well as on a general lack of knowledge about diet and exercise. The fad diets often take some small fact about nutrition and claim that they have uncovered some magic solution to weight loss that wasn't previously known. Consumers often believe the claims because they have a history of failing with past efforts to control their weight.

A common strategy in some fad diets is to warn dieters not to eat carbohydrates. Because water is required to store carbohydrates, reductions in carbohydrate intake leads to reductions in water storage—and weight. The person who restricts carbohydrates may see a reduction in "weight" (not fat!) and assume that the diet worked when it didn't. Regardless of the approach, fad diets provide little hope since they typically can't be maintained over time. Constant losing and gaining, known as "yo-yo" dieting, is actually counterproductive and may lead to negative changes in the person's metabolism and unwanted shifts in sites of fat deposition.

It is also important to avoid diets that require severe caloric restriction and exercise programs that require exceptionally large caloric expenditure. These plans can be effective in fat loss over a short period but are seldom maintained for a lifetime. Studies show that extreme programs for weight control, designed to "take it off fast," result in long-term success rates of less than 5 percent. Research shows one reason extremely low calorie diets are ineffective is that they may promote

i
FEATURE 2 **A combination of physical activity and a healthy diet is the best approach for long-term weight control.** One major advantage of emphasizing both physical activity and dietary changes is that physical activity can help maintain basal metabolic rate and prevent the decline that occurs with calorie sparing. Studies have shown that programs that include both diet and physical activity promote greater loss of body fat than programs based solely on dietary changes. The total weight loss from the programs may be about the same, but a larger fraction of the weight comes from fat when physical activity is included. In contrast, programs based solely on diet result in greater loss of lean muscle tissue. A healthy diet and regular physical activity are the keys for long-term weight control. Small changes, such as eating a few hundred calories less per day or walking for 30 minutes every day, can make a big difference over time. The important point is to strive for permanent changes that can be maintained in a normal daily lifestyle.

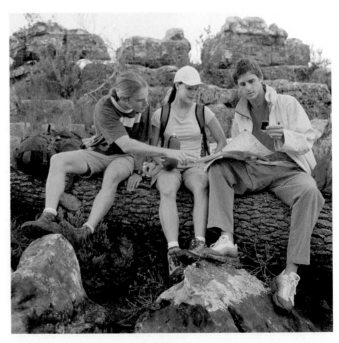

An active, healthy lifestyle is critical for long-term weight control.

Technology Update
Lifestyle Monitoring for Weight Control

New technologies have been developed to make it easier for people to monitor lifestyle behaviors related to weight control. The Sensewear Armband (SWA) monitor (BodyMedia®, Pittsburgh, PA **www.bodymedia.com**) is a wireless multi-sensor monitor that uses motion as well as various heat related sensors to estimate energy expenditure. Studies have demonstrated that the Sensewear monitor provides more accurate estimates of energy expenditure than traditional accelerometers

or pedometers. The monitor can be easily downloaded to provide reports of daily or weekly activity profiles. A particularly novel aspect of the tool is that the data from the monitor can be linked to a detailed dietary analyses tool through the FIT weight management software. The ability to integrate energy intake with estimates of energy expenditure allows users to closely monitor energy balance. Tools such as the Bodymedia FIT system may promote self-monitoring and facilitate weight control. More information is available at the associated Web link.

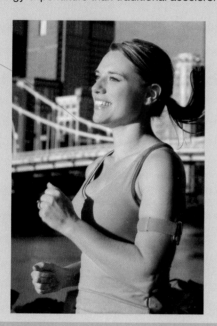

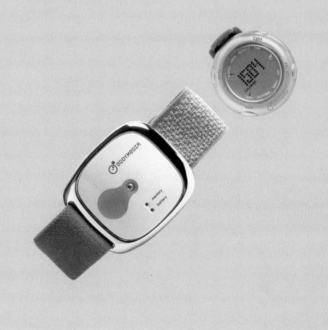

"calorie sparing." When caloric intake is 800 to 1,000 or less, the body protects itself by reducing basal and resting metabolism levels (sparing calories). This results in less fat loss, even though the caloric intake is very low. When in doubt, avoid programs that promise fast and easy solutions, extreme diets that favor specific foods or eating patterns, and any product that makes unreasonable claims about easy ways to stimulate your metabolism or "melt away fat".

Small changes in eating patterns can be effective in fat loss. A number of studies have suggested that individual eating patterns may be associated with obesity. One study found that breakfast skipping, meals eaten away from home, and frequent episodes of eating during the day are associated with obesity—even after controlling for total caloric intake. These results highlight the importance of establishing regular patterns of eating. Another important consideration is to adopt healthy

behaviors that can be maintained over time. The following list highlights a few suggested dietary habits that may be helpful.

- *Make small changes at first.* Small restrictions in caloric intake sustained over time are more effective than drastic short-term changers.
- *Eat less fat.* Research shows that reduction of fat in the diet results not only in fewer calories consumed (fats have more than twice the calories per gram as carbohydrates or proteins) but in greater body fat loss as well.
- *Severely restrict* **empty calories.** Foods that provide little nutrition often account for an excessive proportion of daily caloric intake. Examples of these foods are candy (often high in simple sugar) and potato chips (often fried in saturated fat).

Empty Calories Calories in foods considered to have little or no nutritional value.

Table 2 ▶ Guidelines for Healthy Shopping and Eating in a Variety of Settings

Guidelines for Shopping	• Shop from a list to avoid purchasing foods that contain empty calories and other foods that will tempt you to overeat. • Shop with a friend to avoid buying unneeded foods. For this technique to work, the other person must be sensitive to your goals. In some cases, a friend can have a bad, rather than a good, influence. • Shop on a full stomach to avoid the temptations of snacking on and buying junk food. • Check the labels for contents of foods to avoid foods that are excessively high in fat or saturated fat.
Guidelines for How You Eat	• When you eat, do nothing else but eat. If you watch television, read, or do some other activity while you eat, you may be unaware of what you have eaten. • Eat slowly. Taste your food. Pause between bites. Chew slowly. Do not take the next bite until you have swallowed what you have in your mouth. Periodically take a longer pause. Be the last one finished eating. • Do not eat food you do not want. Some people do not want to waste food, so they clean their plate even when they feel full. • Follow an eating schedule. Eating at regular meal times can help you avoid snacking. Spacing meals equally throughout the day can help reduce appetite. • Leave the table after eating to avoid taking extra, unwanted bites and servings. • Eat meals of equal size. Some people try to restrict calories at one or two meals to save up for a big meal. • Eating several *small* meals helps you avoid hunger (fools the appetite), and this may help prevent overeating. • Avoid second servings. Limit your intake to one moderate serving. If second servings are taken, make them one-half the size of first servings. • Limit servings of salad dressings and condiments (e.g., catsup). These are often high in fat and calories and can amount to greater caloric consumption than expected.
Guidelines for Controlling the Home Environment	• Store food out of sight. Avoid containers that allow you to see food. It is especially important to limit the accessibility of foods that tempt you and foods with empty calories. Foods that are out of sight are out of mouth. • Do your eating in designated areas only. Designate areas such as the kitchen and dining room as eating areas, so you do not snack elsewhere. It is especially easy to eat too much while watching television. • If you snack, eat foods high in complex carbohydrates and low in fats, such as fresh fruits and carrot sticks. • Freeze leftovers. Leftover foods are often tempting to eat. Freezing them so that it takes preparation to eat them will help you avoid temptation.
Guidelines for Controlling the Work Environment	• Take food from home rather than eating from vending machines or catering trucks. • Do not eat while working, but take your lunch as a break. Do something active during other breaks, such as taking a walk. • Avoid sources of food provided by co-workers—for example, food in work rooms, such as birthday cakes, or candy in jars. • Have drinking water or low-calorie drinks available to substitute for snacks.
Guidelines for Eating on Special Occasions	• Practice ways to refuse food. Knowing exactly what to say will help you avoid being talked into eating something you do not want. • Eat before you go out, so you are not as hungry at parties and events. • Do not stand near food sources, and distract yourself if tempted to eat when you are not really hungry. • Limit servings of nonbasic parts of the meal. It is easy to consume large numbers of calories on alcohol, soft drinks, appetizers, and desserts. Limit these items.
Guidelines for Eating at Restaurants	• Make healthy selections from the menu. Choose chicken without skin, fish, or lean cuts of meat. Grilled or broiled options are better than fried. Choose healthier options for dessert, as many decadent desserts can have more calories than the whole dinner. • Limit the use of sauces and condiments, such as butter, margarine, catsup, mayonnaise, and salad dressings. Asking for the condiments on the side allows you to determine how much to put on. • Do not feel compelled to eat everything on your plate. Many restaurants serve exceptionally large portions to try to please the customers. • Order à la carte rather than full meals to avoid multiple courses and servings. • Avoid supersizing your meals if eating at fast-food restaurants, as this can add unwanted calories.

In the News

Use of Social Media for Weight Maintenance and Health Promotion

As noted in this concept, the support of family and friends is very important in weight maintenance and weight loss. Studies show that people who have the support of others are more likely to adhere and benefit from activity and nutrition programs designed to maintain or lose weight. New evidence shows that email feedback can provide social support that encourages healthful behaviors. The more the information is personalized, the better the results in attaining personal goals. Many new behavioral interventions now use various social media (e.g. Facebook and Twitter) to try to facilitate positive norms for health behavior change. Programs may also take advantage of new communication challenges (e.g. text messages and 'tweets' on Twitter) to provide reminders about behavior change. The CDC has recognized the promise (and risks) of social media and has created guidelines to help ensure effective use of these resources in health promotion programming. You will find more on these guidelines (CDC Social Media Tools Guidelines & Best Practices) and information about computer-based social support at the associated Web link.

- *Increase complex carbohydrates.* Foods high in fiber, such as fresh fruits and vegetables, contain few calories for their volume. They are nutritious and filling, and they are especially good foods for a fat loss program.
- *Learn the difference between craving and hunger.* Hunger is a physiological signal that helps promote an organisms drive to eat when energy supply gets low. A craving is simply a desire to eat something, often a food that is sweet or high in calories. When you feel the urge to eat, you may want to ask yourself, Is this real hunger or a craving?
- *Develop better decision making skills.* Making good choices is important when eating at restaurants, at work, special occasions. Making good selections when purchasing and preparing food is also important. See Table 2 for suggestions.

Artificial sweeteners and fat substitutes may help but do not provide a complete weight loss solution. Artificial sweeteners are frequently used in soft drinks and food to reduce the calorie content. Because they have few or no calories, these supplements were originally expected to help people with weight control. However, since they were introduced, the general public has not eaten fewer calories and more people are now overweight than before they were introduced. Studies suggest that people consuming these products end up consuming just as many calories per day as people consuming products with real sugar or sweeteners.

As described in Concept 14, a variety of artificial fat substitutes are now used to reduce fat content in foods. Potato chips and other fried foods cooked in these products as well as baked goods using these products have less fat and fewer calories. If you eat no more food than usual and substitute foods made with these products, you will consume fewer calories and less fat. Experts worry that consumers will not eat the same amount of foods with these fake fats but will feel they can eat more because the fake fats contain fewer calories and less fat."

 A variety of appetite suppressants have been released into the market, but all of FEATURE 3 **them have limitations.** Because long-term weight control is difficult, many individuals seek simple solutions from various nonprescription weight loss products. A common additive in dietary supplements has been the stimulant ephedra (or the herbal equivalent, Ma Huang). Many negative reactions and multiple deaths have been attributed to the use of ephedra, and this led the FDA to ban the sale and use of any products containing this compound. A concern among public health officials is that many products still do not accurately label the contents of their supplements. Manufacturers of supplements have recently started selling "ephedra-free" supplements that use other stimulants, but these have been shown to present similar health risks. Consumers should be wary of dietary supplements, due to the unregulated nature of the industry.

Only two prescription drugs (Sibutramine and Orlistat) have been approved by the FDA to help patients curb appetite and lose weight. Sibutramine (used in the prescription product Meridia) acts by inhibiting the reuptake of the neurotransmitters serotonin and noradrenaline, which regulate hunger. By keeping the levels high, the body doesn't have as high a hunger response. Orlistat (used in Xenical and Alli) enhances weight loss by inhibiting the body's absorption of fat. Studies have confirmed that it can help patients lose more weight, but a limitation is that it also blocks the absorption of important fat-soluble vitamins (A, D, E, and K, as well as betacarotene). Both of these pharmacotherapy treatments are considered to be adjuncts to lifestyle modification and are used only with obese patients (BMI >30) or overweight adults with other comorbidities (e.g., diabetes or hypertension). Xenical is a prescription medication (120 mg.), and Alli is an over-the-counter version of Orlistat with a lower dosage (60 mg.).

Recently the FDA issued MedWatch alerts for Meridia and Alli. The FDA noted that Meridia should not be used by people with heart disease. The manufacturer of Meridia has agreed to including warnings on packages. The FDA also issued a warning that some products sold on the Internet as Alli have counterfeit ingredients. The results demonstrate that there are no shortcuts to weight control. Additional information on appetite suppressants is available at the associated Web link. See Concept 23 to learn how to interpret the diverse array of health information in print and Web media.

Products and procedures claiming to remove fat cells are not safe or effective. A procedure known as "lipodissolve" claims that it is possible to remove fat cells from the body with chemicals. A small amount of a chemical found in lecithin—a food ingredient derived from soybeans—is injected into fatty areas of the body, such as the buttocks or thighs. The fat absorbs the substance (phosphatidylcholine deoxycholate, or PCDC), resulting in an inflammation, followed by a hardening of the fat cells in the area. The fat cells are then allegedly eliminated from the body. The FDA has not approved the procedure, and the safety and effectiveness of the procedure has not been demonstrated by scientific evidence. However, there are reports of the procedure being marketed as a "quick fix" that "burns fat away with an injection." Companies promoting the injections have marketed them as a dietary supplement because the active ingredient (lecithin) has been approved for human consumption by mouth. However, because the PCDC is injected (rather than consumed by mouth), the FDA views the product as a drug and has ordered the manufacturer to stop marketing and distributing the product due to safety concerns. In addition to unproven effectiveness, the procedure can cause permanent scarring, skin deformation, and deep, painful knots under the skin where the lipodissolve treatments are given. This highlights why consumers should be wary of unproven procedures they see on the Internet.

Guidelines for Gaining Muscle Mass

Young people often have difficulty in gaining weight or muscle mass. Typically, those most likely to have difficulty gaining weight are age 10 to 20. This is because more calories are required to maintain weight during the growing years than in adulthood. Young people who want to gain weight have probably been told more than once that they will not have trouble gaining weight when they grow older. Although true for most people, it is of little consolation to those who want to gain weight now.

During adolescence, most people begin to gain weight, including muscle mass that can be enhanced with regular exercise. Excessive eating to gain weight (especially during adolescence) is not without its problems. As noted, the body requires more caloric intake during the teen years because the body is growing. A person who develops a habit of high caloric intake during this time may have difficulty controlling fatness when the demands on the body are less. Most people who want to gain weight want to gain lean body tissue. Only those who have body fat percentages less than what is considered to be essential for good health need to gain body fat.

Changes in the frequency and composition of meals are important to gain muscle mass. To increase muscle mass, the body requires a greater caloric intake. The challenge is to provide enough extra calories for the muscle without excess amounts going to fat. An increase of 500 to 1,000 calories a day will help most people gain muscle mass over time. Smaller, more frequent meals are best for weight gain, since they tend to keep the metabolic rate high. The majority of extra calories should come from complex carbohydrates. Breads, pasta, rice, and fruits such as bananas are good sources. Granola, nuts, juices (grape and cranberry), and milk also make good high-calorie, healthy snacks. Diet supplements are not particularly effective unless used as part of a behaviorally based program. High-fat diets can result in weight gain but may not be best for good health, especially if they are high in saturated fat. If weight gain does not occur over a period of weeks and months with extra calorie consumption, medical assistance may be necessary.

Physical activity is important in gaining muscle mass. Regular strength training can aid in weight gain. The stimulus from this form of exercise causes the body to increase protein synthesis, which allows the body to gain muscle mass. Of course, the body requires higher caloric intake to form this new muscle tissue.

Although some regular aerobic exercise is necessary for health and cardiovascular fitness, excessive aerobic exercise may make gaining weight difficult. Studies have shown that extensive aerobic training can even cause a reduction in muscle mass. When trying to gain weight, aerobic exercise expending no more than 3,500 calories per week is probably best.

Strategies for Action

Knowing about guidelines for controlling body fat is not as important as following them. The guidelines in this concept work only if you use them. In Lab 15A, you will identify guidelines that may help you in the future.

Record keeping is important in meeting fat control goals and making moderation a part of your normal lifestyle. Studies have shown that it is easy to fool yourself when determining the amount of food you have eaten or the amount of exercise you have done. Once fat control goals have been set, whether for weight loss, maintenance, or gain, keeping a diet log and an exercise log can help you monitor your behavior and maintain the lifestyle necessary to meet your goals. A log can also help you monitor changes in weight and body fat levels. But remember, care should be taken to avoid too much emphasis on short-term weight changes. Lab 15B will help you learn about the actual content of fast foods, so you can learn to make better choices when eating out.

The support of family and friends can be of great importance in balancing caloric intake and caloric expenditure. Family and friends can help you adopt and maintain healthy eating practices and follow the guidelines presented in this concept. Sometimes, friends and family can "try too hard" to help. This can have the opposite effect if it is perceived as an attempt to control your behavior. Encouragement and support, rather than control of behavior, are the keys.

Group support can be one of the best reinforcers of proper eating and exercise behavior. Group support is beneficial to many individuals who are attempting to change their behavior. Groups such as Overeaters Anonymous and Weight Watchers help those who need the support of peers in attaining and maintaining desirable fat levels for a lifetime.

Psychological strategies can be useful in eating and exercising to attain and maintain a desirable level of body fat. Adopting healthy lifestyle habits often requires the use of behavioral skills and some degree of discipline. The following list provides tips on maintaining weight control efforts.

- Avoid food fantasies. Sometimes the thought of food is what causes overeating. Practice restructuring your thought process to something other than food fantasies. Use mental imagery to create a mind's-eye view of something you enjoy other than food. When food fantasies occur, you may want to exercise or engage in an activity that refocuses your attention.
- Avoid weight fantasies. Sometimes the thought of being excessively thin or muscular occurs. By itself, this may not be bad. If it causes you to become discouraged and makes your goals seem unattainable, it is bad. When weight fantasies occur, do an activity to redirect your attention or imagine something other than the weight fantasy.
- Avoid **negative self-talk.** One type of negative self-talk occurs when a person starts self-criticism for not meeting a goal. For example, if you are determined not to eat more than one serving of food at a party but fail to meet this goal, you might say, "It's no use stopping now; I've already blown it." It is not too late. Anyone can fail to meet goals. Negative self-talk makes it easy to fail in the future. A more appropriate response is **positive self-talk,** such as, "I'm not going to eat anything else tonight; I can do it."

Web Resources

Additional websites with information related to Concept 15 are available at the associated Web link.

American Dietetic Association **www.eatright.org**
Berkeley Nutrition Sciences **www.nutritionquest.com**
Center for Science in the Public Interest
www.cspinet.org
Nutriwatch (consumer website) **www.nutriwatch.org**
Office of Dietary Supplements **http://ods.od.nih.gov**

STOP Obesity Alliance **www.stopobesityalliance.org**
USDA Food and Nutrition Information Center
www.nal.usda.gov/fnic

Negative Self-Talk Self-defeating discussions with yourself focusing on your failures rather than your successes.

Positive Self-Talk Telling yourself positive, encouraging things that help you succeed in accomplishing your goals.

Suggested Readings

REFERENCES　Selected readings and references are listed below. A more comprehensive list is available at the associated Web link.

Burke, M. A., et al. 2010. From "Overweight" to "About Right": Evidence of a generational shift in body weight norms. *Obesity* 18(6):1226–1234.

Coleman, R. J. 2009. Caloric restriction delays disease onset and mortality in rhesus monkeys. *Science* 325(10):201–204.

Foster-Schubert, K. E., et al. 2009. Effect of diet, exercise, or combined diet and exercise on weight and body composition of overweight to obese post-menopausal women. *Obesity* 17(S-2) Abstract:103.

Harris, J. L., et al. 2009. Priming effects of television food advertising on eating behavior. *Health Psychology* 28(4):404–413.

Hurley, J. and B. Liebman. 2010. Xtreme eating 2010. *Nutrition Action Healthletter*. Available at **http://cspinet.org/nah /articles/xtremeeating2010.html**.

International Food Information Council Foundation. 2010. 2010 Food and Health Survey. Available at **www.foodinsight.org**

Katz, M. H., and R. Katz. 2010. Food surcharges and subsidies: Putting your money where your mouth is. *Archives of Internal Medicine* 170(5):405–406.

Kessler, D. 2009. *The End of Overeating: Taking Control of the Insatiable American Appetite*. New York: Rodale Press.

Kunkel, D., et al. 2009. *The Impact of Industry Self-Regulation on the Nutritional Quality of Foods Advertised on Television to Children*. Oakland, CA: Children Now. Available at **www .childrennow.org/index.php/learn/reports_and_research /article/576**

Lee. I., et al. 2010. Physical activity and weight gain prevention. *Journal of the American Medical Association* 303(12):1173–1179.

Lusk, A. C., et al. 2010. Bicycle riding, walking and weight gain in premenopausal women. *Archives of Internal Medicine* 170(12):1050–1056.

Lynch, F. L., et al. 2010. Cost-effectiveness of guided self-help treatment for recurrent binge eating. *Journal of Consulting and Clinical Psychology* 78(3):322–333.

Lynch, F. L., et al. 2010. Cognitive behavioral guided self-help for the treatment of recurrent binge eating. *Journal of Consulting and Clinical Psychology* 78(3):312–321.

Papalazarou, A., et al. 2010. Lifestyle intervention favorably affects weight loss and maintenance following obesity surgery. *Obesity* 18:1348–1353.

Plotnikoff, R. C., et al. 2010. Six-month follow-up and participant use and satisfaction of an electronic mail intervention promoting physical activity and nutrition. *American Journal of Health Promotion* 24 (4): 255–259.Sacks, F. M., et al. 2009. Comparison of weight-loss diets with different compositions of fat, protein, and carbohydrates. *New England Journal of Medicine* 360(9):859–873.

Schlosser, E. 2006. *Fast Food Nation*. Ventura, CA: Academic Internet Publishers.

Wardlaw, G. M. 2011. *Contemporary Nutrition*. New York: McGraw-Hill Higher Education.

Westcott, W. 2009. ACSM strength training guidelines: Role in body composition and health enhancement. *ACSM's Health and Fitness Journal* 13(4):14–22.

Lab 15A Selecting Strategies for Managing Eating

Name	**Section**	**Date**

Purpose: To learn to select strategies for managing eating to control body fatness

Procedures

1. Read the strategies listed in Chart 1.
2. Check the box beside 5 to 10 of the strategies that you think will be most useful for you.
3. Answer the questions in the Conclusions and Implications section.

Chart 1 ▶ Strategies for Managing Eating to Control Body Fatness

✔	**Check 5 to 10 strategies that you might use in the future.**
	Shopping Strategies
	Shop from a list.
	Shop with a friend.
	Shop on a full stomach.
	Check food labels.
	Consider foods that take some time to prepare.
	Methods of Eating
	When you eat, do nothing but eat. Don't watch television or read.
	Eat slowly.
	Do not eat food you do not want.
	Follow an eating schedule.
	Do your eating in designated areas, such as kitchen or dining room only.
	Leave the table after eating.
	Avoid second servings.
	Limit servings of condiments.
	Limit servings of nonbasics, such as dessert, breads, and soft drinks.
	Eat several meals of equal size rather than one big meal and two small ones.
	Eating in the Work Environment
	Take your own food to work.
	Avoid snack machines.
	If you eat out, plan your meal ahead of time.
	Do not eat while working.
	Avoid sharing foods from co-workers, such as birthday cakes.
	Have activity breaks during the day.
	Have water available to substitute for soft drinks.
	Have low-calorie snacks to substitute for office snacks.

✔	**Check 5 to 10 strategies that you might use in the future.**
	Eating on Special Occasions
	Practice ways to refuse food.
	Avoid tempting situations.
	Eat before you go out.
	Don't stand near food sources.
	If you feel the urge to eat, find someone to talk to.
	Strategies for Eating Out
	Limit deep-fat fried foods.
	Ask for information about food content.
	Limit use of condiments.
	Choose low-fat foods (e.g., skim milk, low-fat yogurt).
	Choose chicken, fish, or lean meat.
	Order á la carte.
	If you eat desserts, avoid those with sauces or toppings.
	Eating at Home
	Keep busy at times when you are at risk of overeating.
	Store food out of sight.
	Avoid serving food to others between meals.
	If you snack, choose snacks with complex carbohydrates, such as carrot sticks or apple slices.
	Freeze leftovers to avoid the temptation of eating them between meals.

Conclusions and Implications

1. In several sentences, discuss your need to use strategies for effective eating. Do you need to use them? Why or why not?

2. In several sentences, discuss the effectiveness of the strategies contained in Chart 1. Do you think they can be effective for people who have a problem controlling their body fatness?

3. In several sentences, discuss the value of using behavioral goals versus outcome goals when planning for fat loss.

Lab 15B Evaluating Fast-Food Options

Name	

Section		Date	

Purpose: To learn about the energy and fat content of fast food and how to make better choices when eating at fast-food restaurants

Procedures

1. Select a fast-food restaurant and a typical meal that you might order there. Then use Appendix C, or one of the food calculators listed at the bottom of this page, to determine total calories, fat calories, saturated fat intake, and cholesterol for each food item.
2. Record the values in Chart 2.
3. Sum the totals for the meal in Chart 2.
4. Record recommended daily values by selecting an amount from Chart 1. The estimate should be based on your estimated needs for the day.
5. Compute the percentage of the daily recommended amounts that you consume in the meal by dividing recommended amounts (step 4) into meal totals (step 3). Record percent of recommended daily amounts in Chart 2.
6. Answer the questions in the Conclusions and Implications section.

Chart 1 ▶ Recommended Daily Amounts of Fat, Saturated Fat, Cholesterol, and Sodium

	2,000 kcal	3,000 kcal
Total fat	65 g	97.5 g
Saturated fat	20 g	30 g
Cholesterol	300 mg	450 mg
Sodium	2,400 mg	3,600 g

Results

Chart 2 ▶ Listing of Foods Selected for the Meal

Food Item	Total Calories	Total Fat (g)	Saturated Fat (g)	Cholesterol (mg)
1.				
2.				
3.				
4.				
5.				
6.				
Total for meal (sum up each column)				
Recommended daily amount (record your values from Chart 1)				
% of recommended daily amount (record your % of recommended)				

Fast Food Calculators

1. Fast Food Nutrition: Meal Calculator www.fastfoodnutrition.org/calc1.php
2. The Fast Food Explorer www.fatcalories.com
3. Fast Food Nutrition Facts Calculator http://pediatrics.about.com/cs/fastfood/l/bl_restaurants.htm
4. Fast Food Charts www.fastfoodnutrition.org/index.php

Conclusions and Implications:

1. Describe how often you eat at fast-food restaurants and indicate whether you would like to reduce how much fast food you consume.

2. Were you surprised at the amount of fat, saturated fat, and cholesterol in the meal you selected?

3. What could you do differently at fast-food restaurants to reduce your intake of fat, saturated fat, and cholesterol?

Stress and Health

Health Goals for the Year 2020

- Promote quality of life, healthy development, and healthy behaviors across all stages of life.
- Increase mental health and wellness of the disabled.
- Increase screening for and treatment of mental health problems.
- Reduce suicide and suicide attempts.
- Increase availability of work-site stress-reduction programs.
- Increase levels of social support among adults.

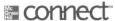 **cOnnect**
|FITNESS AND WELLNESS   http://connect.mcgraw-hill.com

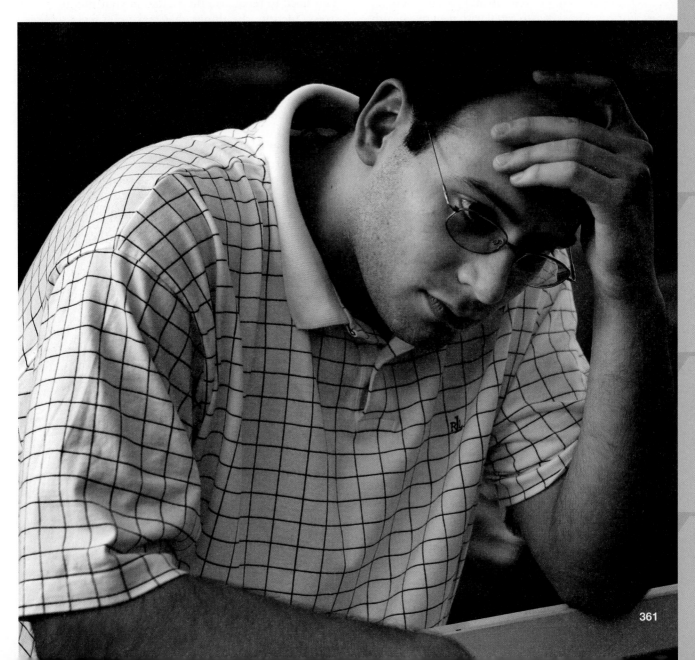

Mental and physical health are affected by an individual's ability to adapt to stress.

Stress affects everyone to some degree. In fact, approximately 75 percent of adults indicate that they have experienced moderate to high levels of stress in the past month, and nearly half report that their level of stress has increased in the past year. **Stressors** come in many forms, and even positive life events can increase our stress levels.

At moderate levels, stress can motivate us to reach our goals and keep life interesting. However, when stressors are severe or chronic, our bodies may not be able to adapt successfully. Stress can compromise immune functioning, leading to a host of diseases of **adaptation.** In fact, stress has been linked to between 50 and 70 percent of all illnesses. Further, stress is associated with negative health behaviors, such as alcohol and other drug use, and to psychological problems, such as depression and anxiety. Although all humans have the same physiological system for responding to stress, stress reactivity varies across individuals. In addition, the way we think about or perceive stressful situations has a significant impact on how our bodies respond. Thus, there are large differences in individual responses to stress.

This concept reviews the causes and consequences of stress. Figure 1 illustrates the many factors involved in individual reactions to stress. First, the sources of stress, (stressors) such as daily hassles and major life events, are described. Then the physiological responses to stress and the impact of these effects on physical and mental health are reviewed. Finally, individual differences in physiological and cognitive responses to stress and the implications of these individual differences for health and wellness are discussed.

Sources of Stress

The first step in managing stress is to recognize the causes and to be aware of the symptoms. You need to recognize the factors in your life that cause stress. Identify the things that make you feel "stressed-out." Everything from minor irritations, such as traffic jams, to major life changes, such as births, deaths, or job loss, can be a stressor. A stress overload of too many demands on your time can make you feel that you are no longer in control. Recognizing the causes and effects of stress is important for learning how to manage it.

Stress has a variety of sources. There are many kinds of stressors. Environmental stressors include heat, noise, overcrowding, pollution, and second-hand smoke. Physiological stressors are such things as drugs, caffeine, tobacco, injury, infection or disease, and physical effort.

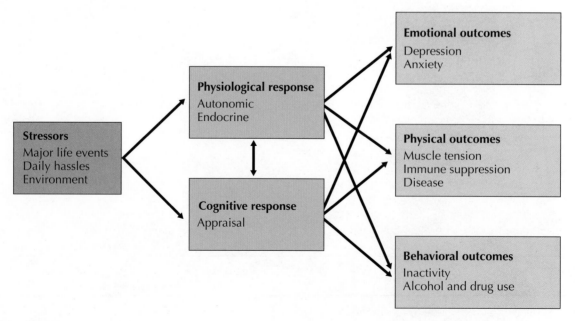

Figure 1 ▶ Reactions to stress.

Table 1 ▶ Ten Common Stressors in the Lives of College Students and Middle-Aged Adults

College Students	Middle-Aged Adults
1. Troubling thoughts about the future	1. Concerns about weight
2. Not getting enough sleep	2. Health of a family member
3. Wasting time	3. Rising prices of common goods
4. Inconsiderate smokers	4. Home maintenance (interior)
5. Physical appearance	5. Too many things to do
6. Too many things to do	6. Misplacing or losing things
7. Misplacing or losing things	7. Yard work or outside home maintenance
8. Not enough time to do the things you need to do	8. Property, investments, or taxes
9. Concerns about meeting high standards	9. Crime
10. Being lonely	10. Physical appearance

Source: Kanner, et al.

Emotional stressors are the most frequent and important stressors. Some people refer to these as *psychosocial stressors.* A national study of daily experiences indicated that more than 60 percent of all stressful experiences fall into a few areas (see Table 1).

Stressors vary in severity. Major stressors create major emotional turmoil or require tremendous amounts of adjustment. This category includes personal crises (e.g., major health problems or death in the family, divorce/separation, financial problems, legal problems) and job/school-related pressures or major age-related transitions (e.g., college, marriage, career, retirement). Daily hassles are generally viewed as shorter-term or less severe. This category includes events such as traffic problems, peer/work relations, time pressures, and family squabbles. In school, pressures such as grades, term papers, and oral presentations would likely fall into this category. Major stressors can alter daily patterns of stress and impair our ability to handle the minor stressors of life, while daily hassles can accumulate and create more significant problems. It is important to be aware of both types of stressors.

Negative, ambiguous, and uncontrollable events are usually the most stressful. Although stress can come from both positive and negative events, negative ones generally cause more distress because negative stressors usually have harsher consequences and little benefit. Positive stressors, on the other hand, usually have enough benefit to make them worthwhile. For example, the stress of starting a new job may be tremendous, but it is not as bad as the negative stress from losing a job.

Ambiguous stressors are harder to accept than are more clearly defined problems. In most cases, if the cause of a stressor or problem can be identified, active measures can be taken to improve the situation. For example, if you are stressed about a project at work or school, you can use specific strategies to complete the task on time. Stress brought on by a relationship with friends or co-workers, on the other hand, may be harder to understand. In some cases, it is not possible to determine the primary source or cause of the problem. These situations are more problematic because fewer clear-cut solutions exist.

Another factor that makes events stressful is a lack of control. Because little can be done to change the situation, these events leave us feeling powerless. If the stressor is something that can be dealt with more directly, efforts at minimizing the stress are likely to be effective.

Americans report high levels of stress. In a 2009 survey conducted by the American Psychological Association, roughly half of respondents indicated that their levels of stress increased in the past year, and nearly one-fourth indicated that they regularly experienced extreme levels of stress. Commonly reported stress responses included both psychological symptoms (e.g., feeling nervous or sad) and physical symptoms (e.g., headaches and fatigue). In 2009, for the first time, the APA included 8- to 17-year-olds in their annual survey about stress. The results were a bit surprising and also concerning. Perhaps the most notable finding was that children seem to be more stressed than their parents realize. For example, among 8- to 12-year-olds, 26 percent reported that their level of worry increased in the past year, whereas only 17 percent of parents believed this to be true for their child. The gap was even larger among teens, with 45 percent of teens reporting increased stress compared to 27 percent of parents reporting increased

Stress The nonspecific response (generalized adaptation) of the body to any demand made on it in order to maintain physiological equilibrium. This positive or negative response results from emotions that are accompanied by biochemical and physiological changes directed at adaptation.

Stressors Things that place a greater than routine demand on the body or evoke a stress reaction.

Adaptation The body's efforts to restore normalcy.

In the News

Rates of mental health problems in the military are increasing dramatically as a consequence of combat stress associated with deployments in Iraq and Afghanistan. Between 2006 and 2007 alone, there was a 50% increase in the incidence of PTSD. A 2010 study of active component and national guard troops following deployment in Iraq confirms the high rates of mental health problems. This study found that, even using the most stringent criteria, rates of depression ranged from 5 to 9 percent and rates of PTSD ranged from 6 to 11 percent. Equally concerning, problems identified at 3 months following return from service were maintained or increased 9 months later. Given the high rates of re-deployment, these persistent problems may lead to impairments in functioning during active deployment and to exacerbation of existing mental health issues. Efforts to provide adequate treatment among this growing population will be a major challenge for the mental health field in the coming years.

stress in their teen. In particular, parents underestimated the extent to which their children experienced financial stress and sleep difficulties.

College presents unique challenges and stressors. For college students, schoolwork can be a full-time job, and those who have to work outside of school must handle the stresses of both jobs. Although the college years are often thought of as a break from the stresses of the real world, college life has its own stressors. Obvious sources of stress include taking exams, speaking in public, and becoming comfortable with talking to professors. Students are often living independently of family for the first time while negotiating new relationships—with roommates, dating partners, and so on. Young people entering college are also faced with a less structured environment and with the need to control their own schedules. Though this environment has a number of advantages, students are faced with a greater need to manage their stress effectively.

In addition to the traditional challenges of college, the new generation of students faces stressors that were not typical for college students in the past. According to the American Council on Education, only 40 percent of today's college students enroll full-time immediately after high school. More students now work, and many go back to school after spending time in the working world. More of today's college students are the first in their family to attend college. Perhaps as a result of some

of these factors and the pressures that they create, rates of mental health problems among college students have increased dramatically in recent years (see Figure 2). In a 2009 survey of campus counseling center directors, 93.4 percent of respondents indicated that they believed that more students today have severe psychological problems. This impression is substantiated by the increasing percentage of students on psychiatric medications (9 percent in 1994 to 25 percent in 2009). Student surveys paint a similar picture. For example, a recent study found that 42 percent of students reported feeling "so depressed it was difficult to function" at some point during the past year. Although counseling centers are doing their best to keep up with increasing demands, increases in funding and staff in college counseling centers have not been sufficient to meet demands.

Some sources of stress are shared by entire communities, cultures, or societies. Although the stresses individuals experience are often unique to their particular circumstances, there are times when entire communities, cultures, or even countries have shared experiences of severe stress. Natural disasters like Hurricane Katrina and acts of terrorism, including the events of September 11, 2001, are prime examples. Most recently, the economic downturn in the United States has been a shared source of stress for everyone in this country. A poll developed by Gallup and Healthways to track the well-being of the U.S. population has documented the effects of shared stressors on well-being. The poll includes daily surveys of 1,000 Americans beginning

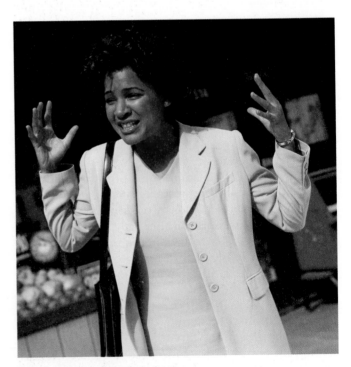

Daily hassles can contribute to stress.

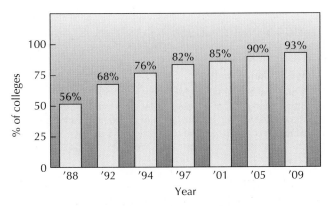

Figure 2 ▶ Colleges reporting increased psychological problems.

Source: R. Gallagher.

Health is available to **EVERYONE** for a Lifetime, and it's Personal

According to a 2008 Associated Press and mtvU survey of college students, 80 percent reported that they "frequently or sometimes experience daily stress." Once a year colleges all over the country participate in a National Stress Out Day where other college students and professionals provide pre-finals stress relief, education about anxiety disorders and help to promote mental awareness among college students. Between classes, finals, jobs and family responsibilities, college students today have a lot on their plate.

Which types of stressors do you think have the most impact on college students?

in January 2008. As the economic downturn worsened in the latter half of 2008, dramatic decreases in well-being were observed, with low levels persisting through the early months of 2009. Although the economic crisis is far from over, Americans have shown themselves to be quite resilient. By June 2009, levels of well-being had returned to levels first assessed in January 2008, and levels have stayed relatively stable since that time.

Reactions to Stress

All people have a general reaction to stress. In the early 1900s, Walter Cannon identified the fight-or-flight response to threat. According to his model, the body reacts to a threat by preparing either to fight or flee the situation. The body prepares for either option through the activation of the **sympathetic nervous system (SNS).** When the SNS is activated, epinephrine (adrenaline) and norepinephrine are released to focus attention on the task at hand. Heart rate and blood

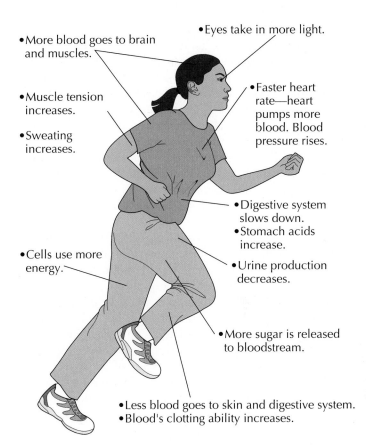

Figure 3 ▶ Physical symptoms of stress.

• More blood goes to brain and muscles.
• Muscle tension increases.
• Sweating increases.
• Cells use more energy.
• Eyes take in more light.
• Faster heart rate—heart pumps more blood. Blood pressure rises.
• Digestive system slows down.
• Stomach acids increase.
• Urine production decreases.
• More sugar is released to bloodstream.
• Less blood goes to skin and digestive system.
• Blood's clotting ability increases.

pressure increase to deliver oxygen to the muscles and essential organs, the eyes take in more light to increase visual acuity, and more sugar is released into the bloodstream to increase energy level. At the same time, nonessential functions like digestion and urine production are slowed. Figure 3 depicts some of the many physiological changes that occur during this process. Once the immediate threat has passed, the **parasympathetic nervous system (PNS)** takes over in an attempt to restore the body to homeostasis and conserve resources. The PNS largely reverses the changes initiated by the SNS (e.g., slows heart rate and returns blood from the muscles and essential organs to the periphery).

Sometimes the fight-or-flight, or SNS, response is essential to survival, but when invoked inappropriately or excessively it may be more harmful than the effects

Sympathetic Nervous System (SNS) The component of the autonomic nervous system that responds to stressful situations by initiating the fight-or-flight response.

Parasympathetic Nervous System (PNS) The component of the autonomic nervous system that helps bring the body to a resting state following stressful experiences.

of the original stressor. Hans Selye, another prominent scientist, was the first to recognize the potential negative consequences of this response. Selye suggested that this system could be invoked by mental as well as physical threats and that the short-term benefits might lead to long-term negative consequences. Based on these ideas, Selye described the general adaptation syndrome, which explains how the autonomic nervous system reacts to stressful situations and the conditions under which the system may break down (Table 2). The term *general* highlights the similarities in response to stressful situations across individuals. Selye's work led him to be referred to as the "father of stress."

Although chronic activation of the SNS is still believed to be important in the development of physical disease, other important systems in the body are also involved. For example, the hypothalamic-pituitary-adrenal (HPA) axis is activated during stress, leading to the release of corticotropin-releasing hormone (CRH) and secondary activation of the pituitary gland. The pituitary releases a chemical called adrenocorticotropic hormone (ACTH), which ultimately causes the release of an active stress hormone called cortisol. With chronic exposure to stress, the HPA system can become dysregulated, and both over- and underactivation of the system are associated with risk for negative health outcomes.

Excessive stress reduces the effectiveness of the immune system. In addition to preparing the body for fight or flight, the stress-related activation of the SNS and the HPA axis slows down the functioning of the immune response. In the face of an immediate threat, mobilizing resources that will help in the moment is more important to the body than preventing or fighting infection. As a result, if the stress response is chronically activated, high levels of adrenaline and cortisol continue to tell the body to mobilize resources at the expense of immune functioning. There are also normative developmental changes in the functioning of the HPA axis. Overall, HPA axis activity increases with age, and a recent study found that the HPA axis becomes more reactive to stress during adolescence. This increased reactivity may contribute to higher rates of negative outcomes during adolescence, including anxiety, depression, and substance use.

Table 2 ▶ The Three Stages in the General Adaptation Syndrome
Stage 1: Alarm Reaction
Any physical or mental trauma triggers an immediate set of reactions that combat the stress. Because the immune system is initially depressed, normal levels of resistance are lowered, making us more susceptible to infection and disease. If the stress is not severe or long-lasting, we bounce back and recover rapidly.
Stage 2: Resistance
Eventually, sometimes rather quickly, we adapt to stress, and we tend to become more resistant to illness and disease. The immune system works overtime during this period, keeping up with the demands placed on it.
Stage 3: Exhaustion
Because the body is not able to maintain homeostasis and the long-term resistance needed to combat stress, we invariably experience a drop in resistance level. No one experiences the same resistance and tolerance to stress, but everyone's immunity at some point collapses following prolonged stress reactions.

Source: Health News Network.

Stress Responses and Health

(i) FEATURE 1 **Chronic or repetitive acute stress can lead to fatigue and can cause or exacerbate a variety of health problems.** Some stress persists only as long as the stressor is present. For example, job-related stress caused by a challenging project generally subsides once that project is complete. In contrast, exposure to chronic stress or repeated exposure to acute stress may lead to a state of fatigue. Fatigue may result from lack of sleep, emotional strain, pain, disease, or a combination of these factors. Both **physiological fatigue** and **psychological fatigue** can result in a state of exhaustion, with resultant physical and mental health consequences. Chronic stress has been linked to health maladies that plague individuals on a daily basis, such as headaches, indigestion, insomnia, and the common cold. In fact, one study concluded that out-of-control stress is the leading preventable source of increased health-care cost in the workforce, roughly equivalent to the costs of the health problems related to smoking.

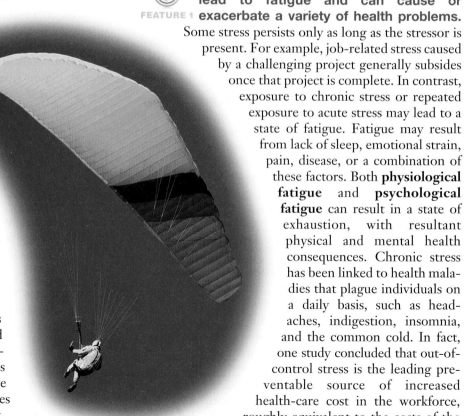

One person's stress is another's pleasure.

The effects of stress on health are not limited to minor physical complaints. Compelling evidence exists linking psychological stress to a host of serious health problems, including cardiovascular disease, cancer, and HIV/AIDS. New evidence suggests that stress may also increase risk for upper respiratory tract infections, asthma, herpes, viral infections, autoimmune diseases, and slow wound healing. Reduced immune function, related to negative emotions and stress, appears to be a principal reason for these health problems. Stress is also associated with increased risk of early death. It is theorized that stress accelerates the aging process by causing a more rapid deterioration of chromosomes (changes in DNA proteins).

Stress can have mental and emotional effects. The challenges caused by psychosocial stress may lead to a variety of mental and emotional effects. In the short term, stress can impair concentration and attention span. Anxiety is an emotional response to stress characterized by apprehension. Because the response usually involves expending a lot of nervous energy, anxiety can lead to fatigue and muscular tension.

Anxiety may persist long after a stressful experience. Both early childhood trauma and recent traumatic experiences have been shown to alter functioning of the HPA axis, contributing to later risk for physical and mental health problems. In some cases, traumatic experiences lead to posttraumatic stress disorder (PTSD). Symptoms of PTSD include flashbacks of the traumatic event, avoidance of situations that remind the person of the event, emotional numbing, and increased level of arousal.

People who are excessively stressed are also more likely to be depressed than people who have optimal amounts of stress in their lives. Research has shown that drugs commonly prescribed to reduce depression can be effective in many cases. However, drugs do not get to the source of the life stressors that cause depression, and many have negative side effects.

 Stress can alter both positive and negative health behaviors. In addition to direct effects FEATURE 2 on health, stress can contribute to negative health outcomes indirectly, through increased engagement in negative behaviors, such as smoking, alcohol use, and overeating. Stress may also decrease engagement in health-protective behaviors like exercise and lead to disruptions in sleep. During periods of increased stress, people may get insufficient sleep due to time constraints and sleep difficulties associated with the causes of stress. For example, an individual experiencing severe stress related to finances may pick up additional shifts at work, leaving less time for sleep. The person may also have difficulty sleeping due to worry associated with the financial situation. Unfortunately, reduced or disrupted sleep may exacerbate the problem. Animal research suggests that chronic sleep deprivation may lead to changes in responses to stress, including dysregulation of the HPA axis. This dysregulation may leave individuals more vulnerable to the negative consequences of future stressors. Studies in humans have also consistently found a link between sleep difficulties and stress-related physical and mental health problems, including cardiovascular disease and depression, and a recent study found a strong link between stress and sleep disturbances among college students.

Individuals respond differently to stress. Individuals exposed to high levels of stress are FEATURE 3 most at risk for negative health consequences. However, not everyone exposed to severe or chronic stress will experience negative outcomes. Those with positive health outcomes despite high levels of stress are said to be "resilient" and have been the subject of study. There is obviously more to the stress-illness relationship than the total number or severity of stressors. What makes an individual more or less susceptible to negative stress-related outcomes?

Two important areas in which individuals differ are stress reactivity and stress appraisals. Stress reactivity is the extent to which the sympathetic nervous system, or fight-or-flight system, is activated by a stressor, whereas

---

Technology Update
Biochemical Markers of Stress

TECH The "stress hormone" cortisol has been implicated in the effects of stress on both physical and mental health outcomes, leading to the development of new tools for assessing cortisol levels. Although early research focused on blood samples, there are now well-established measures of salivary cortisol that can be administered noninvasively. In addition, the Applied Physics Laboratory at Johns Hopkins University is working on a "real-time" measure of cortisol that would allow for repeated measurements during stressful situations. One of their goals is to develop a measure that can be used to assess stress levels among soldiers during combat. Soldiers could wear a hands-free hydration system with the built-in cortisol sensor. Each time they take a drink, their cortisol would be recorded. Such new technology could significantly improve our understanding of the role of cortisol in stress responses.

Physiological Fatigue A deterioration in the capacity of the neuromuscular system as a result of physical overwork and strain; also referred to as true fatigue.

Psychological Fatigue A feeling of fatigue, usually caused by such things as lack of exercise, boredom, or mental stress, that results in a lack of energy and depression; also referred to as subjective or false fatigue.

stress appraisals are an individual's perceptions of a stressor and the person's resources for managing stressful situations. These individual differences are partly due to inherited predispositions and partly due to our unique histories of experiencing and attempting to cope with stress. Recognizing these individual differences has important implications for our well-being because knowledge of our own response to stressful situations can increase our awareness of the impact of stress and can provide information that may lead to more effective stress management.

Everyone has an optimal level of arousal. We all need sufficient stress to motivate us to engage in activities that make our lives meaningful. Otherwise, we would be in a state of **hypostress,** which leads to apathy, boredom, and less than optimal health and wellness. An example of hypostress is a person working on an assembly line. Because the same task is repeated without variation, the level of stimulation is quite low and might lead to a state of boredom and job dissatisfaction. In fact, a certain level of stress, called **eustress,** is experienced positively. In contrast, **distress** is a level of stress that compromises performance and well-being. Each of us possesses a system that allows us to mobilize resources when necessary and that seeks to find a homeostatic level of arousal (see Figure 4). Although we all have an optimal level of arousal, the optimal level varies considerably. What one person finds stressful another may find exhilarating. Stress mobilizes some to greater efficiency, while it confuses others. For example, riding a roller coaster is thrilling for some people, but for others it is a stressful and unpleasant experience.

Reactions to stress depend on one's appraisal of both the event and the subsequent physiological response. Stressors by themselves generally do not cause problems unless they are perceived as stressful. Appraisal usually involves consideration of the consequences of the situation (primary appraisal) and an evaluation of the resources available to cope with the situation (secondary appraisal). If one sees a stressor as a challenge that can be tackled, one is likely to respond in a more positive manner than if the stressor is viewed as an obstacle that cannot be overcome.

The events that occurred on September 11, 2001, provide a vivid example of the very different reactions that people have to the same or similar stressors. Everyone who witnessed these events, in person or on television, was profoundly impacted. At the same time, individual reactions varied dramatically. Most felt overwhelming sadness, many felt extreme anger, others felt hopeless or desperate, and yet others felt lost or confused. Undoubtedly, there were some who were simply too shocked to process their emotional experience at all. With time, most Americans began to experience a wave of additional emotions, such as hope, patriotism,

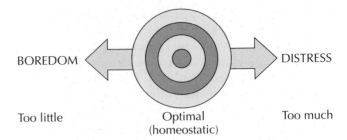

Figure 4 ▶ Stress target zone.

courage, and determination. Others were less quick to experience these positive emotions, and many developed anxiety, depression, or posttraumatic stress disorder. All of these emotions were reactions to the same stressful events. Although a number of factors contributed to these individual differences (e.g., proximity to New York City or personal relationships with individuals who lost their lives), differences in appraisals of the events were probably responsible for much of the variability.

In addition to the appraisal of the event, one's appraisal of the body's response to an event is important. The way in which bodily sensations are interpreted has a significant impact on how one will react emotionally and behaviorally. For example, public speaking is a situation that leads to significant autonomic arousal for most people. Those who handle these situations well probably recognize that these sensations are normal and may even interpret them as excitement about the situations. In contrast, those who experience severe and sometimes debilitating anxiety are probably interpreting the same sensations as indicators of fear, panic, and loss of control. The combination of individual differences in stress reactivity and appraisals may lead to characteristic ways of responding to stress that either confer risk or protect against risk for physical and mental health problems. In fact, several different patterns of behavior (or personality styles) have been clearly identified.

Ⓘ **Type A and Type D personalities may increase risk for negative health** FEATURE 4 **outcomes.** The best-known "personality" style associated with risk for negative health outcomes is the **Type A** behavior pattern. Several decades ago psychologists Friedman and Rosenman identified a subgroup of goal-oriented, or "driven," patients, whom they believed were at increased risk based on their pattern of behavior. These individuals demonstrated a sense of time urgency, were highly competitive, and tended to experience and express anger and hostility under conditions of stress. In contrast, individuals with the Type B behavior pattern were relatively easygoing and less reactive to stress. Although early research on Type A behavior demonstrated increased risk for heart disease, it now appears that certain aspects of the

Type A behavior pattern pose greater risk than others. In particular, hostility and anger appear to be consistently associated with risk for cardiovascular disease. Although most studies have not found time urgency or competitiveness predictive of risk for cardiovascular disease, a recent study found that people who scored high on a measure of impatience were nearly twice as likely to have high blood pressure relative to individuals lower on this trait. At the same time, there is evidence that certain aspects of the Type A behavior pattern (other than hostility) lead to higher levels of achievement and an increased sense of personal accomplishment. Although the Type A behavior pattern has often been referred to as Type A personality, it was not the intention of those who developed the concept to identify a "personality type."

In contrast, the more recently identified **Type D**, or "distressed," personality is associated with two well-defined personality characteristics based on personality theory. Individuals with Type D personality are characterized by high levels of "negative affectivity," or negative emotion, and "social inhibition," or the tendency not to express negative emotions in social interactions. The combination of these characteristics appears to constitute risk for cardiovascular disease and other negative health outcomes. Converging evidence from recent research on both Type A and Type D behaviors has led some to conclude that negative affectivity, in general, is a more important risk for negative health outcomes than any emotion in particular. In other words, anger and hostility (Type A), as well as anxiety and depressed mood (Type D), pose a health risk. Several other well-established personality traits, including neuroticism and novelty seeking, have also been linked to morbidity and mortality.

(i) **Several personality traits are associated with resilience in the face of stress.**
FEATURE 5 **Resilience** is not simply due to an absence of risk factors, but also to the presence of protective factors that lead to adaptive functioning. The experience of positive emotion is one well-established protective factor. Individuals who experience more positive emotion are more likely to adopt healthy lifestyles, and their physical responses to stress are more adaptive than those who experience less positive emotion. For example, patterns of cortisol response, heart rate, and blood pressure under stress are all more favorable among individuals who experience higher levels of positive emotion. Positive emotion may also be an effective coping mechanism for managing acute stress. Positive moods have been shown to undo some of the cardiovascular effects associated with negative emotions. Individuals who have more positive moods are also more socially integrated and report higher levels of social support, both characteristics associated with health benefits. **Optimism** is a personal trait associated with more positive emotional experiences and a more

positive outlook on the future. Extensive research has demonstrated that optimistic individuals have better physical and mental health outcomes than pessimistic individuals.

An individual's **locus of control** can also have a significant impact on how he or she responds to a stressful situation. Research has consistently found that having an internal locus of control is associated with better health outcomes. People with an internal locus of control are more likely to take steps to address the problems that created the stress, rather than avoiding the problem. Those with an external locus of control are more likely to use passive methods for managing stress. In addition, an external locus of control is related to higher perceived levels of stress, lower job satisfaction, and poorer school achievement.

Although an internal locus of control generally promotes health, this is not always the case. This truth is apparent in depressed individuals with a pessimistic explanatory style. They believe that their failures are due to internal factors, squarely placing the control of these events within themselves. Even though they believe stressors are under their control, they don't believe in their ability to initiate change. Thus, for an internal locus of control to be beneficial to well-being, it must be combined with the belief that one is capable of making changes to prevent future problems. The belief in one's ability to reach a desired goal is often referred to as **self-efficacy**. Finally, studies have consistently shown

---

Hypostress Insufficient levels of stress leading to boredom or apathy.

Eustress Positive stress, or stress that is mentally or physically stimulating.

Distress Negative stress, or stress that contributes to health problems.

Type A Personality The personality type characterized by impatience, ambition, and aggression; Type A personalities may be more susceptible to the effects of stress but may also be more able to cope with stress.

Type D Personality The personality type characterized by high levels of negative emotion and the tendency to withhold expression of these emotions.

Resilience Positive outcomes in the face of stress or disadvantage.

Optimism The tendency to have a positive outlook on life or a belief that things will work out favorably.

Locus of Control The extent to which we believe the outcomes of events are under our control (internal locus) or outside our personal control (external locus).

Self-Efficacy The belief in one's ability to take action that will lead to the attainment of a goal.

health benefits of **conscientiousness,** the tendency to be organized, thoughtful, and goal directed. Highly conscientious individuals are at decreased risk for a range of negative outcomes, including asthma, stroke, depression, and panic attacks. It appears that conscientiousness contributes to better health outcomes both through reduced engagement in health risk behaviors like alcohol use and through more adaptive responses to stressful experiences. For example, individuals higher in conscientiousness are more likely to exercise on days that they experience high levels of stress.

As noted earlier, individuals who possess characteristics that protect them from the negative health consequences of stress are said to be resilient. **Hardiness** is one constellation of characteristics associated with resilience. Hardy individuals are strongly committed to their goals, view difficult situations as challenges rather than stressors, and find ways to assume control over their problems.

> **Conscientiousness** A personality style associated with high levels of organization, thoughtfulness, and goal-directed activity.
>
> **Hardiness** A collection of personality traits thought to make a person more resistant to stress.

▶▶ Strategies for Action

Learning stress management skills can help you respond more effectively to stress. Personality characteristics have been associated with both positive and negative health outcomes. Although overall personality structure has proven somewhat resistant to change, it is certainly possible to change both the physiological and the cognitive responses and the resulting emotional, physical, and behavioral outcomes depicted in Figure 1 at the beginning of this concept. Learning and practicing effective stress-management techniques will help you handle stress better and will contribute to improved health and wellness.

Self-assessments of stressors in your life can be useful in managing stress. In Lab 16A you have the opportunity to evaluate your stress levels using the Life Experience Survey. In Lab 16B you can assess your hardiness and locus of control, characteristics associated with coping effectively with stress.

Web Resources

Additional websites with information related to Concept 16 are available at the associated Web link.

American Institute of Stress **www.stress.org**
Gallup-Healthways Well-Being Index **www.well-beingindex.com**
National Center for Post Traumatic Stress Disorder **www.ncptsd.org**
National Mental Health Information Center **www.mentalhealth.samhsa.gov**
Stress and Health **www.stress-and-health.com**
Ulifeline: The online behavioral support system for young adults **www.ulifeline.org**
U.S. Health and Human Services **www.womenshealth.gov/faq/stress.htm**

Suggested Readings

Selected readings and references are listed below. A more comprehensive list is available at the associated Web link.

American College Counseling Association. 2009. *National Survey of Counseling Center Directors*. Alexandria, VA: The International Association of Counseling Services, Inc.
American Psychological Association. 2007. *Stress in America*. Washington, DC: American Psychological Association.
Friedman, H. S. 2008. The multiple linkages of personality and disease. *Brain, Behavior, and Immunity* 22:668–675.
Greenberg, J. S. 2008. *Comprehensive Stress Management*. 10th ed. New York: McGraw-Hill.
Gunner, M. R., et al. 2009. Developmental changes in hypothalamus-pituitary-adrenal activity over the transition to adolescence: Normative changes and associations with puberty. *Development and Psychopathology* 21:69–85.
Lehrer, P. M., R. L. Woolfolk, and W. E. Sime (Eds.). 2008. *Principles and Practice of Stress Management*. 3rd ed. New York: Guilford Publications.
Lund, H. G., et al. 2010. Sleep patterns and predictors of disturbed sleep in a large population of college students. *Journal of Adolescence Health* 46:124–132.
Meerlo, P., A. Sgoifo, and D. Suchecki. 2008. Restricted and disrupted sleep: Effects on autonomic function, neuroendocrine stress systems and stress responsivity. *Sleep Medicine Reviews* 12:197–210.
O'Connor, D. B., et al. 2009. Exploring the benefits of conscientiousness: An investigation of the role of daily stressors and health behaviors. *Annals of Behavioral Medicine* 37:184–196.
Steptoe, A., S. Dockray, and J. Wardle. 2009. Positive affect and psychobiological processes relevant to health. *Journal of Personality* 77:1747–1776.

Lab 16A Evaluating Your Stress Level

Name	Section	Date

Purpose: To evaluate your stress during the past year and determine its implications

Procedures

1. Complete the Life Experience Survey based on your experiences during the past year. This survey lists a number of life events that may be distressful or eustressful. Read all of the items. If you did not experience an event, leave the box blank. In the box after each event that you did experience, write a number ranging from –3 to +3 using the scale described in the directions. Extra blanks are provided to write in positive or negative events not listed. Some items apply only to males or females. Items 48 to 56 are only for current college students.
2. Add all of the negative numbers and record your score (distress) in the Results section. Add the positive numbers and record your score (eustress) in the Results section. Use all of the events in the past year.
3. Find your scores on Chart 1 and record your ratings in the Results section.
4. Interpret the results by discussing the conclusions and implications in the space provided.

Results

Sum of negative scores $\boxed{-4}$ (distress)   Rating on negative scores 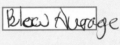 Below Average

Sum of positive scores $\boxed{10}$ (eustress)   Rating on positive scores 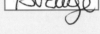 Average

Scoring the Life Experience Survey

1. Add all of the negative scores to arrive at your own distress score (negative stress).
2. Add all of the positive scores to arrive at a eustress score (positive stress).

Chart 1 ▶ Scale for Life Experiences and Stress

	Sum of Negative Scores (Distress)	Sum of Positive Scores (Eustress)
May need counseling	14+	
Above average	9–13	11+
Average	6–8	9–10
Below average	<6	<9

Conclusions and Implications: In several sentences, discuss your current stress rating and its implications.

Life Experience Survey

Directions: If you did not experience an event, leave the box next to the event empty. If you experienced an event, enter a number in the box based on how the event impacted your life. Use the following scale:

Extremely negative impact	= −3
Moderately negative impact	= −2
Somewhat negative impact	= −1
Neither positive nor negative impact	= 0
Somewhat positive impact	= +1
Moderately positive impact	= +2
Extremely positive impact	= +3

1. Marriage ☐

2. Detention in jail or comparable institution ☐

3. Death of spouse ☐

4. Major change in sleeping habits (much more or less sleep) [−1]

5. Death of close family member:
   a. Mother ☐
   b. Father ☐
   c. Brother ☐
   d. Sister ☐
   e. Child ☐
   f. Grandmother ☐
   g. Grandfather ☐
   h. Other (specify) _____ ☐

6. Major change in eating habits (much more or much less food intake) ☐

7. Foreclosure on mortgage or loan ☐

8. Death of a close friend ☐

9. Outstanding personal achievement [+2]

10. Minor law violation (traffic ticket, disturbing the peace, etc.) ☐

11. *Male:* Wife's/girlfriend's pregnancy [−3]

    Female: Pregnancy ☐

12. Changed work situation (different working conditions, working hours, etc.) ☐

13. New job ☐

14. Serious illness or injury of close family member:
   a. Father ☐
   b. Mother ☐
   c. Sister ☐
   d. Brother ☐
   e. Grandfather ☐
   f. Grandmother ☐
   g. Spouse ☐
   h. Child ☐
   i. Other (specify) _____ ☐

15. Sexual difficulties ☐

16. Trouble with employer (in danger of losing job, being suspended, demoted, etc.) ☐

17. Trouble with in-laws ☐

18. Major change in financial status (a lot better off or a lot worse off) [+2]

19. Major change in closeness of family members (decreased or increased closeness) ☐

20. Gaining a new family member (through birth, adoption, family member moving in, etc.) ☐

21. Change of residence ☐

22. Marital separation from mate (due to conflict) ☐

23. Major change in church activities (increased or decreased attendance) ☐

24. Marital reconciliation with mate ☐

25. Major change in number of arguments with spouse (a lot more or a lot fewer arguments) ☐

26. *Married male:* Change in wife's work outside the home (beginning work, ceasing work, changing to a new job) ☐

    Married female: Change in husband's work (loss of job, beginning new job, retirement, etc.) ☐

27. Major change in usual type and/or amount of recreation [+3]

28. Borrowing more than $10,000 (buying a home, business, etc.) ☐

29. Borrowing less than $10,000 (buying car or TV, getting school loan, etc.) ☐

30. Being fired from job ☐

31. *Male:* Wife/girlfriend having abortion

    Female: Having abortion ☐

32. Major personal illness or injury ☐

33. Major change in social activities, such as parties, movies, visiting (increased or decreased participation) ☐

34. Major change in living conditions of family (building new home, remodeling, deterioration of home or neighborhood, etc.) ☐

35. Divorce ☐

36. Serious injury or illness of close friend ☐

37. Retirement from work ☐

38. Son or daughter leaving home (due to marriage, college, etc.) ☐

39. Ending of formal schooling ☐

40. Separation from spouse (due to work, travel, etc.) ☐

41. Engagement ☐

42. Breaking up with boyfriend/girlfriend ☐

43. Leaving home for the first time ☐

44. Reconciliation with boyfriend/girlfriend ☐

Other recent experiences that have had an impact on your life: list and rate.

45. New Fantastic Girlfriend [+3]

46. _____ ☐

47. _____ ☐

For Students Only

48. Beginning new school experience at a higher academic level (college, graduate school, professional school, etc.) ☐

49. Changing to a new school at same academic level (undergraduate, graduate, etc.) ☐

50. Academic probation ☐

51. Being dismissed from dormitory or other residence ☐

52. Failing an important exam ☐

53. Changing a major ☐

54. Failing a course [0]

55. Dropping a course ☐

56. Joining a fraternity/sorority ☐

Source: **Sarason, Johnson, and Siegel.**

Lab 16B Evaluating Your Hardiness and Locus of Control

Name		Section	Date

Purpose: To evaluate your level of hardiness and locus of control and to help you identify the ways in which you appraise and respond to stressful situations

Procedures

1. Complete the Hardiness Questionnaire and the Locus of Control Questionnaire. Make an X over the circle that best describes what is true for you personally.
2. Compute the scale scores and record the values in the Results section.
3. Evaluate your scores using the Rating chart (Chart 1), and record your ratings in the Results section.
4. Interpret the results by answering the questions in the Conclusions and Implications section.

Hardiness Questionnaire

	Not True	Rarely True	Sometimes True	Often True	Score
1. I look forward to school and work on most days.	1	2	3	4	
2. Having too many choices in life makes me nervous.	4	3	2	1	
3. I know where my life is going and look forward to the future.	1	2	3	4	
4. I prefer not to get too involved in relationships.	4	3	2	1	
			Commitment Score, Sum 1–4		
5. My efforts at school and work will pay off in the long run.	1	2	3	4	
6. I just have to trust my life to fate to be successful.	4	3	2	1	
7. I believe that I can make a difference in the world.	1	2	3	4	
8. Being successful in life takes more luck and good breaks than effort.	4	3	2	1	
			Control Score, Sum 5–8		
9. I would be willing to work for less money if I could do something really challenging and interesting.	1	2	3	4	
10. I often get frustrated when my daily plans and schedule get altered.	4	3	2	1	
11. Experiencing new situations in life is important to me.	1	2	3	4	
12. I don't mind being bored.	4	3	2	1	
			Challenge Score, Sum 9–12		

Locus of Control Questionnaire

13. Hard work usually pays off.	1	2	3	4	
14. Buying a lottery ticket is not worth the money.	1	2	3	4	
15. Even when I fail I keep trying.	1	2	3	4	
16. I am usually successful in what I do.	1	2	3	4	
17. I am in control of my own life.	1	2	3	4	
18. I make plans to be sure I am successful.	1	2	3	4	
19. I know where I stand with my friends.	1	2	3	4	
			Locus of Control, Sum 13–19		

373

Results

Hardiness

Commitment score [ ]

Control score [ ]

Challenge score [ ]

Hardiness score [ ]

Locus of Control

Locus of Control score [ ]

Commitment rating [ ]

Control rating [ ]

Challenge rating [ ]

Hardiness rating [ ]

Locus of Control rating [ ]

Chart 1 ▶ Rating Chart

Rating	Individual Hardiness Scale Scores	Total Hardiness Score	Locus of Control Score
High	14–16	40–48	24–28
Moderate	10–13	30–39	12–23
Low	<10	<30	<12

Conclusions and Implications

1. In several sentences, discuss your commitment, control, and challenge ratings, as well as your overall hardiness rating. Are they what you expected? Do you think they are true indications of your hardiness? Explain.

2. In several sentences, discuss your locus of control rating. Is it what you expected (a high rating indicates an internal locus of control)? Do you think your rating is a realistic indicator of your locus of control? Explain.

Stress Management, Relaxation, and Time Management

Health Goals for the Year 2020

- Promote quality of life, healthy development, and healthy behaviors across all stages of life.
- Increase screening and treatment of mental health problems.
- Increase proportion of adults who have social support.
- Reduce suicide and suicide attempts.
- Increase access to employee programs to reduce or prevent stress.

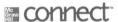 **connect**
|FITNESS AND WELLNESS   http://connect.mcgraw-hill.com

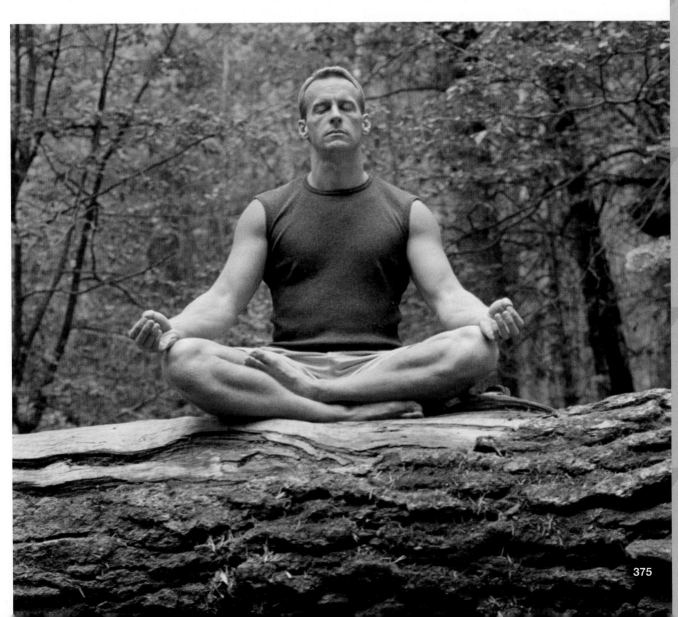

Although stress cannot be avoided, proper stress-management techniques can help reduce the impact of stress in your life.

As outlined in Concept 16, we all experience stress on a daily basis and must find ways to manage stress effectively. We can do many things to prevent excessive levels of stress, including exercising regularly, getting sufficient sleep, and allowing time for recreation. Effective time management is essential for balancing work and other activities. Despite our best efforts, stressful situations will occur, and we must find a way to deal with them. Later in this concept, three effective methods for managing stress are described.

Physical Activity and Stress Management

Regular activity and a healthy diet can help you adapt to stressful situations. An individual's capacity to adapt is not a static function but fluctuates as situations change. The better your overall health, the better you can withstand the rigors of tension without becoming susceptible to illness or other disorders. Physical activity is especially important because it conditions your body to function effectively under challenging physiological conditions.

Physical activity can provide relief from stress and aid muscle tension release. Physical activity has been found to be effective at relieving stress, particularly white-collar job stress. Studies show that regular exercise decreases the likelihood of developing stress disorders and reduces the intensity of the stress response. It also shortens the period of recovery from an emotional trauma. Its effect tends to be short-term, so one must continue to exercise regularly for it to have a continuing effect. Aerobic exercise is believed to be especially effective in reducing anxiety and relieving stress (though other activities are also good). Whatever your choice of exercise, it is likely to be more effective as an antidote to stress if it is something you find enjoyable.

Regular physical activity reduces reactivity to stress. Physical activity is associated with a *FEATURE 1* physiological response that is similar, in many ways, to the body's response to psychosocial stressors. Individuals who are physically fit have a reduced physiological response to exercise. Therefore, it makes sense that someone who is physically fit would also have a reduced response to psychosocial stressors. Research supports this hypothesis indicating that regular exercise reduces physiological reactivity to non-exercise stressors. For example, a recent study found that children's responses to stress are dampened by engagement in exercise. Compared to children who watched television before a stressor, those who exercised showed lower systolic and diastolic blood pressure and reduced heart rate reactivity. Although it is now well established that exercise before a stressor reduces the magnitude of the stress response, a recent study suggests that exercising after a stressor may also be an effective coping mechanism.

Physical activity can improve mental health. The physical health benefits of exer- *FEATURE 2* cise have been well established for some time. Research suggests that the benefits of exercise extend beyond the physical and into the realm of mental health. Exercise can reduce anxiety, aid in recovery from depression, and assist in efforts to eliminate negative health behaviors, such as smoking.

- *Physical activity can reduce anxiety.* Evidence shows that physical activity leads to reductions in anxiety in nonclinical samples. One study found that exercise may also be effective in reducing anxiety among individuals with panic disorder. An aerobic exercise program led to reductions in panic symptoms relative to a control group. Although exercise was not as effective as medication, it may be a useful addition to other treatment methods for anxiety disorders.
- *Physical activity can reduce depression.* A randomized clinical trial compared antidepressant medication and aerobic exercise with a combined antidepressant and exercise condition in the treatment of major depressive disorder. The aerobic exercise group fared as well as the other two at the end of treatment. In addition, the patients who only exercised were less likely to have a remission to depression at a 6-month follow-up.
- *Physical activity can aid in changing behaviors related to health.* One study tested vigorous physical activity as an adjunct to a cognitive-behavioral smoking cessation program for women. Women who received the exercise intervention were able to sustain continuous abstinence from smoking for a longer period relative to those who did not receive the exercise intervention. Women in the exercise program also gained less weight during smoking cessation.

Stress, Sleep, and Recreation

In order to adapt effectively to stressful situations, one must get adequate sleep. *FEATURE 3* Although the number of hours needed varies, the average adult needs between 7 and 8 hours of sleep per night. Research suggests that teenagers and young

Table 1 ▶ Guidelines for Good Sleep

- Be aware of the effects of medications. Some medicines, such as weight loss pills and decongestants, contain caffeine or other ingredients that interfere with sleep.

- Avoid tobacco use. Nicotine is a stimulant and can interfere with sleep.

- Avoid excess alcohol use. Alcohol may make it easier to get to sleep but may be a reason you wake up at night and are unable to get back to sleep.

- You may exercise late in the day, but do not do vigorous activity right before bedtime.

- Sleep in a room that is cooler than normal.

- Avoid hard-to-digest foods late in the day, as well as fatty and spicy foods.

- Avoid large meals late in the day or right before bedtime. A light snack before bedtime should not be a problem for most people.

- Avoid too much liquid before bedtime.

- Avoid naps during the day.

- Go to bed and get up at the same time each day.

- Do not study, read, or engage in other activities in your bed. You want your brain to associate your bed with sleep, not with activity.

- If you are having difficulty falling asleep, do not stay in bed. Get up and find something to do until you begin to feel tired, and then go back to bed.

adults (those in their early 20s) may need slightly more sleep. Unfortunately, many in these age groups do not obtain this extra amount of sleep. With insufficient sleep, many people resort to caffeine to stay awake, leading to an endless cycle of deficient sleep and caffeine usage. This disturbed sleep pattern can compromise health and wellness. Table 1 presents guidelines for good sleep.

All work and no play can lead to poor mental and physical health. Between 1860 and 1990, the number of hours typically spent working in industrialized countries decreased relatively dramatically. While that trend has continued in most countries, work hours in the United States have increased considerably over the past two decades. A major reason for this increase is that more people now hold second jobs than in the past. Also, some jobs of modern society have increasing rather than decreasing time demands. For example, many medical doctors and other professionals work more hours than the 35 to 44 hours that most people work. Nearly three times as many married women with children work full-time now, as compared with 1960.

Experts have referred to young adults as the "over-worked Americans" because they work several jobs and maintain dual roles (full-time employment coupled with normal family chores), or they work extended hours in

Technology Update
Gene-Based Therapies for Stress-Related Conditions

As genetic analyses have become easier to conduct and less costly, research has begun to identify specific genes that contribute to the effects of stress on both health behaviors and health outcomes. For example, a recent study found that a Brain-Derived Neurotrophic Factor (BDNF) gene moderated the relation between physical activity and depressive symptoms. Being physically active was associated with fewer depressive symptoms among adolescent girls with a particular variant of the gene (met), but not for girls without this variant. Such research may ultimately contribute to the ability to tailor interventions to those who are most likely to benefit.

demanding professional jobs. A Gallup poll showed that the great majority of adults have "enough time" for work, chores, and sleep but not enough time for friends, self, spouse, and children. When time is at a premium, the factors most likely to be negatively affected are personal health, relationships with children, and marriage or romantic relationships.

Recreation and leisure are important contributors to wellness (quality of life). **Leisure** is generally considered to be the opposite of work and includes "doing things we just want to do," as well as "doing nothing." In contrast, **recreation** involves the organized use of free time and typically includes social interaction. Leisure and recreation can contribute to stress reduction and wellness, though leisure activities are not done specifically to achieve these benefits.

The value of recreation and leisure in the busy lives of people in Western culture is evidenced by the emphasis public health officials place on the availability and accessibility of recreational facilities in communities.

There are many meaningful types of recreation. If fitness is the goal, recreational activities involving moderate to vigorous physical activity should be chosen. Involvement in nonphysical activities also constitutes recreation. For example, reading is an activity that

Leisure Time that is free from the demands of work. Leisure is more than free time; it is also an attitude. Leisure activities need not be means to ends (purposeful) but are ends in themselves.

Recreation *Recreation* means creating something anew. In this book, it refers to something that you do for amusement or for fun to help you divert your attention and to refresh yourself (re-create yourself).

can contribute significantly to other wellness dimensions, such as emotional/mental and spiritual. Passive involvement (spectating) is a third type of participation.

(i) **Play is critical to development** FEATURE 4 **and a sense of play in adult recreation contributes to wellness.** **Play** is distinct from recreation in that it is typically intrinsically motivated and has an imaginative component. Play has been shown to be important to healthy brain development in humans, and there is considerable evidence for physical, social, and cognitive benefits of play. In children, "free play," or unstructured time for play, seems to be particularly important. This type of play has been linked to a number of positive outcomes, including increased attention in the classroom, better self-regulation, and improved social skills and problem solving. Although much less attention has been given to the value of play in adults, a recent literature review identified benefits of play in adults, including mood enhancement, skill development, and enhanced relationships. Clearly, benefits associated with play have the potential both to prevent stress and to facilitate effective coping with stress.

Time Management

Effective time management helps you adapt to the stresses of modern living. Lack of time is cited by both the general public and experts as a source of stress and a reason for failing to implement healthy lifestyle changes. For college students, managing time is critical to academic success as well as overall well-being. Managing time effectively has become even more of a challenge for college students in recent years, as more and more students are working part- or full-time jobs to support their education (see Figure 1). The following strategies may help you learn to manage your time more effectively.

- *Know how you spend your time.* Where does your time go? The answer to this question is the first step toward better time management. Most of us are not fully aware of how we spend our time. If you carry a notebook and write down what you are doing and how long it takes, you can find out exactly where the time goes. You probably need to do this for at least a week. After you complete this exercise, you will know where you need to spend more time. Just as important, monitoring your time will help you identify where you could spend less

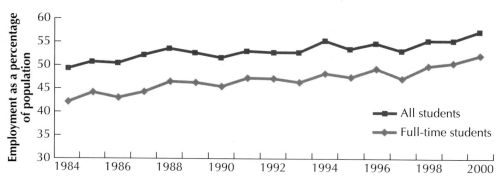

Figure 1 ▶ Employment rates of college students.

Source: Orszag, Jonathan M., Peter R. Orszag, and Diane M. Whitmore, *Learning and Earning: Working in College.* Commissioned by Upromise, Inc., August 2001, and reproduced with permission of Upromise.

time. Some common areas where people spend too much time are socializing (in person, by phone, or via email), watching television, playing video games, surfing the Internet, and doing busywork. Lab 17A will give you a chance to evaluate your current use of time.

- *Set goals and deadlines.* In addition to knowing how you spend your time, it is important to know what things need to get done. This includes everything from small tasks that need to get done today to important long-term goals. When setting goals, make sure they are attainable and that the time frame for completing them is reasonable. Some tasks may be more easily accomplished if they are broken down into a series of smaller tasks, each with its own deadline. Setting deadlines for the completion of goals increases the likelihood that you will follow through.

- *Prioritize.* Many people feel that there are not enough hours in the day to do everything that needs to be done. The truth is, they are probably right. If you think about all the things that have to get done, it can seem unmanageable. That is why it is important to prioritize. Many time-management experts advocate the ABC approach as a way to prioritize tasks effectively. Create three lists of things you need to do, with list A including the most urgent tasks and list C containing the least urgent. See Table 2 for a brief description of the ABC approach.

- *Write it down.* When things are not too busy, it may be possible to remember what you need to do and when you need to do it without writing it down. During busy times, though, trying to remember everything can lead to big problems. One of the most important steps in effective time management is to write things down. This includes keeping a daily planner to remember your schedule, calendars (weekly and/or monthly) to

Play Activity done of one's own free will. The play experience is fun and intrinsically rewarding, and it is a self-absorbing means of self-expression. It is characterized by a sense of freedom or escape from life's normal rules.

Table 2 ► The ABC System for Time Management	
Level of Importance	**Description**
A	*A tasks* are those that *must* be done, and soon. When accomplished, A tasks may yield extraordinary results. Left undone, they may generate serious, unpleasant, or disastrous consequences. Immediacy is what an A priority task is all about.
B	*B tasks* are those that *should* be done soon. While not as pressing as A tasks, they're still important. They can be postponed, but not for too long. Within a brief time, though, they can easily rise to A status.
C	*C tasks* are those that *could* be done. These tasks could be put off without creating dire consequences. Some can linger in this category almost indefinitely. Others—especially those tied to distant completion dates—will eventually rise to A or B levels as the deadline approaches.

Source: Mancini, M.

remember important events and deadlines, and a to-do list (or several, using the ABC approach) to help you remember your goals and priorities. Computers and other digital organizers allow you to keep all of this information in one place.

- *Include recreational activities in your schedule in addition to your responsibilities.* Although it may seem that scheduling fun takes away from the enjoyment, you may not find this to be the case. By scheduling your free time, you can fully enjoy it rather than worrying about other things you "should" be doing.

- *Make the most of the time you have.* To get the most out of your time, know when you do your best work and under what conditions. If you are sharpest in the morning, schedule the most important work to be done during this time. If you study most effectively when you are alone in a quiet place, schedule your studying at a time when you can create that environment. It is also important not to let time that could be productive go to waste. Keep materials with you that will allow you to take advantage of small periods of time (e.g., between classes).

- *Avoid procrastination.* Virtually all of us procrastinate at one time or another, but for many, procrastination can significantly decrease performance and increase stress. A number of causes of procrastination have been identified, including both internal and external influences (see Figure 2). Understanding the causes of procrastination can help you find ways to prevent it in the future. Strategies such as the ABC approach should also help you limit procrastination by getting you to work on the things that are most important first. One of the simplest solutions to procrastination is simply to "get started." The first step toward completing a project is often the most difficult. Once people take the first step, they often find that the task becomes easier, so get started on projects as soon as possible, even if you spend only a short time working.

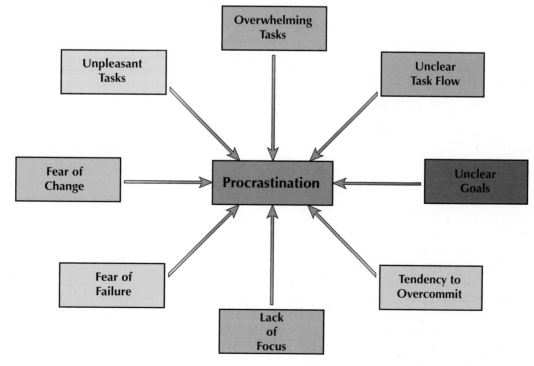

Figure 2 ► Causes of procrastination.
Source: Mancini, M.

- *Self-assessment of time management can help you improve your ability to manage your time effectively.* Monitoring your progress in time management is helpful in two ways. First, it allows you to see the progress you have made. Success is rewarding in and of itself, but you might also consider rewarding yourself with something tangible when you start out. For example, you might treat yourself to a nice dinner if you finish an important project on time. Monitoring also helps you identify areas in need of further improvement, so that you can adapt your plan to improve your chances of success.

Coping with Stress

Stress-management skills can be learned. Although some stressors are short-lived, many persist over a long time. The ability to adapt, or cope with these stressors, largely determines their ultimate effect. If effective **coping** strategies are used, the effects of a stressful situation can be more tolerable. In many cases, reasonable solutions or compromises can be found. On the other hand, if ineffective coping strategies are used, problems may become worse. This can lead to more stress and more severe outcomes. Although stress cannot be avoided, it can be managed. Effective stress management is a skill that contributes to both health and quality of life.

Stress-management training has been shown to improve both physical and mental health outcomes in a variety of populations. For example, a recent study found that stress-management training for patients with ischemic heart disease resulted in improved cardiovascular function, decreased depression, and lower levels of general distress. Similar results were found following

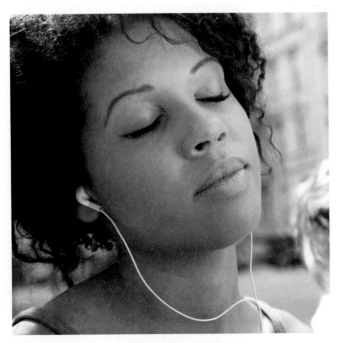

Taking time to relax can help you manage stress.

Health is available to **EVERYONE** for a Lifetime, and it's Personal

Many college campuses have resources available to help students address the various causes of stress. Those resources include academic offices to help with time management, and scholastic difficulties as well as counseling centers for anxiety, depression, relationship, and other problems. Additionally, offices such as housing, the medical clinic, health promotion, financial aid can be a resource for a variety of other stressors that often come up.

Do you take advantage of the resources that your college provides to aid in your stress management? Why or why not? What stress management tactics do you use and how important are they in your lifestyle?

a stress-management intervention provided to women following treatment for breast cancer. Interestingly, and perhaps of more relevance to college students, stress-management training has also been shown to improve academic performance.

One of the most common settings for stress-management training is the workplace. A recent study showed that relaxation training is the most commonly used approach, although cognitive behavioral programs produce the largest benefits. An advantage of cognitive behavioral interventions is that they typically address each of the three types of coping that have been shown to be adaptive. These different coping styles are described in detail in the following section.

Stress-management training focuses on teaching active coping strategies. Active coping strategies are those that attempt to directly affect the source of the stress or to effectively manage the individuals' reactions to stress. In contrast, passive coping strategies attempt to direct attention away from the stressor. Active coping strategies can be classified into three basic categories: **emotion-focused coping, appraisal-focused coping,** and **problem-focused coping.** These coping strategies target the emotional and physiological, behavioral, and cognitive aspects of stress, respectively (see Table 3).

Appraisal-focused coping strategies are based on changing the way one perceives the stressor or changing one's perceptions of resources for effectively managing stress. Emotion-focused coping strategies attempt to regulate the emotions resulting from stressful events. In contrast, problem-focused strategies are aimed at changing the source of the stress. While each of these strategies is effective in various circumstances, **avoidant coping** strategies, such as ignoring or escaping the problem or suppressing negative emotions, are likely to be ineffective for almost everyone.

Concept 16 described the characteristics associated with positive health outcomes, including optimism, an internal

Table 3 ▶ Strategies for Stress Management

Category	Description
Appraisal-Focused Strategies	**Strategies That Alter Perceptions of the Problem or Your Ability to Cope Effectively with the Problem**
• Cognitive restructuring	• Changing negative or automatic thoughts leading to unnecessary distress
• Seeking knowledge or practicing skills	• Finding ways to increase your confidence in your ability to cope
Emotion-Focused Strategies	**Strategies That Minimize the Emotional and Physical Effects of the Situation**
• Relaxing	• Using relaxation techniques to reduce the symptoms of stress
• Exercising	• Using physical activity to reduce the symptoms of stress
• Expressing your feelings	• Talking with someone about what you are feeling or writing about your emotional experiences
• Spirituality	• Looking for spiritual guidance to provide comfort
Problem-Focused Strategies	**Strategies That Directly Seek to Solve or Minimize the Stressful Situation**
• Systematic problem solving	• Making a plan of action to solve the problem and following through to make the situation better
• Being assertive	• Standing up for your own rights and values while respecting the opinions of others
• Seeking active social support	• Getting help or advice from others who can provide specific assistance for your situation
Avoidant Coping Strategies	**Strategies That Attempt to Distract the Individual from the Problem**
• Ignoring	• Refusing to think about the situation or pretending no problem exists
• Escaping	• Looking for ways to feel better or to stop thinking about the problem, including eating or using nicotine, alcohol, or other drugs
• Suppressing	• Actively trying to suppress emotional experiences or emotional expression.
• Ruminating	• Focusing on your negative emotions and what they mean without taking efforts to address the problem

locus of control, self-efficacy and conscientiousness. Not surprisingly, individuals with these characteristics tend to engage more effectively in adaptive coping strategies. Thus, if you want to reap the health benefits of individuals with these characteristics, learning to use appraisal-, emotion-, and problem-focused coping strategies is a good place to start.

Coping with most stress requires a variety of thoughts and actions. Stress forces the body to work under less than optimal conditions, yet this is the time when we need to function at our best. Effective coping may require some efforts to regulate the emotional aspects of the stress and other efforts to solve the problem. For example, if you receive a bad grade on an exam, how you view the situation and interpret its meaning will have a major impact on how you feel. You will have to eventually accept your current grade and manage the emotions that accompany this reality. Then, you will need to take active steps to improve your performance on the next exam. It does no good to worry about past events so it is more important to look ahead for ways to address the problem. Coping with this situation may, therefore, require the use of all three coping strategies.

Emotion regulation is a primary goal of both appraisal- and emotion-focused coping. Emotion regulation refers to efforts to manage initial emotional reactions to stress or the resulting emotions and how they are expressed. Thus, both appraisal- and emotion-focused coping are considered emotion regulation strategies. The difference between the two approaches is in the timing: appraisal-focused coping attempts to change the initial emotional experience, whereas emotion-focused coping attempts to manage the emotional experiences that follow appraisal. Efforts to positively reappraise stressful experiences can reduce initial emotional reactions to a stressor but additional efforts may be needed to manage these emotions. Such efforts can be both adaptive and maladaptive. Adaptive approaches include relaxation and meditation, appropriate emotional expression, and efforts to seek social support. Often the latter two approaches go hand-in-hand, as members of one's social support network provide an outlet for expression of emotional distress. Understanding the difference between appraisal- and emotion-focused coping can help you manage stress.

Coping A person's constantly changing cognitive and psychological efforts to manage stressful situations.

Emotion-Focused Coping The method of adapting to stress based on regulating the emotions that cause or result from stress.

Appraisal-Focused Coping The method of adapting to stress based on changing your perceptions of stress and your resources for coping.

Problem-Focused Coping The method of adapting to stress based on changing the source or cause of stress.

Avoidant Coping Seeking immediate, temporary relief from stress through distraction or self-indulgence (e.g., use of alcohol, tobacco, or other drugs).

Appraisal-Focused Coping Strategies (Cognitive Re-Appraisal)

The way you think about stressful situations can dramatically impact your emotional experiences. Extensive research has demonstrated that cognitive reappraisal leads to down-regulation of the autonomic and endocrine systems, leading to physical and mental health benefits. Fortunately, even those of us who do not typically engage in reappraisal can learn to use this approach. Research on cognitive therapy approaches for treating anxiety and mood disorders has shown that people can readily learn this skill, and learning to change the way you think can reduce emotional distress. Fortunately, the effectiveness of cognitive reappraisal is not limited to people experiencing anxiety or mood disorders. In a study of workplace stress and health, a cognitive-behavioral intervention that targeted appraisal of stress was more effective than a behavioral coping skills intervention that combined emotion- and problem-focused coping strategies. Thus, the way you think about stressful situations can be as important as how you respond to them.

At one time or another, virtually all people have distorted thinking, which can create unnecessary stress. Distorted thinking is also referred to as negative or automatic thinking. To alleviate stress, it can be useful to recognize some common types of distorted thinking (see Table 4). If you can learn to recognize distorted thinking, you can change the way you think and often reduce your stress levels.

If you have ever used any of the 10 types of distorted thinking described in Table 4, you may find it useful to consider different methods of "untwisting" your thinking. Using the strategies for untwisting your thinking can be useful in changing negative thinking to positive thinking.

If you really want to change your way of thinking to avoid stress, you may have to practice the guidelines outlined in Table 5. To do this, think of a recent situation that caused stress. Describe the situation on paper, and see if you used distorted thinking in the situation (see Table 4). If so, write down which types of distorted thinking you used. Finally, determine if any of the guidelines in Table 5 would have been useful. If so, write down the strategy you could have used. When a similar situation arises, you will be prepared to deal with the stressful situation. Repeat this technique, using several situations that have recently caused stress.

Emotion-Focused Coping Strategies

Relaxation techniques and/or coping strategies can help reduce the negative impact of both physical and emotional consequences of stress. These approaches can slow your heart and respiration rate, relax tense muscles, clear your mind, and help you relax mentally and emotionally. Perhaps most

Table 4 ▶ Types of Distorted Thinking

Type	Description
1. All-or-none thinking	You look at things in absolute, black-and-white categories.
2. Overgeneralization	You view a negative event as a never-ending pattern of defeat.
3. Mental filter	You dwell on the negatives and ignore the positives.
4. Discounting the positives	You insist that your accomplishments and positive qualities don't count.
5. Jumping to conclusions	(a) Mind reading—you assume that others are reacting negatively to you when there is no definite evidence of this. (b) Fortune telling—you arbitrarily predict that things will turn out badly.
6. Magnification or minimization	You blow things out of proportion or shrink their importance inappropriately.
7. Emotional reasoning	You reason from how you feel: "I feel like an idiot, so I must be one." "I don't feel like doing this, so I'll put it off."
8. Should statements	You criticize yourself or other people with "shoulds" or "shouldn'ts." "Musts," "oughts," and "have tos" are similar offenders.
9. Labeling	You identify with your shortcomings. Instead of saying, "I made a mistake," you tell yourself, "I am a jerk," "a fool," or "a loser."
10. Personalization and blame	You blame yourself for something that you weren't entirely responsible for, or you blame other people and overlook ways that your own attitudes and behaviors might have contributed to the problem.

Source: Burns, D. D.

Table 5 ▶ Ten Ways to Untwist Your Thinking

Way	Description
1. Identify the distortion.	Write down your negative thoughts, so you can see which of the 10 types of distorted thinking you are involved in. This will make it easier to think about the problem in a more positive and realistic way.
2. Examine the evidence.	Instead of assuming that your negative thought is true, if you feel you never do anything right, you can list several things that you have done successfully.
3. Use the double standard method.	Instead of putting yourself down in a harsh, condemning way, talk to yourself in the same compassionate way you would talk to a friend with a similar problem.
4. Use the experimental technique.	Do an experiment to test the validity of your negative thought. For example, if, during an episode of panic you become terrified that you are about to die of a heart attack, you can jog or run up and down several flights of stairs. This will prove that your heart is healthy and strong.
5. Think in shades of gray.	Although this method might sound drab, the effects can be illuminating. Instead of thinking about your problems in all-or-none extremes, evaluate things on a range from 0 to 100. When things do not work out as well as you had hoped, think about the experience as a partial success, rather than a complete failure. See what you can learn from the situation.
6. Use the survey method.	Ask people questions to find out if your thoughts and attitudes are realistic. For example, if you believe that public speaking anxiety is abnormal and shameful, ask several friends if they have ever felt nervous before giving a talk.
7. Define terms.	When you label yourself "inferior," "a fool," or "a loser," ask, "What is the definition of 'a fool'?" You will feel better when you see that there is no such thing as a fool or a loser.
8. Use the semantic method.	Simply substitute language that is less colorful or emotionally loaded. This method is helpful for "should" statements. Instead of telling yourself, "I *shouldn't* have made that mistake," you can say, "It would be better if I hadn't made that mistake."
9. Use reattribution.	Instead of automatically assuming you are "bad" and blaming yourself entirely for a problem, think about the many factors that may have contributed to it. Focus on solving the problem instead of using up all your energy blaming yourself and feeling guilty.
10. Do a cost-benefit analysis.	List the advantages and disadvantages of a feeling (such as getting angry when your plane is late), a negative thought (such as "No matter how hard I try, I always screw up"), or a behavior pattern (such as overeating and lying around in bed when you are depressed). You can also use the cost-benefit analysis to modify a self-defeating belief, such as "I must always be perfect."

Source: Burns, D. D.

important, these techniques can improve your outlook and help you cope better with the stressful situation. In Lab 17C, you will have the chance to try several relaxation techniques. Performing the exercises in Lab 17C only once will not prepare you to use relaxation techniques effectively. Remember, you must practice learning to relax.

Conscious relaxation techniques reduce stress and tension by directly altering the physical symptoms. When you are stressed, heart rate, blood pressure, and muscle tension all increase to help your body deal with the challenge. Conscious relaxation techniques reduce these normal effects and bring the body back to a more relaxed state. These approaches can also help you manage the negative emotions that result from stressors and your appraisal of those stressors. Most techniques use the "three *R*s" of relaxation to help the body and mind relax: (1) reduce mental activity, (2) recognize tension, and (3) reduce respiration.

Detailed descriptions and examples are available at the associated Web link. Brief descriptions follow.

- *Deep breathing and mental imagery.* One of the quickest ways to experience relaxation is through deep breathing. There are many versions of deep breathing exercises. For example, first inhale deeply through your nose for about 4 seconds, making sure that your abdomen rises when you are inhaling. Next, let the air out slowly through your mouth (for about 8 seconds, or twice as long as the inhalation). Repeating these steps for several minutes can help control the body's reaction to stress. See Lab 17C, Figure 3, for detailed instructions on diaphragmatic breathing. Many relaxation approaches combine deep breathing with mental imagery to maximize the relaxation response. This approach involves imagining a pleasant image or scene that you associate with relaxation, such as a peaceful lake or stream. The goal is to imagine the scene as

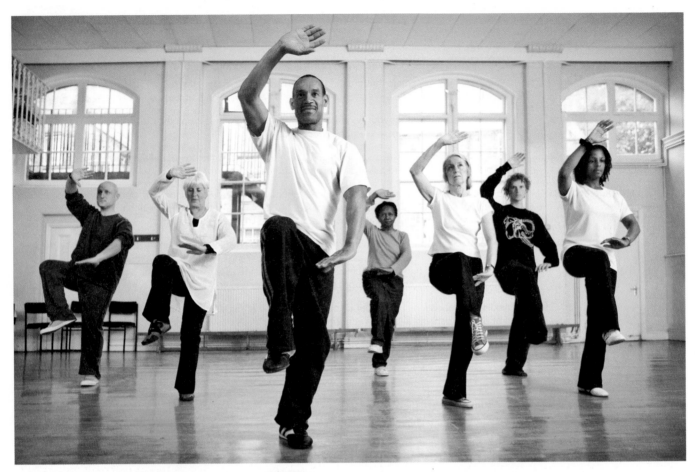

Tai chi has benefits on physical health as well as mental health.

completely as possible using all of your senses. The main advantage of these approaches is that they can be used in any setting, and they take very little time to induce a relaxation response.

- *Jacobson's progressive relaxation method.* You must be able to recognize how a tense muscle feels before you can voluntarily release the tension. In this technique, contract the muscles strongly and then relax. Relax each of the large muscles first and later the small ones. Gradually reduce the contractions in intensity until no movement is visible. The emphasis is always placed on detecting the feeling of tension as the first step in "letting go," or "going negative." Jacobson, a pioneer in muscle relaxation research, emphasized the importance of relaxing eye and speech muscles, because he believed these muscles trigger the reactions of the total organism more than other muscles.

- *Biofeedback.* Biofeedback training uses machines that monitor certain physiological processes of the body and that provide visual or auditory evidence of what is happening to normally unconscious bodily functions. The evidence, or feedback, is then used to help you decrease these functions. When combined with autogenic training, subjects have learned to relax and reduce the electrical activity in their muscles, lower blood pressure, decrease heart rate, change their brainwaves, and decrease headaches, asthma attacks, and stomach acid secretion.

- *Stretching and rhythmical exercises.* People who work long hours at a desk can release tension by getting up frequently and stretching, by taking a brisk walk, or by performing "office exercises." Exercising to music or to a rhythmic beat has been found to be relaxing and even hypnotic. One popular activity that uses stretching and rhythmic exercise (as well as breathing techniques) is yoga. Many find it to be beneficial in reducing stress, and research has found both physical and mental health benefits associated with yoga.

Spirituality and mindfulness can help you cope with stress and daily problems. In addition to managing the body's physical response to stress, one must deal with the impact of stress on thoughts and emotions. Although relaxation strategies may also impact these dimensions, additional approaches may be necessary to adequately manage these aspects of the stress response.

- *Spirituality.* Studies have shown that spirituality can decrease blood pressure and can be a source of internal comfort. It can have other calming effects associated with reduced distress. It can also provide confidence to function more effectively, thereby reducing the stresses associated with ineffectiveness at work or in other situations. The health benefits of spirituality do not appear to be restricted to prayer, however. Using a more global measure of spirituality, one study of college students found that spirituality moderated the relationship between stress and health outcomes. For those low in spirituality, stress was associated with higher levels of negative emotion and physical symptoms of illness. Among those higher in spirituality, the link between stress and health outcomes was much weaker.

- *Mindfulness meditation.* While most relaxation techniques seek to distract attention away from distressing emotions, mindfulness meditation encourages the individual to experience fully his or her emotions in a nonjudgmental way. The individual is encouraged to bring full attention to the internal and external experiences that are occurring "in the moment." Although research on mindfulness is just emerging, results look promising. For example, in a study of medical students, a mindfulness-based stress-reduction program led to significant decreases in mood disturbances. In another study, mindfulness meditation reduced the impact of daily stressors, psychological distress, and medical symptoms. Mindfulness may have particular value for individuals with chronic medical conditions. Benefits have been demonstrated with medical conditions such as fibromyalgia, cancer, and coronary artery disease. The nonjudgmental aspect of awareness in mindfulness is critical to the success of this approach. Increased attention to negative emotion that involves an evaluative component (e.g., this emotion is terrible) is often referred to as rumination. There is considerable evidence that rumination leads to negative psychological adjustment, including increased risk for depression.

Appropriately expressing emotion can help you reduce distress. The ability to control emotional outbursts is an adaptive skill that develops with age. As a society, we socialize our children to develop these skills, as they are critical to adaptive functioning in adulthood. At the same time, complete suppression of emotion has long been recognized as potentially harmful to our health. For example, Freud believed that inhibition of emotion contributed to psychological problems. Although it has taken roughly 100 years since Freud's early writing, recent studies have demonstrated that suppression of emotion leads to negative outcomes. In the laboratory, emotional suppression leads to increased physiological

In the News

In recent years, the hypothalamic-pituitary-adrenal axis (HPA) has received considerable attention as a source of negative health outcomes of stress. Most people are now aware of the hormone cortisol and its negative impact on both physical and mental health. However, not all products of the HPA axis are harmful. Animal studies have shown that the hormone dehydroepiandrosterone (DHEA) has neuroprotective effects and reduces levels of anxiety, depression, and aggression. A recent study extends this evidence to humans. The study examined both performance and psychological reactions to a stressful training procedure among active duty military. Higher levels of DHEA predicted better performance on an underwater navigation exam, and fewer stress-induced symptoms during completion of the task. Although research on DHEA in humans is in its infancy, approaches to increase levels of DHEA in the face of stress may ultimately provide a mechanism for reducing their negative impact.

stress. Among college students, emotional suppression is related to increased anxiety, sensitivity, and depression, and poor social adjustment. Thus, if we want to minimize the potential negative impact of our emotions, we need to find appropriate ways to express them.

We often turn to others who will provide an opportunity for us to "vent" or "get it off our chest." Although this is a perfectly good way to express emotion, there is evidence that we can also benefit from writing about our stressful experiences. Expressive writing has shown benefits for a wide range of outcomes, from faster wound healing to better adaptation following traumatic events. Writing also seems to help mitigate the effects of stress related to discrimination. For example, a recent study of gay male college students found that writing about stresses related to sexual orientation led to better adjustment 3 months later. Interestingly, the writing experience seemed to provide the most benefit to students who had lower levels of social support. Thus, writing about stressful experiences may provide an important outlet when social support is not readily available. In addition, there is some evidence that sharing one's expressive writing with others has further benefits. In fact, a recent study of college students found that, although both private and shared writing improved psychological outcomes, only shared emotional writing showed benefits on physical symptoms.

Problem-Focused Coping Strategies

FEATURE 5 *(i)* **Problem-focused coping is most effective in dealing with controllable stressors.** While appraisal- and emotion-focused coping may be the most effective means for coping with situations beyond one's control, a problem under personal control may best be addressed by taking action to solve the problem.

Problem solving and assertiveness can help you cope. Each stressful situation has unique circumstances and meaning to the individual. For this reason it is impossible to offer specific information about the best stress management strategy without knowing the source of the stress and how it is affecting a specific person. However, it is possible to offer a framework for consistently responding to difficult situations. A technique called "systematic problem solving" provides an excellent framework. This approach has been shown to improve the likelihood of problem resolution.

The first step is brainstorming, generating every possible solution to the problem. During this stage, you should not limit the solutions you generate in any way. Even silly and impractical solutions should be included. After you have generated a comprehensive list, you can narrow your focus by eliminating any solutions that do not seem reasonable. When you have reduced the number of solutions to a reasonable number (four or five), carefully evaluate each option. You should consider the potential costs and benefits of each approach to aid in making a decision. Once you decide on an approach, carefully plan the implementation of the strategy. This includes anticipating anything that might go wrong and being prepared to alter your plan as necessary.

In some cases, directly addressing the source of stress involves responding assertively. For example, if the source of stress is an employer placing unreasonable demands on your time, the best solution to the problem may involve talking to your boss about the situation. This type of confrontation is difficult for many people concerned about being overly aggressive. However, you can stand up for yourself without infringing on the rights of others.

Many people confuse assertiveness with aggression, leading to passive responses in difficult situations. An aggressive response intimidates others and fulfills one's own needs at the expense of others. In contrast, an assertive response protects your own rights and values while respecting the opinions of others.

Once you are comfortable with the idea of responding assertively, you may want to practice or role-play assertive responses before trying them in the real world. With a friend you trust, practice responding assertively. Your friend may provide valuable feedback about your approach, and the practice may increase your self-efficacy for responding and your expectancies for a positive outcome.

Social Support and Stress Management

Social support is important for effective stress management. Social support has been found to play a role in coping with stress, and it has been linked to better physical and mental health outcomes among individuals with chronic stress-related illnesses. For example, in a large group of patients with coronary artery disease, participation in a social support group was associated with lower systolic blood pressure, better social functioning, and better mental health. The improvements in social functioning and mental health were due, at least in part, to improved health behaviors. Social support may also be critical to managing stress in academic settings. A recent study found that a lack of social support from family, teachers, and peers was associated with lack of academic motivation and subsequent academic failure.

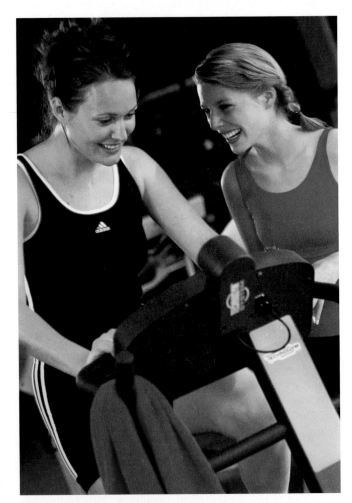

Social support is important for stress management and for maintaining an exercise program.

Social Support The behavior of others that assists a person in addressing a specific need.

Social support may be particularly important for women. Women may be particularly likely to seek and provide social support when stressed. A paradigm called the "tend or befriend" model suggests that women have a unique stress response. Women respond to stress by tending to others (nurturing) and affiliating with a social group (befriending). This response is helpful in protecting offspring and reducing the risk for the negative health consequences of stress.

Social support has various sources. Everyone needs someone to turn to for support when feeling overwhelmed. Support can come from friends, family members, clergy, a teacher, a coach, or a professional counselor. Different sources provide different forms of support. Even pets have been shown to be a good source of social support, with consequent health and quality of life benefits. The goal is to identify and nurture relationships that can provide this type of support. In turn, it is important to look for ways to support and assist others.

There are many types of social support. Social support has three main components: informational, material, and emotional. Informational (technical) support includes tips, strategies, and advice that can help a person get through a specific stressful situation. For example, a parent, friend, or co-worker may offer insight into how he or she once resolved similar problems. Material support is direct assistance to get a person through a stressful situation—for example, providing a loan to help pay off a short-term debt. Emotional support is encouragement or sympathy that a person provides to help another cope with a particular challenge.

Regardless of the type of support, it is important that it fosters autonomy. Social support that helps you to become more self-reliant because of increased feelings of competence is best for developing autonomy. Social support that is controlling or leads to dependence on another person does not lead to autonomy and may increase rather than decrease stress over time.

Obtaining good social support requires close relationships. Although we live in a social environment, it is often difficult to ask people for help. Sometimes the nature and severity of our problems may not be apparent to others. Other times, friends may not want to offer suggestions or insight because they do not want to appear too pushy. To obtain good support, one must develop quality personal relationships. Although having a large social support network is helpful, quality seems to be at least as important as quantity. Many individuals report feeling lonely despite having large social networks, and loneliness is associated with negative health behaviors, including smoking and lack of exercise.

Sometimes professional help is necessary to deal with problems related to stress. FEATURE 3 Although members of your social support network may be able to help you manage many of the stressors you experience, sometimes stress creates problems that require professional help. If you think you might be suffering from posttraumatic stress disorder or depression, there are well-established treatments that can help you function more effectively. Sometimes, professionals can also be helpful in efforts to change negative health behaviors such as alcohol and drug use, or problematic patterns of eating. Thankfully, stigmas associated with these problems have decreased in the past 25 years, leading many more people to seek professional services. In addition, new approaches to treatment are now being developed, including online therapy and mail-based interventions. These approaches have the potential to reach even more people in need of professional help.

Strategies for Action

Several practical steps can help you identify and manage your stress. This concept is dedicated to strategies and skills for preventing, managing, and coping with stress. For strategies to be effective, they must be used regularly. Several practical steps that you can take are described in the following list.

- *Self-assess your stress levels.* Making self-assessments such as those in Labs 16A and 16B can help you identify the sources and the magnitude of stress in your life.
- *Adopt coping strategies.* Consistent with the information presented in this concept, learning about and using a variety of emotion-focused, appraisal-focused,

and problem-focused strategies will help you manage stress in your daily life.

- *Manage time effectively.* Lab 17A can help you understand your current time use patterns and help you develop a schedule that will allow you to focus on your priorities.
- *Evaluate strategy effectiveness.* Lab 17B will help you assess the effectiveness of various coping strategies. It also provides a basis for altering strategies to manage your stress levels more effectively. Lab 17C will help you to relax tense muscles, an emotion-focused coping strategy. Lab 17D will help you evaluate your current social support system.

Web Resources

Additional websites with information related to Concept 17 are available at the associated Web link.

ABC's of Internet Therapy **www.metanoia.org/imhs**
American Institute of Stress **www.stress.org**
American Psychological Association **www.apa.org**
Guide to Online Psychology
   http://allpsych.com/onlinepsychology.html
International Stress Management Association
   www.stress-management-isma.org
Mental Health Resources **www.mentalhealth.about.com**
National Mental Health Information Center
   www.mentalhealth.samhsa.gov
Time Management for College Students
   www.time-management-for-students.com

Suggested Readings

Selected readings and references are listed below. A more comprehensive list is available at the associated Web link.

Blumenthal, J. A., et al. 2006. Effects of exercise and stress management training on markers of cardiovascular risk in patients with ischemic heart disease: A randomized controlled trial. *Journal of the American Medical Association* 293:1626–1634.

Davis, M., M. McKay, and E. R. Eshelman. 2008. *The Relaxation and Stress Reduction Workbook*. Oakland, CA: New Harbinger.

Ginsburg, K. R., et al. 2007. The importance of play in promoting healthy child development and maintaining strong parent-child bonds. *Pediatrics* 119:182–191.

Girdano, D., G. S. Everly, and D. E. Duseck. 2008. *Controlling Stress and Tension*. Needham Heights, MA: Benjamin Cummings.

Goldin, P. R., and J. J. Gross. 2010. Effects of mindfulness-based stress reduction (MBSR) on emotion regulation in social anxiety disorder. *Emotion* 10:83–91.

Greenberg, J. S. 2008. *Comprehensive Stress Management*. 10th ed. New York: McGraw-Hill.

Herman, K. M., et al. 2010. Are youth BMI and physical activity associated with better or worse than expected health-related quality of life in adulthood? The Physical Activity Longitudinal Study. *Quality of Life Research* 19(3):339–349.

Jacobson, E. 1978. *You Must Relax*. New York: McGraw-Hill.

Keogh, E., F. W. Bond, and P. E. Flaxman. 2006. Improving academic performance and mental health through a stress management intervention: Outcomes and mediators of change. *Behaviour Research and Therapy* 44:339–357.

Lehrer, P. M., R. L. Woolfolk, and W. E. Sime (Eds.). 2008. *Principles and Practice of Stress Management*. 3rd ed. New York: Guilford Publications.

Low, C. A., A. L. Stanton, and J. E. Bower. 2008. Effects of acceptance-oriented versus evaluative emotional processing on heart rate recovery and habituation. *Emotion* 8:419–424.

Mancini, M. 2003. *Time Management*. New York: McGraw-Hill.

Needham, B. L. 2010. Trajectories of change in obesity and symptoms of depression: The CARDIA study. *American Journal of Public Health* 100(6):1040–1046.

O'Keefe, E. J., and D. S. Berger. 2007. *Self-Management for College Students: The ABC Approach*. 3rd ed. Hyde Park, NY: Partridge Hill.

Oman, D., et al. 2008. Meditation lowers stress and supports forgiveness among college students: A randomized controlled trial. *Journal of American College Health* 56(5):569–578.

Pachankis, J. E., and M. R. Goldfried. 2010. Expressive writing for gay-related stress: Psychosocial benefits and mechanisms underlying improvement. *Journal of Consulting and Clinical Psychology* 78:98–110.

Penedo, F. J., and J. R. Dahn. 2005. Exercise and well-being: A review of mental and physical health benefits associated with physical activity. *Current Opinion in Psychiatry* 18:189–193.

Richardson, K. M., and H. R. Rothstein. 2008. Effects of occupational stress management intervention programs: A meta-analysis. *Journal of Occupational Health Psychology* 13:69–93.

Roemmich, J. N., et al. 2009. Protective effect of interval exercise on psychophysiological stress reactivity in children. *Psychophysiology* 46:852–861.

Romas, J. A., and M. Sharma. 2007. *Practical Stress Management: A Comprehensive Workbook for Managing Change and Promoting Health*. 4th ed. San Francisco: Benjamin Cummings.

Rugg, G., S. Gerrard, and S. Hooper. 2008. *Stress Free Guide to Studying at University*. Thousand Oaks, CA: Sage.

Seligman, M. E. 1998. *Learned Optimism: How to Change Your Mind and Your Life*. New York: Pocket Books.

Srivastava, S., et al. 2009. The social costs of emotional suppression: A prospective study of the transition to college. *Journal of Personality and Social Psychology* 96:883–897.

Lab 17A Time Management

Name		Section	Date

Purpose: To learn to manage time to meet personal priorities

Procedures

1. Follow the four steps outlined below.
2. Complete the Conclusions and Implications section.

Results

Step 1: Establishing Priorities

1. Check the circles that reflect your priorities in the list below. Add priorities as necessary.
2. Rate each of the priorities you checked. Use a 1 for highest priority, 2 for moderate priority, and 3 for low priority.

Check Priorities	Rating	Check Priorities	Rating	Check Priorities	Rating
◯ More time with family		◯ More time with boy/girlfriend		◯ More time with spouse	
◯ More time for leisure		◯ More time to relax		◯ More time to study	
◯ More time for work success		◯ More time for physical activity		◯ More time to improve myself	
◯ More time for other recreation		◯ Other _____		◯ Other _____	

Step 2: Monitor Current Time Use

1. On the following daily calendar, keep track of daily time expenditure.
2. Write in exactly what you did for each time block.

7–9 A.M.	9–11 A.M.	11 A.M.–1 P.M.	1–3 P.M.

3–5 P.M.	5–7 P.M.	7–9 P.M.	9–11 P.M.

Lab 17A

Time Management

389

Step 3: Analyze Your Current Time Use by Using the ABC Method (See Table 2)

Tasks That *Must* Be Done Soon	Tasks That *Should* Be Done Soon	Tasks That *Could* Be Done

Step 4: Make a Schedule: Write in Your Planned Activities for the Day

Time	Activities	Time	Activities
6:00 A.M.		3:00 P.M.	
7:00 A.M.		4:00 P.M.	
8:00 A.M.		5:00 P.M.	
9:00 A.M.		6:00 P.M.	
10:00 A.M.		7:00 P.M.	
11:00 A.M.		8:00 P.M.	
12:00 P.M.		9:00 P.M.	
1:00 P.M.		10:00 P.M.	
2:00 P.M.		11:00 P.M.	

Conclusions and Implications: In several sentences, discuss how you might modify your schedule to find more time for important priorities.

Lab 17B Evaluating Coping Strategies

Name		Section		Date	

Purpose: To learn how to use appropriate coping strategies that work best for you

Procedures

1. Think of five recent stressful experiences that caused you some concern, anxiety, or distress. Describe these situations in Chart 1. Then use Chart 2 to make a rating for changeability, severity, and duration. Assign one number for each category for each situation.
2. In Chart 3, place a check for each coping strategy that you used in coping with each of the five situations you described.
3. Answer the questions in the Conclusions and Implications section.

Results

Chart 1 ▶ Stressful Situations

Think of five different stressful situations. Appraise each situation and assign a score (changeability, severity, duration) using the scale in Chart 2.

Briefly describe the situation.	Changeability	Severity	Duration
1.			
2.			
3.			
4.			
5.			

Chart 2 ▶ Appraisal of the Stressful Situations

Use this chart to rate the five situations you described in Chart 1. Assign a number for changeability, severity, and duration for each situation in Chart 1.

	1	2	3	4	5
Was the situation changeable?	Completely within my control	Mostly within my control	Both in and out of my control	Mostly out of my control	Completely outside of my control
What was the severity of the stress?	Very minor	Fairly minor	Moderate	Fairly major	Very major
What was the duration of the stress?	Short-term (weeks)	Moderately short	Moderate (months)	Moderately long	Long (months to year)

Chart 3 ▶ Coping Strategies

Directions: Think about your response to the five stressful situations you recently experienced and check the strategies that you used in each situation. List use of other strategies as appropriate.

Coping Strategy	Situation 1	Situation 2	Situation 3	Situation 4	Situation 5
1. I apologized or corrected the problem as best I could.					
2. I ignored the problem and hoped that it would go away.					
3. I told myself to forget about it and grew as a person from the experience.					
4. I tried to make myself feel better by eating, drinking, or smoking.					
5. I prayed or sought spiritual meaning from the situation.					
6. I expressed anger to try to change the situation.					
7. I took active steps to make things work out better.					
8. I used music, images, or deep breathing to help me relax.					
9. I tried to keep my feelings to myself and kept moving forward.					
10. I pursued leisure or recreational activity to help me feel better.					
11. I talked to someone who could provide advice or help me with the problem.					
12. I talked to someone about what I was feeling or experiencing.					
13. Other _____					
14. Other _____					
15. Other _____					

Conclusions and Implications: In several sentences, discuss the coping strategies you used. What were the ones you used the most? Are these the ones you typically use? Were they effective? Would you consider other strategies in the future?

Lab 17C Relaxation Exercises

Name		**Section**	**Date**

Purpose: To gain experience with specific relaxation exercises and to evaluate their effectiveness

Procedures

1. Choose two of the relaxation exercises included in Chart 1 of this lab (see page 394) and read through the written instructions until you have a basic understanding of the exercises. Think through the specific aspects of the exercise until you have the process figured out.
2. Find a quiet place to try one of the exercises and follow the procedures as best you can. It is not possible to provide detailed instructions, but the information should be sufficient to give you a basic understanding of the exercises.
3. On another day try a different exercise.
4. Answer the questions in the Results section. Then complete the Conclusions and Implications section.

Results

1. Which of the two exercises did you try (list them below).

2. Have you done either of the exercises before? ◯ Yes ◯ No

3. Was one relaxation exercise more effective or better suited to you than the others? Which one?

Conclusions and Implications

In several sentences, discuss whether or not you feel that relaxation exercises will be a part of your wellness program. In what ways might you benefit from relaxation training? If you do not think you have a problem with relaxation, explain why.

Chart 1 ▶ Descriptions of Relaxation Exercises

A. Progressive Relaxation

Progressive relaxation uses active (conscious) mechanisms to achieve a state of relaxation. The technique involves alternating phases of muscle contraction (tension) and muscle relaxation (tension release). Muscle groups are activated one body segment at a time, incorporating all regions of the body by the end of the routine. Begin by lying on your back in a quiet place with eyes closed. Alternately contract and relax each of the muscles below—following the procedures described below. Begin with the dominant side of the body first; repeat on the nondominant side.

1. Hand and forearm—Make a fist.
2. Biceps—Flex elbows.
3. Triceps—Straighten arm.
4. Forehead—Raise your eyebrows and wrinkle forehead.
5. Cheeks and nose—Wrinkle nose and squint.
6. Jaws—Clench teeth.
7. Lips and tongue—Press lips together and tongue to roof of mouth, teeth apart.
8. Neck and throat—Tuck chin and push head backward against floor (if lying) or chair (if sitting).
9. Shoulder and upper back—Hunch shoulders to ears.
10. Abdomen—Suck abdomen inward.
11. Lower back—Arch back.
12. Thighs and buttocks—Squeeze buttocks together, push heels into floor (if lying) or chair rung (if sitting).
13. Calves—Pull instep and toes toward shins.
14. Toes—curl toes.

Muscle contraction phase: Inhale as you contract the designated muscle for 3–5 seconds. Use only a moderate level of tension.

Muscle relaxation phase: Exhale, relaxing the muscle and releasing tension for 6–10 seconds. Think of relaxation words such as warm, calm, peaceful, and serene.

Relax every muscle in your body at end of the exercise.

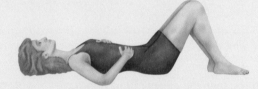

Figure 3 ▶ Diaphragmatic breathing.

B. Diapraghmatic Breathing

This exercise will help improve awareness of using deep abdominal breathing over shallower chest-type breathing. To begin, lie on your back with knees bent and feet on the floor. Place your right hand over your abdomen and left hand over your chest. Your hands will be used to monitor breathing technique. Slowly inhale through the nose by allowing the abdomen to rise under your right hand. Concentrate on expanding the abdomen for 4 seconds. Continue inhaling another 2 seconds allowing the chest to rise under your left hand. Exhale through your mouth in reverse order (for about 8 seconds, or twice as long as inhalation). Relax the chest first, feeling it sink beneath the left hand and then the abdomen, allowing it to sink beneath the right hand. Repeat 4–5 times. Discontinue if you become light-headed.

C. Show Gun

This is a form of chi gun, a Chinese meditation technique. The basic principles of tai chi are to maintain balance, use the entire body to achieve movement, unite movement with awareness (mind) and breathing (chi), and to keep the body upright. Tai chi involves holding the body in specific positions, or "forms." To execute the basic form, stand straight, feet shoulder-width apart and parallel with one another. Your knees should be bent and turned outward slightly with knees over the foot. Your hands are on belly button with palms facing body (men place hands right on left and women left on right), fingers are straight, spread slightly and relaxed.

1. Bring arms in front of body at a 30-degree angle to the plane of the back, palms face downward. Reach up to shoulder height with arms moving up and to the sides. (Breathe in, allowing belly to move out as you raise arms upward.)
2. When hands reach shoulder height, turn palms up and move hands to head, allowing wrists to drop down. Imagine energy (chi) flowing from palms to top of head. (Continue breathing in.)
3. Imagine energy flowing down through a central line of the body. Follow the energy with hands, point fingers toward one another, palms down, move arms downward in front of the midline of face and chest. (Breathe out as arms lower.)
4. Two inches bellow belly button stop, cross palms, and move hands together.
5. Lower hands toward sides. (Complete breathing out.)
6. Repeat.

Lab 17D Evaluating Levels of Social Support

Name		**Section**	**Date**

Purpose: To evaluate your level of social support and to identify ways that you can find additional support

Procedures

1. Answer each question in Chart 1 by placing a check in the box below Not True, Somewhat True, or Very True. Place the number value of each answer in the score box to the right.
2. Sum the scores (in the smaller boxes) for each question to get subscale scores for the three social support areas.
3. Record your three subscores in the Results section on the next page. Total your subscores to get a total social support score.
4. Determine your ratings for each of the three social support subscores and for your total social support score using Chart 2 on the next page.
5. Answer the questions in the Conclusions and Implications section.

Chart 1 ► Social Support and Locus of Control Questionnaire

The first nine questions assess various aspects of social support. Base your answer on your actual degree of support, not on the type of support that you would like to have. Place a check in the space that best represents what is true for you.

Social Support Questions	Not True 1	Somewhat True 2	Very True 3	Score
1. I have close personal ties with my relatives.				
2. I have close relationships with a number of friends.				
3. I have a deep and meaningful relationship with a spouse or close friend.				
Access to social support score:				
4. I have parents and relatives who take the time to listen and understand me.				
5. I have friends or co-workers whom I can confide in and trust when problems come up.				
6. I have a nonjudgmental spouse or close friend who supports me when I need help.				
Degree of social support score:				
7. I feel comfortable asking others for advice or assistance.				
8. I have confidence in my social skills and enjoy opportunities for new social contacts.				
9. I am willing to open up and discuss my personal life with others.				
Getting social support score:				

Results

Scores and Ratings

(Use Chart 2 to obtain ratings.)

Access to social support score [ ]   Rating [ ]

Degree of social support score [ ]   Rating [ ]

Getting social support score [ ]   Rating [ ]

Total social support score
(sum of three scores) [ ]   Rating [ ]

Chart 2 ► Rating Scale for Social Support

Rating	Item Scores	Total Score
High	8–9	24–27
Moderate	6–7	18–23
Low	Below 6	Below 18

Conclusions and Implications

1. In several sentences, discuss your overall social support. Do you think your scores and ratings are a true representation of your social support?

2. In several sentences, describe any changes you think you should make to improve your social support system. If you do not think change is necessary, explain why.

The Use and Abuse of Tobacco

Health Goals for the Year 2020

- Reduce secondhand smoke among nonsmokers.
- Increase the success of smoking cessation efforts.
- Reduce smoking during pregnancy.
- Increase the percentage of smoke-free homes.
- Increase insurance coverage of smoking cessation programs.
- Increase state taxes on tobacco products.
- Reduce the percentage of adolescents exposed to tobacco advertising and promotions.
- Increase tobacco screening in health-care settings.

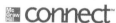 **connect**™ |FITNESS AND WELLNESS http://connect.mcgraw-hill.com

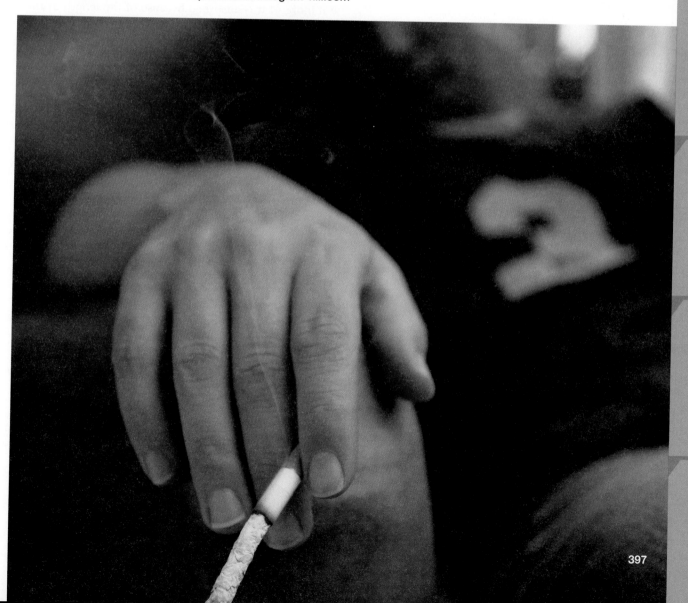

Tobacco use is the number 1 cause of preventable disease and is associated with the leading causes of death in our culture.

Tobacco is the number 1 cause of preventable mortality in the United States. It is linked to most of the leading causes of death, and it leads to various other chronic conditions. Rates of smoking in the United States have decreased in recent decades due to better awareness and a changed social norm concerning smoking and tobacco use. Despite the progress, smoking is still a major public health problem. Today, 46 million adults in the United States smoke (approximately 23 percent of men and 18 percent of women). Worldwide, an estimated 5 million people die annually from smoking, with an estimated 8 million by the year 2030. According to a recent Gallup poll, the majority of smokers (74 percent) would like to quit but find freeing themselves from the grip of nicotine addiction too difficult. This concept reviews the health risks of tobacco use and provides practical guidelines for quitting.

Tobacco and Nicotine

Tobacco and its smoke contain over 400 noxious chemicals, including 200 known poisons and 50 carcinogens. Tobacco smoke contains both gases and particulates. The gaseous phase includes a variety of harmful gases, but the most dangerous is carbon monoxide. This gas binds onto hemoglobin in the bloodstream and thereby limits how much oxygen can be carried in the bloodstream. As a result, less oxygen is supplied to the vital organs of the body. While not likely from smoking, overexposure to carbon monoxide can be fatal. The particulate phase of burning tobacco includes a variety of carbon-based compounds referred to as tar. Many of these compounds found in tobacco are known to be **carcinogens.** Nicotine is also inhaled during the particulate phase of smoking. Nicotine is a highly addictive and poisonous chemical. It has a particularly broad range of influence and is a potent psychoactive **drug** that affects the brain and alters mood and behavior.

Nicotine is the addictive component of tobacco. When smoke is inhaled, the nicotine reaches the brain in 7 seconds, where it acts on highly sensitive receptors and provides a sensation that brings about a wide variety of responses throughout the body. At first, heart and breathing rates increase. Blood vessels constrict, peripheral circulation slows down, and blood pressure increases. New users may experience dizziness, nausea, and headache. Then feelings of tension and tiredness are relieved.

After a few minutes, the feeling wears off and a rebound, or **withdrawal,** effect occurs. The smoker may feel depressed and irritable and have the urge to smoke again. **Physical dependence** occurs with continued use. Nicotine is one of the most addictive drugs known, even more addictive than heroin or alcohol.

Smokeless chewing tobacco is as addictive (and maybe more so) as smoking and produces the same kind of withdrawal symptoms on quitting. Chewing tobacco comes in a variety of forms, including loose leaf, twist, and plug forms. Rather than being smoked, the dip, chew, or chaw stays in the mouth for several hours, where it mixes well with saliva and is absorbed into the bloodstream. Smokeless tobacco contains about seven times more nicotine than cigarettes, and more of it is absorbed because of the length of time the tobacco is in the mouth. It also contains a higher level of carcinogens than cigarettes.

Snuff, a form of smokeless tobacco, comes in either dry or moist form. Dry snuff is powdered tobacco mixed with flavorings, designed to be sniffed, pinched, or dipped. Moist snuff is used the same way, but it is moist, finely cut tobacco in a loose form or in a tea-bag-like packet.

The Health and Economic Costs of Tobacco

Tobacco use is the most preventable cause of death in our society. Four decades FEATURE 1 after the landmark surgeon general's report on smoking, a new surgeon general's report draws four major conclusions. First, tobacco use affects all organs of the body, reducing the health of smokers. Second, quitting smoking has immediate and long-term benefits. Third, smoking cigarettes low in tar and nicotine provides no clear benefit to health. Finally, the number of diseases resulting from tobacco is much more extensive than previously thought (see Figure 1). Tobacco use is the leading cause of death in the United States, accounting for nearly one in five of all deaths (over 440,000 per year, according to the CDC). Deaths from smoking are preventable and are linked to 7 of the 10 leading causes of death. It is estimated that between 80 and 90 percent of all deaths related to lung cancer and obstructive lung disease are caused by smoking, and risk for coronary disease and stroke is two to four times higher among smokers.

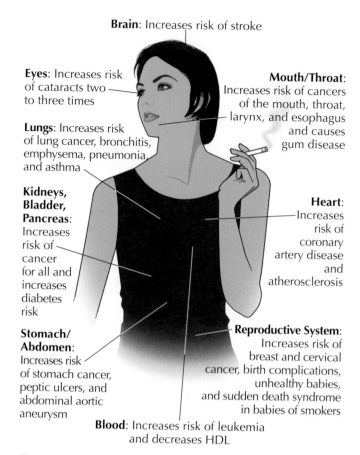

Brain: Increases risk of stroke

Eyes: Increases risk of cataracts two to three times

Lungs: Increases risk of lung cancer, bronchitis, emphysema, pneumonia, and asthma

Kidneys, Bladder, Pancreas: Increases risk of cancer for all and increases diabetes risk

Stomach/ Abdomen: Increases risk of stomach cancer, peptic ulcers, and abdominal aortic aneurysm

Mouth/Throat: Increases risk of cancers of the mouth, throat, larynx, and esophagus and causes gum disease

Heart: Increases risk of coronary artery disease and atherosclerosis

Reproductive System: Increases risk of breast and cervical cancer, birth complications, unhealthy babies, and sudden death syndrome in babies of smokers

Blood: Increases risk of leukemia and decreases HDL

Figure 1 ▶ Unhealthy effects of smoking.

One way to highlight the health risks associated with smoking is to examine the health benefits associated with smoking cessation. Estimates suggest that reducing serum cholesterol to recommended levels can increase life expectancy by about 1 week to 6 months. In contrast, smoking cessation may increase life expectancy by 2½ to 4 ½ years. The earlier people quit, the more years of life they save, with roughly 3 years saved for those who quit at 60 years of age, 6 years for those who quit at 50, and 9 years for those who quit at 40. The most effective way to reduce health risks associated with smoking is clearly to quit; however, reducing how much one smokes also makes a difference. In one study, rates of lung cancer dropped by 27 percent among those who reduced their smoking from 20 or more to less than 10 cigarettes a day.

(i) **Smoking has tremendous economic costs.** In addition to the cost of human life, FEATURE 2 smoking in the United States causes more than $193 billion in annual health-related economic losses ($97 billion in productivity losses and $96 billion in health-care expenditures). Over and above the costs at the societal level, there are significant financial costs for the individual, particularly with increased taxes on

tobacco products. In an effort to help smokers appreciate the financial burden of smoking, the American Cancer Society has a tool on its website that allows users to see how much they spend on cigarettes. For someone who smokes a pack a day for 10 years, the total would be nearly $18,000 based on current average cigarette prices.

The health risks from tobacco are directly related to overall exposure. In past years, tobacco companies denied there was conclusive proof of the harmful effects of tobacco products. Now, in the face of overwhelming medical evidence, tobacco officials have finally conceded that tobacco is harmful to health. It is now clear that the more you use the product (the more doses), the greater the health risk. Several factors determine the dosage: (1) the number of cigarettes smoked; (2) the length of time one has been smoking; (3) the strength (amount of tar, nicotine, etc.) of the cigarette; (4) the depth of the inhalation; and (5) the amount of exposure to other lung-damaging substances (e.g., asbestos). The greater the exposure to smoke, the greater the risk.

While risks clearly increase with the amount of exposure, recent studies suggest that even low levels of smoking have negative consequences. Unfortunately, while overall rates of smoking have decreased in recent years, rates of nondaily smoking have increased. These "chippers" or "social smokers" have lower risk relative to regular smokers, but there are negative health consequences of even low levels of smoking. For example, one study found that smoking one to four cigarettes per day nearly triples the risk of death from heart disease. Social smoking may also set the stage for the development of nicotine dependence and increased use later in life. Short-term physical consequences of smoking include increased rates of respiratory infections and asthma, impairment of athletic performance, and reduced benefits and enjoyment associated with recreational exercise. Smoking also causes shortness of breath and increases in phlegm production leading to a subjectively negative state.

Carcinogens Substances that promote or facilitate the growth of cancerous cells.

Drug Any biologically active substance that is foreign to the body and is deliberately introduced to affect its functioning.

Withdrawal A temporary illness precipitated by the lack of a drug in the body of an addicted person.

Physical Dependence A drug-induced condition in which a person requires frequent administration of a drug in order to avoid withdrawal.

(i) FEATURE 3 **Cigar and pipe smokers have lower death rates than cigarette smokers but are still at great risk.** Cigar and pipe smokers usually inhale less and, therefore, have less risk for heart and lung disease, but cigarette smokers who switch to cigars and pipes tend to continue inhaling the same way. As the number of cigars smoked and the depth of smoke inhalation increase, the risk for death from cigar smoking approaches that of cigarette smoking. Cigar and pipe smoke contains most of the same harmful ingredients as cigarette smoke, sometimes in higher amounts. It may also have high nicotine content, leading to no appreciable difference between cigarette and pipe/cigar smoking with respect to the development of nicotine dependence. Cigar and pipe smokers also have higher risks for cancer of the mouth, throat, and larynx relative to cigarette smokers. Pipe smokers are especially at risk for lip cancer.

Secondhand smoke poses a significant health risk. When smokers light up they expose those around them to **secondhand smoke.** Secondhand smoke is a combination of **mainstream smoke** (inhaled and then exhaled by the smoker) and **sidestream smoke** (from the burning end of the cigarette). Because sidestream smoke is not filtered through the smoker's lungs, it has higher levels of carcinogens and is therefore more dangerous. Although the negative health consequences of secondhand smoke have been known for some time, a new report (*The Health Consequences of Involuntary Exposure to Tobacco Smoke: A Report of the Surgeon General*) establishes in detail the health dangers of secondhand smoke. The following are the six major conclusions from the report (see Surgeon General's website):

- Millions in the United States are exposed to secondhand smoke despite progress in tobacco control.
- Secondhand smoke exposure leads to disease and early death.
- Infants and children are especially at risk of illnesses related to secondhand smoke.
- Adult secondhand smoke exposure contributes strongly to heart disease and lung cancer risk.
- Even brief secondhand exposure is harmful.
- Eliminating secondhand smoke indoors protects against harm, while separation of smoking and non-smoking spaces does not.

Women and children are especially susceptible to the negative effects of secondhand smoke. Evidence suggests that adolescents exposed to secondhand smoke are at five times the risk of developing metabolic syndrome, which increases risk for heart disease, stroke, and diabetes, and they are also at increased risk of becoming smokers themselves. Finally, there is evidence that secondhand smoke can have a negative impact even when smokers try to protect children from exposure. A recent study found that babies of parents who only smoked outdoors had levels of cotinine (a nicotine by-product) seven times higher than babies of nonsmokers. This has been attributed to "thirdhand" smoke that may cling to clothing and hair. These findings have led to public health efforts to involve pediatricians in smoking cessation efforts. Pediatricians are in a unique position to influence parental smoking because parents generally see their child's pediatrician more often than their own doctor. Parents may also be more responsive to the message if they learn that smoking can hurt their children.

While not technically considered secondhand exposure, smoking during pregnancy harms a developing fetus. Children of smoking mothers typically have lower birth weight and are more likely to be premature, placing them at risk for a host of health complications. There is also a well-established relation between maternal smoking and risk for sudden infant death syndrome (SIDS). Finally, children of mothers who smoke are at increased risk for later physical problems (respiratory infections and asthma) and behavioral problems (attention deficit disorder). The best way to reduce risk for pregnant mothers and their children is for women to quit smoking

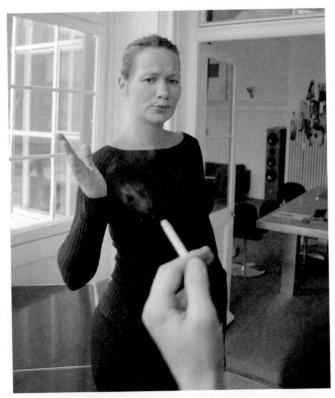

Awareness about the risks of secondhand smoke has contributed to changed social norms.

altogether. However, there is some evidence that reductions in smoking also have benefits.

Secondhand smoke exposure may also negatively impact mental health. In addition to the physical health consequences, there is now evidence of mental health consequences of secondhand smoke exposure. A recent study using a national survey found a significant relation between cotinine levels, an indicator of secondhand smoke exposure, and depression. Among those who never smoked, risk for depression was substantially increased for those exposed to cigarette smoke in their home or at work. Other recent studies show that secondhand smoke increases the risk of memory problems among the elderly.

The health risks of smokeless tobacco are similar to those of other forms of tobacco. Some smokers switch to smokeless tobacco because of the misconception that it is a safe substitute for cigarette, cigar, and pipe smoking. While smokeless tobacco does not lead to the same respiratory problems as smoking, the other health risks may be even greater because smokeless tobacco has more nicotine and higher levels of carcinogens. Because it comes in direct contact with body tissues, the health consequences are far more immediate than those from smoking cigarettes. One-third of teenage users have receding gums, and about half have precancerous lesions, 20 percent of which can become oral cancer within 5 years. Some of the health risks of smokeless tobacco are listed in Table 1.

Table 1 ▶ Health Risks of Smokeless Tobacco
Smokeless tobacco increases the risk for the following:
• Oral cavity cancer (cheek, gum, lip, palate); it increases the risk by 4 to 50 times, depending on length of time used
• Cancer of the throat, larynx, and esophagus
• Precancerous skin changes
• High blood pressure
• Rotting teeth, exposed roots, premature tooth loss, and worn-down teeth
• Ulcerated, inflamed, infected gums
• Slow healing of mouth wounds
• Decreased resistance to infections
• Arteriosclerosis, myocardial infarction, and coronary occlusion
• Widespread hormonal effects, including increased lipids, higher blood sugar, and more blood clots
• Increased heart rate

The Facts about Tobacco Usage

 FEATURE 4 At one time, smoking was an accepted part of our culture, but the social norm has changed. While smoking has always been a part of our culture, the industrialization and marketing in the middle of the 20th century led to tremendous social acceptance of smoking. As odd as it may sound, cigarettes were once provided free to airline passengers when they boarded planes. The release of the Surgeon General's report on smoking in 1964, aggressive and well-funded antismoking campaigns, and increases in cigarette prices have contributed to reductions in smoking in the United States.

Since the 1950s, the prevalence of smoking has steadily declined from a high of 50 percent. Based on data from the National Health Interview Survey, rates of smoking in the United States dropped from 25 percent in the late 1990s to 20 percent in 2007. Unfortunately, rates have begun to climb over the past 2 years with a prevalence of 20.8 percent in 2009. Fortunately, rates of smoking among adolescents have continued to decline since peak rates in the mid-1990s. Although much progress has been made in the United States, smoking remains a global public health threat, with prevalence rates in Europe and China that far exceed those in the United States. The use of smokeless tobacco is not as prevalent as smoking, but the National Institute on Drug Abuse estimates that 22 million Americans (mostly males) have used it. Young people are also among the most frequent users. The nationwide prevalence of smokeless tobacco use among 8th- to 12th-graders ranges from 3.7 to 6.1 percent.

 FEATURE 5 Most tobacco users begin "using" during adolescence and find it hard to quit. The initiation of smoking is viewed as a pediatric problem by most public health experts. Data from the National Survey on Drug Use and Health indicate that roughly 3,800 adolescents initiate cigarette use each day, with over 1,000 becoming daily smokers by the age of 18. Most adult smokers began smoking before the age of 21, and this group finds it particularly difficult to break the habit later in life.

Secondhand Smoke A combination of mainstream and sidestream smoke.

Mainstream Smoke Smoke that is exhaled after being filtered by the smoker's lungs.

Sidestream Smoke Smoke that comes directly off the burning end of a cigarette/cigar/pipe.

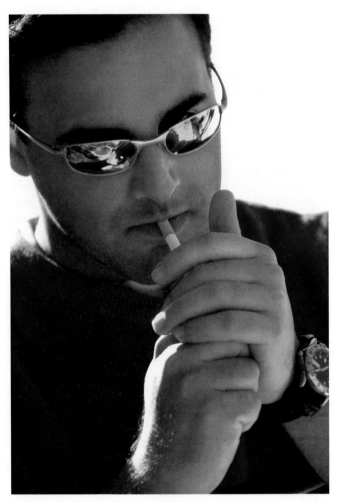

Like fashion, attitudes change with the times. The majority of people now view smoking very negatively.

Although most regular smokers begin in adolescence, a significant number start later in life, particularly during early adulthood (18–25). Unfortunately, the number of new smokers over age 18 increased from 600,000 in 2002 to 1 million in 2008. Smoking rates among college students are slightly lower than rates among high school seniors (18 versus 20 percent reported that they smoked in the past 30 days), and the rate is dramatically lower than the overall rate among young adults (about 25 percent). Smokeless tobacco use also begins early in life. Almost 50 percent of users report that they started before the age of 13, and initiation of smokeless tobacco use has nearly doubled between 2002 and 2008. The media play a role in promoting and preventing tobacco use (Figure 2). Much of the blame for tobacco use among youth is attributed to media campaigns of tobacco companies that target this age group. Lawsuits filed against tobacco companies have played an important role in decreased smoking rates in the United States. Money from state settlements have helped to fund smoking prevention programs and public education campaigns. The

lawsuits also prevented companies from direct marketing to anyone under the age of 18. These lawsuits have also had an impact on public opinions of tobacco companies. Documents uncovered from the files of tobacco companies, during litigation against the companies, have contained incriminating evidence that has undermined the reputation of tobacco companies and contributed to unfavorable public attitudes.

(i) **Public policy can affect tobacco use.** As a matter of public policy, several states have
FEATURE 6 passed special tax laws to fund anti-tobacco efforts. In addition to efforts at the state level, in 2009 federal taxes were raised from $.39 to $1.01 a pack. These tax increases have contributed to the dramatic decreases in smoking in recent years. There is, however, wide variability in state taxes resulting in prices of nearly $10 a pack in areas of New York, compared to prices of about $5 a pack in many other states. It is clear that state tax rates are tied to rates of smoking. A recent study identified only four states in which there was no clear evidence of decreases in smoking between 1998 and 2007. Recent statistics indicate that these states rank 47th, 44th, 39th, and 11th in cigarette excise taxes.

Public health campaigns by several state agencies have also been very effective in reducing smoking. Four states

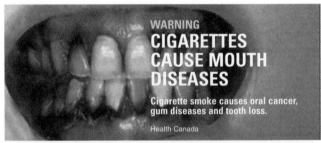

Source: Health Canada.

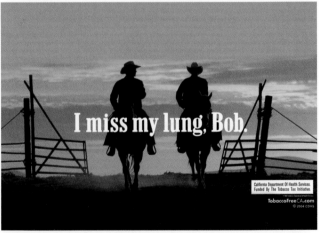

Source: TobaccoFreeCA.com.

Figure 2 ▶ Antismoking messages.

that have aggressive anti-tobacco campaigns reported a 43 percent decrease in tobacco use—double that reported by other states. According to the Substance Abuse and Mental Health Services Administration (SAMHSA), recent efforts to cut down on tobacco sales to minors have also been extremely effective. Rates of selling to minors decreased dramatically between 1997 and 2008, falling from 40.1 to 9.9 percent. These changes have been accompanied by significant reductions in rates of smoking among minors. In addition, a number of states have implemented indoor smoking bans. A total of 31 states now ban smoking in all restaurants, 28 ban smoking in bars, and 28 ban smoking in the workplace. A total of 22 states plus the District of Columbia are now smoke-free in all three settings. Including local bans by cities and counties, there are now over 17,000 indoor smoking laws in the United States. Information on smoking bans is regularly updated by Americans for Non-smokers' Rights (www.no-smoke.org/).

Fortunately, recent efforts to limit exposure to secondhand smoke seem to be paying off. A recent review confirms that public smoking bans decrease rates of heart attacks. Researchers reviewed studies conducted in the United States, Canada, and Europe, and found that heart attack rates fell 17 percent within a year after implementing smoking bans. Presumably, the immediate results are related to reductions in smoke exposure by individuals with underlying heart disease for whom exposure to smoke may trigger a heart attack. Although workplace smoking bans have focused on keeping smokers from smoking at work, employers have begun to encourage employees who smoke to quit altogether. Smokers suffer from more physical and mental health problems at a cost to employers via higher health-care premiums. The CDC estimates the cost for smoking at over $3,000 per smoker per year, including lost productivity and medical bills. Many employers, including the World Health Organization, now refuse to hire smokers, and many companies include smoking cessation in employee assistance programs to encourage smokers to quit. Recent evidence suggests that such programs can pay off for employers in as little as 2 years.

In the News

The Family Smoking Prevention and Tobacco Control Act

The FDA was recently given the authority to regulate tobacco products as part of the Family Smoking Prevention and Tobacco Control Act. As one of their first actions, the FDA banned candy, fruit, and clove-flavored cigarettes due to concerns that they attract young smokers. Some experts have argued that the regulation is not strict enough, as it does not ban menthol cigarettes. Menthol cigarettes are disproportionately used by young people, and some have argued that newer low-menthol cigarettes were developed specifically to attract young smokers. According to recent reports, menthol cigarettes and tobacco pills are at the top of the priority list of issues the committee is currently evaluating.

Tobacco companies are finding new ways to recruit smokers. As expected, the tobacco industry has fought back after the many legal settlements. Since that time, the industry has nearly doubled its budget for advertising and promotions, spending over $13 billion on advertising in 2005. Tobacco companies have also begun providing discounts to offset increased taxes and introducing new products and packaging to entice young smokers. New alternative products include tobacco pills and electronic, or e-cigarettes. Early in 2009, Camel introduced the Camel Orb, a small tobacco pill that dissolves in the mouth, in three test markets. Several companies have introduced "e-cigarettes", electronic cigarettes that produce a puff of vapor containing nicotine and other additives. Critics have argued that e-cigarettes contain known carcinogens and should have the similar warning labels and regulations. A number of state and local ordinances banning the sale of e-cigarettes or banning their use in public places have already been initiated. With a ban on obvious

HELP
Health is available to Everyone for a Lifetime, and it's **PERSONAL**

Thirty-nine states and the District of Columbia have each passed laws that ban smoking in workplaces, restaurants and/or bars. Additionally, in California specifically there are more than 20 cities that have enacted park and beach smoking bans.

What do you think about the formalized bans on smoking in most public places?

Table 2 ▶ Why Young People Start Using Tobacco
• Peer influence
• Social acceptance
• Desire to be "mature"
• Desire to be "independent"
• Desire to be like their role models
• Appealing advertisements

marketing to adolescents, tobacco companies' best legal target for promoting their products is now college students and other young adults. One approach they use to reach this audience is industry-sponsored parties at bars and nightclubs. In a national study of college students, nearly 1 in 10 reported attending industry-sponsored events. Students who had not smoked in high school but attended industry-sponsored events where free cigarettes were provided were nearly twice as likely to begin smoking.

Various factors influence a person's decision to begin or quit smoking. The reasons for starting smoking are varied, but are strikingly similar to reasons given for using alcohol and other drugs (see Table 2). Once a person starts, he or she will typically find it difficult to quit. Although a variety of smoking cessation programs are available, several studies have found that increasing the price of cigarettes is the most successful method of reducing smoking in youth.

Many young women begin smoking because they believe it will help them control their weight and negative mood states. Some current smokers feel they are unable to quit because they fear gaining weight. There is also evidence that stress and negative emotion play important roles in smoking behavior. Those who smoke report higher levels of stress, and stress has been shown to be a maintaining factor among current smokers and a barrier to quitting among those who want to stop smoking. The stress-management approaches introduced in the previous concept may help with managing stress more effectively during attempts to quit.

People who smoke cigarettes also tend to use alcohol, marijuana, and hard drugs. Alcohol has often been considered a gateway to other drug use, and marijuana is often thought of as a gateway to the use of other drugs, such as cocaine and heroine. Although tobacco use has been studied less extensively as a gateway drug, there is strong evidence that smoking is associated with increased risk for the use of both alcohol and illicit drugs. The combination of smoking and drinking is particularly common in college students. Results of a nationally representative study of college students indicated that 97 percent of college smokers drink, while other national data report that 80 percent of all college students. Those who drink also report higher levels of drinking. Rates of smoking among college drinkers range from 44 to 59 percent (compared with a national average rate of under 30 percent). The combination of alcohol use and smoking poses an even greater risk to physical health.

The addictive nature of nicotine makes it difficult to quit using tobacco. Salient examples of the power of nicotine addiction are high rates of continued use among those with serious smoking-related health consequences and low rates of success for quit attempts. In a study in 15 European countries, over half of adults who suffered from serious medical problems known to be associated with smoking (e.g., heart attack, bypass surgery) continued to smoke 1 year later. Data from the CDC found that 13 million adult smokers in the United States stopped for at least 1 day during the past year in an attempt to quit. Unfortunately, most of these attempts were unsuccessful. Most people make many attempts before they succeed. Withdrawal symptoms and associated cravings for nicotine are often cited reasons for failed quit attempts. Many former smokers report continued nicotine craving months and even years after quitting. The important thing is to keep trying to quit, because most people eventually succeed (47 million adults in the United States are former smokers).

Technology Update
Promising Medical Advancements

TECH Researchers are working hard on developing a nicotine vaccine to help smokers quit. The vaccine is not yet available, but like all vaccines, it stimulates the production of antibodies, which in this case block nicotine from passing through the blood-brain barrier. As a result, smokers no longer get the reinforcing effects of the drug and are left with the negative effects associated with smoke inhalation. Although the vaccine shows promise, those using it would need to be highly motivated to quit, as the vaccine will likely require five or six vaccine shots over the course of roughly 6 months. The vaccine is designed to help smokers get through the difficult first 6 months, after which they will have to rely on their own motivation to stay smoke free.

Strategies for Action

Some techniques and strategies increase the probability of breaking the nicotine FEATURE 7 **addiction.** A number of national organizations provide telephone hotlines to help those trying to quit smoking. These include the American Cancer Society (1-877-YES-QUIT), the National Cancer Institute (1-877-44U-QUIT), and the CDC (1-800-QUIT-NOW). In addition, an online smoking program sponsored by several federal agencies is now available at **www.smokefree.gov.** The U.S. Public Health Service (USPH) has published a consumer's guide to quitting smoking. It has determined that the following five factors are associated with the likelihood of success:

1. Get ready.
2. Get support.
3. Learn new skills and behaviors.
4. Get medication and use it correctly.
5. Be prepared for relapse and difficult situations.

The following are some more specific strategies that are consistent with these five basic keys to quitting:

- You must want to quit. The reasons can be for health, family, money, and so on.
- Remind yourself of the reasons. Each day, repeat to yourself the reasons for not using tobacco.
- Decide how to stop. Methods to stop include counseling, attending formal programs, quitting with a friend, going "cold turkey" (abruptly), and quitting gradually. More succeed "cold turkey" than with the gradual approach.
- Remove reminders and temptations (ashtrays, tobacco, etc.).
- Use substitutes and distractions. Substitute low-calorie snacks or chewing gum, change your routine, try new activities, and sit in nonsmoking areas.
- Do not worry about gaining weight. If you gain a few pounds, it is not as detrimental to your health as continuing to smoke.
- Get support. Try a formal "quit smoking program." Examples include "Freedom from Smoking" (American Lung Association) and "Fresh Start" (American Cancer Society). Many state, county, and local health departments, as well as colleges and universities, have programs. Seek support from friends and relatives.
- Assess your current behavior (see Lab 18A).
- You may want to consider a product that requires a prescription, such as a nicotine transdermal patch (Zyban) or nicotine chewing gum.
- Develop effective stress-management techniques. The single most frequently cited reason for difficulty in quitting smoking is stress.

- Set up a system of rewards for your success (e.g., use the money you would have spent on cigarettes to do something nice for yourself).

The USPHS consumer guide also provides a list of questions you may want to ask yourself as you prepare to quit. This exercise may help you increase your motivation to change and decrease the likelihood of a relapse. You may want to talk about your answers with your health-care provider.

1. Why do you want to quit?
2. When you tried to quit in the past, what helped and what did not?
3. What will be the most difficult situations for you after you quit? How will you plan to handle them?
4. Who can help you through the tough times? Your family? Friends? Your health-care provider?
5. What pleasures do you get from smoking? In what ways can you still get pleasure if you quit?

Exercise and medication can also help you quit. Recent studies suggest that regular physical activity can reduce the health risks of smoking in two important ways. First, among smokers, those who regularly exercise may be at decreased risk for the development of cardiovascular disease due to improved peripheral blood flow. Perhaps more importantly, physical activity reduces the likelihood of relapse among those who quit. Nicotine replacement products (patches, gum, nasal sprays) and medications such as Zyban, have helped some smokers quit, but others fail to benefit from their use. Luckily, new options are becoming available. The drug Chantix, recently approved by the FDA, works differently than other products on the market by partially activating nicotinic receptors in the brain, which helps reduce the rewarding properties of smoking and decreases craving for nicotine. In one clinical trial, relative to a placebo, participants who received Chantix were roughly 2.5 times more likely to sustain abstinence for 6 months.

The good news is that when you quit you may feel better right away and your body will eventually heal. You will feel more energetic, the coughing will stop, you will suddenly begin to taste food again, and your sense of smell will return. Your lungs will eventually heal and look like the lungs of a nonsmoker. Your risk for lung cancer will return to that of the nonsmoker in about 15 to 20 years. There is life after smoking!

Web Resources

Additional websites with information related to Concept 18 are available at the associated Web link.

American Cancer Society **www.cancer.org**

American Heart Association **www.americanheart.org**

Americans for Non-smokers' Rights **www.no-smoke.org**

Campaign for Tobacco Free Kids **www.tobaccofreekids.org**

Dr. Koop—Tackling Tobacco Abuse **www.drkoop.com-search tobacco**

National Center for Chronic Disease Prevention and Health Promotion: Tobacco Information and Prevention Source **www.cdc.gov/tobacco**

Quitnet—a Free Resource to Quit Smoking **www.quitnet.org**

Smoking Cessation Health Center from WebMD **www.webmd.com/smoking-cessation**

Tobacco News and Information from Tobacco.org **www.tobacco.org**

You Can Quit Smoking, Consumer Guide, June 2000. U.S. Public Health Service **www.surgeongeneral.gov/tobacco**

You Can Quit Smoking Now **www.smokefree.gov**

Suggested Readings

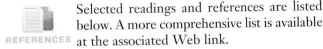

Selected readings and references are listed below. A more comprehensive list is available at the associated Web link.

Bandiera, F. C., et al. 2010. Secondhand smoke exposure and depressive symptoms. *Psychosomatic Medicine* 72:68–72.

Hahn, D. B., et al. 2011. *Focus on Health.* 10th ed. New York: McGraw-Hill Higher Education, Chapter 8.

Johnston, L. D., et al. 2009. *Monitoring the Future: National Survey Results on Drug Use, 1975–2008* (Vol. I). (NIH Publication No. 09-7402). Bethesda, MD: National Institute on Drug Abuse.

Kaczynski, A. T., et al. 2008. Smoking and physical activity: A systematic review. *American Journal of Health Behavior* 32(1):93–110.

Meyers, D. G., J. S. Neuberger, and J. He. 2009. Cardiovascular effect of bans on smoking in public places: A systematic review and meta-analysis. *Journal of the American College of Cardiology* 54:1249–1255.

Office of the Surgeon General. 2004. *The Health Consequences of Smoking: A Report of the Surgeon General.* Atlanta, GA: U.S. Department of Health and Human Services.

Paul, S. L., et al. 2008. Parental smoking and smoking experimentation in childhood increase the risk of being a smoker 20 years later: The childhood determinants of adult health study. *Addiction* 103(5): 846–853.

Perkins, K. A., C. A. Conklin, and M. D. Levine. 2008. *Cognitive-Behavioral Therapy for Smoking Cessation: A Practical Guidebook to the Most Effective Treatments.* New York: Routledge/Taylor & Francis Group.

Rubin, R. 2009, September 29. FDA: Sweet-flavored cigarettes cannot be sold. *USA Today.*

Schane, R. E., S. A. Glantz, and P. M. Ling. 2009. Nondaily and social smoking: An increasingly prevalent pattern. *Archives of Internal Medicine* 169:1742–1744.

Substance Abuse and Mental Health Services Administration. 2009. *Results from the 2008 National Survey on Drug Use and Health: National Findings* (Office of Applied Studies, NSDUH Series H-36, HHS Publication No. SMA 09-4434). Rockville, MD.

Teague, M. L., et al. 2009. *Your Health Today: Choices in a Changing Society.* 2nd ed. New York: McGraw-Hill Higher Education, Chapter 13.

Tonstad, S., et al. 2006. Effects of maintenance therapy with Varenicline on smoking cessation: A randomized controlled trial. *Journal of the American Medical Association* 296:64–71.

U.S. Department of Health and Human Services. 2006. *The Health Consequences of Involuntary Exposure to Tobacco Smoke: A Report of the Surgeon General.* Atlanta, GA: U.S. Department of Health and Human Services, Center for Disease Control and Prevention, Coordinating Center for Health Promotions, National Center for Chronic Disease Prevention and Health Promotion, Office on Smoking and Health.

Warner, K.E., et al. 2010. Tobacco control policy in developed countries: Yesterday, today, and tomorrow. *Nicotine & Tobaccio Research* 12(9):876–887.

World Health Organization. 2009. WHO report on the global tobacco epidemic, 2009: Executive summary. Accessed on 5/15/10 at **www.who.int/tobacco/mpower/2009/mpower _report_2009_executive_summary_EN_11b.pdf**

Lab 18A Use and Abuse of Tobacco

Name	**Section**	**Date**

Purpose: To understand the risks of diseases (such as heart disease and cancer) associated with the use of tobacco or exposure to tobacco by-products

Procedure

1. Read the Tobacco Use Risk Questionnaire (Chart 1).
2. Answer the questionnaire based on your tobacco use or exposure.
3. Record your score and rating (from Chart 2) in the Results section.

Results

What is your tobacco risk score? [   ] (total from Chart 1)

What is your tobacco risk rating? [   ] (see Chart 2)

Chart 1 ▶ Tobacco Use Risk Questionnaire

Circle one response in each row of the questionnaire. Determine a point value for each response using the point values in the first row of the chart. Sum the numbers of points for the various responses to determine a Tobacco Use Risk score.

	Points				
Categories	**0**	**1**	**2**	**3**	**4**
Cigarette use	Never smoked		1–10 cigarettes a day	11–40 cigarettes a day	>40 cigarettes a day
Pipe and cigar use	Never smoked	Pipe— occasional use	Cigar— infrequent daily use	Cigar or pipe— frequent daily use	Cigar—heavy use
Smoking style	Don't smoke		No inhalation	Slight to moderate inhalation	Deep inhalation
Smokeless tobacco use	Don't use	Occasional use: not daily	Daily use: one use per day	Daily Use: multiple use per day	Heavy use: repetitious, multiple use daily
Secondhand or sidestream smoke	No smokers at home or in workplace	Smokers at work-place but not at home	Smokers at home but not workplace	Smokers at home and at workplace	
Years of tobacco use	Never used	1 or less	2–5	6–10	>10

Note: Different forms of tobacco use pose different risks for different diseases. This questionnaire is designed to give you a general idea of risk associated with use and exposure to tobacco by-products.

Chart 2 ▶ Tobacco Use Risk Questionnaire Rating Chart	
Rating	**Score**
Very high risk	16+
High risk	7–15
Moderate risk	1–6
Low risk	0

Conclusions and Implications

1. In several sentences, discuss your personal risk. If your risk is low, discuss some implications of the behavior of other people that affect your risk, including what can be done to change these risks. If your risk is above average, what changes can be made to reduce your risk?

2. In several sentences, discuss how you feel about public laws designed to curtail tobacco use. Discuss your point of view, either pro or con.

The Use and Abuse of Alcohol

Health Goals for the Year 2020

- Reduce substance abuse to protect the health, safety, and quality of life for all, especially children.
- Reduce deaths and injuries caused by alcohol-related motor vehicle crashes.
- Reduce number of adolescents who rode with a drinking driver in the past 30 days.
- Reduce alcohol-related injuries and hospital emergency room visits.
- Reduce the frequency of driving while intoxicated.
- Increase age and proportion of adolescents who remain alcohol free.
- Reduce binge drinking and average alcohol consumption.
- Reduce cirrhosis deaths.

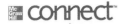

Mc Graw Hill **connect**™
| **FITNESS AND WELLNESS**   http://connect.mcgraw-hill.com

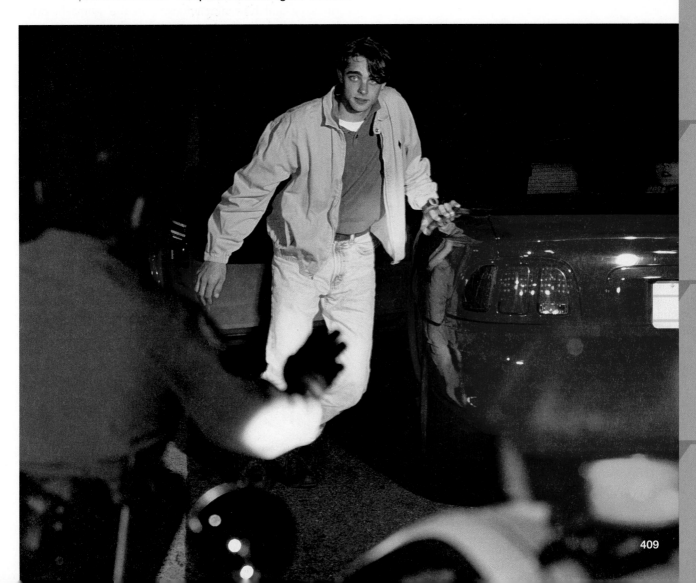

Alcohol is among the most widely used and destructive drugs and ranks high among causes of health problems and death in our culture.

Alcohol is the most widely used and destructive drug in the United States. If all of the deaths caused by this drug are counted, it is the third leading health problem and cause of early death in the United States. Only tobacco and inactivity/poor nutrition rank ahead of alcohol use. Some consider alcohol use to be the most destructive because of the devastating results of drinking and driving (or operating other vehicles) and because of the consequences of increased crime, physical and sexual abuse, and destroyed family relationships that are often associated with overindulgence in alcohol. It is estimated that over 17 million people in the United States, representing over 8 percent of the total population, meet the criteria for some type of alcohol-related diagnosis.

Alcohol and Alcoholic Beverages

Alcoholic beverages contain ethanol (ethyl alcohol), an intoxicating and addictive drug that is often misused. The active **drug** in alcoholic beverages (ethanol) is a toxic chemical, but unlike methanol (wood alcohol) and isopropyl (rubbing alcohol), it can be consumed in small doses. As a drug, it is classified as a depressant. However, this classification does not capture the full range of alcohol effects. The effects experienced by the drinker depend, in part, on whether blood alcohol concentration is rising or falling. The sedative effects of alcohol as blood alcohol levels fall are consistent with its classification as a depressant drug. In contrast, primarily stimulant effects are experienced by the user as blood alcohol concentration rises.

Humans have consumed alcoholic beverages for thousands of years. Unfortunately, many people in our culture (particularly college students) view drunkenness as a rite of passage and an expectation. Indeed, there are more synonyms for the word *drunk* or *intoxication* than for any other word in the English language. This illustrates the importance we give to overconsumption. Fortunately, as people mature, they tend to reduce their consumption, as responsibilities such as work and family become more important.

Alcoholic beverages have varying concentrations of alcohol, but many have similar amounts per serving. Beverages are usually served in proportions such that a drink of any one of the three categories (beer, wine, or liquor) contains the same amount of alcohol. Beer is usually served in a 12-ounce can, bottle, or mug. A typical glass of wine holds 5 ounces, and a shot of liquor is 1.5 ounces. Even though the percentage of alcohol in the beverages differs, the drinks would be equivalent in alcohol because each would contain about 14 gm of alcohol (see Figure 1). Although the amount of alcohol is equivalent across these different drink types, differences in the way they are consumed may lead to differences in blood alcohol concentrations. For example, because liquor is often consumed more quickly than beer or wine, blood alcohol concentrations rise more quickly.

Alcohol's effect on the body depends on many factors. Alcohol is absorbed directly into the bloodstream, primarily in the small intestine, though some absorption occurs in the mouth, esophagus, and stomach. It then concentrates in various organs in proportion to the amount of water each contains. The brain has a high water content, so much of the alcohol goes there. The rate and magnitude of the effects on an individual depend on what and how much food is in the stomach; other drugs and medications consumed; body size/weight; rate of consumption; individual body chemistry and genetic predisposition; individual beliefs about the effects of alcohol; and the context in which drinking occurs. In general, the more and faster one drinks, the greater the effect. Differences in effects are apparent between genders even when differences in body size are considered. One reason for this is that women have lower amounts of body water, so a given amount of alcohol represents a greater percentage of the volume of the blood in their bloodstream. Another factor is that women have lower amounts of the enzymes needed to process alcohol. Thus, alcohol stays in the bloodstream longer before being broken down.

The body usually cannot process alcohol as quickly as it is consumed. Alcohol in the bloodstream is eventually oxidized in the liver. An enzyme in the liver, called

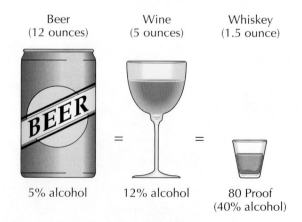

Beer
(12 ounces)

Wine
(5 ounces)

Whiskey
(1.5 ounce)

5% alcohol

12% alcohol

80 Proof
(40% alcohol)

Figure 1 ▶ Alcohol content of drinks.
Source: National Institute on Alcohol Abuse and Alcoholism.

Table 1 ▶ Terms and Criteria for Patterns of Alcohol Use

Term	Criteria
Moderate drinking (NIAAA)	Men: ≤2 drinks/day Women: ≤1 drink/day Over 65: ≤1 drink/day
At-risk drinking (NIAAA)	Men: >14 drinks/week or >4 drinks/occasion Women: >7 drinks/week or >3 drinks/occasion
Heavy-episodic drinking (NIAAA)	Men: 5 or more alcoholic drinks consumed in a row Women: 4 or more alcoholic drinks consumed in a row
Alcohol abuse (APA)	Maladaptive pattern of alcohol use leading to clinically significant impairment or distress, manifested within a 12-month period by one or more of the following: • Failure to fulfill role obligations at work, school, or home • Recurrent use in hazardous situations • Legal problems related to alcohol • Continued use despite alcohol-related social or interpersonal problems
Alcohol dependence (APA)	Maladaptive pattern of alcohol use leading to clinically significant impairment or distress, manifested within a 12-month period by three or more of the following: • Tolerance (either increasing amounts used or diminished effects with the same amount) • Withdrawal (withdrawal symptoms or use to relieve or avoid symptoms) • Use of larger amounts over a longer period than intended • Persistent desire or unsuccessful attempts to cut down or control use • Great deal of time spent obtaining, using, or recovering from use • Important social, occupational, or recreational activities given up or reduced • Use despite knowledge of alcohol-related physical or psychological problems

Note: NIAAA, National Institute on Alcohol Abuse and Alcoholism; APA, American Psychiatric Association.

Source: O'Conner and Schottenfeld.

alcohol dehydrogenase (ADH), converts alcohol to acetaldehyde, which is then converted by acetate and other enzymes into carbon dioxide and water. Individuals differ with respect to their ability to metabolize alcohol, but a healthy adult takes 1 to 2 hours to metabolize one standard drink. Because the rate of alcohol consumption is typically greater than the rate at which it is processed, the alcohol concentration in the bloodstream begins to increase. The blood alcohol concentration (BAC) is measured as a percentage and is used by law enforcement officials to determine if a driver is legally intoxicated.

A BAC of .10 percent used to be the level at which driving became illegal in most states. Due to evidence of impairment at much lower doses and the extreme social and economic costs associated with drinking and driving, all 50 states have now reduced the legal limit to .08 percent.

Alcohol Consumption and Alcohol Abuse

Risks and benefits of alcohol use depend on the amount and pattern of consumption. Making statements about the consequences of alcohol consumption is difficult because the consequences vary depending on the amount consumed and the pattern of consumption. Moderate alcohol consumption has been shown to

provide some benefits for reducing risks of heart disease, but considerable risks occur when consumed in excess. Risks for alcohol consumption are not the same for everyone, so it is important to understand the relative risks and benefits of various levels of alcohol consumption.

ⓘ FEATURE 1 **Patterns of alcohol consumption are characterized in a variety of ways.** Roughly half (50.9 percent) of the U.S. population over the age of 12 report alcohol consumption in the past 30 days. This makes alcohol the most widely used drug of abuse in this country. Most who choose to drink develop a pattern of light or moderate drinking. Although various definitions of *moderate drinking* have been proposed, perhaps the most widely used is that of the National Institute on Alcohol Abuse and Alcoholism (NIAAA). According to the NIAAA, moderate consumption is characterized as one drink per day or less for women and two drinks per day or less for men (see Table 1). Those who exceed

Drug Any biologically active substance that is foreign to the body and is deliberately introduced to affect its functioning.

Intoxication Also referred to as drunkenness; a blood alcohol level of .08.

these standards are often described as at-risk drinkers. Heavy-episodic drinking (commonly referred to as binge drinking) is common among at risk drinkers. It is generally defined as five or more standard alcoholic drinks consumed in a row (four or more for women). Approximately 23 percent of the U.S. population (57 million people) report heavy-episodic drinking in the past 30 days. Thus, nearly half of those who drink report having five or more (four or more for women) drinks at least occasionally.

Heavy-episodic drinkers are 14 times more likely to drink and drive, and they are at increased risk for a host of negative outcomes, including development of **alcohol abuse** and **alcohol dependence** (see Table 1 for characteristics of these conditions). Two key signs of alcohol dependence (the diagnosis most people refer to as alcoholism) are **tolerance** and **withdrawal.** Tolerance is a reduced response to alcohol—in other words, more alcohol is needed to get similar effects. Unfortunately, many people seem to think that tolerance is a good sign, as evidenced by statements such as "I can hold my liquor" and "I'm not a lightweight." The reality is that tolerance has mostly negative implications. There is also recent evidence that those who have a natural, or "innate," tolerance to alcohol effects are at increased risk for developing alcohol use disorders. With the heavier use that comes with the development of tolerance, withdrawal symptoms may develop when alcohol is not administered regularly. Withdrawal symptoms include anxiety, increased heart rate, sweating, hand tremor, nausea, and vomiting. In more severe cases, withdrawal can lead to hallucinations and seizures.

Health and Behavioral Consequences of Alcohol Use

Heavy alcohol use is associated with an increased risk for a variety of negative health and social outcomes. The most well-established health risk associated with alcohol consumption is liver disease. Alcohol is the leading cause of disease and death from liver dysfunction, with an estimated 2 million Americans suffering from alcohol-induced liver disease. Although the liver is capable of metabolizing moderate amounts of alcohol on a regular basis, persistent, heavy drinking may lead to swollen liver cells, a condition called **fatty liver.** If drinking is stopped or significantly reduced at this point, the damage to the liver is likely reversible. With continued heavy drinking, the individual is likely

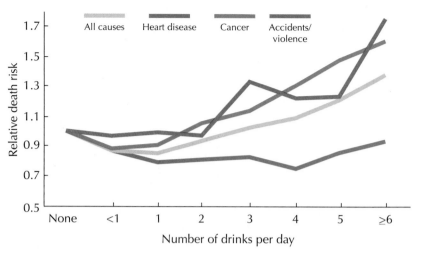

Figure 2 ▶ Alcohol consumption and death risk.
Source: American Cancer Society.

to develop **alcoholic cirrhosis,** or permanent scarring of the liver.

Heavy drinking is also a risk factor for other life-threatening diseases (see Figure 2). FEATURE 2 Although moderate alcohol consumption may protect against coronary heart disease (CHD), as outlined later in the concept, heavier use of alcohol may increase the risk for CHD and other cardiovascular disease. Specifically, heavy drinking is associated with increased risk for hypertension, cardiomyopathy, cardiac arrhythmia, and congestive heart failure. There is considerable evidence that alcohol consumption increases the risk for cancer, including cancer of the oral cavity and pharynx, esophagus, liver, larynx, and female breast. The risk for certain types of stroke (hemorrhagic) is also increased by alcohol, and there is evidence that heavy drinking may impair immune functioning, leading to increased risk for infectious diseases, including pneumonia and tuberculosis. Heavy alcohol use also has both acute and long-term effects on cognitive functions including memory, and increases risk for psychiatric disorders that often co-occur with alcohol problems (e.g., mood and anxiety disorders).

Although many health risks of alcohol use are directly related to the effects of alcohol on the body, others are related to the intoxicated behavior of the drinker. For example, heavy episodic drinking increases risk for motor vehicle crashes, falls, burns, drownings, interpersonal violence, and sexually transmitted diseases. The overall impact of drinking on other members of society is particularly troubling. Ambitious public health goals have been set for curtailing heavy episodic drinking in the United States, but rates have remained relatively stable.

Women appear to be especially susceptible to the negative health consequences of heavy drinking. At similar levels of alcohol consumption, women are more likely than men to experience liver, cardiovascular, and brain damage from drinking. Alcohol also increases risk of breast cancer and negatively impacts the reproductive system. Women who are pregnant should avoid alcohol because drinking during pregnancy can lead to fetal alcohol effects, including fetal alcohol syndrome (FAS), which is associated with low birth weight, physical defects, mental retardation, and stunted growth. In summary, the health risks of alcohol consumption are extensive, and must be considered in relation to the potential benefits.

While excessive drinking presents many risks, moderate consumption can provide some health benefits. There is substantial evidence that moderate alcohol consumption (one drink per day for women, up to two drinks per day for men) is associated with decreased risk for coronary heart disease (CHD), Type II diabetes, and certain types of stroke. At this point, it is not entirely clear the extent to which moderate drinking "causes" reduced risk for cardiovascular disease. It may be that moderate drinkers are at lower risk based on other characteristics, such as higher education and income, better diet, and more regular exercise. Still, mechanisms for a causal role of alcohol use in protection against CHD are plausible and have been studied extensively. Evidence suggests that decreased risk for CHD and stroke may be due to reductions in blood clotting and increased levels of high-density lipoproteins (HDL), or "good cholesterol." Recent evidence suggests that moderate alcohol use may also protect against cognitive declines with aging. Although the health benefits of moderate alcohol consumption have largely been attributed to wine consumption, beer appears to have similar benefits. In addition, there is some evidence that beer consumption may benefit bone strength because it has high levels of dietary silicon, which contributes to bone density. Beers with high levels of barley and hops are particularly good sources of silicon.

Although the protection against health risks by moderate alcohol consumption is significant, particularly given the impact on CHD risk, it is important to keep in mind that moderate alcohol consumption may not be safe for everyone. Age, gender, health status, and a family history of alcoholism are just a few of the individual differences that contribute to the relative safety of alcohol consumption for any individual. Certain groups are best off not drinking at all, despite potential health benefits (see Table 2). Also note that the pattern of drinking is as important as the absolute level. A woman who has seven drinks one time each week consumes an average of one drink per day but does not receive the same health benefits as a woman who consumes one drink each day. Moderate consumption of alcohol can be safely

Table 2 ▶ People Who Should Consider Abstaining from Alcohol Use
• People under age 21 (legal age)
• Athletes striving for peak performance
• Women trying to get pregnant or who are pregnant or nursing
• Alcoholics and recovering alcoholics
• People with a family history of alcoholism
• People with a medical or surgical problem and/or on medications
• Psychiatric patients or persons experiencing severe psychosis
• People driving vehicles, operating dangerous machinery, or involved in public safety
• People conducting serious business transactions or study

incorporated into a healthy lifestyle, but heavy episodic drinking cannot.

The greatest danger of alcohol occurs when the drinker gets behind the wheel of a motor vehicle. Alcohol-related traffic crashes are the leading cause of death and spinal cord injury for young Americans. Approximately 37 percent of fatal injury traffic accidents are alcohol-involved. The driver's likelihood of causing a highway accident increases at a BAC of .04 percent. When BAC reaches .10 percent, the chances increase by 600 percent. The effects of different BAC values on physical and driving performance are summarized in Table 3.

In addition to risks associated with traffic accidents, those who drink and drive face significant legal, financial,

Alcohol Abuse Use of alcohol in hazardous situations or continued alcohol use in hazardous situations or despite significant negative consequences.

Alcohol Dependence Severe form of alcohol abuse that is often characterized by physical symptoms of dependence.

Tolerance The phenomenon of requiring more and more alcohol over time to achieve the desired effect.

Withdrawal Symptoms that occur when alcohol is withdrawn after a period of prolonged heavy use. Symptoms include sweating, anxiety, tremors, and seizures.

Fatty liver Swelling of the cells of the liver.

Alcoholic Cirrhosis Permanent scarring of the liver, resulting in reduced blood flow and buildup of toxins in the body.

Table 3 ▶ The Effects of Blood Alcohol Concentration (BAC) on Driving Performance and Function

BAC 0.02%
- Vision is impaired: less ability to see objects in motion; less ability to monitor multiple objects.
- Attention span is lower.
- Reaction time slows.
- Less critical of own actions.

BAC 0.05–0.06%
- Inhibitions are reduced (unnecessary chances may be taken).
- Visual abilities decrease; side vision is impaired by 30%.
- Superficial feelings of relaxation.
- Judgment is the first function to be impaired.
- Braking distance is extended.
- Diminished ability to maneuver through narrow spaces.
- Coordination is impaired.
- Information processing is impaired.
- Driving performance is impaired at moderate speed.

BAC 0.08%
- Vision is seriously impaired, especially at night.
- Overconfidence in driving ability.
- Emotions are exaggerated.
- Thinking and reasoning powers are impaired.
- Less ability to concentrate.
- Judgments are dulled; driver is more careless.
- Muscle control and coordination are hindered.
- Distances are misjudged.
- Driving performance is impaired at low speeds.
- Possible steering inaccuracy.
- Driver increases the use of the accelerator and brake.

BAC .15%
- Gross motor impairment and lack of physical control.
- Blurred vision and loss of balance.
- Increased risk of hangovers.

BAC .20%
- Disorientation and difficulty walking.
- Nausea and vomiting.
- Anesthesia.
- Impaired gag reflex.
- Blackouts.

BAC .30%
- Stupor and decreased respiration.
- Loss of consciousness.

BAC .40%
- Coma.
- Death is possible, due to respiratory arrest.

Source: Mothers Against Drunk Driving.

Technology Update
Alcohol Consumption Detection

TECH Current alcoholo detection systems can only detect very recent use (breath or blood alcohol levels). A new method based on ethyl glucoronide (EtG) shows promise for detecting long term alcohol consumption. Elevated levels of EtG can be detected for several days following heavy alcohol consumption, and lower levels of consumption can be detected within a 24-hour period. To date, EtG has been used primarily for forensics or other law enforcement applications, but it also offers potential for monitoring progress in centers designed to treat alcohol abuse and dependence. Remaining issues include a lack of established cutoffs for defining a positive test, and concerns about positive readings caused by use of non-beverage products that contain ethanol (e.g., mouthwash and hand sanitizers). Although more research is needed, EtG may ultimately prove to be a valuable tool for providers of treatment services for individuals with alcohol use disorders.

immediate financial burden. Having an offense on your record can lead to problems with schools, family, and future employers. Despite the potential short- and long-term costs, in a government survey 70 percent of college students reported driving while under the influence of alcohol at least once in the past year, and 22 percent said they had done it five times or more.

Understanding the effects of alcohol at various blood alcohol levels and being able to estimate your own blood alcohol level can help prevent you from driving when impaired. Table 4 provides estimated BACs for men and women at various weights. Lab 19A will provide the formula necessary to calculate BAC for your precise weight.

Increased prevention efforts and changing attitudes have led to dramatic FEATURE 3 **decreases in alcohol-related traffic fatalities.** Although alcohol-related traffic fatalities remain a major public health concern, rates have decreased dramatically during the past three decades, down from 60 percent of all traffic fatalities in 1982 to 37 percent in 2008. Many factors have contributed to the decrease, but lowering the legal limit for intoxication to .08 and raising the legal drinking age to 21 are two important contributing factors. One of the most recent approaches involves the use of ignition interlock devices for those arrested for driving under the influence. These devices do not allow drivers to start their cars unless they provide a breath

and social costs. There were approximately 1.46 million arrests for driving under the influence in 2006, and penalties have become increasingly severe. Although the short-term costs are significant, the long-term costs of a drunk driving arrest typically far outweigh the

Number of drinks	Females		Males	
	120-Pound	180-Pound	140-Pound	200-Pound
1	.04	.03	.03	.02
2	.08	.05	.05	.04
3	.11	.08	.08	.06
4	.15	.10	.11	.08
5	.19	.13	.13	.09
6	.23	.15	.16	.11
7	.27	.18	.19	.13
8	.30	.20	.21	.15

Table 4 ▶ Approximate BAC Values (%) Based on the Number of Drinks Consumed over a One-Hour Period

Source: U.S. Department of Health and Human Services, Substance Abuse and Mental Health Services Administration.

sample showing no or low alcohol content. Although these devices have limitations, they do seem to deter repeat offending. Most states now have mandatory ignition interlock laws for at least some offenders, though the laws differ in terms of who is mandated to use them. Some states mandate their use for all offenders, whereas others mandate their use only for repeat offenders or only for those with high BACs (.15, for example). A federal law that would require all states to use ignition interlock devices for all DUI offenders is currently being considered. States that fail to comply with the law would risk losing federal highway funding. Perhaps in response to stricter laws, many people are making the decision to test their own blood alcohol levels before getting behind the wheel. Sales of blood-alcohol self-tests have increased dramatically (over 700 percent) in the past 5 years.

Risk Factors for Alcohol-Related Problems

Early age of drinking onset increases risk for later problems. Studies have consistently demonstrated that those who begin drinking at an earlier age are at risk for the development of alcohol abuse and dependence. Although the nature of the relation between age of onset and later problems is not yet clear, many believe that early use interferes with a critical period of brain development. Studies have shown that the part of the brain involved in emotion regulation and impulse control (the frontal lobe) is not fully developed until the mid-20s, so, although physical maturation may be complete by the age of 18, cognitive abilities are still developing during

this period. Use of alcohol and other drugs during this important period of brain development may have long-term negative consequences for young people.

Having a family member with an alcohol problem places you at increased risk for developing a problem yourself. Experts have known for some time that the development of alcohol abuse and dependence has a genetic component. Alcohol problems run in families, and it is estimated that genetics account for roughly half of the risk for alcohol dependence. In the future, we may find out exactly how genetic differences contribute to risk, but for now we know that genetics are important. Thus, if you have a family history of alcoholism, you should be especially careful about your drinking behavior.

Environment also plays a role in the initiation and escalation of alcohol use. During childhood, parents play a significant role in the socialization process, which includes socialization regarding alcohol use. Parents who talk to their kids about alcohol use, provide social support, and monitor their children's behavior are less likely to have children who drink excessively during adolescence. During adolescence, peers take on a powerful role in the development of alcohol problems. One of the best predictors of adolescent alcohol use patterns is the pattern of alcohol use among their close friends.

Broader environmental influences also play a key role in the development of alcohol use. The promotion of alcohol as a social lubricant leads to the development of positive beliefs about the effects of alcohol, referred to as "alcohol expectancies." These beliefs have been shown to develop even before personal experience with alcohol. Media portrayals of the benefits of drinking are believed to play an important role in the development of positive expectancies. Adolescents are bombarded with these messages from an early age. Between 2001 and 2006, youth were 287 times more likely to see a TV commercial promoting alcohol than to see an industry-sponsored "responsibility" ad. Of the $5.6 billion spent by the

Health is available to Everyone for a Lifetime, and it's **PERSONAL**

According to the most recent National Survey on Drug Use and Health, young adults enrolled in college full time are more likely than those not attending college to use alcohol, binge drink and participate in heavy drinking. It was also reported that alcohol use decreases with increasing age.

Do you think alcohol consumption in college has an impact on your drinking patterns and lifestyle later in life? Explain.

alcohol industry during this period, only 2.2 percent was devoted to "responsibility" ads.

Alcohol on Campus

(i) **College students drink more than the rest of society and are at increased risk**
FEATURE 4 **for alcohol problems.** The problem of college drinking has gained increased attention over the past 20 years. The vast majority of college students have consumed alcohol in the past year (roughly 80 percent), and drinking among college students is a significant public health problem. It is estimated that drinking by college students is associated with 696,000 physical assaults, 599,000 injuries, 400,000 instances of unsafe sexual behavior, 97,000 sexual assaults, and 1,700 deaths annually. About 25 percent of college students report academic problems caused by drinking, including lower grades, poor performance on exams and papers, and missed classes. Grade point average has also been found to be inversely related to the amount of alcohol consumed (see Figure 3). Rates of heavy-episodic drinking are particularly high among college students, with rates of roughly 40 percent reported across several large nationally representative studies. Roughly 20 percent of college students report engaging in frequent heavy-episodic drinking, defined as three or more occasions in a 2-week period (see Table 5).

The college environment plays a key role in heavy alcohol use among college students. College attendance for most students means putting off some of the adult responsibilities historically associated with this period of development. For example, marriage and full-time jobs are not common among college students. Because of the lack of traditional adult responsibilities, some have argued that college has become a period of extended adolescence. Others refer to this period between adolescence and adulthood as "emerging adulthood." Regardless of the terminology, the early 20s are clearly a period of heightened risk for engagement in risky behaviors, including alcohol and other drug use. It has been suggested that flexible schedules for college students contribute to this problem. In contrast to emerging adults in the work sector, college students can often avoid morning classes and Friday classes to extend the weekend. In fact, a recent study found that the later students' Friday classes began, the more they drank on Thursday nights, with the heaviest drinking among those with no Friday classes. The authors argue that offering more Friday classes and requiring students to take them may help reduce alcohol use on college campuses.

Some have argued that the legal drinking age of 21 contributes to drinking problems in college. In August 2008, 100 university presidents joined forces to urge lawmakers to lower the drinking age from 21 to 18. Among the institutions whose presidents are represented in the movement (called the Amethyst Initiative) are Colgate, Duke, Dartmouth, Ohio State University, and Syracuse. Those leading the movement argue that current laws are routinely evaded and encourage dangerous binge drinking on campus. The presidents indicate that their movement is designed to stimulate public debate. Some student groups have supported the movement, suggesting that if they are old enough to fight in wars, they are old enough to drink. On the other hand, the organization Mothers Against Drunk Driving (MADD) has argued that lowering the drinking age would lead to more car crashes. In fact, alcohol-related traffic fatalities have decreased dramatically since the legal drinking age was raised to 21. There is also concern that allowing 18-year-olds to possess alcohol legally will facilitate access to those who are under the age of 18, and an earlier age of alcohol use is a well-known risk factor for later problems with alcohol. The debate over the legal drinking age will no doubt continue. As noted in this concept, there are many factors to be considered.

Drinking games place college students at high risk for negative consequences. Drinking games, such as "quarters," "three-man," and "beer pong" (or "Beirut"), are common on college campuses, and recent studies have shown that students who engage in drinking games reach dangerously high blood alcohol concentrations and experience more negative consequences. Younger students are more likely to play drinking games and to

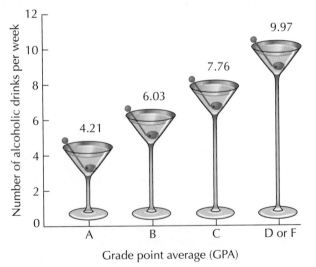

Figure 3 ▶ Average number of alcoholic drinks per week by GPA.

Source: Adapted from Core Institute.

Table 5 ▶ Alcohol-Related Problems among College Students

Problems	All students	Nonheavy-Episodic Drinkers (%)	Occasional Heavy-Episodic Drinkers (%)	Frequent Heavy-Episodic Drinkers (%)
Did something you regret	36.1	18.0	39.6	62.0
Missed a class	29.9	8.8	30.9	62.5
Drove after drinking	28.8	18.6	39.7	56.7
Forgot where you were or what you did	27.1	10.0	27.2	54.0
Argued with friends	22.5	9.7	23.0	42.6
Got behind in schoolwork	24.1	9.8	26.0	46.3
Engaged in unplanned sexual activities	21.6	7.9	22.3	41.5
Got hurt or injured	12.4	3.9	10.9	26.6
Damaged property	10.8	2.3	8.9	22.7
Had unprotected sex	10.3	3.7	9.8	20.4

Source: Wechsler, et al.

experience negative consequences as a result. This may be due to the fact that younger drinkers have less tolerance and are therefore more impaired at comparable blood alcohol levels.

Female college students are at particularly high risk for negative behavioral consequences of drinking. Women are at increased risk for a variety of acute negative behavioral outcomes of drinking, though unprotected or unwanted sexual behavior is perhaps the greatest concern. Risks are particularly high for young women in situations where high blood alcohol levels are likely. For example, women experience more negative consequences of drinking games because they drink at similar levels to men, leading to higher blood alcohol concentrations. Women are also at very high risk for negative consequences during Spring Break. In a recent online survey, 83 percent of women reported that Spring Break involved heavier than usual drinking, and 74 percent said sexual activity was increased. Thirteen percent of women said they had sex with more than one partner, and 10 percent said they regretted engaging in public or group sexual activity.

Misperceptions of peer attitudes and drinking behavior contribute to heavy drinking in college. Although increased attention to college drinking problems has led to increased education and prevention, rates of heavy use have changed little. One contributing factor may be that attention to heavy drinking has led to the perception by college students that their peers are drinking more than they actually are. Research has shown that college students routinely overestimate use by their peers and that these misperceptions are associated with increases in drinking. In theory, students drink more to keep up with what they perceive to be the norm on campus. In addition to overestimating how much alcohol their peers consume, college students appear to overestimate how much alcohol their peers want them to consume. This may be particularly true for women. A recent study found that 71 percent of women believed men wanted them to consume alcohol excessively, and 17 percent thought that men would find them more sexually attractive if they had five or more drinks. In truth, the percentage of men who endorsed these beliefs was about half of what women perceived it to be. Together, beliefs that peers engage in and condone heavy drinking serve to promote excessive consumption on college campuses.

_(i)_ **New approaches to preventing heavy drinking among college students are** FEATURE 5 **showing promise.** Efforts to prevent heavy drinking among college students have traditionally focused on education. Unfortunately, a task force developed by the National Institute on Alcohol Abuse and

Alcoholism (NIAAA) found that these approaches are largely ineffective. Confrontational approaches do not work well either, particularly with young people. Effective strategies include motivational and skills-based approaches. These approaches encourage young people to examine how their drinking behavior impacts their lives, and to consider ways that changing their behavior might benefit them. Skills training focuses on teaching young people strategies to moderate their consumption or to maintain abstinence in the face of social pressure to drink. Another promising approach that is increasingly used on college campuses addresses students' misperceptions of drinking behavior on campus. This approach focuses on the high percentage of students who *do not* drink heavily. One study found that 66.2 percent of college students reported any alcohol use in the past 30 days. Those who did report drinking had an average of 4.22 drinks over an average of 2.75 hours the last time they "partied." This amount of alcohol over this time frame would result in relatively low levels of intoxication. Figure 4 provides an example of a media campaign designed to counter misperceptions about campus drinking.

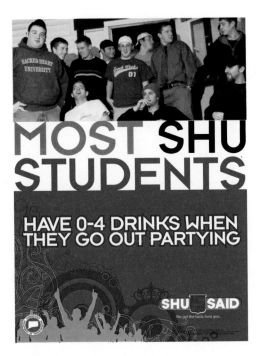

Figure 4 ▶ Knowledge of peer behavior can reduce peer pressure.

 In the News

Drinking Problems in the Military

Rates of alcohol use and abuse in the military are high, and the stresses of repeated deployments have led to recent increases in treatment seeking. Young men as a group are at high risk for heavy drinking and related problems, and the military is a major employer of this demographic (roughly 86 percent of active duty military are male, and roughly 67 percent are between the ages of 18 and 30). This risk is exacerbated by the stress associated with deployment, and ongoing conflicts have led to repeated deployments for many young men and women in the military. As a result, the number of Army soldiers in treatment for alcohol abuse or dependence has nearly doubled since 2003. Although less dramatic, recent increases in alcohol problems have also been found among members of the Marine Corps. For many of these soldiers, alcohol may be used as a means to cope with the stresses of war or with symptoms of posttraumatic stress disorder related to their experiences in the field.

 Strategies for Action

Determining if a problem exists is an important strategy for taking action. Moderate alcohol consumption is safe for many people and may even have some health benefits. However, many people who drink do so beyond safe levels. If you drink, experts recommend no more than one drink per day for women and no more than two drinks per day for men.

Additional information about safe levels of drinking is available on a new website developed by the NIAAA. The "Rethinking Drinking" website is designed to provide a mechanism for evaluating your alcohol use and risk for the development of alcohol-related problems. The site also provides resources for those who wish to change their drinking behavior. The site is specifically targeted toward young adults with the goal of reducing harm associated with heavy drinking.

If you consume more than the recommended amount, you may have a problem. The term *alcoholism* is widely used to define individuals with alcohol problems, but this label best corresponds to alcohol dependence and therefore does not adequately define the range of alcohol-related problems depicted in Table 1. For example, one study indicated that only one of every four hazardous drinkers is alcohol dependent. The remainder would be classified as at-risk drinkers or alcohol abusers. Although the problems experienced by these at-risk drinkers may be less severe than the problems experienced by those with alcohol dependence, much of the societal costs associated with alcohol are attributable to these groups.

If you currently exceed safe levels of consumption, you can take steps to control your drinking.

- Make a list of reasons to stop drinking or cut down.
- Set a goal for yourself and make plans to meet it.
- Monitor your drinking so you know exactly when, where, and how much you are drinking.
- Use self-monitoring to identify situations that trigger strong urges to drink.
- Limit the amount of time you spend drinking by drinking slowly, by alternating between alcoholic and nonalcoholic drinks, and by spending less time in drinking settings, such as bars or parties.
- Practice drink refusal skills by establishing nondrinking days. If friends offer you a drink, explain to them that you are not drinking that day. You can offer to be the designated driver on your nondrinking days.
- Don't try to keep up with your friends, and avoid drinking games that promote excessive use.

If you are giving a party at which alcohol will be served, be a responsible host.

- Encourage guests to bring a designated driver.
- Secure safe transportation for those who are intoxicated. Do not let them drive.
- Have plenty of nonalcoholic beverages and high-protein and starchy foods available for the guests.
- Tactfully remove alcoholic beverages from the hands of guests who overindulge.
- Close the bar an hour or two before the party ends.

ⓘ **If you think you may have a problem with alcohol, help is available.** If you think you (or someone you know) has a problem with alcohol, a number of options are available. Self-help groups, such as Alcoholics Anonymous (AA) and Rational Recovery, are widespread in the United States. Treatment centers are also readily available. Most treatment centers focus on abstinence-based treatment, but some help nonalcohol-dependent drinkers control their drinking. The options for treating alcohol dependence have expanded in recent years.

FEATURE 6

The NIAAA conducted a multisite clinical trial demonstrating the effectiveness of 12-step programs (based on the principles of AA). This type of empirical evidence provides confidence in the effectiveness of this approach. The AA program has a strong religious component, which may prevent some people from seeking out (or following through with) the program. Fortunately, there are alternatives to the standard12-step AA programs. The multisite trial mentioned previously (Project MATCH) demonstrated that two other behavioral programs are also effective in treating alcoholism. These programs use different approaches (motivational enhancement and cognitive-behavioral therapy) but appear to be just as effective and can often be implemented in less time. They also place more emphasis on personal control over behavior. The different approaches provide flexibility in treatment and increase the chance for long term succes.The medication naltrexone has also been shown to help those trying to abstain or reduce their alcohol consumption, providing yet another alternative or adjunct to behavioral treatment.

Web Resources

Additional websites with information related to Concept 19 are available at the associated Web link.

Alcohol: A Women's Health Issue, from **NIAAApubs** **.niaaa.nih.gov/publications/brochurewomen/women.htm**
Alcohol: Problems and Solutions **www2.potsdam.edu/** **hansondj/index.html**

Alcoholics Anonymous **www.alcoholics-anonymous.org**
Center on Alcohol Marketing and Youth **http://camy.org/**
Join Together: Advancing Effective Alcohol and Drug Policy, Prevention, and Treatment **www.jointogether.org**
Marin Institute **www.marininstitute.org**
National Clearinghouse for Alcohol and Drug Information (NCADI) **www.health.org**

National Institute on Alcohol Abuse and Alcoholism (NIAAA)
    College Drinking **www.collegedrinkingprevention.gov**

Rational Recovery **www.rational.org**

Rethinking Drinking, from NIAAA **www.rethinkindrinking**
    .niaaa.nih.gov

Smart Recovery **www.smartrecovery.com**

Suggested Readings

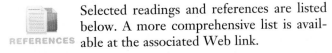

Selected readings and references are listed below. A more comprehensive list is available at the associated Web link.

Anton, R. F., et al. 2007. Combined pharmacotherapies and behavioral interventions for alcohol dependence. *Journal of the American Medical Association* 295:219–220.

Bjerre, B., and Thorsson, U. 2008. Is an alcohol ignition interlock programme a useful tool for changing the alcohol and driving habits of drink-drivers? *Accident Analysis & Prevention* 40:267–273.

Brick, J. (Ed.). 2008. *Handbook of the Medical Consequences of Alcohol and Drug Abuse.* 2nd ed. New York: The Haworth Press/Taylor and Francis Group.

Brown, S. A., et al. 2008. A developmental perspective on alcohol and youths 16 to 20 years of age. *Pediatrics* 121(Suppl4):S290–S310.

Fairlie, A. M., et al. 2010. Fraternity and sorority leaders and members: A comparison of alcohol use, attitudes, and policy awareness. *American Journal of Drug and Alcohol Abuse* 36(4):187–193

Casey, T. R., and Bamforth, C. W. 2010. Silicon in beer and brewing. *Journal of the Science of Food and Agriculture* 90:784–788.

Jacobson, I. G., et al. 2008. Alcohol use and alcohol-related problems before and after military combat deployment. *Journal of the American Medical Association* 300:663–675.

Jatlow, P., and O'Malley, S. S. 2010. Clinical (nonforensic) application of ethyl glucuronide measurement: Are we ready? *Alcoholism: Clinical and Experimental Research* 34:968–975.

Kinney, J. 2008. *Loosening the Grip: A Handbook of Alcohol Information.* 9th ed. New York: McGraw-Hill Higher Education.

LaBrie, J. W., et al. 2009. What men want: The role of reflective opposite-sex normative preferences in alcohol use among college women. *Psychology of Addictive Behaviors* 23:157–162.

Lackey, K. 2009, December 18. Blood-alcohol self-tests spiking. *USA Today.*

Lee, C. M. 2010. The social norms of alcohol-related negative consequences. *Psychology of Addictive Behaviors* 24(2):342–348.

Linton, J. M. 2008. *Overcoming Problematic Alcohol and Drug Use: A Guide for Beginning the Change Process.* New York: Routledge/Taylor & Francis Group.

Outside the Classroom and NASPA. 2009, March 11. College students spend more time drinking than studying. Press release at **www.outsidetheclassroom.com/Upload/images/ PDF/NaspaRelease.pdf.**

Willenbring, M. L. 2007. Medications to treat alcohol dependence: Adding to the continuum of care. *Journal of the American Medical Association* 298:1691–1692.

Wood, P. K., K. J. Sher, and P. C. Rutledge 2007. College student alcohol consumption, day of the week, and class schedule. *Alcoholism: Clinical and Experimental Research* 31:1195–1207.

Zoroya, G. 2009, June 19. Alcohol abuse by GIs soars since '03. *USA Today.*

Lab 19A Blood Alcohol Level

Name **Section** **Date**

Purpose: To learn to calculate your (or a friend's) blood alcohol concentration (BAC)

Procedures

1. Assume a drink is a 12-ounce can or bottle of 5 percent beer or a 5-ounce glass (a small glass) of 12 percent alcohol (wine), or a mixed drink with a 1½-ounce shot glass (jigger) of 80 proof liquor.
   Case A: Assume you consumed two drinks within 40 minutes.
   Case B: Assume you consumed two drinks over a period of 1 hour and 20 minutes.
   Case C: Assume you had two six-packs of beer (12 cans) over 5 hours.
   Case D: Same as C, but, if you weigh less than 150 pounds, assume you weigh 50 pounds more than you now weigh, and, if you weigh more than 150 pounds, assume you weigh 50 pounds less.

2. Divide 3.8 by your weight in pounds to obtain your "BAC maximum per drink," or refer to Table 4 (page 000). You should obtain a number between 0.015 and 0.04 (based on one drink in 40 minutes). Use the formula below to determine BAC over time.

$$\text{Approximate BAC over time} = \frac{(3.8 \times \text{\# of drinks})}{(\text{body weight})} - \frac{[0.01 \times (\text{\# min.} - 40)]}{40}$$

3. After 40 minutes have passed, your body will begin eliminating alcohol from the bloodstream at the rate of about 0.01 percent for each additional 40 minutes. Multiply the number of drinks you've had by your "BAC maximum per drink" and subtract 0.01 percent from the number for each 40 minutes that have passed since you began drinking— but don't count the first 40 minutes. Compute your BAC for cases A, B, C, and D.

   Example: Case A. Mary weighs 100 pounds. $\dfrac{3.8 \times 2}{100} = \dfrac{7.6}{100} = 0.076\%$ BAC

   Case B. Mary takes 80 minutes. $0.076\% - \dfrac{[0.01 \times (80 - 40)]}{40} = 0.066\%$ BAC

4. Record your results below by writing the formula and computing the BAC for each case.

Results

Case A $\dfrac{(3.8 \times \underline{\quad} \text{\# of drinks})}{\underline{\quad} \text{lbs}} = \underline{\quad} \%$ BAC

Case B $\dfrac{(3.8 \times \underline{\quad}\text{\# of drinks})}{\underline{\quad} \text{lbs}} - \dfrac{[0.01 \times (\underline{\quad}\text{\# min.} - 40)]}{40} = \text{BAC} (\quad) - (\quad) = \underline{\quad}\%$ BAC

Case C $\dfrac{(3.8 \times \underline{\quad}\text{\# of drinks})}{\underline{\quad} \text{lbs}} - \dfrac{[0.01 \times (\underline{\quad}\text{\# min.} - 40)]}{40} = \text{BAC} (\quad) - (\quad) = \underline{\quad}\%$ BAC

Case D $\dfrac{(3.8 \times \underline{\quad}\text{\# of drinks})}{\underline{\quad} \text{lbs}} - \dfrac{[0.01 \times (\underline{\quad}\text{\# min.} - 40)]}{40} = \text{BAC} (\quad) - (\quad) = \underline{\quad}\%$ BAC

1. Would you (or your friend) be able to drive legally according to your state laws? Place an X over your answer.

Case A   (Yes) (No)

Case B   (Yes) (No)

Case C   (Yes) (No)

Case D   (Yes) (No)

2. Would you (or your friend) be able to drive legally if the Health Goals for the Year 2020 (.08) were put into effect? Place an X over your answer.

Case A   (Yes) (No)

Case B   (Yes) (No)

Case C   (Yes) (No)

Case D   (Yes) (No)

Conclusions and Implications: In several sentences, discuss what you have learned from doing this activity.

Lab 19B Perceptions about Alcohol Use

Name		Section	Date

Purpose: To better understand perceptions about drinking behaviors

Procedures

1. Think of a person you care about. Do not identify this person on this lab report.
2. Answer each of the questions in the questionnaire below as honestly as possible, evaluating the behavior of the person you have identified. Calculate a total score and determine a rating (see Chart 1).
3. At another time, when you do not have to submit your results, you should answer the questions about yourself.
4. Answer the questions in the Conclusions and Implications section.

Results

Question	Never	Sometimes	Frequently	Too Often	Add Score
1. How often does the person drink?	0	1	2	3	
2. How often does the person have six or more drinks on one occasion?	0	1	2	3	
3. How often do friends of the person drink?	0	1	2	3	
4. How often has the person been unable to stop after starting to drink?	0	1	2	3	
5. How often does the person need a drink to get started in the morning?	0	1	2	3	
6. How often has the person been unable to remember previous events after drinking?	0	1	2	3	
7. How often does the person miss class or work associated with drinking?	0	1	2	3	
8. How often does the person have social or personal problems associated with drinking?	0	1	2	3	
9. How often does the person deny drinking too much (only for those who you consider to drink too much)?	0	1	2	3	

Total Score _____

Chart 1 ▶ Drinking Behavior Rating Scale

Rating	Score
Alcohol abuse*	18+
Drinking problem	12–17
Potential problem	8–11
Low risk of problem	<8

*Professional help recommended.

_____ **Rating**

Conclusions and Implications

1. In several sentences, discuss the drinking behavior of the person you identified. Do you think your ratings give an accurate picture of the person? Do you think the person you rated has a problem with alcohol?

2. In several sentences, discuss the drinking behavior of the person's friends. Do the friends promote drinking, or not?

3. In several sentences, discuss things that you could do to help a friend or loved one solve a drinking problem.

The Use and Abuse of Other Drugs

Health Goals for the Year 2020

- Reduce substance abuse to protect the health, safety, and quality of life for all, especially children.
- Reduce deaths and injuries caused by drug-related motor vehicle crashes.
- Reduce past-month use of illicit substances.
- Increase effectiveness of drug abuse treatment programs.
- Reduce proportion of youth offered drugs or sold drugs at school.
- Reduce nonmedical use of prescription drugs.
- Increase age of onset and proportion of young people who remain drug free.
- Reduce inhalant use.

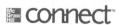

| FITNESS AND WELLNESS   http://connect.mcgraw-hill.com

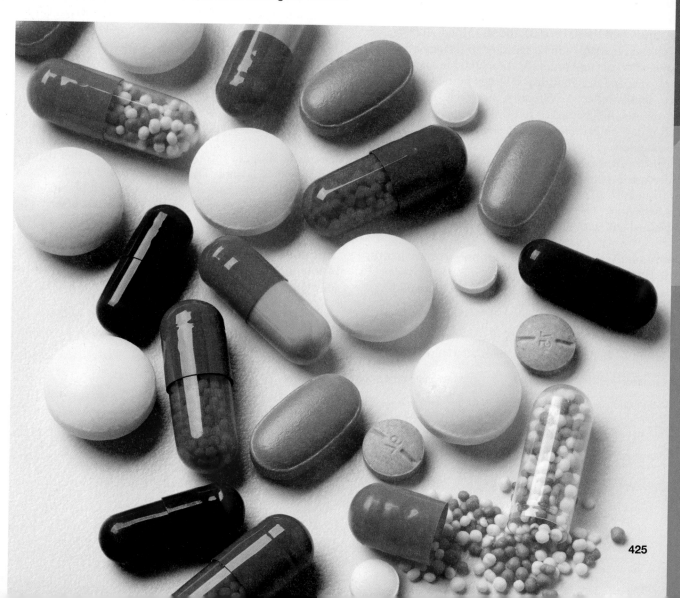

Drug abuse has serious health consequences and enormous personal, social, and economic costs.

About 35 percent of college students reported using illegal drugs in the past year, up from a low of 29 percent in 1991 but far below the 56.2 percent who used illicit drugs in 1980. Of serious concern are rates of illicit drug use among 12th-graders (37 percent), which are even higher than among college students and represent the peak rate for any age group. Millions of people are arrested each year for drug offenses—including sale, distribution, and possession. This has a tremendous cost to society. This concept discusses **drug abuse** and misuse with an emphasis on illegal, so-called, street drugs.

Classification of Illicit and Prescription Drugs

Drugs can be classified in several ways, but the mood-altering, or psychoactive, drugs are the ones we hear about most. Mood-altering, or **psychoactive drugs** can be classified in six major groups: depressants, opiate narcotics, stimulants, hallucinogens, marijuana, and designer drugs. Drugs in the same group have similar effects. Narcotics, however, are actually depressants, but because the word *narcotics* is so widely used in law enforcement and in society in general, they are generally given their own category. Each of the six categories of drugs is discussed in this concept. Their effects are classified as either physiological or psychological (primarily affecting the body versus primarily affecting behavior). The effects of drugs can vary with each individual and with different doses.

Depressant drugs include alcohol, tranquilizers, and barbiturates. Depressants come in the form of pills, liquids, and injectables (see Table 1). In small doses, they slow heart rate and respiration. In larger doses, they act as a poison and damage every organ system in the body. In large enough doses, they can dramatically depress heart rate and respiration enough to cause death, if quick intervention is not available. In terms of their effect on behavior, the user might at first feel stimulated, despite their depressant effects. Depression, loss of coordination, drop in energy level, mood swings, and confusion occur after prolonged use. Alcohol is the most widely used depressant; it is discussed in detail in Concept 19.

Opiate narcotics include heroin, codeine, morphine, and methadone. Narcotics are either smoked, injected, sniffed, or swallowed (see Table 2). Narcotics are often used clinically to treat pain; however, heroin has no legal medical use in the United States and has a high rate of addiction. It is three times stronger than other medicinal narcotics and induces different physiological effects. Narcotics are all opium poppy derivatives or synthetics that emulate them. The *narco-* part of the word derives from the Greek word for sleep, because of its sleep-inducing properties.

Every narcotic, legal or illegal, is a potential poison. A single dose can be fatal, although this is rare. Deaths related to narcotic abuse are typically caused by overdose, impurities of the drug, or mixing of the drug with other depressants, such as alcohol. The mixing of drugs in the same or similar categories can produce a heightened physiological effect known as synergism, or the **synergistic effect.** The combined use makes drug taking far more dangerous.

Some effects of stimulants are described in Table 3. One of these stimulants—cocaine—comes in powder form (coke) and a rocklike form (crack). The

---

Table 1 ▶ Depressants ("Downers," Sedatives)

Examples	Physiological Effects	Psychological Effects
• Tranquilizers (e.g., Valium, Xanax, meprobamate, sleeping pills, methaqualone) are also called tranks, downers, or candy	• In large doses, act as a poison and damage every organ system	• After prolonged use: depression, loss of coordination, drop in energy level, mood swings, confusion, euphoria
• Barbiturates (e.g., Mebaral, Nembutal)	• Quick sedation: vomiting; loss of motor and neurological control; combined with alcohol, can lead to coma and death	• Amnesia

Table 2 ▶ Opiate Narcotics

Examples	Physiological Effects	Psychological Effects
• Codeine • Morphine • Synthetic opiates (e.g., Vicodin, Oxycontin) • Methadone	• Narcotics: blockage of pain, chronic constipation, depressed respiration, redness and irritation of nostrils, nausea, lowered sexual drive, impaired immune system	• Narcotics (including herion): euphoria and feeling of pleasure; nontherapeutic doses may result in mental distress, such as fear and nervousness; in heavy users, drowsiness and apathy may occur
• Heroin (also called brown sugar, junk, or smack)	• Heroin: blood clots, bacterial endocarditis, serum hepatitis, brain abscess, HIV infection (from shared needles); in pregnant users, high risk of miscarriage, stillbirths, birth defects, toxemia, addicted babies	

Table 3 ▶ Stimulants

Examples	Physiological Effects	Psychological Effects
• Cocaine (also called coke, blow, snow, or crack)	• Cocaine: sore throat, hoarseness, shortness of breath (leads to bronchitis and emphysema), dilated pupils, "lights" seen around objects	• Powder Cocaine: initial rush of energy, feeling of confidence; as it wears off: depression, moodiness, irritability, severe mental disorders • Crack: intense euphoria, then crushing depression, intense feeling of self-hate; as it wears off: depression and sadness, intense anxiety about where to get more drugs, aggressiveness, paranoia
• Amphetamines and powder methamphetamines (also called speed, uppers, or black beauties); diet and pep pills, Ritalin	• Excite central nervous system; increase blood pressure, respiration, and heart rate (sometimes resulting in convulsions and stroke); reduce appetite; highly addictive; overdose is fatal; with increased use: dizziness, headaches, sleeplessness; with long-term use: progressive brain damage, malnutrition	• Initially, feeling of being invincible, alertness, excitement; with increased use: feeling of anxiety; with long-term use: hallucinations, psychosis
• Crystal methamphetamine (also called meth, crystal, crank, or ice)	• Extreme energy, sleeplessness, seizures, flushed skin, constricted pupils	• Major effect is toxic psychosis; euphoria, delusions of grandeur, feelings of invincibility, violent when provoked
• Caffeine	• Increased metabolism, heart rate, respiration, and urine output; decreased sleep time and quality; headache and fatigue on withdrawal	• Increased energy level, reduced fatigue, and improved performance on simple tasks; irritability on withdrawal

timing and magnitude of effects of cocaine vary depending on whether it is inhaled, injected, or smoked. The low cost of crack has contributed to its abuse. Combining cocaine and alcohol use leads to production of cocaethylene, which increases risk for overdose. Amphetamines and methamphetamines are also classified as stimulants due to their effects on the central nervous system. Stimulants are often included in diet pills to reduce appetite; others (e.g., Ritalin) are used clinically to treat attention deficit disorder.

Crystal methamphetamine (also known as ice, meth, or crystal) is a purified methamphetamine that also comes

Drug Abuse The use of a drug to the extent that it impairs social, psychological, or physiological functioning.

Psychoactive Drug Any drug that produces a temporary change in the physiological functions of the nervous system, affecting mood, thoughts, feelings, or behavior.

Synergistic Effect The joint actions of two or more drugs that increase the effects of each.

in rock form or powder. As a powder, it is usually smoked in a glass pipe or cigarette. It is a powerful stimulant, with an effect that lasts 8 to 30 hours. Much like crack cocaine, ice is a concentrated form of an already potent stimulant drug that is either smoked or injected. Also like crack, ice causes an intense "rush" or "flash," which is experienced as highly pleasurable. Because the initial rush lasts for only a few minutes, users need to administer the drug frequently to maintain the effects. Tobacco, which contains the powerful stimulant nicotine, is discussed in detail in Concept 18.

Drugs that cause the user to have hallucinations are called hallucinogens, or psychedelics. PCP and LSD are among the psychedelic drugs that cause **hallucinations** (see Table 4). Less-known drugs in this category include mushrooms, or "shrooms," which are chewed, and peyote cactus buttons. They are used legally by some American Indians in religious rites.

Inhalants are sometimes classified separately from other hallucinogens because their effects are so serious. They reach the brain in seconds, and the effect lasts only a few minutes. They come in three types: (1) solvents, such as glue, gasoline, paints, paint thinner, typewriter correction fluid, lighter fluid, shoe polish, and liquid wax; (2) aerosols, such as hair spray, air fresheners, insect spray, and spray paint; and (3) nitrites, including amyl nitrite, nitrous oxide (laughing gas), and butyl nitrite (a room odorizer or liquid incense).

Marijuana is classified as a hallucinogenic, but its effects are less dramatic than those of other drugs in this class. The active ingredient in marijuana (delta-9-tetrahydrocannabinol—THC) is technically a hallucinogen (see Table 5). Marijuana use became widespread in the 1960s and, despite decreased use over time, is still the most widely used illicit substance in the United States. Marijuana use

Table 4 ▶ Hallucinogens (Psychedelics)

Examples	Physiological Effects	Psychological Effects
• Lysergic acid diethylamide (LSD, also called acid, boomers, or cubes)	• Changes chromosomes and may result in birth defects of babies of users; bad trips, confusion, flashback	• Vivid hallucinations, feelings of overlapping/merging of the senses, expanded consciousness and mystical experiences, stimulated awareness and desire, confusion, flashback
• Phencyclidine (PCP)	• Accumulates in fat cells and may remain in body longer than most drugs; impaired immune system, poor coordination, weight loss, speech problems, heart and lung failure, irreversible brain damage, convulsions, coma, death	• Insensitivity to pain can lead to death; euphoria, depersonalization, hallucinations, delirium, amnesia, tunnel vision, loss of control, violent behavior
• Inhalants (solvents, aerosols, and nitrites, also known as poppers, rush)	• Slow reaction time, headache, nausea, vomiting, seizure, brain damage, suffocation, heart attack, death, double vision, sensitivity to light, dizziness, loss of coordination, weakness, numbness; irregular heartbeat, liver and kidney failure, bone marrow damage	• Giddiness, overexcitement, less inhibition, feelings of being all-powerful; powerfulness soon fades and leaves irritability

Table 5 ▶ Marijuana (Subclass of Hallucinogens)

• Marijuana (containing tetrahydrocannabinol, or THC) is also called pot, grass, weed, blunt, or herb	• Long-term use: bronchitis, emphysema and lung cancer, bloodshot eyes, heart disease, infertility, sexual dysfunction, permanent memory loss (brain damage)	• May not hallucinate; pleasant, relaxed feeling; giddiness; self-preoccupation; less precise thinking; impaired task performance; inertia; with prolonged use: may be withdrawn and apathetic, have anxiety reactions, paranoia; eventually, decreased motivation and enthusiasm, reduced ability to absorb and integrate effectively, profoundly impaired scholastic performance

Table 6 ▶ Designer Drugs

Examples	Effects
Date Rape Drugs Rohypnol Gamma hydroxy butyrate (GHB) is also called Georgia homeboy or liquid ecstasy Ketamine (also called Special K)	Predominantly central nervous system depressants; Rohypnol incapacitates, may cause amnesia; GHB can cause comas, seizures, insomnia, anxiety, tremors, nausea, and sweating; Ketamine can cause delirium, amnesia, impaired motor function, high blood pressure, depression, and potentially fatal respiratory problems
3-4 methylenedioxymethamphetamine (MMDA, also called ecstasy, or X)	May cause irregular heart beat, intensified heart problems, exhaustion, liver and brain damage, nervousness, muscle tension, and dry mouth; initial feelings of calm may be followed by psychosis and/or psychological burnout

leads to a range of experiences, which differ from person to person. Marijuana is generally smoked in a pipe, joint, or bong, although it can also be eaten and is also smoked in hollowed-out cigars called blunts.

(i) FEATURE 1 **Designer drugs, which are made in laboratories, have many of the same properties as the drugs they simulate, such as pain relievers, anesthetics, and amphetamines.** Designer drugs (see Table 6) are modifications of illegal or restricted drugs made by chemists working illicitly to create street drugs that are not specifically listed as controlled. They change the molecular structure of an existing drug to create a new substance. Since new drugs are being created all the time, their potential effects are unknown.

Criminal justice (law enforcement, private legal cases, property destruction, etc.) (72%)

Treatment (2.7%)

Early death (3%)

Reduced productivity (7.2%)

Social programs and other costs (14%)

Figure 1 ▶ The estimated cost of drug abuse (percentage of total costs).

Source: National Institute on Drug Abuse.

The Consequences of Drug Use

(i) FEATURE 2 **Drug use takes a human toll in terms of increased morbidity and mortality and lost productivity.** Over 1.7 million drug-related visits to the emergency room (ER) are reported annually. Also annually, over 38,000 people die of drug-induced causes, including poisonings and deaths related to prescription drug use. This does not take into account the indirect effects of drug use on mortality, including deaths from accidents, homicides, and AIDS (acquired via intravenous drug use). Because of problems with low productivity in the workplace, a large percentage of American businesses now conduct employee drug tests.

Drug use also has significant economic costs. The economic costs of illicit drug abuse are estimated at approximately $180 billion a year. Approximately 22.5 million people abuse or are dependent on illicit drugs, but most of the national economic burden is not related to treatment (3 percent). More than half of the costs are

associated with drug-related crime. Figure 1 illustrates the proportion of societal costs resulting from factors such as law enforcement expenditures, social programs, and reduced productivity.

(i) FEATURE 3 **Drug use can lead to significant legal problems, resulting in jail time and substantial fines.** State laws regarding the possession and sale of illicit drugs vary considerably, and penalties within states vary based on the amount of the drug, the type of drug, and the type of offense (possession, sales, or production). Penalties for the possession of small amounts are the least severe, with penalties for the sale or production of large amounts the most severe. Still, the penalties for the possession of even small

Hallucinations Imaginary things seen, felt, or heard or things seen in a distorted way.

amounts of illicit drugs are substantial. In most states, the maximum jail time for possession ranges from 6 months to a year for marijuana and from 1 to 7 years for cocaine, methamphetamine, and ecstasy. In addition, fines between $500 and $1,000 for marijuana and between $5,000 and $25,000 for other illicit drugs are typical of most states.

Use and Abuse of Drugs

Drug use generally begins with cigarette smoking and alcohol use. Of course, most people who smoke or drink will not go on to use illegal drugs, but it is rare for people who do not smoke or drink to use illegal drugs. The average age for starting to smoke cigarettes is 12; for alcohol and marijuana, about 13. In general, the younger a person is when he or she starts using drugs, including nicotine and alcohol, the more likely that person is to use illegal drugs and the more likely he or she is to become physically dependent on drugs.

Most experts agree that drug use and abuse are complex phenomena that must be understood within a biopsychosocial model. The biopsychosocial model suggests that biological, psychological, and social factors must all be considered in understanding substance use and abuse. From this perspective, the potential for **addiction** depends on a host of factors, including genetic vulnerability, the type of drug used, the route of administration, attitudes toward drug use, expectations regarding drug effects, peer use, and ease of access.

Genetics play a role in susceptibility to drug addiction. Research has suggested that genetic factors explain as much as 50 percent of alcohol and nicotine addiction, and the same is likely true for other drugs of abuse. The effect of genetics (and susceptibility to addiction) depends on how the drug is used and how it impacts the brain. Some drugs act on receptors in the brain that are specific to that drug (e.g., cannabanoid receptors for marijuana; opioid receptors for heroin and prescription narcotics); whereas others act on more general neurotransmitters associated with reward (e.g., effects of cocaine and methamphetamine on the dopamine system) and the regulation of mood and behavior (e.g., MDMA effects on the serotonin system). Because both the dopamine and opioid systems are directly related to the experience of reward, drugs like heroin and cocaine that impact these systems are particularly addictive. The route of administration also affects risk for addiction. For example, the likelihood of becoming addicted to cocaine is much higher if it is smoked as crack than if it is inhaled as powder.

Psychological factors such as personality traits, attitudes, perceptions of risk, and expectations of benefits can influence drug use. Individuals with higher levels of sensation seeking and impulsivity have been shown to be at increased risk for use of a range of illicit drugs. Those who believe drug use is acceptable and affiliate with others with similar views are also more likely to use drugs and to develop problems. These attitudes are influenced by both parental and peer attitudes as well as the attitudes of the broader culture. Perceptions of risk are also a strong predictor of drug use. In fact, national studies have consistently found that shifts in perceptions of risk related to specific drugs precede changes in rates of use of those drugs. Much like alcohol, those who believe drugs will have strong positive effects are more likely to use and abuse them. This is

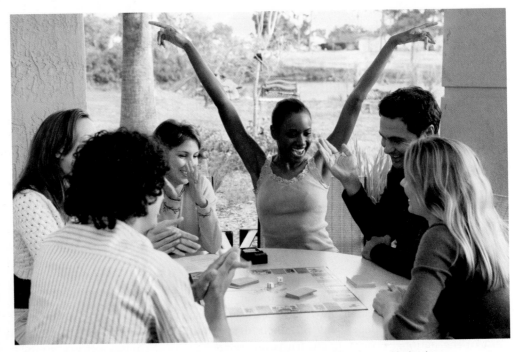

Connecting with the right social group can help you adopt positive lifestyles and behaviors.

particularly true for those who believe that drug use is an effective way to cope with stress.

Social factors and social norms have important effects on drug use. People who live in areas where drugs are readily available are at increased risk for both use and abuse. Another major influence on drug use in young people is the extent to which their social group engages in drug use. Those who perceive that most of their peers use drugs are likely to use drugs themselves.

Although use of most illicit substances has decreased in the past decade, rates of use remain high among adolescents and young adults. In the United States, rates of illicit drug use peaked in the 1970s followed by sharp decreases during the 1980s (see Figure 2). Overall drug use by adolescents spiked upward in the early 1990s, primarily as a result of two- to threefold increases in marijuana use. Rates of illicit drug use then began a steady but gradual decline during the first decade of the new century. Unfortunately, rates of illicit drug use in the United States increased in 2008 for both 8th- and 10th-graders. In addition, prescription drug use has been the one exception with respect to the overall decreases in drug use in the past decade. Use of these drugs hit a historical peak in 2001 and has remained relatively stable since. Among adolescents and young adults, rates of use of prescription narcotics (7 to 9 percent) and tranquilizers (5 to 7 percent) exceed those of all illicit drugs other than marijuana.

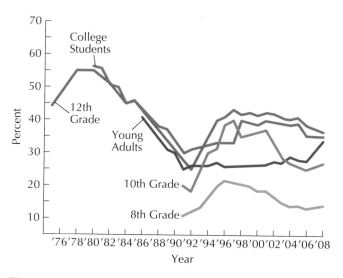

Figure 2 ▶ Trends in annual prevalence of an illicit drug use index across five populations.

Notes: Use of "any illicit drugs" includes any use of marijuana, LSD, other hallucinogens, crack, other cocaine, or heroin, or any use that is not under a doctor's orders of other opiates, stimulants, barbiturates, methaqualone (excluded since 1990), or tranquilizers.

Source: National Institute on Drug Abuse.

Technology Update
Epigenetic Effects of Cocaine Identified

A new area of genetic research called "epigenetics" is shedding new light on the process of addiction. Epigenetics is the study of processes that affect gene expression without actually changing the genetic structure. A recent study in mice found that repeated cocaine administration repressed an enzyme (G9a) that is critical in gene expression in the nucleus accumbens, an area of the brain associated with pleasure and desire. The suppression of this enzyme was associated with increased preference for cocaine, and reversing this suppression reduced cocaine preference. This type of epigenetic research may identify mechanisms that can be targeted in the development of new medications to treat addictions.

Rates of illicit drug use among college students are among the highest of any age group. High rates of drug use in college are associated with a host of negative consequences, including impaired cognitive abilities and academic performance, increased risk of accidents and injuries, greater incidence of high-risk sexual behavior, and increased risk for substance abuse or dependence. Students who use drugs have less academic motivation and report lower involvement in religion, community service, and extracurricular activities on campus.

Much like alcohol, both direct and indirect peer influences are important predictors of use among college students. Students with friends who use marijuana are more likely to use it themselves. Misperceptions of normative behavior may also influence personal behavior. One study found that 98 percent of students incorrectly believed that the typical student on campus used marijuana at least once per year, despite the fact that most of the students reported no personal use of marijuana. Although both direct and indirect peer influences may contribute to drug use, these same influences can also deter use. One study found that peers exposed to a peer group with strong anti-drug attitudes were likely to conform to this norm.

The development of new drugs contributes to the maintenance of drug use in the United States. New drugs are always being manufactured, and new

---

Addiction A drug-induced condition in which a person requires frequent administration of a drug in order to avoid withdrawal; also referred to as physical dependence.

ways of administering old drugs often lead to a resurgence in use. Club drugs provide examples of new drugs, and crack cocaine and crystal methamphetamine are examples of old drugs that became popular in new forms. When these new drugs become available, information about their benefits is generally spread immediately by word of mouth. In contrast, the risks associated with use are often unknown until the drug has been used for a number of years. This gives new drugs time to become popular before information that might deter their use is available. Ecstasy is a good example of this phenomenon. Fortunately, public campaigns by the National Institute on Drug Abuse and other agencies to provide information about risks helped curb levels of use relatively quickly. Ecstasy use declined dramatically after peaking at the turn of the 21st century. In addition to the introduction of new drugs, there seems to be a "generational forgetting" of the risks associated with older drugs that leads to a resurgence in their use after years of reduced prevalence. Increases in the use of drugs that have been decreasing or stable for a period of time are first identified in the youngest users. Increases in usage are then noted in other (older) age groups as the young users age.

Marijuana is the most widely used [illicit] drug in the United States and is associated with a host of physical health and social consequences. FEATURE 4 In a national survey, over 15 million Americans, or roughly 6 percent of people over the age of 12, reported the use of marijuana in the past month (see Figure 3). Although many believe it is a relatively safe drug, and some favor decriminalization or legalization, a number of risks are associated with marijuana use. With respect to health, chronic marijuana use leads to many of the negative consequences associated with cigarette smoking, including cardiovascular disease and lung cancer. One study showed that marijuana use also increases risk for stroke. Another

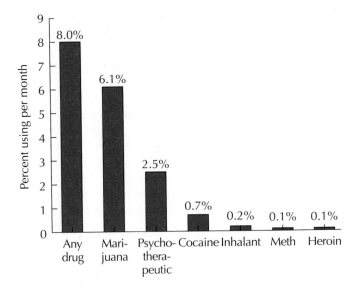

Figure 3 ▶ Illicit drug use among persons 12 and older, by drug (% per month).
Source: Substance Abuse and Mental Health Services Administration.

study found that marijuana use leads to nearly a fivefold increase in acute risk for a heart attack, especially among those with existing cardiovascular risk. Marijuana use is also associated with impaired cognitive abilities. For example, adolescents who use marijuana heavily have been shown to have deficits in attention, learning, and processing speed. There is also direct evidence from neuroimaging studies for differences in brain function. In particular, areas of the brain associated with processing of emotional information appear to be affected. These findings are cause for concern, given evidence for increased risk of emotional problems among individuals who use marijuana. For example, a recent study found that marijuana use increased risk for experiencing panic attacks.

Although the debate is ongoing regarding the addictive (physical dependence) potential of marijuana, it is clear that one can become psychologically addicted to the drug. Psychological dependence is characterized by craving for the drug and continued use despite negative consequences. There is also emerging evidence that those who try to quit using marijuana experience withdrawal symptoms. For example, a recent study found that smokers of marijuana experienced withdrawal symptoms that were quite similar to those of tobacco smokers, including irritability, anxiety, and sleep difficulties.

Stimulants, including cocaine and methamphetamine, are the second most commonly used illicit drugs. FEATURE 5 Cocaine and methamphetamine are both stimulant drugs, and they share a number of other characteristics. First, both come

HELP HEALTH is available to Everyone for a Lifetime, and it's Personal

Patterns of use of specific drugs among young adults seem to go up and down in cycles, while overall rates of illicit drug use remain relatively stable. Declines in use of one drug appear to be offset by increases in other drugs (often new ones). The patterns suggest that new drugs and drug trends influence exploration in young adults.

Do you think there is sufficient warning about dangers of drug use or do warnings only attract students to try them?

in powder form as well as more concentrated crystal (ice) or rock (crack) forms. Crack cocaine was one of the most abused drugs in the United States during the peak rates of use in the early to mid-1980s, and crystal methamphetamine was at the center of the more recent but less dramatic increase in illicit drug use in the early 1990s. Crack and ice also share the characteristic of being highly addictive. Because of the intense, short-lived high associated with using these drugs, patterns of repeated use are developed quickly, leading to rapid development of dependence. Both drugs are also known to damage dopamine neurons in the brain and lead to a host of short- and long-term health consequences. Short-term effects that occur after the initial high include irritability, anxiety, and paranoia. In terms of long-term risk, cocaine and methamphetamine use lead to increased risk for stroke, respiratory problems (including respiratory failure), irregular heartbeat, heart attacks, and psychiatric symptoms.

Unique physical consequences of methamphetamine use include poor complexion and tooth loss, which is costly and extremely distressing. Ice has added risks associated with its production. Because some of the products used to produce meth (e.g., pseudoephedrine) have legitimate pharmaceutical uses, policies have been put in place to monitor their sale. If you go to your pharmacy to purchase an over-the-counter decongestant, you may be asked to provide identification and a signature.

Caffeine is used by over 80 percent of the population on a daily basis. Many believe that caffeine allows them to function more effectively, particularly when sleep-deprived. Although there is evidence of improved performance on certain types of tasks, caffeine does not appear to improve negative mood states among those who are sleep-deprived, and there is evidence for a number of negative effects of caffeine. For example, caffeine intake (particularly in the evening) can negatively impact sleep length and quality. There is also evidence of increased risk for cardiovascular disease among chronic users due to associated increases in blood pressure and cortisol. Caffeine use may also negatively impact mental health. For example, caffeine has been found to increase anxiety levels among vulnerable individuals.

The continued use of club drugs is a concern, given strong evidence of their harmful effects. Club drugs include ecstasy (MDMA), Rohypnol, GHB, Ketamine, DOM, DOB, and NEXUS. Ecstasy, a hallucinogen, is inhaled, injected, or swallowed. The drug was initially popular at all-night dance parties called raves, but its use quickly expanded beyond the club scene. Ecstasy alters brain levels of serotonin, negatively

impacts memory, and affects the brain regions that regulate sleep, mood, and learning. Recently, a more potent form of ecstasy sold in capsules or as powder has been a major concern in several areas of the country. This type of ecstasy is often referred to as "Molly." The negative effects of ecstasy may last as long as 7 years. Dealers often pass off other drugs as ecstasy, and they are often even more dangerous.

Rohypnol and GHB are predominately central nervous system depressants, like the other sedative drugs described previously. These drugs are odorless, colorless, and tasteless, so they can be added to food or beverages without the consumer detecting their presence. Because of these properties, Rohypnol and GHB are known as drug-assisted assault or date-rape drugs. In addition to incapacitating the user, these drugs lead to anterograde amnesia, or the inability to remember events that occur after consumption. Women should be especially careful not to leave their drinks unattended or to accept drinks from strangers.

ⓘ **FEATURE 6** **Inhalant use poses a serious risk to physical health, including risk for sudden death.** Those who use inhalants are at risk for what is known as "sudden sniffing death." Sniffing inhalants can lead to irregular and rapid heart rhythms that can cause heart failure and rapid death. This can occur from a single episode of sniffing in an otherwise healthy adolescent.

Misuse and abuse of prescription and over-the-counter (OTC) drugs has become an increasing problem. Prescription drugs are often used inappropriately. Examples include using prescriptions written for other people and using medicines for purposes other than prescribed. Users may also obtain prescription drugs without prescriptions via the Internet, though most who misuse prescription drugs indicate that they obtain them for free from friends or family members. Many fail to recognize the potential risks of prescription drug use, assuming that anything prescribed by a physician must be safe. The more commonly abused prescription drugs among college students include Ritalin, Valium, Xanax, Percoset, Vicodin, and Oxycontin. Sometimes called "hillbilly heroin," Oxycontin is a painkiller that has received much attention because of its misuse by celebrities and its link to many deaths nationwide. However, Vicodin is by far the most widely misused prescription narcotic in the United States. Methadone use without a prescription also appears to be increasing. Methadone has been approved in the United States for the treatment of opiate dependence (primarily heroin) since 1972, but it is increasingly making its way into the hands of those without prescriptions. Although nonprescription use of methadone has not been systematically tracked, methadone-related overdoses have been. Recent data from the CDC indicate a sevenfold increase in methadone-related deaths in less than a decade. With a street value of about $20 a pill, methadone is considerably cheaper than many of the other prescription opiates, which may have led to its increased popularity.

Rates of misuse of ADHD drugs like Ritalin and Adderall are particularly high among young people, particularly college students who often use the drug in an effort to enhance academic performance. The most recent national data indicate that over 3 percent of college students report using the drug without a prescription in the past year.

Accidental misuse is another common problem. Examples of unwitting misuse of drugs include taking a medicine twice, taking the wrong medicine from unlabeled bottles, and using outdated medicines. Another cause of unintentional misuse is taking multiple medications that negatively interact with one another. Thus, it is important to understand the nature of all the medications you are taking (including supplements, prescription drugs, and OTC drugs) and how they interact. Women who are pregnant, are nursing, or want to get pregnant should avoid drug use, including many prescription drugs. The most recent results of the National Pregnancy and Health Survey, conducted by the National Institute on Drug Abuse (NIDA), estimated that 5.5 percent of the 4 million women who give birth each year in the United States used illegal drugs while they were pregnant.

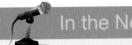

In the News

Risks from Misuse of Prescription Drugs

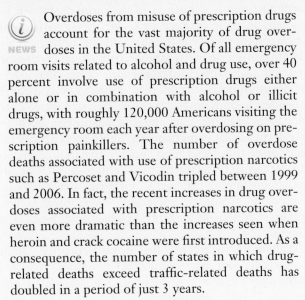

Overdoses from misuse of prescription drugs account for the vast majority of drug overdoses in the United States. Of all emergency room visits related to alcohol and drug use, over 40 percent involve use of prescription drugs either alone or in combination with alcohol or illicit drugs, with roughly 120,000 Americans visiting the emergency room each year after overdosing on prescription painkillers. The number of overdose deaths associated with use of prescription narcotics such as Percoset and Vicodin tripled between 1999 and 2006. In fact, the recent increases in drug overdoses associated with prescription narcotics are even more dramatic than the increases seen when heroin and crack cocaine were first introduced. As a consequence, the number of states in which drug-related deaths exceed traffic-related deaths has doubled in a period of just 3 years.

Taking drugs during pregnancy can result in various conditions, including premature separation of the placenta from the womb, fetal stroke, miscarriage, birth defects, low birth weight babies, babies born addicted to substances, and postnatal risks, including SIDS and learning disabilities.

Strategies for Action

The best way to avoid problems associated with drug use is not to try illegal drugs and to be careful in the use of legal drugs. The information presented in this concept clearly indicates that starting to take a drug for reasons other than managing your own good health increases the risk of taking more drugs in the future. Most readers of this book have already made the decision not to take illegal drugs. However, most people will take medication sometime in their lives. Be continually aware of what you are taking and why. Monitor the use of medications to be sure that you are using them as directed and not with other medications that may result in dangerous synergistic effects.

Learning skills to cope with problems and stress is also essential (see Concept 17). Making responsible decisions is another skill that needs to be learned. Knowing the effects and risks of drugs should help you to make more responsible decisions. To combat peer pressure, the ability to clearly and effectively say no is necessary. Be assertive. And finally, you need to choose friends whose values support, rather than undermine, your own.

People who have a problem with drugs typically will need help to develop skills and personal characteristics to quit using them. For people with a problem, the first step is recognizing that help is needed. In Lab 20A, you will have the opportunity to evaluate the behavior of a friend or loved one to determine if the person needs help. People who need help need to talk to someone they can trust, perhaps a friend or relative. You may be able to help the person seek help from a referral source, such as an employee assistance program, a family or university physician or hospital, or your city or county health department. These sources help get the person into a treatment program or support group. Some of the better-known nationwide programs include Alcoholics (or Narcotics or Cocaine) Anonymous and Al-Anon Family Groups. Another option is to look in the yellow pages of the telephone book for programs operated by public and private agencies. Still another possibility is to call a hotline, and someone will direct you to help in your area. You might try one or more of these three sources:

- National Institute on Drug Abuse (NIDA) Hotline (1-800-662-HELP)
- Cocaine Helpline (1-800-COCAINE)
- Just Say No International (1-800-258-2766)

If you think a fellow student might have a problem with illicit or prescription drugs, help is probably available within the counseling center at your school. Most colleges and universities have information about available substance abuse services on their website. At a later time, it would be wise to answer the questions in Lab 20A for yourself rather than for a friend or loved one. This will allow you to determine if you need help.

Web Resources

Additional websites with information related to Concept 20 are available at the associated Web link.

American Council for Drug Education **www.acde.org**

Federal Drug Data Sources
www.whitehousedrugpolicy.gov/drugfact/sources.html

Help Guide.org
**http://helpguide.org/mental/drug_substance_abuse
_addiction_signs_effects_treatment.htm**

Join Together **www.jointogether.org**

Marin Institute **www.marininstitute.org**

National Clearinghouse for Alcohol and Drug Information
www.health.org

National Institute on Drug Abuse **www.nida.nih.gov**

Office of National Drug Control Policy (ONDCP)
www.whitehousedrugpolicy.gov

The Partnership for a Drug Free America **www.drugfree.org**

The President's National Drug Control Strategy
www.whitehousedrugpolicy.gov/publications/policy/ndcs07

Suggested Readings

Selected readings and references are listed below. A more comprehensive list is available at the associated Web link.

Becker, W. C. 2008. Non-medical use, abuse and dependence on prescription opioids among U.S. adults: Psychiatric, medical and substance use correlates. *Drug and Alcohol Dependence* 94(1–3):38–47.

Budney, A. J., et al. 2008. Comparison of cannabis and tobacco withdrawal: Severity and contribution to relapse. *Journal of Substance Abuse Treatment* 35:362–368.

Centers for Disease Control and Prevention. 2007. Unintentional poisoning deaths—United States, 1999–2004. *Morbidity and Mortality Weekly Reports* 56:93–96.

Gruber, S. A., J. Rogowska, and D. A. Yurgelun-Todd. 2009. Altered affective response in marijuana smokers: An fMRI study. *Drug and Alcohol Dependence* 105:139–153.

Homer, B. D., et al. 2008. Methamphetamine abuse and impairment of social functioning: A review of the underlying neurophysiological causes and behavioral implications. *Psychological Bulletin* 134(2):301–310.

Jacobus, J., et al. 2009. Functional consequences of marijuana in adolescents. *Pharmacology, Biochemistry and Behavior* 92:559–565.

Johnston, L. D., et al. 2009. *Monitoring the Future: National survey results on drug use, 1975-2008* (Vol. II). *NIH Publication No. 09-7403.* Bethesda, MD: National Institute on Drug Abuse.

Ksir, C. J., et al. 2010. *Drugs, Society, and Human Behavior.* 14th ed. New York: McGraw-Hill Higher Education.

Maze, A., et al. 2010. Essential role of the histone methyltransferase G9a in cocaine-induced plasticity. *Science* 327:213–216.

McCabe, S. E. 2008. Misperceptions of non-medical prescription drug use: A web survey of college students. *Addictive Behaviors* 33(5):713–724.

Partnership for a Drug Free America. 2009 Partnership/ MetLife Foundation Attitude Tracking Survey. Available at **www.drugfree.org/Portal/DrugIssue/Research/Teen _Study_2009/National_Study**

Schepis, T. S., and S. Krishnan-Sarin. 2009. Sources of prescriptions for misuse by adolescents: Differences in sex, ethnicity, and severity of misuse in a population-based study. *Journal of the American Academy of Child and Adolescent Psychiatry* 48:828–836.

Setlick, J., J. R. Bond, and M. Ho. 2009. Adolescent prescription ADHD medication abuse is rising along with prescriptions for these medications. *Pediatrics* 124: 875–880.

Substance Abuse and Mental Health Services Administration. 2009. *Results from the 2008 National Survey on Drug Use and Health: National Findings.* (Office of Applied Studies, NSDUH Series H-36, HHS Publication No. SMA 09-4434). Rockville, MD.

Warner, M., L. H. Chen, and D. M. Makuc. 2009. Increase in fatal poisonings involving opioid analgesics in the United States, 1999–2006. *NCHS Data Brief, No 22.* Hyattsville, MD: National Center for Health Statistics.

Wilson, H. T. 2009. *Annual Editions: Drugs, Society and Behavior.* 23rd ed. New York: McGraw-Hill.

Zvolensky, M. J., et al. 2010. Marijuana use and panic psychopathology among a representative sample of adults. *Experimental and Clinical Psychopharmacology* 18:129–134.

Lab 20A Use and Abuse of Other Drugs

Name		Section	Date

Purpose: To evaluate a friend or family member's behavior and potential for becoming an abuser of drugs; if this report is submitted to an instructor, be sure *not* to identify by name the person you are evaluating

Procedure: Answer these questions to determine if the person you are evaluating is an abuser of medications. Place an X over the answer that applies.

A. Prescription Drug Abuse

(Yes) (No) 1. Does he/she take more medicine than prescribed per dosage?

(Yes) (No) 2. Does he/she feel more nervous than ever when the medicine wears off?

(Yes) (No) 3. Does he/she hoard medicine?

(Yes) (No) 4. Does he/she gulp pills?

(Yes) (No) 5. Does he/she hide the amount of medicine taken from friends, family, or his/her doctors?

(Yes) (No) 6. Does his/her doctor know he/she has other doctors, and does the doctor have a list of all the medications he/she is taking from all sources (dentist, family physician, specialists)?

The more questions to which you answered "yes," the more likely he/she is a drug abuser.

B. Risk Factors for Becoming Addicted

(Yes) (No) 1. Have any members of his/her family ever abused drugs?

(Yes) (No) 2. Was he/she abused as a child, or did he/she go through other trauma during childhood?

(Yes) (No) 3. Is he/she now undergoing unusual stress or mental pain?

(Yes) (No) 4. Does he/she have easy access to drugs?

(Yes) (No) 5. Has he/she used or does he/she use drugs recreationally?

(Yes) (No) 6. If he/she has used or now uses drugs recreationally, did or does he/she choose the fastest method of getting a hit?

The more "yes" answers, the greater his/her risk of addiction. (Remember that alcohol is a drug, too.)

C. Signs and Symptoms That a Problem with Drugs Exists

(Yes) (No) 1. Does he/she use drugs as an escape or to cope with a stressful situation?

(Yes) (No) 2. Does he/she become depressed easily?

(Yes) (No) 3. Does he/she use drugs the first thing in the morning?

(Yes) (No) 4. Has he/she ever tried to quit and resumed using again?

(Yes) (No) 5. Does he/she do things under the influence of a drug that he/she would not normally do?

(Yes) (No) 6. Has he/she had any drug-related "close calls" with the police or any arrests?

(Yes) (No) 7. Does he/she think a party or social gathering isn't fun unless drugs are served?

(Yes) (No) 8. Does he/she feel proud of an increased tolerance to drugs?

(Yes) (No) 9. Does he/she use drugs when alone?

(Yes) (No) 10. Has or does he/she use a wide variety of drugs?

(Yes) (No) 11. Is he/she constantly thinking about being high?

(Yes) (No) 12. Does he/she avoid people or places that oppose usage?

(Yes) (No) 13. Has his/her friends, family, teachers, or employer expressed concern about his/her use?

(Yes) (No) 14. Is his/her usage causing him/her to neglect responsibilities?

(Yes) (No) 15. Has he/she ever had blackouts or lack of memory of drug use or other events?

(Yes) (No) 16. Has he/she stolen to get money for drugs?

(Yes) (No) 17. Has he/she seriously considered that he/she might have a drug problem?

The more "yes" answers, the more likely he/she is to have a serious problem with drugs.

Results

A. Does he/she abuse prescription drugs?   (Yes) (No)
   (Questions A: 1–6)

B. Is he/she at considerable risk for addiction?   (Yes) (No)
   (Questions B: 1–6)

C. Does he/she have a serious problem with drugs? (Yes) (No)
   (Questions C: 1–17)

Conclusions and Implications: In several sentences, discuss a plan of action that could be taken by a person who has a problem with the misuse of over-the-counter drugs, prescription drugs, or illegal drugs. Discuss specific things you could do to help a person with a problem. At some point, you may want to answer the questions about yourself.

Preventing Sexually Transmitted Infections

Health Goals for the Year 2020

- Promote responsible sexual behaviors to prevent sexually transmitted infections (STIs) and their complications.

- Reduce incidence of chlamydia, gonorrhea, syphilis, genital herpes, human papillomavirus (HPV), pelvic inflammatory disease (PID), and hepatitis B.

- Increase percentage of family planning agencies with emergency contraception.

- Increase proportion of young people who abstain from sexual intercourse, use condoms during sexual activity, and avoid risky sexual behaviors.

- Increase effective vaccine coverage universally.

- Increase proportion tested for HIV.

- Increase percentage of adolescents who receive formal instruction on reproduction before age 18.

- Increase percentage of sexually active women who receive reproductive health services.

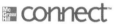

FITNESS AND WELLNESS   http://connect.mcgraw-hill.com

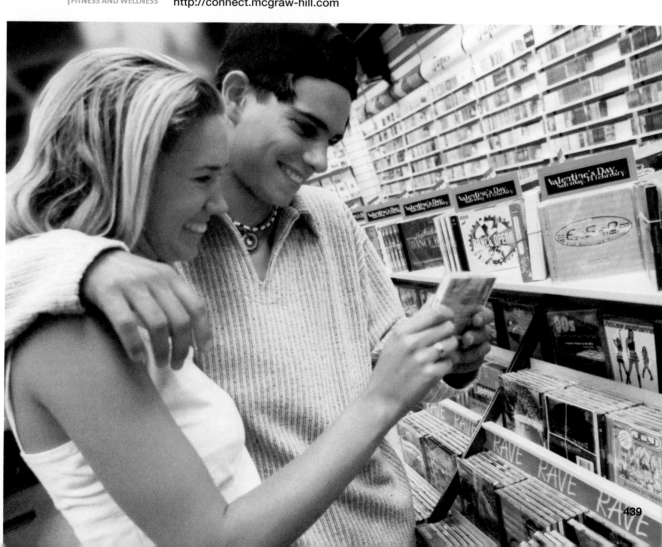

Safe sex and sound information about sexually transmitted infections are important to health and wellness.

The sexual experience is an interpersonal one that influences our actions and behaviors. It is basic to family life and fundamental to the reproduction of the human species. Approached responsibly, the human sexual experience contributes to wellness and quality of life in many ways. When approached irresponsibly, it can result in disease and personal and interpersonal suffering. Learning and adopting safe sex practices are important aspects of a healthy lifestyle. Safe sex is critical for avoiding unwanted pregnancies and for reducing risks for various infections and diseases. This concept provides information about the symptoms, causes, and treatments of various infections and diseases transmitted through sexual contact.

The term *sexually transmitted disease (STD)* has been used to refer to these conditions, but the broader term of **sexually transmitted infection (STI) is now more accepted.** The term STI better reflects the fact that a period of infection typically occurs prior to the emergence of any associated disease symptoms. HIV/AIDS is an example of this, as one can be infected for many years before signs of disease begin to occur. In other cases, STIs never result in identifiable disease symptoms. Human papillomavirus (HPV) is an example of this type of STI. Although HPV can lead to cervical cancer in women, most women infected with HPV never experience disease symptoms. Because *STI* better captures the range of outcomes, this term will be used throughout the remainder of the concept.

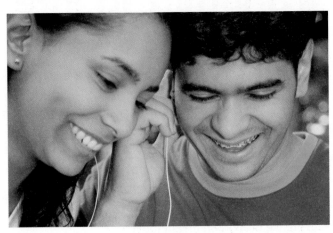

Shared interests can help build healthy relationships with friends.

General Facts

The healthy sexual experience can contribute to wellness in many ways. All five wellness dimensions are involved in decisions concerning participation in, the meaningfulness of, and the long-term consequences of the sexual experience. The healthy sexual experience requires sensitive and thoughtful consideration of the consequences. When approached responsibly, sexual behavior can enhance quality of life in important ways. This fact is evident in a recent study of the reasons that college students have sex. The study of over 1,500 college students identified 237 different reasons for engaging in sexual behavior. Although women tended to report more intimacy reasons and men tended to report more reasons related to physical pleasure, 20 of the top 25 reasons overlapped for men and women. The most common reasons across the full sample were attraction, pleasure,

affection, love, romance, emotional closeness, arousal, the desire to please, adventure, excitement, experience, connection, celebration, curiosity, and opportunity. Although antisocial reasons for sexual behavior were less common, they have the potential for severe negative consequences. For example, one of the very infrequently endorsed reasons for sex was to intentionally infect a partner with an STI, and another was to break up a rival's relationship. Thus, as stated previously, sexual behavior can have both rewarding and costly effects.

Good physical health contributes to an active and satisfying sex life. Two population-based studies in the United States found that individuals who were in good or excellent health were more likely to be sexually active. Among those who were sexually active, good health was associated with greater interest in sex, more frequent sex, and a better-quality sex life. On average, being in good health increased the sexual life expectancy for men by 5 to 7 years and for women by 3 to 6 years.

Unsafe sexual activity can result in disease, poor health, and much pain and suffering. Until the 1940s, STIs were a leading cause of death. The discovery of penicillin and other antibiotics, and improved public health practices, lowered the death rate from STIs, but they have remained a significant health problem. In 1991, STIs became one of the 10 leading causes of death in the United States, principally because of the high death rate from **acquired immune deficiency syndrome (AIDS)** caused by the **human immunodeficiency virus (HIV). The development of** more effective treatments have reduced deaths from HIV/AIDS and moved STIs off the top ten list.

HIV/AIDS

Of all the STIs, HIV/AIDS poses the greatest health threat to the world. Health experts remind us that we are still in the midst of a worldwide HIV/AIDS epidemic. Currently, over 56,000 people in the United States are infected with HIV annually, with a total of over 1.1 million people currently infected. Worldwide, the problem is even more profound, with roughly 1.7 million people infected each year and a total of more than 33 million people currently living with HIV. The problem of HIV/AIDS is particularly bad in sub-Saharan Africa, which accounts for roughly 67 percent of the global prevalence of HIV. Rates vary considerably across countries, with a high of 27 percent in Swaziland. International health agencies have been working to address the gap in awareness and the limited access to treatments in these parts of the world. Fortunately, these efforts are starting to pay off, with a 25 percent decrease in new HIV infections in 2008 relative to the peak in 1995.

Women and minorities are populations in which the incidence of HIV/AIDS is increasing disproportionately. What was once thought to be a disease of males, especially gay men, is now increasingly a female condition. Women now represent roughly 27 percent of those living with HIV in the United States and roughly half of the global cases of HIV. Ethnic minority groups in the United States are also disproportionately affected, with roughly 45 percent of new cases occurring among African Americans and another 17 percent occurring among Hispanics. This discrepancy is largest among women, with African American women accounting for 66 percent of new cases among women.

(i) **HIV attacks the immune system and can lead to AIDS.** A test of **serostatus** can indicate

FEATURE 1 if a person is seropositive. When a person tests seropositive for HIV, it means that a blood test has indicated the presence in the body of the HIV. HIV invades the body's immune system cells, even killing them. This results in damage to the immune system and the body's ability to fight infections. One of the principal problems is that HIV causes immune suppression by directly invading and killing **CD4+ helper cells.** When too many of these cells (also called **T helper cells**) are destroyed, the body cannot fight **opportunistic infections** effectively.

When T cell counts are low and the **viral load** is high, the immune system can not function properly, thereby making the seropositive person more susceptible to various types of diseases and disorders. **Antibodies** in the blood that normally fight infections are ineffective in stopping the HIV from invading the body.

HIV comes in many forms, creating unique challenges for treatment. There are two primary types of HIV (HIV1 and HIV2). HIV2 appears to be less contagious and to have a longer latency between infection and disease, but the vast majority of cases of AIDS are due to HIV1. There are three groups of HIV1 (M, N, and O), with the M, or "Major," type accounting for most cases. Within the M group, there are at least nine different subtypes, though type B (predominant in the United States and Europe) and type C (predominant in south and east Africa) account for the majority of the global epidemic.

An individual has AIDS when he or she is infected with HIV and develops opportunistic diseases because of impairment of the immune system. Examples of opportunistic diseases associated with AIDS are pneumonia, tuberculosis, **Kaposi's sarcoma,** yeast infections, and cervical cancer. Other symptoms include

Sexually Transmitted Infection (STI) An infection for which a primary method of transmission is sexual activity.

Acquired Immune Deficiency Syndrome (AIDS) An HIV-infected individual is said to have AIDS when he or she has developed certain opportunistic infections (for example, pneumonia, tuberculosis, yeast infections, or other infections) or when his or her CD4+ cell count drops below 200.

Human Immunodeficiency Virus (HIV) A virus that causes a breakdown of the immune system in humans, resulting in the body's inability to fight infections. It is a precursor to AIDS.

Serostatus A blood test indicating the presence of antibodies the immune system creates to fight disease. A seropositive status indicates that a person has antibodies to fight HIV and is HIV positive.

CD4+ Helper Cells (T Helper Cells) Cells that protect against infections and activate the body's immune response. HIV kills these cells, so a high count usually means better health.

Opportunistic Infections Infections that typically do not affect healthy people, but may lead to diseases in people whose immune systems have been compromised.

Viral Load The level of virus (HIV) in the blood.

Antibodies Proteins in the bloodstream that react to overcome bacterial and other agents that attack the body.

Kaposi's Sarcoma A type of cancer evidenced by purple sores (tumors) on the skin.

fatigue, swollen glands, rashes, weight loss, and loss of appetite. Once a person receives a diagnosis of AIDS, the diagnosis is maintained even if the individual becomes nonsymptomatic.

There are three mechanisms for most HIV transmission. The three primary mechanisms responsible for the transmission of HIV are sexual activity, contact with infected blood (needle sharing), and transmission from an infected mother to her child. Among men in the United States, the greatest number of new cases result from men having sex with men, though a significant number of cases result from heterosexual sex. Among women, risk of transmission is most frequent in heterosexual sex. Worldwide, two-thirds of all AIDS cases are transmitted by heterosexual sex.

More than 10 percent of new cases worldwide are the result of using contaminated needles to inject drugs, but another 11 percent of cases are caused by transmission from HIV-infected mothers to their children. The latter mode of transmission could be largely prevented through the use of a specific drug (nevirapine) and with a cesarean delivery. It is important to understand that HIV is not transmitted through the air or in saliva, sweat, or urine. It does not spread by hugging, sharing foods or beverages, or casual kissing. Contact with phones, silverware, or toilet seats does not cause the spread of HIV. Although people who had blood transfusions before 1985 had an increased risk of HIV transmission, the safety of the blood supply has increased dramatically since that time, resulting in extremely low rates of risk from transfusion.

The risk of acquiring HIV/AIDS is reduced if exposure to HIV and to the methods of transmission is avoided. Experts from the National Institutes of Health have concluded that HIV transmission could be reduced if legislative barriers to needle exchange programs were lifted, if greater emphasis were given to youth education programs about HIV/AIDS, if greater funding were available for the treatment of people who abuse drugs, and if educational efforts among high-risk populations were increased. Worldwide, the money expended on treatment far exceeds the amounts spent on prevention. Taking personal responsibility for reducing risky behaviors is important for prevention on a personal level. Increasing awareness of and education about these risks is important for national and international prevention. Steps that can be taken to lower your risk of HIV infection are presented in Table 1.

Early detection is critical for controlling the spread of AIDS. Unfortunately, the majority of adults in the United States have

---

Table 1 ▶ Factors Associated with Reducing Risk for HIV/AIDS

- Abstain from sexual activity.

- Limit sexual activity to a noninfected partner. A lifetime partner who has never had sex with other people and has never used injected drugs (other than medically administered) is the only safe partner.

- Avoid sexual activity or other activity that puts you in contact with another person's semen, vaginal fluids, or blood.

- Use a new condom (latex) every time you have sex, especially with a partner who is not known to be safe. Know how to use it properly.

- Use a water-based lubricant with condoms because petroleum-based lubricants increase risk for condom failure.

- Abstain from risky sexual activity, such as anal sex and sex with high-risk people (prostitutes, people with HIV or other STIs).

- Do not inject drugs.

- Never share a needle or drug paraphernalia.

- Get tested for STIs, and seek proper treatment.

- Use a condom or dental dam when engaging in oral sex.

- Talk with your partner about his or her and your own sexual history before initiating sexual behavior.

- Remember that condoms are for STI prevention as well as pregnancy prevention. Even if your partner is using another form of birth control, use condoms if your partner has not been tested or you do not know his or her sexual history.

---

never been tested for HIV. Although rates have gradually increased over the past decade, only 4 in 10 adults in 2009 reported having been tested for HIV. Even in a sample of people at high risk for HIV, about 30 percent reported that they had not been tested. Further, the CDC estimates that about 25 percent of individuals with HIV are unaware that they are infected. To facilitate early identification of HIV, the CDC in 2006 revised its guidelines for HIV screening in medical settings, suggesting that testing should be routine for every person over the age of 15. In 2009, the American College of Physician's joined the CDC, recommending that physicians encourage all of their patients to get tested for HIV, regardless of their level of risk.

Testing for HIV and other STIs can be either confidential or anonymous. When a test is confidential, there is a written record of the test results, but there is also assurance that this information will be kept private by the health-care provider. An anonymous test is one for which there is no written record, and the results cannot be connected to a name or other identifiable information. Clinics throughout the country provide both confidential and anonymous (in most states) testing at no cost. In the past, HIV tests required blood samples and had to be completed in the presence of a health-care provider. In addition, the wait for test results lasted for weeks. Much has changed in the past decade. There are now self-testing kits that can be mailed to labs for analysis so the individual does not have to see a health-care provider. Some of these tests are noninvasive, requiring the use of a swab to collect cells from the inside of the mouth.

 There is no cure for AIDS, but treatments have improved. For those infected with
FEATURE 4 HIV/AIDS, there is no known cure. However, treatments have been developed to suppress or slow the progress of the disease process. Several medications are used in combination to target different stages in the progression of HIV infection. In the first stage, the virus must enter T cells in the body. Once HIV enters these cells, HIV RNA is translated into DNA through a process called reverse transcription. Once the HIV RNA has been converted, an enzyme called integrase facilitates the integration of HIV DNA into the host DNA of the cell. The HIV DNA is then able to generate new protein sequences necessary to create new copies of the virus. In the final step, the HIV protein called protease separates the protein sequence into its components so these proteins can combine to form new viruses.

Fusion inhibitors are a class of drugs that operate in the first stage of the process by interfering with the virus's ability to enter the host cell. Reverse transcriptase inhibitors disrupt reverse transcription so that HIV RNA cannot be converted into DNA or integrated into the DNA of the host cell. Finally, protease inhibitors interfere with the protease enzyme, which prevents the HIV DNA from being separated into its components. This prevents the development of new viruses within the host cell. These combination treatments are referred to as highly active antiretroviral therapy (HAART), or the "HIV cocktail."

A three-drug "cocktail" has been the most common treatment, but the FDA recently approved a new "once a day" pill for treating HIV. The advent of this new medication greatly simplifies the treatment and is considered by experts to be a big forward step.

Early treatment dramatically reduces death rates. A review of 22 studies in Canada and the United States found a 70 percent reduction in mortality for those who received earlier treatment for HIV, and several other studies have provided support for earlier treatment. These studies support new recommendations from both the CDC and the World Health Organization (WHO).

> ## Technology Update
> **HIV-Resistant Gene Provides Possible**
> TECH **Clues to Prevention and Treatment**
>
> Early in the fight against HIV and AIDS, researchers became interested in a small group of individuals for whom HIV infection rarely leads to disease symptoms associated with AIDS, even without treatment. In the late 1990s, researchers identified a gene (HLA B57) that seems to contribute to protection among this group. Most recently, researchers have gained insight into the role of this type of gene in protecting individuals from infection. This research suggests protective genes like HLA B57 may allow the body to generate more cross-reactive T cells, the cells that help defend the body from infection. These cross-reactive T cells are better able to recognize HIV infected cells, providing greater protection from their effects. The knowledge gained through this research may lead to the development of new vaccines that target the types of T cells that seem to be particularly effective in fighting HIV.

The CDC has shifted the CD4 count for initiating treatment from less than 500 to between 350 and 500, and the WHO has shifted from a count of 200 to a count of 350.

Early treatment with ART may also decrease rates of HIV transmission. Although antiretroviral treatment (ART) does not eliminate the risk for HIV among partners of individuals who are HIV positive, one study found over a 90 percent reduction in risk for infection among the sexual partners of individuals started on ART, relative to those who did not begin ART. Combining the approaches of routine testing and early treatment may have a particularly dramatic impact. A recent mathematical model of this approach, called "test and treat," proposed universal voluntary testing combined with immediate ART for those infected with HIV. Using South Africa as a basis for calculations, the mathematical model suggested that the incidence and mortality associated with HIV could be reduced to 1 in 1,000 cases within 10 years of full implementation. Current incidence rates in South Africa are roughly 1 in 20. The researchers acknowledge that their model makes a number of assumptions and that this approach would be costly. Nonetheless, the study raises intriguing possibilities, ones that are currently being explored by the CDC.

Improvements in drug therapies raise concerns about increases in high-risk sexual behavior. Strides in reducing new cases of HIV infection have largely been driven by decreases among men having sex with men, but there is concern that the availability of effective drug therapies will lead to an increase in rates of infection in this group. According to the CDC, rates of new infections transmitted via male-to-male sexual contact increased about 9 percent between 2001 and 2006 during a time when overall rates of new infections were decreasing. These recent trends suggest it is critical that we continue to devote adequate resources to prevention with this high-risk group.

The search for a vaccine for HIV is well under way, though no vaccine is currently available. More than 100 vaccines have been tested in humans or animals, and many vaccines are currently undergoing clinical trials in the United States and abroad. Unfortunately, the search for an AIDS vaccine took a serious blow when a clinical trial of a promising vaccine developed by Merck was discontinued in 2007 due to heightened risk of HIV among those receiving the vaccine. The authors of the study suggest that the failure may have been due to the adenovirus, which served as the "shell" through which the vaccine was delivered. Many lost hope for the successful development of a vaccine, at least in the near future.

More promising results emerged in September 2009, when a U.S.-funded study conducted in Thailand found a significant reduction in new cases of HIV among those receiving a combination of two vaccines that had been ineffective on their own. Presumably, the combination might work better because one vaccine serves to prime the immune system, while the second serves to boost its response. The study found a 31 percent reduction of new HIV cases for participants receiving the vaccine relative to those receiving a placebo. Although the results are encouraging, the effects were modest, and it is not yet clear how the vaccine actually works. Nonetheless, these new findings have provided renewed hope.

Common Sexually Transmitted Infections

STIs infect about 19 million people in the United States each year. Although HIV is the deadliest of the sexually transmitted infections, it is not among the most common in the United States. Table 2 lists some of the most common STIs in terms of both incidence (new cases) and prevalence (cumulative number of cases). Although rates of human papillomavirus (HPV) have not been tracked by the CDC because the vast majority of individuals with HPV are unaware that they are infected, it is estimated that over 50 percent of sexually active adults will be infected with HPV at some point in their lifetime. A recent study found a current prevalence of 27 percent among women between 14 and

Table 2 ▶ Rankings of Incidence and Prevalence of Common STIs

STI	Rank of Incidence (Number of New Cases of the Condition)	Rank of Prevalence (Number of People with Condition)
Chlamydia	2	3
Gonorrhea	4	4
Hepatitis B	5	5
Herpes	3	1
Human papillomavirus (HPV)	1	2
Syphilis	6	6

Source: Cates et al.

59 years of age, with a high of 45 percent among women between the ages of 20 and 24 years. Thus, HPV is by far the most common STI.

Of the STIs that are tracked by the CDC, **chlamydia** has been the most commonly reported for the past decade. With improved methods of screening and efforts by the CDC and other agencies to increase screening, rates of identified cases have increased dramatically in the past 25 years despite the fact that most experts believe that rates of infection are not increasing. Gonorrhea was the most commonly reported STI until the early 1990s and is now the second most common. Rates of gonorrhea infection in the United States have decreased dramatically over the past 25 years. Syphilis rates are much lower, though recent increases are cause for concern, particularly among men who have sex with men (MSM). Figure 1 provides a graphic depiction of the trends in STI rates over the past 40 years.

ⓘ **The human papillomavirus (HPV) is a very common STI in young people.** An estiFEATURE 5 mated 6 million people become infected with HPV each year, making this the most commonly transmitted STI. The virus is responsible for the development of genital warts, but most people do not develop them and are therefore unaware that they are infected. Although the disease is asymptomatic in the short term, it leads to significantly increased risk for cervical cancer in women. In fact, HPV is the leading cause of cervical cancer. Certain strains of HPV are particularly dangerous, accounting for approximately 80 percent of cases of cervical cancer.

Although it has now been 3 years since federal health officials recommended that young girls routinely receive the HPV vaccine Gardisil, only the state of Virginia and

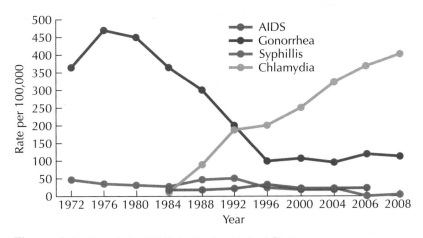

Figure 1 ▶ Trends in STI Rates in the United States.
Based on data from the annual CDC Sexually Transmitted Disease Surveillance reports and HIV/AIDS Surveillance reports.

Washington D.C. require the shots, and parents can opt out of the vaccination for any reason. A recent study of girls between the ages of 13 and 17 in six U.S. states found that only one-third had been vaccinated. Although the percentage was much higher in a study of college students, only half of college women had been vaccinated. This is concerning in the face of evidence for very high rates of HPV in young adults. A recent study found that over half of young adults in a new relationship were infected with HPV, and nearly half were infected with a type known to increase risk for cancer. It is important to note that the vaccine will not help those already infected with HPV. However, routine Pap tests can identify the early cell changes associated with HPV and help to prevent the development of cervical cancer.

(i) **Chlamydia is a common STI, but it is often difficult to detect.** About 1.2 million FEATURE 6 new cases of chlamydia are reported in the United States each year. Chlamydia is known as the "silent" STI because about three-fourths of infected women and about half of infected men have no symptoms. Thus, routine screening is essential for detecting most cases of chlamydia. If symptoms do occur, it is typically in the first three weeks following infection. For men who experience symptoms, the most common are discharge from the penis and a burning sensation when urinating. Common symptoms in women include abnormal vaginal discharge, a burning sensation when urinating, lower abdominal or back pain, pain during intercourse, and bleeding between menstrual periods. If chlamydia is left untreated, the health consequences can be extensive, particularly for women. The disease has been linked to increased risk of **pelvic inflammatory disease (PID),** as well as a number of other secondary health problems, including urethritis, cervicitis, ectopic pregnancy, infertility, and chronic pelvic pain.

As a result of the high levels of risk for young women (over half of cases in women are among those under age 25), guidelines from the U.S. Preventive Services Task Force suggest that sexually active women under the age of 25 undergo routine screening for chlamydia. Although rates of screening have increased, less than half of women in this age group are screened annually. Fortunately, chlamydia is very treatable, and its long-term health consequences can be prevented if the infection is identified quickly. Treatment with antibiotics can clear up the infection within a week to 10 days.

(i) **Early detection is critical for effective treatment of gonorrhea. Gonorrhea** is a FEATURE 7 bacterial infection that can be treated with modern antibiotics if detected early. Sexual activity is the principal method of disease transmission. Penile and vaginal gonorrhea are the most common types. Symptoms usually occur within 3 to 7 days after bacteria enter the system. Among men, the most common symptoms are painful urination and penile drip or discharge. Symptoms are less apparent among women, though painful urination and vaginal discharge are not uncommon. Other types of gonorrhea often have fewer symptoms. Chills, fever, painful bowel movements, and sore throat are the most common. Early detection by a culture or smear test at the site or sites of sexual contact is how the disease is diagnosed. Early cure is especially important for females because gonorrhea can lead to pelvic inflammatory disease, which can result in infertility.

Hepatitis B is considered to be an STI. Like other STIs, hepatitis B (HPB) is typically spread through unprotected sex with an infected partner, IV drug use, or transmission from an infected mother to her baby.

Chlamydia A bacterial infection, similar to gonorrhea, that attacks the urinary tract and reproductive organs.

Pelvic Inflammatory Disease (PID) An infection of the urethra (urine passage), which can lead to infertility among women.

Gonorrhea A bacterial infection of the mucous membranes, including the eyes, throat, genitals, and other organs.

Although rare, HPB can be spread through blood transfusion or any other contact with infected blood. Symptoms of HPB include jaundice, fatigue, abdominal pain, loss of appetite, and nausea. Among those chronically infected with the virus, chronic liver disease typically develops, leading to premature death in 15 to 25 percent of cases. Fortunately, a vaccine for HPB has been available since 1982, and rates have decreased since then from over 260,000 cases to less than 43,000 cases in 2007.

(i) **Genital herpes is among the most commonly spread STIs because of a lack of awareness of infection. Genital herpes,** one of the most commonly reported STIs, is caused by the herpes simplex virus (HSV). Although fewer new cases of genital herpes are reported annually than cases of HPV and chlamydia, the number of individuals currently infected is much higher. This is because chlamydia is treatable and HPV typically goes away on its own. In contrast, once someone contracts genital herpes, he or she will always carry the virus. Genital herpes causes lesions or blisters on the penis, vagina, or cervix usually occurring 2 to 12 days after infection and typically lasting a week to a month. Swollen glands and headache may also occur.

No cure exists for genital sores caused by HSV, though some prescription drugs can help treat the disease symptoms. Episodic antiviral therapy is taken at the first sign of an outbreak, and suppressive antiviral therapy is taken daily to prevent outbreaks from occurring. HSV can remain dormant in the body for long periods, and as a result, symptoms can recur at any time, especially after undergoing stress or illness.

Genital herpes is especially contagious when blisters are present. Condom use or abstinence from sexual activity when symptoms are present can reduce the risk of transmission of the disease. Although genital herpes is less infectious when there are no symptoms present, the infection can still be spread to other partners. In addition, although condoms provide some protection, they are not totally effective in preventing infection because they do not cover all genital areas. Herpes is more dangerous for women than men because of the association between genital herpes and cervical cancer and the risk of transmitting the disease to the unborn.

(i) **Syphilis is another serious but less commonly contracted STI. Syphilis** was a serious national health problem in the 1940s, when it was 10 times more prevalent than it is now. Cases of syphilis declined 84 percent nationwide during the 1990s. Although progress toward the national health goal of reducing the number of syphilis cases has been made, recent increases are cause for concern. In the past 8 years, rates of syphilis have more than doubled in the United States. In addition, the CDC reports that syphilis continues to have a disproportionate effect on African Americans and people living in the South.

Like gonorrhea, syphilis is a bacterial infection that can be effectively treated with antibiotics. The symptoms of syphilis include **chancre** sores that generally appear at the primary site of sexual contact, then change from a red swelling to a hardened ulcer on the skin. Even if not treated, the sores disappear after 1 to 5 weeks. It is important to get treatment even after this primary phase of the disease because the disease is still present and contagious. After several weeks or longer, secondary symptoms occur, such as a rash, loss of hair, joint pain, sore throat, and swollen glands. Even after these symptoms go away, untreated syphilis lingers in a latent phase. Serious health problems may result, including blindness, deafness, tumors, and stillbirth.

Early detection is important and can be diagnosed from chancre discharge or a blood test several weeks after the appearance of chancres. There is an association between syphilis and the spread of HIV. Evidence suggests that the presence of chancres increase the risk of transmitting HIV during sexual activity.

In the News

Sexually Explicit Media and Teen Sexual Behavior

(i) There has been considerable concern about the impact of explicit sexual content in the media (music, magazines, television, movies, and Internet) on teen sexual behavior, and there appears to be good reason. A recent study found that adolescents exposed to sexually explicit content on the Internet had more permissive attitudes toward sex, and were more likely to have multiple sexual partners and to have engaged in anal sex. Another study evaluating exposure to sexually explicit content in several forms of media (magazines, movies, and Internet) found that early exposure predicted more permissive sexual norms and an increased likelihood of oral sex and sexual intercourse 2 years later. Most recently, "sexting" has gained considerable media attention. A recent study found that 1 in 5 teens had "sexted"—defined as sending or receiving sexually suggestive, nearly nude, or nude photos by text message or email. Although most reported sending sexts to boyfriends or girlfriends, more than 10 percent reported sending them to strangers. Also of concern, 40 percent of teens indicated that they tell their parents little or nothing about what they do online.

Some lesser-known STIs are significant health problems. Genital warts, pubic crab lice, and **chancroid** are examples of lesser-known but prevalent STIs (see Table 3). Genital warts are caused by the strains of the human papillomavirus, discussed earlier. Fortunately, the strains of HPV associated with genital warts tend to be relatively low risk. The most significant consequence to the individual is often psychological, due to concern about the appearance of the warts and the potential consequences associated with them. Because HPV is so common, the chance of developing genital warts is relatively high, even with a small number of sexual partners. Fortunately, there are several effective treatments for genital warts, including remedies that can be self-administered by

patients in their own homes. Pubic lice also tends to be highly distressing to the individual, but effective over-the-counter treatments are available to eliminate pubic lice in a matter of days. Although individuals with genital warts and pubic lice may have few long-term effects from these infections, studies have found that both groups tend to have more sexual partners and to be at higher risk for other STIs, including gonorrhea and chlamydia. Therefore, these individuals should be routinely tested for other STIs. Chancroid is most common in developing countries, with very low rates in the United States. Most patients with chancroid in the United States contract it during travels to countries where it is more common. Although rare, chancroid is a known risk factor for transmission of HIV and should therefore be treated promptly, typically with antibiotics.

Table 3 ▶ Facts about Lesser-Known STIs

Genital Warts (Condylomas)

- Constitute approximately 5 percent of all reported STIs
- Are most prevalent in ages 15 to 24
- Are caused by the human papillomavirus (HPV)
- Are hard and yellow or gray on dry skin
- Are soft and pink, red or dark on moist skin
- Are treated by the prescription drug Podophyllin

Pubic Crab Lice

- Are pinhead-sized insects (parasites) that feed on the blood of the host
- Are transmitted by sexual contact and/or contact with contaminated clothes, bedding, and other washable items
- Have symptoms that include itching, but some people have no symptoms
- Can be controlled by using medicated lotion and shampoos and by washing contaminated bedding
- Do *not* transmit other STIs

Chancroid

- Is caused by bacteria
- Is more commonly seen in men than in women, particularly uncircumcised males
- Has symptoms including one or more sores or raised bumps on the genitals
- Can result in progressive ulcers occurring on the genitals; sometimes the ulcers persist for weeks or months
- Can be successfully treated with certain antibiotics

Genital Herpes A viral infection that can attack any area of the body but often causes blisters on the genitals.

Syphilis An infection, caused by a corkscrew-shaped bacteria, that travels in the bloodstream and embeds itself in the mucous membranes of the body, including those of the sexual organs.

Chancre Sore or lesion commonly associated with syphilis.

Genital Warts Warts, caused by a virus, that grow in the genital/anal area (also called condyloma).

Pubic Crab Lice Lice that attach themselves to the base of pubic hairs.

Chancroid A bacterial infection resulting in sores or ulcers on the genitals; different from chancres associated with syphilis.

Strategies for Action

Many young people engage in unsafe sex because they perceive that they are not at risk or they lack knowledge about effective strategies for safe sex. Roughly two-thirds of all STIs occur in people under the age of 25. Both teens and college students are at high risk, although they often fail to recognize their level of risk. In Lab 21A, you will have the opportunity to evaluate the risk of a friend or loved one. You may also want to evaluate your own risk using the STI Risk Questionnaire. Adequate knowledge of risk is likely to increase use of the behaviors outlined in Table 1, reducing risk for STIs.

Inaccurate perceptions that "everyone is doing it" may drive early sexual behavior. Many teens engage in sex because they believe that "everybody is doing it." A recent study suggests that this perception may be fueled by inaccurate information about actual behavior, especially from boys. In a study of boys between the ages of 15 and 22, 45 percent reported that they were virgins, though 23 percent indicated that they told others they were not. Overall, 60 percent reported that they lied about something related to sex. Participants indicated that they thought appearing more sexually experienced would make them more popular. Interestingly, they said that girls who were more sexually experienced were perceived as less popular. Young people need to be aware of the true norms for sexual behavior and not get caught up in perceptions that may be based on inaccurate information.

Early prevention can increase understanding of risk and strategies for practicing safe sex. Some argue that abstinence-only education is best, while others believe that young people also need to be educated about ways to protect themselves in the event that they are or will become sexually active. Between 2001 and 2009, the federal government allocated over a billion dollars to abstinence-only sex education programs. Proponents of this strategy point to recent decreases in sexual activity among teenagers as signs of success. Rates of sexual intercourse decreased from 54 to 47 percent between 1991 and 2005, and rates of teen pregnancy were also at an all-time low in 2005. Unfortunately, increases in teen birth rates were found in 2006 and 2007, raising concerns about a reversal of the trend, despite continued funding for abstinence-based sex education. In addition, a review study published in 2007 did not find any evidence for the efficacy of abstinence-based sex education.

In contrast, after reviewing 83 studies of sex education programs, a CDC task force recently concluded that comprehensive sex education programs that both promote abstinence and teach safer sex practices are effective. The CDC report has been used to support legislation proposed by the current administration to discontinue funds specified for abstinence-only sex education, instead devoting funds to programs with demonstrated scientific evidence. This does not rule out funding for abstinence-based programs if they can demonstrate evidence of effectiveness, and a recent study shows promise. Among 6th- and 7th-grade African American girls, an abstinence-based sex education program significantly increased rates of sexual abstinence.

College students are at risk for HIV and other STIs due to the practice of serial monogamy. Many college students are sexually active, yet most do not use condoms on a consistent basis. This is, in part, due to perceptions that they are in committed relationships and, therefore, are at low risk for infection. Such perceptions are problematic for several reasons. First, college students typically define a regular partner as someone they have been with for as little as 1 month, with most defining a regular partner as someone they have been with for less than 6 months. Second, most college students do not get tested on a regular basis, if at all. Third, when students perceive that they are in a committed relationship, the likelihood of condom use decreases dramatically. This is particularly true when an alternative form of birth control, primarily birth control pills, is being used. For example, one study found that 93.7 percent of sexually active college women were using contraception to prevent pregnancy, but only 23 percent reported that they also used contraception to prevent STIs. The common result is unprotected sexual intercourse between two people who have known one another for a relatively short time and who are unaware of their own and each other's STI status. Many students go through multiple committed relationships during the college years. This type of serial monogamy places college students at increased risk for HIV and other STIs, even though they may not believe they are engaging in high-risk behavior.

Low perceived risk of oral sex contributes to STIs. Although oral sex puts individuals at much lower risk for contracting STIs than do vaginal and anal sex, this behavior is not without risk.

Regular screening and notification of partners who may be infected can reduce the spread of STIs. Regular screening for sexually transmitted infections can reduce rates of new infections. In addition, because many STIs are treatable with antibiotics, catching them early can reduce the negative health consequences associated with infection. For those who are sexually active with partners of unknown STI status, yearly testing is a good idea. Even more frequent

testing may be appropriate for those at very high risk (e.g., IV drug users and those previously diagnosed with an STI). When an individual is identified with a sexually transmitted infection, it is important that he or she notify his or her sexual partners so they can also receive treatment. This helps reduce the spread of the infection. Hotlines are available to help people who want information concerning STIs, including HIV/AIDS. A recent publication from the Henry J. Kaiser Family Foundation provides a list of resources available for those concerned about STIs. The publication is available at **www.kff.org/youthhivstds/upload/MTV_Think_IYSL_Booklet.pdf.**

Web Resources

Additional websites with information related to Concept 21 are available at the associated Web link.

AVERT: Averting HIV and AIDS **www.avert.org**

CDC—Division of Sexually Transmitted Diseases
www.cdc.gov/STD/

Cells Alive! Human Immunodeficiency Virus
www.cellsalive.com/hiv5.htm

Center for Young Women's Health Information on STDs
www.youngwomenshealth.org/std-general.html

National Institutes of Health Aids Information
http://aidsinfo.nih.gov/

WHO Sexually Transmitted Diseases Information
www.who.int/topics/sexually_transmitted_infections/en

X-Plain.com, the Patient Education Institute Online Tutorial on STDs **www.nlm.nih.gov/medlineplus/tutorials/sexuallytransmitteddiseases/htm/index.htm**

National AIDS and STI Hotlines

AIDS hotline (English): 1-800-342-AIDS (2437)
AIDS hotline (Spanish): 1-800-344-SIDA (7432)
CDC STD (STI) hotline: 1-800-232-4636

Suggested Readings

Selected readings and references are listed below. A more comprehensive list is available at the associated Web link.

Benlahrech, A., et al. 2009. Adenovirus vector vaccination induces expansion of memory CD4 T cells with a mucosal homing phenotype that are readily susceptible to HIV-1. *Proceedings of the National Academy of Sciences* 106:19940–19945.

Branson B. M., et al. 2006. Revised recommendations for HIV testing of adults, adolescents, and pregnant women in health-care settings. *Morbidity and Mortality Weekly Reports* 55(RR14):1–17.

Braun–Courville, D. K., and M. Rojas. 2009. Exposure to sexually explicit web sites and adolescent sexual attitudes and behaviors. *Journal of Adolescent Health* 45:156–162.

Brown, J., and K. L. L'Engle. 2009. X-rated: Sexual attitudes and behaviors associated with U.S. early adolescents' exposure to sexually explicit media. *Communication Research* 36:129–151.

Cates, J. R. 2008. Education on sexually transmitted infections: Finding common ground among youth, parents, providers and policy advocates. *Sex Education* 8(2):129–143.

CDC. 2009. *Sexually Transmitted Disease Surveillance, 2008.* Atlanta, GA: Department of Health and Human Services.

Donnell, D., et al. 2010. Heterosexual HIV-1 transmission after initiation of antiretroviral therapy: A prospective cohort analysis. *Lancet.* Early online publication doi:10.1016/S0140-6736(10)60705-2.

Granich, R. M., et al. 2009. Universal voluntary HIV testing with immediate antiretroviral therapy as a strategy for elimination of HIV transmission: A mathematical model. *Lancet* 373:48–57.

Jemmott, J. B., L. S. Jemmott, and G. T. Fong. 2010. Efficacy of a theory-based abstinence-only intervention over 24 months: A randomized controlled trial with young adolescents. *Archives of Pediatrics and Adolescent Medicine* 165:152–159.

Kitahata, M. M. 2009. Effect of early versus deferred anti-retroviral therapy for HIV on survival. *New England Journal of Medicine* 360:1815–1826.

Kosmrlj, A., et al. 2010. Effect of thymic selection of T-cell repertoire on HLA class I associated control of HIV infection. *Nature*. Advance online publication doi:10.1038/nature08997.

Leinwand, D. 2009, June 24. Survey: 1 in 5 teens "sext" despite risks. *USA Today*.

Lindau, S. T., and N. Gavrilova. 2010. Sex, health, and years of sexually active life gained due to good health: Evidence from two US population based cross sectional surveys of ageing. *British Medical Journal* 340:c810. Available at **www.bmj.com**

Meston, C. M., and D. M. Buss. 2007. Why humans have sex. *Archives of Sexual Behavior* 36:477–507.

The National Campaign to Prevent Teen and Unplanned Pregnancy and Seventeen Magazine. 2010. That's what he said: What guys think about sex, love, contraception, and relationships. Available at **www.thenationalcampaign.org**

Panel on Antiretroviral Guidelines for Adults and Adolescents. 2009, December 1. Guidelines for the use of antiretroviral agents in HIV-1-infected adults and adolescents. Department of Health and Human Services, 1-161. Available at **www.aidsinfo.nih.gov**

Qaseem, A., et al. 2009. Screening for HIV in health care settings: A guidance statement from the American College of Physicians and HIV Medicine Association. *Annals of Internal Medicine* 150:126–131.

Rerks-Ngarm, S., et al. 2009. Vaccination with ALVAC and AIDSVAX to prevent HIV-1 infection in Thailand. *New England Journal of Medicine* 361:2209–2220.

Trenhom, C., et al. 2007. Impacts of four Title V, Section 510 abstinence education programs. Mathematica Policy Research, Inc. Available at **www.mathematica-mpr.com**

UNAIDS. 2009. AIDS epidemic update 2009. Geneva, World Health Organization. Available at **http://data.unaids.org/pub/Report/2009/JC1700_Epi_Update_2009_en.pdf**

WHO. 2009. Rapid advice: antiretroviral therapy for HIV infection in adults and adolescents. Geneva: World Health Organization. Available at **www.who.int**

Lab 21A Sexually Transmitted Infection Risk Questionnaire

Name	Section	Date

Purpose: To help you understand the risks of contracting a sexually transmitted infection

Procedure

1. Read the Sexually Transmitted Infection Risk Questionnaire.
2. Answer the questionnaire based on information about someone you know who might be at high risk of contracting an STI.
3. Record the scores in the Results section for the person for whom the questionnaire was answered but do *not* include the person's name on the lab sheet. Use the scores to make a rating (Chart 2) and draw conclusions.
4. You may also wish to answer the questionnaire based on your own information but do *not* record your personal results on the lab sheet. Use these scores strictly for your own personal information.

Chart 1 ▶ Sexually Transmitted Infection Risk Questionnaire

Directions: Mark an X over one response in each row of the questionnaire. Determine a point value for each response using the values in the circles. Sum the numbers of points for the various responses to determine an STI risk score.

	Points				
Categories	**0**	**1**	**3**	**5**	**8**
Feelings about prevention	Able to talk with future partner about STIs ⓪	Finds it hard to discuss STIs with a possible partner ①			
Behaviors	Never engages in sexual activity ⓪		Sexual activity with one partner, well known to him or her ③	Sexual activity with one partner, not well known to him or her ⑤	Sexual activity with multiple partners and/or high-risk individuals ⑧
Behavior of friends	Most friends do not engage in unsafe sexual activity ⓪	Many friends engage in unsafe sexual activity ①			
Contraception	Not sexually active ⓪	Would use condom to prevent STI ①		Would sometimes use condom to prevent STI ⑤	Would never use condom to prevent STI ⑧
Other	Does not use drugs ⓪				Uses injected drugs in unsafe manner ⑧

451

Chart 2 ▶ Risk Questionnaire Rating Chart

Rating	Score
High risk	9+
Above average risk	7–8
Moderate risk	4–6
Low risk	0–3

Results

What is the person's STI risk score?   (Total from STI Risk Questionnaire)

What is the person's STI rating?   (See STI Risk Questionnaire Rating Chart.)

Conclusions and Implications: Of course, risk varies with different types of STIs. However, this questionnaire will give you an idea of an individual's "general" risk for most STIs. Answer the following questions about the risk of the person you scored and rated.

1. In several sentences, explain which STI you think this person should be especially concerned about. Why?

2. What specific recommendations would you have for the person for whom you filled out this questionnaire?

Cancer, Diabetes, and Other Health Threats

Health Objectives for the Year 2020

- Reduce overall cancer death rate and increase cancer patient longevity.
- Reduce rate of sunburn among young people (tanning).
- Increase quality of life among cancer survivors.
- Increase screening and counseling for cancer, diabetes, depression, and other health threats.
- Reduce diabetes death rates and new cases.
- Increase diagnosis and reduce complications of diabetes.

- Increase percentage of diabetics receiving care for symptoms.
- Increase aspirin use among diabetics.
- Increase education for health threats such as cancer and diabetes.
- Reduce injuries and accidental deaths (automobile, assault, drowning, firearms-related, homicides, motorcycle, pedestrian, poisonings).
- Reduce suicide and suicide attempts.
- Increase access to emergency medical services.
- Achieve health equity, eliminate disparities, and improve the health of all groups.

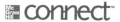

FITNESS AND WELLNESS   http://connect.mcgraw-hill.com

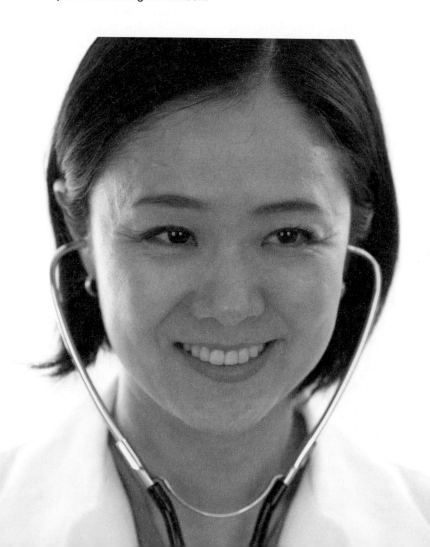

Many health problems that cause pain, suffering, and premature death are associated with unhealthy lifestyles.

The broad vision of Healthy People 2020 is to create a society in which all people live long, healthy lives. Every year, many deaths and much pain and suffering could be prevented by altering lifestyles associated with various diseases and health threats. Heart disease, the leading cause of death; stroke (third leading cause of death); and osteoporosis were discussed in Concept 4, on health benefits of physical activity, so they are not discussed here. Among the conditions discussed in this concept are cancer, diabetes, bronchitis/emphysema, injuries, diabetes mellitus, and emotional disorders (including suicide). As noted in Concept 4, cancer is second only to heart disease among the leading causes of death. Cancer deaths have decreased in recent years, but new cases have remained steady. Diabetes, injuries, and suicide all rank among the top 10 leading causes of death in our society.

Cancer

Cancer is a group of more than 100 different diseases. According to the American Cancer Society, cancer is a group of many different conditions characterized by abnormal, uncontrolled cell growth that will ultimately invade the blood and lymph tissues and spread throughout the body if not treated. Throughout the body, new cells are constantly being created to replace older ones. For reasons unknown, abnormal cells capable of uncontrolled growth sometimes develop. **Benign tumors** are generally not considered to be cancerous because a protective membrane restricts their growth to a specific area of the body. Treatment is important

because any tumor can interfere with normal bodily functioning. Once removed, a benign tumor typically will not return.

Malignant tumors are capable of uncontrolled growth that can cause death to tissue. Approximately 85 percent of malignant tumors are carcinomas, or tumors of the epithelial cells of the inner and outer linings of the body (e.g., lungs, skin). Other malignant tumors include adenocarcinomas (glands such as breast tissue) and sarcomas (bones, muscles, connective tissue, and blood). Malignant cells invade healthy tissues, deplete them of nutrition, and interfere with a multitude of tissue functions. In the early stages of cancer, malignant tumors are located in a small area and can be more easily treated or removed. In advanced cancer, the cells invade the blood or lymph systems and travel throughout the body **(metastasize).** When this occurs, cancer becomes much more difficult to treat.

Figure 1 provides a more detailed illustration of the stages in the spread of cancer. It illustrates how an abnormal cell can divide to form a primary tumor (a), get nourishment from new blood vessels (b), invade the blood system (c), and escape to form a new (secondary) tumor (d). The four stages of cancer range from I to IV, with I being the early stage and IV being most advanced. The early stage is characterized by containment only in the layers of cells where they developed. When cancer spreads beyond the original layers (see Figure 1), it is considered to be invasive and is rated at a higher stage. Early detection is very important in the treatment and cure of cancer. One method of detecting a tumor is to take a **biopsy** of suspicious lumps in the breasts, testicles, or other parts of the body.

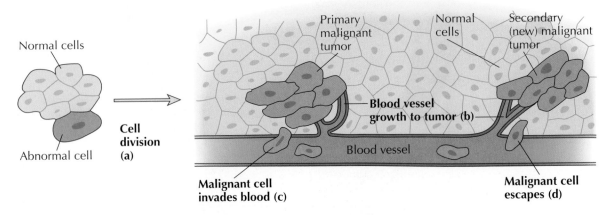

Figure 1 ▶ The spread of cancer (metastasis).

Cancer Type

Deaths Rank/%	Incidence Rank/%	Cancer Type
1. 30%	2. 15%	lung/bronchus
2. 9%	1. 25%	prostate
3. 9%	3. 10%	colon/rectal
4. 6%	8. 3%	pancreas
5. 4%	8. 3%	leukemia
6. 4%	*	liver
7. 4%	*	esophagus
8. 3%	4. 7%	urinary/bladder
9. 3%	5. 5%	non-Hodgkin's lymphoma
10. 3%	5. 5%	kidney
*	5. 5%	skin
*	8. 3%	oral

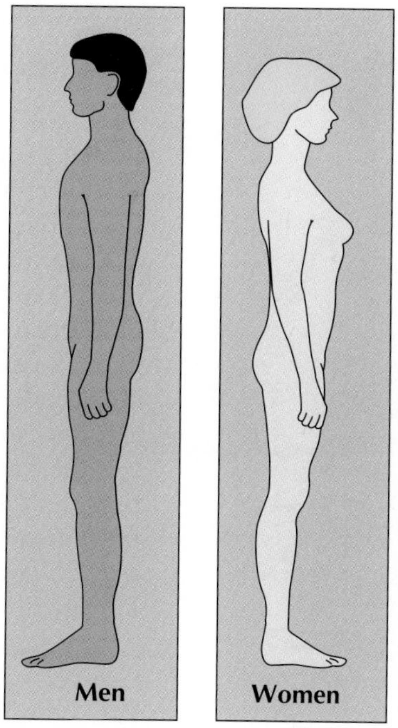

Men

Deaths Rank/%	Incidence Rank/%	Cancer Type
1. 26%	2. 14%	lung/bronchus
2. 15%	1. 27%	breast
3. 9%	3. 10%	colon/rectal
4. 6%	10. 3%	pancreas
5. 5%	9. 3%	ovary
6. 4%	*	leukemia
7. 3%	5. 4%	non-Hodgkin's lymphoma
8. 3%	4. 6%	uterine
9. 2%	*	brain/nerve
10. 2%	*	multiple myeloma
*	6. 4%	skin
*	7. 4%	thyroid
*	8. 3%	kidney

Women

Figure 2 ▶ Cancer incidence (new cases) and death by site and sex (percent).
Source: American Cancer Society.

Cancer is not only a leading killer but a cause of much suffering. One of every four deaths in the United States is caused by some form of cancer. Slightly more than one in three women and slightly less than one in two men will have cancer at some time in his or her life. It is the cause of much suffering and accounts for a large portion of the money spent on health care. Cancer death rates (all forms of cancer) have decreased 2 percent for men and 1.6 percent for women each year since the beginning of this century. Much of the decrease is attributed to decreases in tobacco use and improved screening and treatment. Of the over 100 forms of cancer, 4 of them (sometimes referred to as the Big 4) account for more than half of all illness and death (see Figure 2). Because of the high incidence of these types of cancers (lung, colon-rectal, breast, and prostate), they are discussed in more detail here. In addition, three forms of cancer for which college students have relative high risk—skin, ovary, and uterus—are discussed.

While some forms of cancer are equally threatening to both sexes (e.g., lung and colon-rectal), others are more specific to one sex or the other (see Figure 2). It is also important to note that incidence rates are different from death rates. Skin cancer is an example of a form of cancer that is high in incidence (fifth for men and sixth for women) but relatively low in death rate (not in the top 10 for men or women). This is because it can be treated with early detection, and steps can be taken to prevent it. In Lab 22A you will have the opportunity to assess your risk for the major forms of cancer.

Breast Cancer

Breast cancer is the most prevalent form of cancer among women, but lung cancer causes more deaths. There are fewer deaths from breast cancer partly because of improved early diagnosis resulting from screening and more effective treatments. Though breast cancer is not as common among men, both men and women should do regular screening. Like

Benign Tumors Slow-growing tumors that do not spread to other parts of the body.

Malignant Tumors *Malignant* means "growing worse." A malignant tumor is one that is considered to be cancerous and will spread throughout the body if not treated.

Metastasize The spread of cancer cells to other parts of the body.

Biopsy The removal of a tissue sample that can be checked for cancer cells.

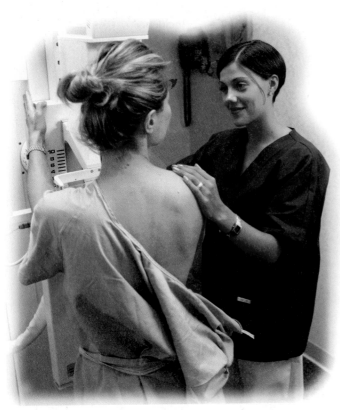

Cancer risk can be reduced by periodic medical tests and self-screening.

colon-rectal and lung cancers, breast cancer is most prevalent among African Americans (more than twice as frequent) and least prevalent among Asians and Hispanics.

Symptoms of breast cancer include lumps and/or thickening or swelling of the breasts. In many cases, lumps are present before they can be detected with self-exams. This is one reason for regular **mammograms** (breast X-rays). A recent report from a government prevention task force (see In the News) recommended changes in mammogram schedules. To date, the recommendations of the American Cancer Society, as noted in Table 1, have not changed. However, the task force's recommendations have provoked much debate.

Breast pain may also exist but is more often a symptom of benign tumors. Risk becomes greater as you grow older. Other risk factors include gender (females have higher risk), family history of disease, early menstruation, hormone supplementation, use of oral contraceptives, late childbirth or no children, excessive use of alcohol, poor eating habits, and sedentary living. The discovery of a breast cancer "gene" provides

In the News

Mammograms

The American Cancer Society recommends an annual mammogram and a breast exam by a physician beginning at age 40 (see Table 1). A U.S. Preventive Services Task Force, however, recently recommended "against screen mammography in women aged 40 to 49 years." The task force noted that "the decision to start regular, biennial mammography screening before age 50 should be an individual one and take patient context into account, including the patient's values regarding specific benefits and harms." This recommendation and others in the report have drawn criticisms from members of the medical community and from women's groups (see associated Web link for more information).

a possible explanation of the hereditary risks. Research has demonstrated that both breast implantation and hormone replacement therapy may increase risk of breast cancer. Because a number of factors influence breast cancer risk, it is important to follow appropriate screening procedures to detect the possible presence of the disease.

Early detection steps include regular self-exams of the breasts (see Lab 22B), breast exams by a physician, and regular mammograms. While there is some debate (see In the News) among experts as to the frequency with which women should have a mammogram, the American Cancer Society (ACS) recently reaffirmed the recommendation that "women age 40 and older have a screening mammogram every year." In spite of this recommendation, a recent study showed a decrease in mammograms by women aged 50 to 70 in the past 5 years. Another study showed that only two-thirds of college-educated women had mammograms as often as every 2 years. There is evidence that digital mammography may be more effective than traditional film mammography. Digital mammography is still quite rare but will no doubt become more common in the future.

Mammograms X-rays of the breast.

Table 1 ▶ Cancer Screening Guidelines

Test or Procedure	Sex	Age	Frequency
General Cancer-Related Checkup			
Exam for thyroid, oral cavity, skin, lymph nodes, testes, and ovaries as part of periodic health exam	Both	20+	With health exam
Breast Cancer[a]			
Breast self-exam (see Lab 22B) Know how breasts look and feel, report changes	Women	20+	Optional
Clinical breast exam (by physician)	Women	20–40	Every 3 years
	Women	40+	Every year
Mammogram	Women	40+	Every year
Breast MRI for those with high risk	Women		Consult physician
Colon-Rectal Cancer[a, b]			
Fecal occult blood test (gFOBT), or fecal immunochemical test (FIT), or stool DNA test (interval uncertain)	Both	50+	Every year (except stool DNA)
Flexible sigmoidoscopy, or double-contrast barium enema, or CT colonography (virtual colonoscopy), or colonoscopy (every 10 years)	Both	50+	Every 5 years (except colonoscopy)
Testicular Cancer[c]			
Self-exam	Men	20+	Monthly
Prostate Cancer[c]			
Consult with physician	Men	50+	Consult physician
African American/family history	Men	45+	
Digital rectal exam	Men		Consult physician
PSA test	Men		Consult physician
Cervical Cancer[a]			
Pelvic exam and Pap test	Women	21 or earlier	Yearly
Pelvic exam and liquid-based Pap		Some 30+	Every 2–3 years[d]
Uterine Cancer[a]			
Physician consultation	Women	Menopause	Consult physician
Skin Cancer			
Self-exam	Men and women	Any age	Monthly
Exam by physician	Men and women	Any age	With symptoms

[a]Frequency varies based on family history, genetics, etc. Physician consultation is recommended and additional tests may be required.

[b]A colonoscopy should be performed if other tests are positive.

[c]The ACS has no current recommendation but many doctors recommend monthly self-exams.

[d]Exams should begin three years after vaginal intercourse, those with three years of normal tests may be tested less often (see ACS website).

Standard treatments for breast cancer include lumpectomy (removal of the tumor and surrounding lymph nodes), mastectomy (removal of breast and surrounding lymph nodes), chemotherapy, radiation, and/or hormone therapies. Tamoxifen, or other drugs, may be prescribed for those at high risk.

Colon-Rectal Cancer

Colon-rectal cancer is tied for second as a killer of men and is third for women. There has been a consistent but small decline in colon-rectal cancer among men and women over the past two decades. Like lung cancer, risk is highest among African Americans. Whites have slightly less risk. Risk among Asians and Hispanics is less than half that of blacks. Lifestyle risk factors include diet, use of alcohol, family history, physical activity patterns, and smoking (see Lab 22A). A high-fiber diet and physical activity can decrease the risk. It is most common among those over 50 years of age. When caught early, 90 percent of colon-rectal cancers can be cured.

Symptoms include cramping in the lower stomach, change in the shape of the stool, urge to have a bowel movement when there is no need to have one, and blood in the stool. Because observable blood in the stool could indicate an advanced problem, consult your physician about an appropriate stool sample test (see Table 1). A six-sample stool test (including an available in-home test) is better than a one-sample test. Other tests to find colon-rectal cancer include the following: barium enema, sigmoidoscopy, virtual colonoscopy, and a colonoscopy. The colonoscopy is considered to be the "gold standard" because it checks for polyps and lesions in the entire colon. If polyps are found during a colonoscopy, they can be removed immediately without an additional procedure. The sigmoidoscopy tests only the lower one-third of the colon, and if polyps are found, a follow-up colonoscopy is recommended. Still, a recent study found that having one sigmoidoscopy between the ages of 55 and 64, as opposed to no screening test, cuts risk of colon cancer by 43 percent.

The virtual colonoscopy uses a CT scan rather than a more invasive rectal probe. A recent study showed that the procedure identified 90 percent of large polyps. The advantages of the procedure are that it is much less invasive than a traditional colonoscopy and for this reason may encourage more people to do the test. Two major disadvantages are that the procedure requires exposure to radiation, and if a positive test occurs (polyps found), a regular colonoscopy must be done to remove them. Other information about colon-rectal cancer screening is available at the associated Web link.

All of the tests are designed to detect either the presence of polyps that can turn into cancer or polyps (or cancers) that are bleeding. Any or all of the tests may be recommended by a physician, especially after age 50. The frequency of screening recommended by the ACS is shown in Table 1.

Studies show that the frequency of screening should vary, depending on symptoms and heredity. For example, people with a family history of colon-rectal cancer and those who have found a polyp in previous exams should schedule a procedure more frequently than listed in Table 1. People who smoke and drink should also begin screening earlier. Polyps can occur as many as 8 years earlier among this group than among nonsmokers and nondrinkers.

Several innovations in testing for colon cancer are being pioneered. One is a probe-free colonoscopy that uses either two-dimensional or three-dimensional CT scans. The 3-D version may be more effective than the colonoscopy and is much less invasive. It does involve radiation exposure equal to that of a chest X-ray, however. A gene test (APC) offers promise for the future. It involves examination of stool samples for damaged genes that trigger cancer. The most common treatments are surgery for cancer or polyp removal, radiation, and/or chemotherapy.

Lung Cancer

Lung cancer is the leading cause of cancer death in men and women. Lung cancer rates have dropped in the past decade, and this has been attributed, in part, to declines in smoking. In the past decade, smoking rates among youth and young adults have increased, however, suggesting that lung cancer deaths may increase in the years ahead. Incidence and death rates are much higher among African Americans than whites, with considerably lower rates among Asians and Hispanics.

By far, the greatest risk factor for lung cancer is smoking. Environmental tobacco smoke (ETS) has been shown to be a potent risk factor. According to the American Cancer Society, nonsmoking spouses of smokers have a 30 percent greater risk of developing lung cancer than do spouses of nonsmokers. A number of other carcinogens, including radon, asbestos, and pollution, have been linked to lung cancer, so nonsmokers can also get lung cancer.

Symptoms of lung cancer include persistent cough, chest pain, recurring pneumonia or bronchitis, and sputum (spit) streaked with blood. Lung cancer can spread to other organs and tissues before symptoms are evident, so it is important to pay attention to possible symptoms rather than to disregard them.

Early detection steps include monitoring for symptoms, chest X-rays, and analyses of sputum samples. Standard treatments include radiation and chemotherapies.

Prostate Cancer

(i) FEATURE 4 Prostate cancer is one of the most common forms of cancer in men. One of every six men will get prostate cancer. Deaths from prostate cancer account for 9 percent of all cancer deaths in men (3 percent of all deaths). The death rate among African Americans is five times higher than among Asians, more than three times higher than Hispanics, and more than twice as high as whites.

Risks of prostate cancer increase dramatically after age 50, so current guidelines recommend that men begin annual screening between the ages of 45 and 50. Symptoms of prostate cancer are urination problems (weak or interrupted stream, inability to start or stop, pain, high frequency of urination at night and/or presence of blood in the urine). The two principal screening techniques include a digital rectal exam by a physician (to detect an enlarged prostate gland) and a prostate-specific antigen (PSA) blood test. Previously the ACS recommended that these two tests be done yearly beginning at age 50. Because research has shown that there is "little proof" of the effectiveness of these two procedures, the ACS has modified its screening guidelines to encourage men to begin a dialogue with their physician at age 50, or at age 45 for African American men and men with a blood relative who had prostate cancer before 65. A PSA threshold of 4 nanograms per milliliter was previously used as an indicator of potential risk, but other screening criteria are now being used. Research suggests that year-to-year changes in PSA are a better predictor, even if the score is lower than 4. A single PSA test misses as many as 15 percent of cancers, so regular testing is advised. A new "autoantibody signatures" test has promise for the future. If future research verifies early findings, this test may be used instead of, or in addition to, the PSA test. Preliminary studies with the new test show that it identifies 82 percent of cancers correctly.

Current treatments for prostate cancer have been shown to be highly effective, and death rates due to prostate cancer have decreased. In spite of the progress in reducing deaths from prostate cancer, the ACS points out that there is no uniform agreement on treatment. Among the most common treatments are "watchful waiting" with no immediate treating since prostate cancer progresses slowly in some patients; surgery to remove the prostate; hormone therapy; radiation therapy, including implanting of radioactive seeds to kill the tumor; and chemotherapy. Early in 2010 the FDA approved a treatment called Provenge, "a vaccine that uses a patient's own immune system to fight advanced prostate cancer that is no longer responding to hormone therapy (see Suggested Readings).

Uterine and Ovarian Cancers

Combined, uterine and ovarian cancers account for 10 percent of all cancer cases and 7 percent of all deaths among women. Uterine cancer is of two different types: cervical cancer occurs when cancers develop in the cervix, or opening to the uterus, and endometrial cancer occurs when a tumor develops in the inner wall of the uterus. Ovarian cancer occurs when a cancer develops in an ovary. Symptoms of ovarian cancer include abdominal swelling and digestive disturbances. Vaginal bleeding can be a symptom of either uterine or ovarian cancer. Other vaginal discharge may be a symptom of uterine cancer. Understanding the risk factors for these female reproductive system cancers is important for prevention.

Established risk factors for cervical cancer include having sex at an early age, having sex with many partners, and a history of smoking. However, the most important risk factor for cervical cancer is infection by human papillomavirus (HPV), a sexually transmitted infection. As noted in Concept 21, the FDA recently approved a "cervical cancer" vaccine (Gardasil) that acts to prevent precancerous genital lesions and genital warts due to HPV among those not previously infected. While it is not effective against all forms of HPV, it is effective against the form implicated in most cervical cancers. A very recent study has also shown the HPV vaccine to be effective in preventing vaginal and vulvar cancer.

The other form of uterine cancer, endometrial cancer, is less common and has a different mechanism of causation. The primary risk factors (early menarche, late menopause, infertility) are all associated with increased exposure to estrogen during the life span. However, other risks include obesity and a high-fat diet.

Risk factors for ovarian cancer include age, family history, and lack of pregnancy during the lifetime. One study showed that risk is considerably higher among those who have taken estrogen-progestin therapy, especially those who have taken it for 10 years or more. Those who have had breast cancer or who are at high risk for breast cancer have a relative high risk for ovarian cancer.

A periodic and thorough pelvic exam is the best method of screening for cervical and ovarian cancers. A **Pap test** is an important part of the exam for

Pap Test A test of the cells of the cervix to detect cancer or other conditions.

detecting cervical cancer. This test—named for Dr. George Papanicolaou, who pioneered it—involves taking scrapings (samples) from the cervix and analyzing them under a microscope. Liquid-based Pap testing (sometimes referred to as ThinPrep) was thought to be more effective than previous Pap testing procedures, but recent research has shown the methods to be equally effective. The liquid-based test is more expensive but is preferred by labs because of the speed and ease of assessment. For this reason, some labs have stopped using the more conventional method. The liquid-based method allows for HPV testing from the same sample, and the ACS indicates that it can be done less frequently. Some home Pap smear kits are available, but these have not been shown to provide accurate information. As noted in Table 1, women should begin Pap testing within 3 years after they begin having intercourse and no later than age 21.

Treatments include surgery to remove one or both of the ovaries and fallopian tubes and/or removal of the uterus (hysterectomy). Radiation and chemotherapy are other options. DNA tests to find cancer-specific genes have been found to predict this form of cancer in a small percentage of the population, but this test has yet to receive governmental approval.

Skin Cancer

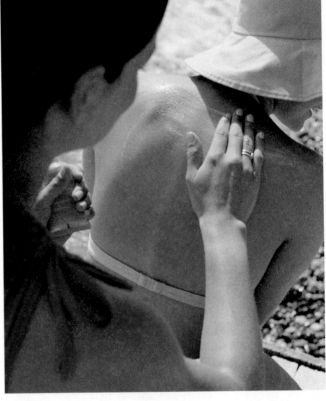

Using sunscreen can protect the skin and reduce the risk of skin cancer.

Skin cancer incidence is increasing, and at least one study indicates that the increase in use of tanning salons is one reason. Each year, more than 1 million people get basal or squamous cell cancer. This curable form is not included in the overall incidence statistics in Figure 2. **Melanoma,** on the other hand, is a deadly cancer if not treated early. Melanoma is 10 times more frequent in whites than African Americans. Unlike many other forms of cancer, it is not necessarily a disease of older adults. Young people who do not take preventive measures are at risk.

Symptoms include darkly pigmented growths, changes in size or color of moles, changes in other nodules on the skin, skin bleeding or scaliness, and skin pain. The principal risk factor is exposure to ultraviolet light, such as sun exposure. Some feel that tanning lights are safe, but research has shown the opposite. Other risk factors include family history, pale skin, exposure to pollutants, and radiation.

Early detection is essential to treatment, so regular screening is important. Screening techniques include self-exams of the skin followed by a physician's exam of suspicious lesions. The ACS recommends that you

follow the ABCD rule for self-exams (see Figure 3). *A* is for asymmetry: does one-half of a growth look different from the other half? *B* is for border irregularity: are the edges notched, rugged, or blurred? *C* is for color: is the color uniform, not varying in shades of tan, brown, and black? *D* is for any lesion with a diameter greater than 6 millimeters (about 1/4 inch). Beware of sudden or progressive growth of any lesion. Some experts have recommended adding *E* and *F* to the list. *E* stands for evolution of a lesion (changes in shape or elevation of a lesion, scaliness, pain, itching, or bleeding), and *F* stands for friend (attentive friends may see changes before you do).

Nonmalignant basal and squamous cell cancers can be treated in a doctor's office using freezing, heat, or laser

A. Asymmetry	B. Border Irregularity	C. Color	D. Diameter
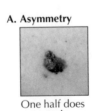	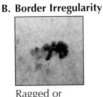		
One half does not match other half	Ragged or notched edges	Color uneven shades of tan, brown, or black and sometimes red, white or blue	Diameter larger than 1/4 inch (diameter of a pencil eraser) Note: some cancers can be smaller

Figure 3 ▶ The ABCD rule for skin cancer self-examination.

procedures. These milder forms of cancer have become more common among younger people in recent years. They occur on the head and neck in 90 percent of cases; however, with the increase in total body exposure and tanning practices, they are now much more common on other parts of the body. Once you have had one of these cancers, your risk of having another is high. Treatment for early melanoma involves the removal of affected cells and surrounding lymph tissues. Advanced cases require chemo and/or radiation therapies. Immunotherapy is another option.

Important preventive measures include limiting exposure to the sun or tanning devices, reducing exposure during midday hours, covering the skin when exposed to the sun (hat, long pants, long-sleeve shirts, high collars on shirts, sunglasses), and using sunscreen that screens for both UVA and UVB. Those with a family history of skin cancer and a history of sunburn or extensive sun exposure should be especially careful.

The ACS uses the slogan "Slip, Slop, Slap and Wrap" to encourage safe practices in the sun: slip on a shirt, slop on sunscreen, slap on a hat, and wrap on sunglasses to protect your eyes. For sunscreen, apply it 20 to 30 minutes before going outside, apply it generously (a palmful), cover all body parts, and reapply every 2 hours and after swimming, sweating heavily, or using a towel.

The FDA has proposed new sunscreen regulations that would require a five star rating system (five stars equal best rating). For now the ACS recommends a sunscreen with an SPF factor of 15 or higher. According to the ACS ". . . using an SPF 15 and applying it correctly, you get the equivalent of 1 minute of UVB rays for each 15 minutes you spend in the sun." So, 1 hour in the sun wearing SPF 15 sunscreen is the same as spending 4 minutes totally unprotected. Many experts recommend a higher SPF factor. Chemical blocks, such as benzophenone and octocrylene, are effective in blocking UVB rays, and mexoryl is effective in blocking UVA rays. Physical blocks are good for people with allergies to chemicals. They contain substances, such as zinc oxide and titanium dioxide, that reflect UVA and UVB rays.

Testicular Cancer

While not a leading cause of death, testicular cancer is a threat to men of all ages, including young men. As noted in Table 1, a monthly testicular self-exam is recommended (see Lab 22B for more information).

(i) FEATURE 6 **Many factors are associated with increased risk for cancer; unhealthy lifestyles are among them.** The malfunction of genes that control cell growth and development is responsible for all cancers. From 5 to 10 percent of cancers result from an inherited faulty gene. Although

genetics can't be altered, a variety of lifestyle and environmental factors are also known to influence cancer. Some risks are hard to avoid, but by being aware of potential risks, you can reduce your exposure. Environments or exposures that may be harmful include exposure to carcinogens at work (e.g., secondhand smoke, coal dust), exposure to geophysical factors (e.g., radon and radiation), exposure to polluted environments (e.g., poor air and water), exposure to certain industrial products (e.g., polychlorinated biphenyls [PCBs] produced in making plastics), and exposure to medical procedures (e.g., X-rays, CT scans). Minimizing exposure to the carcinogens related to environmental factors is an effective strategy for cancer prevention.

Making changes in lifestyles can also be important to cancer prevention. The World Cancer Research Fund and the American Institute for Cancer Research recently released a definitive source of information concerning nutrition and physical activity in cancer prevention (see Suggested Readings). The primary recommendations of this report are included in Table 2. Table 3 summarizes relevant lifestyle changes other than nutrition and physical activity.

Many forms of cancer can now be effectively treated. Many people have lived long, healthy lives after breast, skin, and many other forms of cancer. These

---

Table 2 ▶ Recommendations for Nutrition and Physical Activity to Prevent Cancer

- Be as lean as possible within the normal range of body weight. A BMI in the healthy range is recommended (see Concept 13).

- Be physically active as part of everyday life. At least 30 minutes of moderate activity per day is recommended, with an increase to 60 minutes of moderate activity or 30 minutes of vigorous activity per day as fitness improves.

- Limit consumption of energy-dense foods (including fast foods), and avoid sugary drinks.

- Eat mostly foods from plant origin. Eat five to nine servings of nonstarchy vegetables and fruits every day.

- Limit intake of red meat and avoid processed meat (no more than 30 g per week).

- Limit alcoholic drinks to no more than two drinks a day for men and one for women.

- Limit consumption of salt (less than 1.5 g a day). Avoid moldy foods.

- Aim to meet nutritional needs through diet alone. Dietary supplements are not recommended for cancer prevention.

Source: Adapted from WCRF/AICR.

Melanoma Cancer of the cells that produce skin pigment.

Table 3 ▶ Other Lifestyle Changes for Cancer Prevention

- Eliminate tobacco use (smoke and smokeless).
- Reduce sun and ultraviolet light exposure: use sunscreen, wear protective clothing, and avoid excess sun and tanning lights.
- Do regular self-screening and medical testing.
- Avoid excessive X-rays.
- Avoid breathing polluted air (e.g., exercise away from free-ways and polluted air, check for pollution advisories).
- Minimize occupational and environmental pollutants (as described above) when possible.

people die from other causes, and some would consider them to be "cured." Still, what constitutes a cure is elusive. The 5-year survival rate for all forms of cancer is 62 percent. Though people who survive for 5 years after detection may not be considered cured, the high survival rate illustrates that cancer can be treated, even for those with inherited faulty genes.

Because of the prevalence of cancer, the chances are high that someone you know and care about will get cancer in your lifetime. It is important that you learn to help others who have cancer, as well as those who have survived cancer. There is evidence that some cancer survivors have problems after initial treatment. The National Academy of Sciences has prepared a booklet to help cancer survivors.

ⓘ **Medical consultation is essential when considering hormone replacement therapy.** TECH For years, hormone replacement therapy (HRT) was prescribed to women to help reduce the symptoms of menopause, prevent loss of bone density, and reduce risk for heart disease. However, it has been known for some time that HRT increases the risk for some forms of cancer, is not effective in reducing heart disease, and increases the risk for blood clots. Some experts still support HRT as a method of relieving menopausal symptoms, such as hot flashes, sleep disturbances, fatigue, poor concentration, and disruption of work and recreational activities. Very recent evidence suggests that HRT delivered by gels, patches, and creams is reasonably effective in treating symptoms of menopause and is less likely to cause clotting than oral forms. One recent study indicates that women who stopped HRT had markedly lower risk 2 years after non-use. Each case should be considered individually, with patient and doctor weighing all risks and benefits before choosing a course of action. Those who do not continue HRT should discuss alternate methods of preventing bone loss and reducing post-menopausal symptoms with their physician.

Recognizing early warning signals can help reduce the risk of cancer. The acronym CAUTION will help you remember these early warning signs. Look for the following:

C	=	Changes in bowel or bladder habits
A	=	A sore that does not heal
U	=	Unusual bleeding or discharge
T	=	Thickening or lump (e.g., breast)
I	=	Indigestion or difficulty swallowing
O	=	Obvious change in a wart or mole
N	=	Nagging cough or hoarseness

Diabetes

Several classifications of diabetes cause health risks for many individuals. Glucose, a source of energy, is a sugar in the blood. Diabetes mellitus, typically referred to as diabetes, is a disease that occurs when the blood sugar is abnormally high. Normally, glucose levels range from 50 to 100 mg per 100 ml of blood based on a fasting plasma glucose (FPG) test. According to the American Diabetes Association (ADA), **pre-diabetes** exists when blood glucose levels range from 101 to 125, and diabetes exists when blood glucose levels regularly exceed 125 using the FPG test. An oral glucose tolerance test can also be used to detect diabetes, but different values are used to indicate its prevalence. The ADA recommends the FPG test because it is "easier, faster, and less expensive to perform."

There are as many as 30 different reasons for high blood sugar, therefore diabetes is really many different diseases, not just one. There is no cure for diabetes, but with proper medical treatment and healthy lifestyle modifications, the condition can be managed effectively.

Insulin, a hormone produced by the pancreas, regulates the glucose in the blood. When a person's body fails to produce adequate insulin and the individual needs to take insulin (oral or injection) to regulate blood glucose levels, he or she is said to have **Type I diabetes.** About 5 percent of all diabetics have Type I diabetes, and this condition is typically diagnosed before the age of 30.

Type II diabetes (fasting blood glucose >126) is typically noninsulin dependent and can often be controlled with significant lifestyle changes and drugs other than insulin. Nearly 95 percent of all diabetics have Type II diabetes. Nearly 21 million people have been diagnosed with diabetes, and more than 6 million are diabetic and do not know it. Type II diabetes was referred to as "adult-onset diabetes" in the past because it was a disease that occurred later in life. In the past decade, children and adolescents have begun to develop the disease. This development is closely tied to the epidemic of obesity among youth, thought to be caused primarily by excessive caloric intake and sedentary living.

According to the ADA, before people develop diabetes, they almost always have a condition referred to as pre-diabetes. This condition was formerly known as "impaired glucose tolerance," but the name was changed to help focus attention on the seriousness of this condition. Recent research has shown that pre-diabetes can result in long-term damage to the body similar to that of diabetes. People who do screening and take steps to control pre-diabetes can delay or even prevent the development of Type II diabetes. A third and relatively rare form of diabetes is referred to as "gestational diabetes mellitus." This occurs when high blood sugar levels occur in pregnant women previously not known to have diabetes. This condition is present in about 3 percent of all pregnancies, can have implications for the fetus, and may or may not result in a diabetic state after pregnancy. Other forms of diabetes are rare.

People have a familial predisposition to Type I and Type II, though the predisposition is greater for Type I diabetes. Some people with Type II diabetes do not produce enough insulin to regulate their blood sugar levels. More commonly, they are insensitive to insulin, so the body cannot effectively regulate blood sugar.

Diabetes and related conditions are a leading cause of death in our society.
As noted in Concept 1, diabetes is the sixth leading cause of death, and it is a leading killer in other Western nations, including Canada. People with diabetes have a shortened life span, as well as many short-term and long-term complications associated with the disease. A study of people in the Netherlands, England, and the United States indicated that longevity after 50 years of age is decreased by 7.5 years for men and 8.2 years for women for diabetics as opposed to nondiabetics.

African Americans and Native Americans are especially at risk for diabetes. Not only is the death rate higher among these groups but so are the health problems associated with the disease. Unlike heart disease and cancer that have shown recent decreases in incidence, the incidence of diabetes has increased in the last decade, with little progress being made in accomplishing national health goals for this disease.

Diabetes is associated with other health problems.
People with diabetes have an increased risk for additional health problems. For example, diabetes is considered to be a risk factor for heart disease and high blood pressure. Diabetics have a higher rate of kidney failure (including the need for kidney transplants and kidney dialysis), a high incidence of blindness, and a high incidence of lower limb amputation. Women with diabetes also have a high rate of pregnancy complications. A national health goal is to increase the rate of diagnosis

and to increase the number of diabetics who get regular blood lipid assessments, blood pressure checks, and eye examinations.

Lifestyle changes can help reduce the symptoms and complications associated with diabetes.
National health goals for the year 2010 reflect lifestyle changes that can help reduce health problems associated with diabetes. Table 4 illustrates these and other ways of preventing and controlling diabetes.

Screening for pre-diabetes and diabetes is essential for diagnosis and treatment.
The symptoms of diabetes include frequent urination, excessive thirst, extreme

Table 4 ▶ Lifestyle Changes for Diabetes Prevention and Control

- Maintain a healthy body fat level. For many, achieving a healthy body fat level is effective in preventing or reducing Type II diabetes symptoms.
- Maintain healthy blood sugar levels. For diabetics, regular testing is necessary.
- Eat well. Limit fats and simple carbohydrates in the diet. Increase complex carbohydrates. Keep total calorie consumption at a level that keeps the body weight at a healthy level.
- Exercise regularly. Physical activity expends calories and helps regulate blood sugar levels.
- Learn to recognize symptoms of diabetes and seek screening.
- If you are diabetic, are pre-diabetic, or have symptoms, seek and adhere to medical advice. Many pre-diabetics do not know that they have a problem. Diabetics need to adhere to a plan for blood sugar regulation.
- Learn stress-management skills to reduce stress and maintain a healthy sleep schedule.

Pre-diabetes A condition in which fasting blood glucose levels are higher than normal but not high enough to be clinically diagnosed as diabetes.

Insulin A hormone that regulates blood sugar levels.

Type I Diabetes A chronic metabolic disease characterized by high blood sugar (glucose) levels associated with the inability of the pancreas to produce insulin; also called insulin-dependent diabetes mellitus (IDDM) or juvenile-onset diabetes.

Type II Diabetes A chronic metabolic disease characterized by high blood sugar, usually not requiring insulin therapy; also called noninsulin dependent diabetes mellitus (NIDDM) or adult-onset diabetes.

hunger, unusual weight loss, increased fatigue, irritability, and blurry vision. Those who have recently gained large amounts of weight are also at risk. Early diagnosis as a result of attention to the symptoms can expedite treatment. Guidelines recommend screening for pre-diabetes and diabetes using either of two blood tests: a fasting plasma glucose (FPG) test, which measures levels of glucose in the blood after an overnight fast, or a 2-hour **oral glucose tolerance test (OGTT),** which includes the FPG test but also tests glucose levels 2 hours after a person drinks a standard glucose solution. Guidelines recommend regular screening beginning at age 45. Because African Americans, Hispanics, Asians, American Indians, and Pacific Islanders have especially high risk, some experts recommend testing at age 30 or earlier for these groups. Others with diabetes risk factors and those with a BMI over 25 should also consider testing at an earlier age. Consider using the ADA diabetes risk calculator to see what your risk is (**www.diabetes.org/ diabetesphd/default.jsp**).

Once diabetes is recognized, adherence to a treatment program is essential to prevent related conditions. Type I diabetics typically test blood samples regularly and self-administer insulin as needed. Type II diabetics, depending on the severity of their condition, may need to do similar testing and insulin administration. Consultation with a physician is essential to determine the best treatment plan. The lifestyle recommendations presented in Table 4 are appropriate for diabetics, for pre-diabetics, and for prevention of diabetes. A *Healthy People 2020* goal is to increase aspirin use by diabetics. Diabetes is a risk factor for heart disease, and taking low doses of aspirin can reduce heart disease risk among those in high-risk categories. Before taking aspirin, diabetics are urged to discuss the medication with their health-care professionals (see Web Resources).

Other Health Threats

Injuries are a major cause of death and suffering. Not only are injuries the fifth leading cause of death among people of all ages, but they also claim more lives than chronic and infectious diseases among people aged 40 and younger. According to the U.S. Public Health Service, the major causes of injuries are motor vehicle crashes, falls, poisoning, drowning, and residential fires.

Injuries also account for much pain and suffering. Of all hospital stays, one in six results from a nonfatal injury. Injury rates are higher among males than females, and they are quite high among ethnic and racial minority groups. In the past decade, the number of deaths caused by unintentional injuries and by work-related injuries has decreased.

Changes in lifestyles can reduce injury rates. A major conclusion of the Public Health Service is that the prevention of injuries requires the combined efforts of many fields, including health, education, transportation, law, engineering, architecture, and safety science.

The second major conclusion of the Public Health Service is that alcohol is "intimately associated" with the causes and severity of injuries. Other lifestyle behaviors are also associated with reducing injury incidence, and steps that can be taken to reduce these injuries are listed in Table 5.

Prompt emergency medical care is critical for saving lives. Paramedics and emergency medical teams work hard to provide emergency medical service (EMS) when needed. Emphasis is placed on reducing the average time required to reach the majority of residents in different areas. Where you live can have a lot to do with whether you get good medical treatment. A survey of medical directors conducted over an 18-month period in the nation's 50 largest cities shows that treatment effectiveness for those needing emergency medical care

Technology Update
Genetic Testing

Recent news headlines attest to the current interest in genetic testing as a potentially useful medical technique. Preliminary results suggest that genetic testing may be useful in determining which patients are susceptible to certain diseases and which patients will benefit from certain medicines. While researchers are optimistic about the use of genetic testing, they are also quick to point out that applications for genetic testing are still in the early stages. Home kits for genetic testing are available online and were to be sold at Walgreens until the FDA ruled that genetic testing is a "medical device" that requires FDA approval. Whether home genetic testing is approved, or not, the applications are not fully understood and medical experts are concerned about their use. The potential for quackery exists as unscrupulous doctors now use the Internet to tout genetic testing and other miracles (e.g., stem cell treatments). Experts advise that you consult your regular physician or a well-known specialist before considering gene testing and related treatments. For more information on the headlines below go to the associated Web link

Oral Glucose Tolerance Test (OGTT) A test used to diagnose diabetes. It consists of a blood sugar measurement following the ingestion of a standard amount of sugar (glucose) after a period of fasting.

Table 5 ▶ Steps to Reduce Injuries

Reduce Motor Vehicle Accidents

- Do not drive while under the influence of alcohol.
- Use shoulder seat belts and air bags.
- Reduce driving speed.
- Use motorcycle helmets.
- Increase safety programs for pedestrians and cyclists.
- Establish more effective licensing for very young and older drivers.

Improve Home and Neighborhood Environments

- Require safety controls on handguns.
- Require sprinkler systems in homes with high risk of fire.
- Increase presence of functional smoke detectors in homes.
- Increase injury and poison education in schools.
- Wear effective safety gear in sports.
- Improve pool and boat safety education.
- Learn cardiopulmonary resuscitation.
- Properly mark poisons and prescription drugs.
- Require childproof packaging for poisons and prescription drugs.

varies, depending on where you live. In many cities, the EMS responses were slow and less than effective. The study estimates that about 1,000 lives a year could be saved with more effective systems. Figure 4 provides information concerning which of the 50 cities had the most effective EMS, according to the survey.

Improved occupational safety could help reduce injury rates. Many of the nation's health goals focus on improving occupational safety, especially among construction, health-care (e.g., nurses), farm, transportation, and mine workers.

Many mental disorders pose threats to health and wellness. The health goals for the nation identify suicide, schizophrenia, and depression as the most serious mental disorders needing attention. Although the Public Health Service uses the term *mental disorders,* they are sometimes called emotional disorders. Other common mental disorders are panic disorders, alcohol and other drug problems, personality disorders, and phobias.

Mental disorders result in loss of life, injury, and inability to function, and they cost the public millions of dollars annually. More than one in four adults (26 percent) suffer from a diagnosed mental

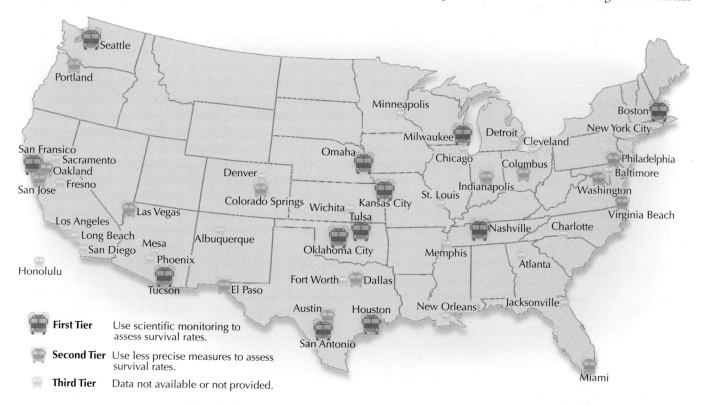

First Tier   Use scientific monitoring to assess survival rates.

Second Tier Use less precise measures to assess survival rates.

Third Tier   Data not available or not provided.

Figure 4 ▶ Emergency medical treatment effectiveness in major cities.
Source: USA Today EMS survey.

disorder that limits the ability to function effectively and requires special assistance. Depression (see Web Resources) and other mood disorders affect nearly one in five people, and anxiety disorders affect about one in five. These disorders cost $150 billion annually, primarily from loss of productivity. A depressed worker's medical costs average $1,038 a year, while non-depressed workers' costs average $325. The most serious outcome of mental disorders is suicide (30,000 annually).

Reducing the incidence of suicide and serious injury from suicide attempts is an important national health goal. Progress has been made in reducing suicide, but it is still far too common. Women are about three times more likely to attempt suicide than men, but men are four times more likely to complete a suicide attempt. Among male teenagers, it is the second leading cause of death, and male teenagers with antisocial personality disorders are especially susceptible.

Depression is closely associated with suicide, as are alcohol and other drug abuse. Inability to cope with stressful life events may contribute to suicide. Examples of precipitating events are divorce, separation, loss of a loved one, unemployment, and financial setbacks.

The best chance for reducing suicides appears to be early detection and treatment of mental disorders such as depression. Professional help should be sought, and as many concerned people as possible should be recruited to help the suicidal individual seek professional assistance. Experts suggest that threats of suicide must be taken seriously.

Depression, a common mental disorder, can usually be treated effectively. Most people occasionally feel depressed or sad. This type of depression is usually not a mental disorder. People with clinical depression (classified as a mental disorder) have chronic feelings of guilt, hopelessness, low self-esteem, and dejection. They might have trouble sleeping, loss of appetite, lack of interest in social activities, lack of interest in sex, and inability to concentrate.

Among the lifestyle changes that can help relieve symptoms are exercising regularly, increasing social contact, setting realistic goals, using stress-management techniques (see Concept 17), and removing oneself from situations that contribute to depression. These changes, however, may need to be accompanied by professional therapy and/or medication.

Sleep disorders can often be helped by lifestyle changes. Sleep disorders, especially insomnia (long-term problems with sleep), can result in depression and other dysfunctions. Physiological problems in the brain can cause sleep disorders, but depression, stress, chronic pain, or abuse of alcohol or other drugs are often the source of the problem. Some sleep disorders require professional help; however, you can take action to prevent insomnia. Creating a healthy sleeping environment, avoiding excessive caffeine or alcohol, exercising regularly, and establishing a regular routine for sleeping can help you avoid sleep disorders.

Various health threats put the public's health at risk. The health threats outlined in *Healthy People 2020* are too numerous to be dealt with in depth in this book. More information concerning health threats such as chronic kidney disease, hepatitis, asthma, and arthritis can be found at the HP 2020 website (see Web Resources).

HELP

HEALTH is available to Everyone for a Lifetime, and it's Personal

Students often think that they are not susceptible to health conditions such as cancer and diabetes. Challenges with insurance and transportation often make it difficult to get regular check ups. Students may also ignore warning signs (e.g. skin cancer) and dismiss symptoms of depression. See Table 6 for common reasons for skipping regular check ups.

Have you made regularly scheduled medical checkups or health screenings part of your lifestyle? Why or why not?

Table 6 ▶ Types of People Who Avoid Medical Checkups

- *Gamblers.* These people do not think about their health until a serious problem occurs.

- *Martyrs.* These people are so busy taking care of others that they fail to take care of themselves.

- *Economists.* These people think the cost of preventive exams is too high for the benefits received.

- *Shamans.* These people buy in on the latest health fad and self-diagnose, while avoiding regular medical care.

- *Informers.* These people have an ax to grind with health-care professionals and avoid health care for this reason.

- *Queens of denial (Cleopatra syndrome).* These people do not believe something could be wrong with them or do not want to know if there is.

- *Busy bees.* These people feel they are too busy to take the time to get regular medical care.

Adhering to sound medical advice is important for disease prevention and treatment. Many conditions described in this concept, especially cancer and diabetes, can be managed or cured with early diagnosis and proper treatment. Many people ignore early warning signs or symptoms, hoping that problems go away on their own. Some people fear disease and avoid medical advice because of this fear. An important key to good health is to note any irregularities in your health and to seek expert advice when needed. Establishing a regular habit of getting scheduled checkups and/or health screens is part of a healthy lifestyle because it helps ensure that your health is where it should be.

Periodic checks can also help detect early signs of heart disease, cancer, diabetes, and other health threats, and this allows for more effective treatment. These checks become increasingly important with advancing age because people become vulnerable to a wider array of chronic conditions.

The Cooper Clinic in Dallas, Texas, specializes in preventive medical care. A staff physician (Dr. Tedd Mitchell) has categorized the types of people by the reasons they give for not seeing a doctor or getting a regular medical checkup (see Table 6). According to Dr. Mitchell, "there is no good reason to avoid your annual visit to the doctor."

Strategies for Action

Self-assessments and regular medical exams can help you determine if you need help with various health problems. Just as the fitness assessments you completed earlier in this book helped you build a profile that will help you improve your fitness, regular self-assessments can help you identify and prevent common health problems. Regular medical exams that include the tests outlined in Table 1 as well as those described in other sections of this concept will help you identify problems that can be treated and cured with early diagnosis. In Lab 22A, you will have the opportunity to assess your cancer risk. In Lab 22B, you will learn

to do self-exams to help you resist breast and testicular cancer. Web addresses for self-assessments are provided in Lab 22B.

Staying current with new health information can help you identify and get treatment for health problems. Information about various health problems changes rapidly as new methods of treatment and prevention become available. It is important to learn ways to stay current on health topics. Addresses for the Web sites of reputable health organizations that will help you stay abreast of current information are included in *Web Resources*.

Web Resources

Additional websites with information related to Concept 22 are available at the associated Web link.

WEB

American Cancer Society **www.cancer.org**

American Diabetes Association **www.diabetes.org**

Environmental Protection Agency (EPA) **www.epa.gov**

EPA Table of Toxic Environmental Assessment
   www.epa.gov/ttn/atw/nata2002/tables.html#table1

Healthy People 2020 **www.healthypeople.gov/hp2020**

National Cancer Institute **www.nci.nih.gov**

National Center for Environmental Health **www.cdc.gov/nceh**

National Center for Health Statistics **www.cdc.gov/nchs**

National Institute of Mental Health (NIMH)
   www.nimh.nih.gov/health/topics/depression/index.shtml

Suggested Readings

Selected readings and references are listed below. A more comprehensive list is available at the associated Web link.

REFERENCES

American Cancer Society. 2010. *Stories of Hope.* Available at **www.cancer.org/docroot/fps/fps_0.asp?from=fast**

American Diabetes Association. 2010. *Diabetes Basics.* Available at **www.diabetes.org/diabetes-basics**

Atkins, W. S., et al. 2010. Once-only flexible sigmoidoscopy screening in prevention of colorectal cancer: A multicentre randomised controlled trial. *Lancet* 375(9726):1624–1633.

Berrington de González, A., et al. 2009. Projected cancer risks from computed tomographic scans performed in the United States. *Archives of Internal Medicine* 169(22): 2071–2077.

Chebowski, R. T., et al. 2009. Breast cancer after use of estrogen plus progestin in postmenopausal women. *New England Journal of Medicine* 360(6):573–587.

Curkendall, S., et al. 2010. Productivity losses among treated depressed patients relative to healthy controls. *Journal of Occupational and Environmental Medicine* 52(2):125–130.

Fletcher, R. H. 2008. Colorectal cancer screening on stronger footing. *New England Journal of Medicine* 359 (12): 1285–1287

Hamann, B. P. 2007. *Disease: Identification, Prevention and Control.* 3rd ed. New York: McGraw-Hill Higher Education.

Johnson, C. D., et al. 2008. Accuracy of CT colonography for detection of large adenomas and cancers. *New England Journal of Medicine* 359(12):1207–1217.

Mayo Clinic (Collazo-Clavel, M., medical editor). 2009. *Mayo Clinic Essential Diabetes Book.* New York: Time Inc.

National Institute of Mental Health. Accessed May 2010. *Depression.* Available at **www.nimh.nih.gov/health /publications/depression-easy-to-read/index.shtm**

U.S. Preventive Services Task Force. 2009. Screening for breast cancer: U.S. Preventive Services Task Force recommendation statement. *Annals of Internal Medicine* 151(10):716–726. Information available at **www.preventiveservices.ahrq.gov**

World Cancer Research Fund/American Institute for Cancer Research. 2007. *Food, Nutrition, Physical Activity and the Prevention of Cancer: A Global Perspective.* Washington, DC: American Institute for Cancer Research.

Lab 22A Determining Your Cancer Risk

Name	Section	Date

Purpose: To become aware of your risk for various types of cancer

Procedures

1. Answer the questions in the six-part questionnaire for the various forms of cancer.
2. Record the number of "yes" answers for each form of cancer in the Results section.
3. Use Chart 1 to determine ratings and record the ratings in the Results section.
4. Answer the questions in the Conclusions and Implications section.

Results: Mark an X over your answer to each question.

Skin Cancer Risk Factors

Do you frequently work or play in the sun for long periods? (Yes) (No)

Do you work or have you worked near industrial exposure (coal mine, radioactivity)? (Yes) (No)

Do you have a family history of skin cancer? (Yes) (No)

Do you have fair skin? (Yes) (No)

Lung Cancer Risk Factors

Do you smoke? (Yes) (No)

Do you work or have you worked near industrial exposure (coal mine, radioactivity)? (Yes) (No)

Do you have a family history of cancer? (Yes) (No)

Do you work in a place that allows smoking, such as a bar, or live in a home with smokers? (Yes) (No)

Colon-Rectal Cancer Risk Factors

Do you eat poorly, abuse alcohol, or smoke? (Yes) (No)

Are you African American or over 50? (Yes) (No)

Do you have a family history of colon or rectal cancer? (Yes) (No)

Have you noticed blood in your stool? (Yes) (No)

Breast Cancer Risk Factors

Do you have a family history of breast cancer? (Yes) (No)

Are you sedentary, do you eat poorly, or do you abuse alcohol? (Yes) (No)

Are you a female over 35 who has not had children? (Yes) (No)

Have you ever detected lumps or cysts in your breasts? (Yes) (No)

Uterine/Cervical Cancer Risk Factors* (Females)

Do you regularly have bleeding between periods? (Yes) (No)

Is your body fat level high? (Yes) (No)

Did you have early intercourse and multiple sexual partners? (Yes) (No)

Have you had viral infections of the vagina, such as HPV? (Yes) (No)

Prostate Cancer Risk Factors (Males)

Do you eat a high-fat or low-fiber diet? (Yes) (No)

Are you a male over 50 years of age or African American? (Yes) (No)

Have you had a regular PSA test? (Yes) (No)

Has a digital rectal exam shown an enlargement of the prostate? (Yes) (No)

*Because of the personal nature of several questions, do not record results if turned in to an instructor.

Cancer Type	Score	Rating
Breast		
Uterine/cervical (women)*		
Colon-rectal		
Skin		
Lung		
Prostate (men)		

*Do not record results if handed in to an instructor.

Chart 1 ▶ Cancer Risk Ratings

Rating	Score
High risk	4
Relatively high risk	3
Lower risk	2
Low risk	0–1

Conclusions and Implications: In several sentences, discuss the type or types of cancer for which you are at greatest risk and why. Also, discuss the lifestyles you could modify to reduce your risk.

Lab 22B Breast and Testicular Self-Exams

Name **Section** **Date**

Purpose: To learn to do breast or testicular self-exams

Procedures

1. If you are female, read the procedures for breast self-exams. Note: Males should also be aware of abnormal lumps in their breasts.
2. If you are male, read the procedures for testicular self-exams.
3. After reading the directions, perform the self-exam. If you find lumps or nodules, contact a physician.
4. This procedure should be done monthly. The breast exam is best done a day or two after the end of menstrual flow. For this lab, it can be done at any time.
5. It is not necessary to record your results here. Do answer the questions in the Conclusions and Implications section.

Lying Breast Self-Exam (Men and Women)*

1. Lie down with one arm behind your head (see illustration). You can more easily detect lumps when lying as compared to standing or sitting because when lying the breast tissue is spread more evenly.

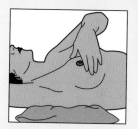 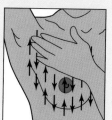

2. With the tips of the middle three fingers (see illustration) of the hand opposite the one behind your head, feel for lumps in the breast on the side of the raised arm. Use overlapping, dime-sized, circular motions of the finger pads to feel the breast tissue.
3. Identify the spot for the overlapping, dime-sized, circular motions and feel for lumps using three levels of pressure. First apply light pressure to feel for lumps closest to the skin. Then apply medium pressure to feel for lumps deeper below the skin. Finally, to find lumps near the ribs and chest cavity, apply firm pressure. Then move to another spot and repeat the same procedure, applying all three levels of pressure. A firm ridge in the lower curve of each breast is normal. If you have questions about this procedure and how hard to press, talk with your doctor or medical professional.
4. To assure full coverage of each breast, use an up-and-down pattern (see illustration), starting at an imaginary line drawn straight down your side from the underarm and moving across the breast to the middle of the chest bone (sternum, or breastbone). Be sure to check the entire breast area, going down until you feel only ribs and up to the neck or collarbone (clavicle).
5. Repeat the exam on the other breast, using the finger pads of the opposite hand.

Standing Breast Self-Exam (Women)*

1. Stand in front of a mirror. Press down firmly on your hips with your hands. Look for any changes of size, shape, contour, or dimpling or redness or scaliness of the nipple or breast skin. (Pressing down on the hips contracts the chest wall muscles and enhances any breast changes.)
2. Examine each underarm with your arm slightly raised, so that you can easily feel in this area. Raising your arm straight up (too high) tightens the tissue in this area and makes it harder to examine.

Testicular Self-Exam (Men)*

1. Using both hands, grasp one testicle between the thumb and first finger.
2. Roll the testicle gently with the thumb and first finger, feeling for lumps or nodules.
3. Examine the other testicle using the same procedure.
4. If you find a lump or nodule, consult a physician. Note: a lump or nodule may not be a result of disease, but this can only be determined by a physician.

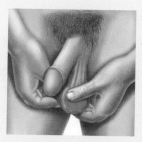

*Adapted from American Cancer Society.

Conclusions and Implications: In several sentences, discuss the effectiveness of the procedure you performed. Do you think the directions provided were adequate for you to perform the self-exam effectively? Do you think you will perform this self-exam on a regular basis? Do you believe the screening procedures described in the lab are effective? Why or why not? What could be done to motivate you and others to do regular self-exams?

Additional Self-Exam Information

Several national health agencies maintain websites that include detailed breast and testicular self-exam information. These sites contain both written and pictorial descriptions of both self-exam procedures. For more information, visit the sites listed below.

American Cancer Society
www.cancer.org

Mayo Clinic
www.mayohealth.org

National Cancer Institute
www.nci.nih.gov

Early detection is critical for effective cancer treatment. The ACS notes that a "breast self exam is an option for women starting in their 20s. Women should be told about the benefits and limitations of BSE. Women should report any changes in how their breasts look or feel to a health expert right away." Men should also be aware of changes in breast tissue. The ACS indicates that many physicians recommend a BSE each month. For those who do a BSE it is wise to review the technique with a physician or medical professional. The ACS indicates that finding a lump in the testicles at an early stage is important. They recommend a regular testicular exam by a physician and indicate that many doctors recommended testicular self-exams

Evaluating Fitness and Wellness Products: Becoming an Informed Consumer

Health Goals for the Year 2020

- Improve the health literacy of the population.
- Increase percentage of high-quality health-related websites.
- Increase percentage of college students receiving information on priority risk behavior areas. (D)
- Create social and physical environments that promote good health for all.
- Promote quality of life, healthy development, and healthy behaviors across all stages of life.
- Increase policies that give retail food outlets incentives to carry foods that meet dietary guidelines.
- Increase number of work sites that offer nutrition and weight management classes and counseling.

- Increase physician counseling on nutrition and weight management.
- Increase food safety (variety of areas).
- Increase percentage of people with health-care providers who involve them in decisions about health care.
- Reduce adverse events from medical products.
- Reduce medical emergencies that occur from adverse events associated with medicines.
- Increase counseling by physicians.
- Increase comprehensive school health education.
- Increase number of adults who meet guidelines for physical activity.

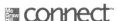

connect
|FITNESS AND WELLNESS**   http://connect.mcgraw-hill.com

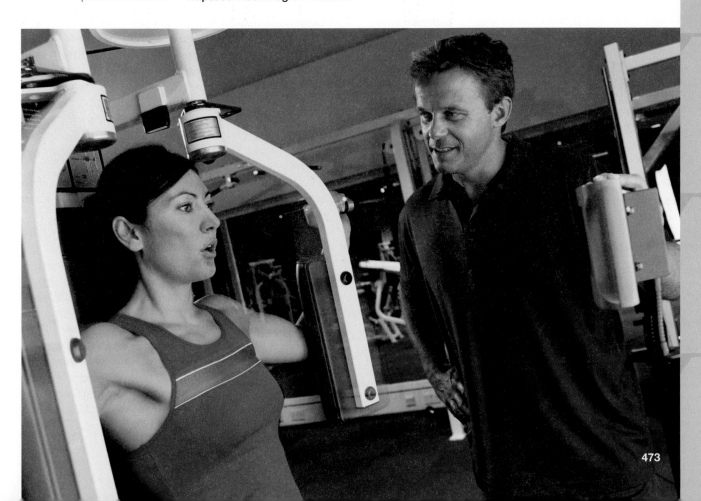

"Let the buyer beware" is a good motto for the consumer seeking advice or planning a program for developing or maintaining fitness, health, or wellness.

People have always searched for the fountain of youth and an easy, quick, and miraculous route to health and happiness. In current society, this search often focuses on fitness, nutrition, weight loss, or appearance. A variety of products are available that promise weight loss, improved health, or improved fitness with little or no effort. The sale of these products can typically be classified as either quackery or fraud, since most do not work.

The dictionary definition of *quack* is "a pretender of medical skill" or "one who talks pretentiously without sound knowledge of the subject discussed." These definitions imply that the promotion of quackery involves deliberate deception, but quacks often believe in what they promote. A consumer watchdog group, called Quackwatch, defines quackery more broadly as "anything involving overpromotion in the field of health." This definition encompasses questionable ideas as well as questionable products and services. The word *fraud* is reserved for situations in which deliberate deception is involved. This concept discusses common myths and provides guidelines to help you be a more informed consumer of fitness, health, and wellness products.

Quacks and Quackery

Quacks can be identified by their unscientific practices. Some of the ways to identify quacks, frauds, and rip-off artists are to look for these clues:

- They do not use the scientific method of controlled experimentation, which can be verified by other scientists.
- To a large extent, they use testimonials and anecdotes to support their claims rather than scientific methods. There is no such thing as a valid testimonial. Anecdotal evidence is no evidence at all.
- They have something to sell, and they advise you to buy something you would not otherwise have bought.
- They claim everyone can benefit from the product or service they are selling. There is no such thing as a simple, quick, easy, painless remedy for conditions for which medical science has not yet found a remedy.
- They promise quick, miraculous results. A perfect, no-risk treatment does not exist.

- Their claims cover a wide variety of conditions.
- They may offer a money-back guarantee. A guarantee is only as good as the company.
- They claim the treatment or product is approved by the Food and Drug Administration (FDA), but federal law does not permit mentioning the FDA to suggest marketing approval.
- They may claim the support of experts, but the experts are not identified.
- The ingredients in the product are not identified.
- They claim there is a conspiracy against them by "bureaucrats," "organized medicine," the FDA, the American Medical Association (AMA), and other groups. Never believe a doctor who claims the medical community is persecuting him or her or that the government is suppressing a wonderful discovery.
- Their credentials may be irrelevant to the area in which they claim expertise.
- They use scare tactics, such as "If you don't do this, you will die of a heart attack."
- They may appear to be a sympathetic friend who wants to share a new discovery with you.
- They misquote scientific research (or quote out of context) to mislead you; they also mix a little bit of truth with a lot of fiction.
- They cite research or quote from individuals or institutions with questionable reputations.
- They claim it is a new discovery (often originated in Europe). There is never a great medical breakthrough that debuts in an obscure magazine or tabloid.
- The person or organization named is similar to a famous person or credible institution (e.g., the Mayo diet had no connection with the Mayo Clinic).
- They often sell products through the mail, which does not allow you to examine the product personally.

Experts have a good education, have a good scientific base, and meet other professional criteria. Unlike quacks, experts base their work on the scientific method. Some characteristics of professional experts are an extended education, an established code of ethics, membership in well-known associations, involvement in the profession as an intern before obtaining credentials, and a commitment to perform an important social service. Some experts require a license. Examples of experts in the fitness, health, and wellness area are medical doctors, nurses, certified fitness leaders, physical educators, registered dietitians, physical therapists, and clinical psychologists. In most cases, you can check if a person has the credentials to be considered an expert before obtaining services. The following list includes some things that can be done to determine a person's expertise.

- Determine the source of the person's education and the nature of the degree and/or certification.
- Check with the person's professional association or with a government board, licensing agency, or certifying agency to see if there are any complaints against the person; for example, you can check with the medical board in your state to check complaints against physicians.
- Check if the person has credentials to provide the service you are seeking (e.g., a registered dietician is qualified to give nutrition advice but not medical advice).

You can reduce your susceptibility to quackery by being an informed consumer. The three key characteristics that predispose people to health-related quackery are a concern about appearance, health, or performance; a lack of adequate knowledge; and a desire for immediate results. Understanding the principles of exercise and nutrition presented in this book will help you know when something sounds "too good to be true."

When evaluating health-related products or information, carefully consider the quality of your source. Common sources of misinformation are magazines, health food stores, and TV infomercials. These entities all have an economic incentive in promoting the purchase and use of exercise, diet, and weight loss products. Because of freedom of speech laws, it is legal to state opinion through these media. Note, however, that few companies make claims on product labels, since this is false advertising. Follow these additional guidelines to avoid being a victim of quackery:

- Read the ad carefully, especially the small print.
- Do not send cash; use a check, money order, or credit card so you will have a receipt.
- Do not order from a company with only a post office box, unless you know the company.
- Do not let high-pressure sales tactics make you rush into a decision.
- When in doubt, check out the company through your Better Business Bureau (BBB).

Scientific research is a systematic search for truth. Occasionally, companies will mention that their product or program has been scientifically tested, but this does not necessarily mean that the results were positive. Even if a study did show positive results, the study may have been flawed. An article in a prominent scientific journal documented that results of studies, especially small studies that are not well controlled, are often found to be

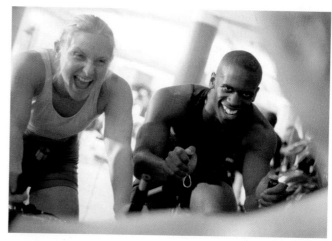

Changing your lifestyle, rather than quick solutions, is the key to health, fitness, and wellness.

wrong or the effects are not as large as originally thought. The media often highlight the results of novel or unusual findings, and this leads some people to conclude that experts simply "can't make up their minds." In actuality, scientists typically take a cautious approach with any new finding and wait for other studies to confirm the results. Beware of news reports that denounce established evidence based on a single study or "preliminary research." With accumulating evidence, even the most established beliefs may change. But it takes many confirming studies to provide the best evidence. Consider this before making quick consumer judgments.

Physical Activity Quackery

There is no "effortless" way to get the benefits from physical activity. Advertisements for exercise that claim to "get you totally fit in 10 minutes" or that their program "will get you fit with little effort" are false. The only way to get fit is to follow the FIT formula for the type of exercise that you choose for meeting specific fitness goals. Claims for exercise that will effortlessly reduce weight or produce significant health benefits are equally false. As noted in previous concepts, there are specific guidelines for physical activity designed for weight loss or maintenance and for achieving health benefits. Beware of those who claim otherwise.

Claims for many forms of exercise are overstated or unsubstantiated. New exercise programs or routines are often promoted as the complete answer for total fitness or a **panacea** for health. Claims for hatha yoga suggest it will help you lose weight, trim inches,

Panacea A cure-all; a remedy for all ills.

strengthen glands and organs, or cure health problems, such as the common cold or arthritis. Hatha yoga can be useful in reducing stress, promoting relaxation, and improving flexibility, but the other claims are overstated.

Similar hype may be used for promoting new pieces of exercise equipment. Each piece of equipment claims to be fun, easy to use, and more effective than other forms of exercise. The benefits from exercise depend on the relative intensity and duration of the activity—and whether it is done regularly over time. The best form of exercise is clearly the one that you are willing and able to do.

Contrary to claims, passive exercises do not provide any benefits for fitness or weight loss. For exercise to be beneficial, the work must be done by contracting skeletal muscles. A variety of **passive exercise** forms have been promoted to try to reduce the effort required to perform regular exercise. Some passive devices have value for people with special needs, when used by a qualified person, such as a physical therapist. However, passive devices sold for use by the general public are ineffective. The goal of sellers is to convince people that there is an effortless way to exercise—there is not. The fallacies associated with many past forms of passive exercise, such as fat rolling machines (purported to break up and redistribute fat), seem obvious today, but new approaches come out all the time with different marketing and promotions. The list that follows highlights some of the common forms of passive exercise.

- *Vibrating belts.* These wide canvas or leather belts are driven by an electric motor, causing loose tissue of the body part to shake. They have no beneficial effect on fitness, fat, or figure. They are potentially harmful to the back and if used on the abdomen (especially if used by women during pregnancy, during menstruation, or while an IUD is in place).
- *Vibrating tables and pillows.* Contrary to advertisements, these passive devices (also called toning tables) will not improve posture, trim the body, reduce weight, or develop muscle **tonus.**
- *Continuous passive motion (CPM) tables.* The motor-driven CPM table, unlike the vibrating table, moves body parts repeatedly through a range of motion. Tables are designed to do such things as passively extend the leg at the hip joint and raise the upper trunk in a sit-up-like motion. Advocates claim that the tables remove cellulite, increase circulation and oxygen flow, and eliminate excess water retention. All of these claims are false. Hospitals and rehabilitation centers use a similar machine to maintain range of motion in the legs of knee surgery patients, maintain integrity of the cartilage, and decrease the incidence of blood clots. Certainly, a healthy person has nothing to gain from using such a device.
- *Motor-driven cycles and rowing machines.* Like all mechanical devices that do the work for the individual, these motor-driven machines are not effective in a fitness program. They may help increase circulation, and some may even help maintain flexibility, but they are not as effective as active exercise. *Nonmotorized cycles and rowing machines* are good equipment for use in a fitness program.
- *Massage.* Whether done by a certified or licensed massage therapist or by a mechanical device, massage is passive, requiring no effort on the part of the individual. It can help increase circulation, induce relaxation, prevent or loosen adhesions, retard muscle atrophy, and serve other therapeutic uses when administered in the clinical setting for medical reasons. However, massage has no useful role in a physical fitness program and will not alter your shape. There is no scientific evidence that it can hasten nerve growth, remove subcutaneous fat, or increase athletic performance. Some athletes (e.g., cyclists) find that it aids in recovery from exercise.
- *Magnets.* The law requires magnets marketed with medical claims to obtain clearance from the FDA. To date, the FDA has not approved the marketing of any magnets for medical use, and sellers making medical claims for magnets are in violation of the law.
- *Electrical muscle stimulators.* Neuromuscular electrical stimulators cause the muscle to contract involuntarily. In the hands of qualified medical personnel, muscle stimulators are valuable therapeutic devices. They can increase muscle strength and endurance selectively and aid in the treatment of edema. They can also help prevent atrophy in a patient who is unable to move, and they may decrease muscle spasms, but in a healthy person they do not have the same value as exercise. The Federal Trade Commission (FTC) has filed false advertising claims against several firms that market exercise stimulators that promise to build *"six-pack abs"* and tone muscles without exercise. These devices, worn over the abdomen, are heavily advertised in infomercials and have been shown to be ineffective and potentially hazardous to health. Electrical stimulators placed on the chest, back, or abdomen can interfere with the normal rhythm of the heart, even for normally healthy people. For those with heart, gastrointestinal, orthopedic, kidney, and other health problems, such as epilepsy, hernia, and varicose veins, they can be especially dangerous. Beware of spas and clinics that use these devices and make claims of fitness enhancement for healthy people.
- *Weighted belts.* Claims have been made that these belts reduce waists, thighs, and hips when worn under the

clothing. In reality, they do none of these things and have been reported to cause physical harm. However, when used in a progressive resistance program, wristlet, anklet, or laced-on weights can help produce an overload and, therefore, develop strength or endurance.

- *Inflated, constricting, or nonporous garments.* These garments include rubberized inflated devices (sauna belts and sauna shorts) and paraphernalia that are airtight plastic or rubberized. Evidence indicates that their girth-reducing claims are *unwarranted.* If exercise is performed while wearing such garments, the exercise, not the garment, may be beneficial. You cannot squeeze fat out of the pores, nor can you melt it.
- *Body wrapping.* Some reducing salons, gyms, and clubs advertise that wrapping the body in bandages soaked in a magic solution will cause a permanent reduction in body girth. This so-called treatment is pure quackery. Tight, constricting bands can temporarily indent the skin and squeeze body fluids into other parts of the body, but the skin or body will regain its original size within minutes or hours. The solution is usually similar to Epsom salts, which can cause fluid to be drawn from tissue. The fluid is water, not fat, and is quickly replaced. Body wrapping may be dangerous to your health; at least one fatality has been documented.

Exercise Equipment

Exercise machines are very useful, but be careful when determining the type of machine to use. Most health and fitness clubs have many types of machines. When deciding which machines are best for you, ask yourself these questions.

- *What is your current state of fitness and your current activity level?* Beginners and people with low fitness will want to choose a different piece of equipment than a more advanced exerciser. For example, exercise on a spinning bike would be appropriate for an advanced exerciser. The beginner might choose a regular exercise bicycle instead.
- *What are your goals?* Make sure the machine will help you meet your goals. For example, a resistance machine would be a good choice for building muscle fitness, and a treadmill or an elliptical machine would be a good choice for building cardiovascular fitness.
- *Will you enjoy it?* One limitation of exercise machines is that they are not as fun as doing sports and some other activities. But some machines may be more fun for you than others. Try several machines and consider one that you enjoy the most.
- *Will you stick with it?* Choose a machine that you think you can use consistently. Enjoyment is a factor, but so is difficulty. Find a machine that allows you to easily adjust the intensity. This allows you to find a

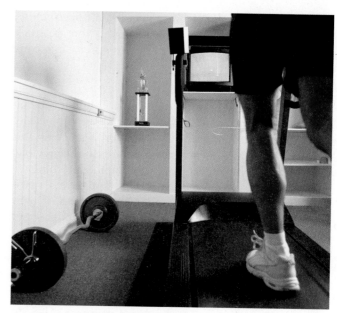

Ask import questions before buying home exercise equipment. Will you use it? Do you need it? Will it last?

comfortable intensity and to gradually increae it over time.

- *Is it safe?* Recent research has shown that exercise machines are the source of more than a few injuries. People with limitations (e.g., knee problems) may choose a bicycle rather than a treadmill. Make sure to get proper instruction on how to use the machine before trying it. Some suggestions for avoiding injury are included in a recent Consumer Reports article (see Suggested Readings).
- *Can it be adjusted to fit your body?* Before you begin exercising, adjust the machine to fit your body. For example, adjust the seat on an exercise bicycle. If you are short or tall, some equipment may not fit you.

Home exercise machines can be very useful, but research your options before making a purchase. Research by the Consumer's Union (Consumer Reports) has shown that well-designed and manufactured exercise machines can be used as an effective means to achieving good health-related physical fitness (see Suggested Readings). When using a piece of equipment at a health

Passive Exercise Exercise in which no voluntary muscle contraction occurs; an outside force moves the body part with no effort by the person.

Tonus The most frequently misused and abused term in fitness vocabularies. Tonus is the tension developed in a muscle as a result of passive muscle stretch. Tonus cannot be determined by feeling or inspecting a muscle. It has little or nothing to do with the strength of a muscle.

club, you can change machines if you don't like the one you are using. If you buy the equipment, you are stuck with it even if you don't like it. Before purchasing, consider the questions provided in the previous section, but also consider the following questions.

- *Is this the best piece of equipment for you?* Should you buy a resistance machine, a treadmill, an exercise bicycle, or some other equipment? Consider your goals and fitness needs, and answer the questions in the previous section to help you decide what equipment to buy.

- *Do you have space for it?* If you do not have a space where you can put the equipment and leave it, you will probably not use it regularly. Some equipment is "portable" so that it can be stored when not in use. Be aware that "portable" equipment is less likely to be used regularly than equipment that is readily available. The more difficult it is to move equipment, the less likely it is to be used. Be sure to consider ceiling height, room width, other uses for the space. Also, do you have space to have a TV to watch?

- *Is the space appropriate?* More than a few people have bought equipment thinking they will put it in the TV room or the garage. Be sure all members of the family approve of the location of the equipment before purchasing it. Garages may be appropriate for some machines in some locales, but may be unusable in some climates (e.g., too hot, too cold). Also remember that some equipment such as free weights may take up extra space.

- *Will you use it?* The best time to buy used exercise equipment is in February or March. This is because many people buy equipment in January to fulfill a New Year's resolution to be more active. They don't carefully consider the reasons for their purchase and find that they don't use what they have bought. Try out the equipment before you buy, especially when considering expensive machines.

- *Do you need it?* Are there cheaper alternatives? Can you do the same thing less expensively? Consider these questions.

- *Have you considered information from a source such as Consumer Reports?* Consumer Reports does regular evaluations of exercise equipment. Consider their ratings and ratings of fitness experts to determine the quality, reliability, and repair records of various machines. Price is also a consideration. In some cases, if you cannot afford a quality machine, it might be wise to wait rather than to buy something that may not last. Finally, consider the product warranty and the cost of repairs if you do not get a warranty (see Suggested Readings for ratings of treadmills, elliptical trainers, and stationary bikes).

- *Is the dealer reputable?* Select a company or store that has been in business for a while and is a member of the Better Business Bureau. Compare prices for similar equipment. Beware of dealers who try to sell you extra attachments or accessories that you won't use.

- Consider the limitations of exercise machines described in the section that follows.

Be aware of the limitations of exercise machines and devices. As discussed in the previous sections, exercise machines can be useful in carrying out your personal exercise plan. However, machines are not without limitations. Some of these limitations are described here.

- *Many pieces of equipment are for a single purpose.* A machine that builds cardiovascular fitness may do little for muscle fitness or flexibility.

- *Monitors on machines are often inaccurate.* Studies have shown that machines that provide feedback often overestimate energy expenditure (calories expended).

- *Claims for the benefits of some machines are exaggerated.* Claims that machines can get you in the "fat burning zone" or that promise high calorie expenditure with "low effort" are examples of quackery and should be discounted.

- *Some home equipment is not cost effective.* Be sure that you will get significant benefits for high-cost items. Consider low-cost equipment, such as exercise bands, exercise balls, and low-cost weights (see Suggested Readings).

The use of hand weights and wrist weights while walking, running, dancing, or bench-stepping can increase the energy expended but require caution. Various devices have been marketed as aids for increasing the energy expenditure in activities such as walking, running, and other forms of aerobic exercise. Examples include wrist, arm, or ankle weights and small, handheld weights. Step benches are another device that can be used to increase energy expenditure for aerobic exercise.

The practice of carrying weights is controversial. Carrying weights (not more than 1 to 3 pounds) while doing aerobic dance, walking, and other aerobic activities has been shown to increase energy expenditure, but the effect is negligible unless the arms are pumped (bending the elbow and raising the weight to shoulder height and then extending the elbow as the arm swings down). When the arms are pumped, the energy output is comparable to a slow jog. Some experts caution that pumping the arms using weights can increase the risk for injury and suggest that the benefit of added energy expenditure is not worth the added risk for injury. Also, gripping weights while exercising can cause an increase in blood pressure.

Those who choose to use weights while doing aerobic activity are at less risk for injury if they use wrist weights rather than handheld weights. Arm movements should be limited to a range of motion below the shoulder level. Coronary patients and people with shoulder or elbow joint problems are advised not to use hand or wrist weights. Ankle weights are not recommended because they may alter your gait and stress the knees.

Health Clubs and Leaders

(i) FEATURE 2 **Consider the credentials of a fitness leader or personal trainer before making a selection.** Individuals with a college degree in physical education, physical therapy, exercise science, or kinesiology are recommended. Certifications from reputable organizations, such as the American College of Sports Medicine (ACSM), are also recommended. The ACSM offers several certifications with differing levels of expertise and education ranging from certified personal trainer to registered clinical exercise physiologist. Be aware that not all certifications are equal. Some unreputable and unethical organizations require little more than an application and a fee payment.

Consider a number of factors before making decisions about a health or fitness club. Consider the following factors when making your decisions.

- Is access to the facility really essential for you to begin or maintain a program?
- Is the facility convenient? The distance of a facility from home or work will greatly influence whether you use it regularly.
- Determine the qualifications of the personnel, especially of the individual responsible for your program. Is he or she an expert, as defined previously?
- Observe staff conduct to determine if they are available and efficient in day-to-day operations.
- Check to see if your membership can be sold or transferred if you move. Check if you can cancel the contract if you prove you are moving away.
- Choose a no-contract or monthly payment option if it is available so you can change your mind. Be prepared to resist options for long-term contracts.
- Check for hidden costs associated with membership (e.g., costs for testing, use of personal training).

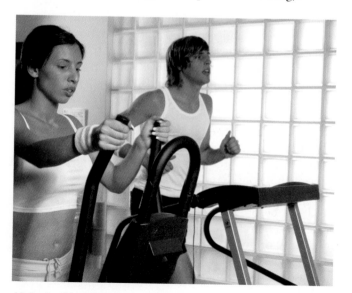
Visit a health club before you join.

- Do not be swayed by promises of quick results.
- Check if the equipment is up to date and maintained.
- Check for cleanliness. Is the facility clean?
- Are quack products sold and pushed? If so, it does not speak well of the professionalism of the staff.
- Check to see if unproven products, such as supplements, are sold or pushed to gain income.
- Check to see that towels are provided to wipe machines after use and that weights are replaced after use. If not, it is a good indication that supervision is not adequate.
- Check to see if rules are posted. For example, is there a time limit for using machines and is there a dress code?
- Speak with other members to get an insider's perspective on how they have been treated.
- Make a trial visit during the hours when you would expect to use the facility to determine if it is overcrowded, and if you would enjoy the atmosphere.
- Make certain the club is a well-established facility that will not disappear overnight.
- Check its reputation with the Better Business Bureau. Be aware that the BBB can only tell you if complaints have been made. It does not endorse companies and may lack information on new companies.
- Investigate programs offered by the YMCA/YWCA, local colleges and universities, and municipal park and recreation departments. These agencies often have excellent fitness classes at lower prices than commercial establishments and usually employ qualified personnel.

Body Composition

Getting rid of cellulite does not require a special exercise, diet, cream, or device, as some books and advertisements insist. Cellulite is ordinary fat with a fancy name. You do not need a special treatment or device to get rid of it. In fact, it has no special remedy. To decrease fat, reduce calories and do more physical activity.

Spot-reducing, or losing fat from a specific location on the body, is not possible. When you do physical activity, calories are burned and fat is recruited from all over the body in a genetically determined pattern. You cannot selectively exercise, bump, vibrate, or squeeze the fat from a particular spot. If you are flabby to begin with, local exercise can strengthen the local muscles, causing a change in the contour and the girth of that body part, but exercise affects the muscles, not the fat on that body part. General aerobic exercises are the most effective for burning fat, but you cannot control where the fat comes off.

Surgically sculpting the body with implants and liposuction to acquire physical beauty will not give you physical fitness and may be harmful. Rather than doing it the hard way, an increasing number of people are having their *"love handles"* removed surgically and fake calf and pectoral muscles implanted to improve their physique. Liposuction is not a weight loss technique but, rather, a contouring procedure. Like any surgery, it has risks. There are risks for infection, hematoma, skin slough, and other conditions, and there have been fatalities. As noted in Concept 15, a widely advertised product that claims to dissolve fat (Lipodissolve) has not been approved as safe by the FDA, and the FDA has issued a letter to sellers warning them to stop making unsubstantiated claims. Muscle implants give a muscular appearance, but they do not make you stronger or more fit. The implants are not really muscle tissue but, rather, silicon gel or saline, such as that used in breast implants or a hard substitute. Some complications can occur, such as infection and bleeding, and some physicians believe that calf implants may put pressure on the calf muscles and cause them to atrophy. A better way to improve physique and fitness is to engage in proper exercise.

Nutrition

Diets are a major source of quackery. Basic guidelines for sound eating were described in Concepts 14 and 15. Beware of diets that do not follow these guidelines. Diets that emphasize one nutrient at the expense of others (unbalanced diets), diets that require the purchase of special products, especially products that make claims inconsistent with established guidelines, and diets that are proposed by people lacking sound credentials should be avoided.

It is not true that if a little of something is "good," more is "better." The marketing of nutrition products often relies on convincing people that additional vitamins, minerals, or enzymes are beneficial. It is true that deficiencies of certain compounds may be harmful, but extra amounts don't always provide added protection or improved health. The myth that vitamin C can cure the common cold is based on the fact that deficiencies of vitamin C can lead to scurvy. The same hype is used to sell consumers many other unnecessary supplements. For example, protein supplements are marketed with convincing (and honest) claims that the body needs amino acids to form muscle. The hidden truth is that the body cannot store or use more than it needs.

Beware of energy drinks with "boosts" sold at smoothie shops and fitness clubs. Many restaurants and shops now promote drinks contain "boosts" (a tablespoon or two of a food supplement). Health clubs that sell drinks with supplements are susceptible to the claim that they are selling products for financial gain rather than the best interests of clients. Even if supplements are effective, which most are not, taking one dose in a drink would be ineffective and a waste of money.

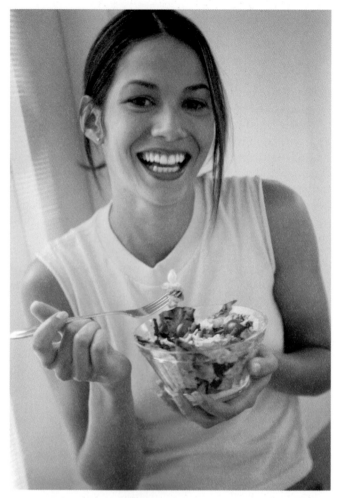

Eating a healthful diet is the best way to get necessary vitamins and minerals and other essential nutrients.

(i) **Current legislation does not protect food supplement customers.** According to the FEATURE 3 FDA, a dietary supplement is a product taken by mouth that contains a "dietary ingredient" intended to supplement the diet. These ingredients include vitamins, minerals, herbs and other botanicals, amino acids, and other substances, such as enzymes, organ tissues, glandulars, and metabolites. Supplements come in many forms, including powders, tablets, softgels, capsules, gelcaps, and liquids. The passage of the Dietary Supplements Health and Education Act (DSHEA) in 1994 shifted the burden of providing assurances of product effectiveness from the FDA to the food supplement industry, which really means it shifted to you—the consumer. Food supplements are typically not considered to be drugs, so they are not regulated. Unlike drugs and medicines, food supplements need not be proven effective or even safe to be sold in stores. To be removed from stores, they must be proven ineffective or unsafe. This leaves consumers vulnerable to false claims. Many experts suggest that quackery has increased significantly since 1994, when the act was passed.

When the DSHEA was passed in 1994, there were no provisions for assuring that dietary supplements contained the ingredients they claimed to contain. In 2007, the FDA instituted a new rule requiring supplement manufacturers to provide labels to "insure a consistent product free of contamination, with accurate labeling." This is important because more than a few cases of product contamination have been reported (see Table 2 later in the concept). Under the new regulations, the manufacturer, not the FDA, will test products to be sure that they are pure and accurately labeled. Consumers need to know that the FDA monitors the safety of supplements through "adverse events monitoring." This means that the FDA relies on consumers to report problems, or adverse events, rather than performing tests on the contents of products. When reports of problems are filed, the FDA investigates. For this reason, the only way that dangerous products and unscrupulous manufacturers can be identified is if consumers report problems to the FDA. Reports can be made at **www.fda.gov/medwatch/ how.htm**. As noted in Table 1, there are other steps that can be taken to help determine if specific supplements contain what they say they contain.

When informed that the FDA does not regulate supplements, more than 80 percent of adults indicate that the FDA should review supplements before they are offered for sale. More than half of adults want more regulation on advertising of supplements and better rules to ensure purity and accurate dosage. In spite of the problems associated with the lack of regulation of supplements, one study indicated that nearly half of Americans routinely take supplements and slightly more than half believe in the value of supplements. Interestingly, 44 percent believe that physicians know little or nothing about supplements. More than a few critics point out that self-regulation within the industry has not worked well. They suggest that the public would have more

confidence in supplements if the FDA were watching out for their best interests. Table 1 presents some questions that should be asked about food supplements.

 Consumers should review the evidence carefully before using supplements. In
FEATURE 4 2006 a review panel of the National Institutes of Health (NIH) prepared a report concerning vitamins/minerals and chronic disease prevention. The report noted the value of some vitamin and mineral supplements while not recommending others. It endorsed folic acid supplements for women of childbearing age, calcium and vitamin D to protect against osteoporosis for postmenopausal women, and several other supplements for those with an eye condition called macular degeneration. The board found that there was not enough evidence to support taking a daily multivitamin. The board did not suggest, however, that those already

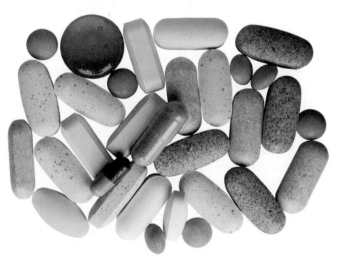
Good consumer skills are important for evaluating health products and for interpreting health claims.

Table 1 ▶ Summary of Important Facts about Food Supplements
The government does not test food supplements to ensure effectiveness or safety. This means that dietary supplements do not need approval of the FDA before they are marketed, and products are not prevented from reaching the market even if no evidence exists as to effectiveness.
Beginning in 2007, the FDA began requiring manufacturers to accurately label the content of supplements and to assure that products are what the manufacturer claims they are. However, the FDA does not test these products and, as noted in the text, relies on consumers to report problems with supplements.
Supplements can have side effects and interact with medicines (see Table 2 for examples).
U.S. Pharmacopia (USP) is a private, nonprofit organization that tests supplements to assure the quality, purity, and strength of a standard unit (dose size and strength). The USP label ensures that a product is what it says it is and that a dose is in the amount advertised. USP periodically tests products and removes its label from those who fail to meet its standards.
Informed-Choice is another nonprofit organization that provides information about dietary supplements. A list of supplements tested by the organization can be found at **www.informed-choice.org/tested-products**.
Little is known about the long-term effects of most supplement use. For example, melatonin is a hormone that is used for insomnia. Hormones can have strong side effects, and little is known about melatonin's long-term effects. Consider alternative solutions to long-term use of unstudied supplements.
People who sell supplements are not required to have special training. Beware of people who use tactics such as those described this concept to sell supplements. Avoid verbal information about products, especially information from sellers. Be wary of "third-party" information that cites research out of context or inaccurately.

In the News

Supplements: Research, Warnings, and Recalls

As noted in the previous section, the FDA does not regulate supplements. Some popular supplements have recently been shown to be ineffective. Others could be dangerous. The FDA posts warnings about supplements that have caused problems and that have dangerous ingredients. Listed below are some recent headlines related to supplement research, warnings, and recalls.

- "FDA Hydroxycut warning" (*USA Today*). A supplement company (Innovate Health Sciences) agreed to recall a variety of weight loss and other supplements after 1 death and 23 severe liver problems were reported.
- "Steroids disguised as supplements" (*USA Today*). Testimony before a Senate subcommittee on crime and drugs investigating sports supplements noted that 23 of 31 supplements purchased on the Internet from bodybuilding.com contained anabolic steroids.

- "Popular supplement fails second arthritis test" (*USA Today*). A popular supplement that combines glucosamine and chondroitin was touted as a treatment for arthritis and joint pain. Two large-scale studies have now shown this supplement to be no more effective than sugar pills. The article provided warnings, but the FDA can't stop the company from selling the product, because it causes no harm.
- "High risk of supplements gets exposed—yet again" (USA Today). This article details findings from Consumer Reports (see suggested readings) about abuses of the supplement industry. It names 12 ingredients that have serious side effects and should be avoided: aconite, bitter orange, chaparral, colloidal silver, coltsfoot, comfrey, country mallow, germanium, greater celandine, kava, lobelia, and yohimbe.

These are provided as examples of recent headlines related to supplements. Additional detail on these headlines is provided at the associated Web link along with other news clips.

---

taking a multivitamin stop doing it and did not find evidence that daily multivitamins are harmful. The review board did take a position against beta-carotene (a form of vitamin A), saying there was no evidence that it is effective. Also, board members warned against taking very high levels of vitamins and minerals (megadoses), noting that they are not beneficial and can be dangerous.

Many other supplements, such as herbals, have not been as well studied. Part of the problem is that there are thousands of products and few resources to support studies. Herbals are made from one plant or plant parts, or a mixture of plants and plant parts. Herbs are sometimes assumed to be safer or better than other supplements because they are purported to be "natural." However, a large percentage of medicines are extracted from plants. The fact that it "comes from nature" does not mean that it is safe. One herbal on which there is considerable evidence is ephedra, which was removed from the market in 2004 after 155 deaths and thousands of adverse reactions to it. It was widely used in weight loss supplements.

Saw Palmetto is another herbal supplement, which is widely used as a preventive for prostate cancer, and preliminary studies supported its use. Echinacea is an herbal widely used to reduce symptoms of the common cold. Subsequent studies have not supported claims for these supplements.

Some supplements are not made from plants. Glucosamine, for example, is made from shellfish, and chondroitin is made from the cartilage of sharks and/or cattle. Glucosamine and chondroitin are two of the most widely used supplements other than vitamins and minerals. They are often used to relieve symptoms and pain from osteoarthritis. Results of one large clinical trial suggested that the two supplements, taken together or separately, were no more effective than a placebo; however, a small group of people who had moderate to severe pain did experience some relief after using the supplements.

The effectiveness of supplements is in question. Also in question is the safety of supplement use. Some of the problems that you should be aware of when considering the use of supplements are described in Table 2. Some other incidents illustrate that supplements are not always what they appear to be:

- A former food supplement executive admits false statements. The founder and former president of Metabolife recently pled guilty to federal charges that he gave false statements to the FDA. He claimed he had received no complaints about a diet pill containing ephedra (prior to FDA ban of ephedra). In his plea, he admitted the company received thousands of complaints about adverse effects.

- Fines have been levied for misleading claims. Hi Health, a major supplier of supplements, was fined by the FTC ($450,000) for false and misleading claims for one of its products (Ocular Nutrition). Producers of Airborne, a supplement purporting to help the body fight germs in public places, have agreed to pay $23.3 million when a lawsuit exposed the fact that no scientists participated in studies cited by the company.
- Weight loss products top the list in consumer fraud. A one-year FTC study found that 30.2 million adults bought fraudulent products; nearly 7 million people bought fraudulent weight loss products.
- Sex enhancement supplements are a big source of fraud. A major supplement company was found guilty of selling bogus pills (e.g., to increase height, breast size, and penis size) that do not work. The company took in more than $77 million, but will pay only $4 million in refunds to customers.

The cost of supplements is substantial. Since the Dietary Supplements Health and Education Act was passed in 1994, the annual sales of food supplements nearly tripled, totaling more than $20 million each year. The cost of food supplements in a bottle (e.g., pills, capsules, powders) is typically very high. For example, a protein supplement can cost as much as $1 per gram. The cost per gram in good food, such as in a chicken breast, is typically a few cents per gram. Also, "protein bars" have a high cost per gram of protein and are sometimes high in empty calories (simple sugars) and/or fat.

In addition to the dollars spent on supplements and the high relative cost of supplements as opposed to food, there are costs to people who experience health problems associated with the use of some supplements. Over the past few years, the FDA has received thousands of complaints of adverse events (resulting in approximately 200 deaths). An editorial in a leading national newspaper suggests that "troubling side effects mount" and that "putting customers' health at risk is a high price to pay for a free market in diet supplements." Among the adverse effects reported are lead poisoning, nausea, vomiting, diarrhea, abnormal heart rhythm, fainting, impotence, and lethargy. Over a 6-year period, 2,621 adverse events were reported to the FDA, and 184 resulted in death. Also, one study showed that 15 to 20 percent of over 1,600 supplements tested included substances that would cause a positive test for drugs banned by sports organizations.

Be wary of claims made for supplements. The DSHEA has had at least one positive effect. Food supplement labeling must now be truthful. Claims concerning disease prevention, treatment, or diagnosis must be substantiated in order to appear on the product. Unfortunately, the act did not limit false claims if they are not on the product label. The result has been the removal of claims from labels in favor of claims on separate literature, often called third-party literature, because the label makes no claims and the seller (the second party) makes no written claims. Rather, the seller provides claims in literature by other people (a third party). The literature is distributed separately from the product, thus allowing sellers to make unsubstantiated claims for products. Also, the law does not prohibit unproven verbal claims by salespeople. Many medical experts feel that "alternative treatments" should be subjected to the same type of rigorous scientific testing used to evaluate other medicines. However, as things currently stand, it is up to the consumer to make decisions about the safety and effectiveness of food supplements, so it is especially important to be well informed.

Table 2 ▶ Problems Associated with Supplements
Postsurgical problems, including bleeding, irregular heartbeat, and stroke—examples: echinacea, ephedra, ginkgo, kava, St. John's wort, ginseng
Dangerous interactions with medicines—examples: ephedra, St. John's wort (interact with birth control pills and HIV pills)
FDA warnings concerning unsubstantiated claims about herbs added to foods, such as energy bars and water—examples: ginkgo, ginseng, echinacea
Allergic and other physiological reactions; negative effect on decision making—example: GHB
Known ill effects to health—examples: comfrey (kidneys), kava (liver), ephedra (multiple deaths)
Recall because of dangerous effects associated with contamination—examples: PC SPES, Lipokinetix
Action by the FTC because of deceptive advertisements—examples: Exercise in a Bottle, Fat Trapper
Banned by several sporting groups, including the International Olympic Committee, NCAA, and NFL—examples: steroids, androstendione, ephedra (illegal in doses above 10 mg), THC
Contents may not be what they appear to be and dosage information is unknown—example: the International Olympic Committee studied 240 different supplements and found that 18.8 percent of the products contained steroids.

Other Consumer Information

Saunas, steam baths, whirlpools, and hot tubs provide no significant health benefits, and guidelines must be followed to ensure safety. Baths do not melt off fat; fat must be metabolized. The heat and humidity from baths may make you perspire, but it is water, not fat, oozing from the pores.

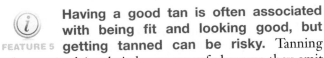

In the News

Vitamin Supplements and Disease Prevention

NEWS 2 During the 1990s and early 2000s, vitamin supplements were touted as a good way to ward off disease. Now reports are accumulating that vitamin supplements are not as effective as many thought. The following headlines from the national newspaper *USA Today* are based on well-documented studies. The research on which these headlines were based is found at the associated Web link.

- Vitamins get "F" in cancer prevention.
- Study: Vitamin E doesn't prevent heart "events."
- Folic acid, B vitamins offer no cancer protection, study reaffirms.
- Study doubts benefits of multivitamins.

The effect of such baths is largely psychological, although some temporary relief from aches and pains may result from the heat. The same relief can be had by sitting in a tub of hot water in your bathroom. The following guidelines and precautions should be considered when using a sauna, steam bath, whirlpool, or hot tub:

- Take a soap shower before and after entering.
- Do not wear makeup or skin lotion or oil.
- Wait at least an hour after eating before bathing.
- Cool down after exercise before entering the bath.
- Drink plenty of water before or during the bath.
- Do not wear jewelry.
- Do not sit on a metal stool; do sit on a towel.
- Do not drink alcohol before bathing.
- Get out immediately if you become dizzy; feel hot, chilled, or nauseous; or get a headache.
- Get approval from your physician if you have heart disease, low or high blood pressure, a fever, kidney disease, or diabetes; are obese; are pregnant or think you might be pregnant; or are on medications (especially anticoagulants, stimulants, or tranquilizers).
- Limit use for the elderly and for children.
- Do not exercise in a sauna or steam bath.
- Skin infections can be spread in a bath; make certain it is cleaned regularly and that the hot tub or whirlpool has proper pH and chlorination.
- Follow appropriate guidelines:
  Sauna: should not exceed 190°F (88°C) and duration should not exceed 10 to 15 minutes
  Steam bath: should not exceed 120°F (49°C) and duration should not exceed 6 to 12 minutes
  Whirlpool/hot tub: should not exceed 100°F (37°C) and duration should not exceed 5 to 10 minutes

FEATURE 5 **Having a good tan is often associated with being fit and looking good, but getting tanned can be risky.** Tanning salons may claim their lamps are safe because they emit only UVA rays, but these rays can age the skin prematurely, making it look wrinkled and leathery. They may also increase the cancer-producing potential of UVB rays and cause eye damage. Since there is no warning sign of redness, overdosing can occur. Thirty minutes of exposure to UVA can suppress the immune system. Tanning devices can also aggravate certain skin diseases. The Food and Drug Administration advises against the use of any suntan lamp. It is dangerous to use tanning accelerator lotions with the lamps because they can promote burning of the skin. Tanning pills are an even worse choice. They can cause itching, welts, hives, stomach cramps, and diarrhea and can decrease night vision. Tanning in the sun is also hazardous because it damages the skin, making it age prematurely, and it is a cause of skin cancer. It is worth repeating that wearing sunscreen with at least a 15 SPF (sun protection factor), wearing sunglasses, and wearing protective clothing (including a hat) are good ideas when exposed to the sun.

Books, Magazines, and Articles

Not all books provide scientifically sound, accurate, and reliable information. Some material is published on the basis of how popular, famous, or attractive the author is or how sensational or unusual his or her ideas are. Very few movie stars, models, TV personalities, and Olympic athletes are experts in biomechanics, anatomy and physiology, exercise, and other foundations of physical fitness. Having a good figure or physique, being fit, or having gone through a training program does not, in itself, qualify a person to advise others.

After reading the facts presented in this book, you should be able to evaluate whether or not a book, a magazine, or an article on exercise and fitness is valid, reliable, and scientifically sound. To assist you further, Lab 23A lists 10 guidelines.

The Internet

FEATURE 6 **Not all websites provide scientifically sound, accurate, and reliable information.** Currently, approximately three-fourths of all teen and young adult computer users seek health information on the Web. But many health websites contain misinformation. Studies show that Wikipedia is the most common source of health information for the general public. One report showed that as many as one-half of doctors surveyed used Wikipedia for health information. Many consumers, and some physicians, do not realize

that Wikipedia can be edited by anyone and for this reason can contain erroneous information.

A recent study compared prescription drug information from Wikipedia and Medscape Drug Reference and found that Wikipedia had incomplete answers, incorrect information about dosage, and errors of omission about side effects. The authors of the study noted that Wikipedia should be used only as a supplemental source for drug information.

Recently there have been efforts to improve the quality of health information on the Internet. The FTC is charged with making sure that advertising claims for products are not false or misleading. Several years ago the FTC initiated "Operation Cure-All" in an effort to help "clean up" websites that provide false information. If you find incorrect or misleading information on the Web, you can file a complaint with the FTC at the "cure-all" site (**www.ftc.gov/cureall**). In spite of the FTC efforts, the Web still contains much health misinformation, leading one FTC official to suggest that "miracle cures, once thought to have been laughed out of existence, have now found a new medium . . . on the Internet." Clearly, Internet users must be careful in selecting websites for obtaining fitness, health, and wellness information.

Improving health literacy is a key public health goal for 2020. The Internet has made an almost unlimited amount of health information accessible, but it has proven difficult to ensure that the information is used wisely. The public health service has established key goals to improve public health literacy and the quality of health information on the Internet. The two goals are designed to work together: consumers need access to accurate information, but they also need to know how to interpret and use the information (health literacy). The content presented in this concept provides a foundation for interpreting health information, but some additional guidelines are provided for effectively using the Internet.

One general rule is to consult at least two or more sources to confirm information. Getting confirmation of information from non-Web sources is also a good idea. Perhaps the most important recommendation is to consider the source of information. In general, government sites are valid sources that contain sound information prepared by experts and based on scientific research. Government sites typically include ".gov" as part of the address. Professional organizations and universities can also be good sources of information. Organizations typically have ".org" and universities typically have ".edu" as part of the address. However, caution should still be used with organizations because starting an organization and obtaining an ".org" address is easy. Your greatest trust can be placed in the sites of stable, credible organizations (see *Web Resources* in this book). The great majority of websites

Technology Update
Health Websites

As noted in this section of the book, many health websites are lacking in quality. Some of the best are listed below and at the associated Web link.

- National Institutes of Health—Health Information is a comprehensive and reliable source of health information from the U.S. government's medical research agency: **http://health.nih.gov**
- Health on the Net (HON) recently received special consultative status with the Economic and Social Council of the United Nations. It includes MedHunt, a search engine for medical and health information, and other tools for gaining access to health information: **www.hon.ch**
- Medwatch, an FDA website that includes safety alerts for drugs, supplement information, and health advisories: **www.fda.gov./medwatch**
- The American Psychological Association has developed a site called Psychology Matters: Psychological Applications in Daily Life that offers sound advice concerning "how to be a wise consumer of psychological research": **www.psychologymatters.org**
- Google Health is a free website that allows you to build a medical profile online, store your medical records, and send them to others, including your physician. It also directs you to medical sources. Because there are many sources listed, it is impossible to endorse the available sites. Use the guidelines in this book if you choose Internet links from Google Health (**www.google.com/health**).

promoting health products have ".com" in the address because these are commercial sites, which are in business to make a profit. Thus, although some contain good information, they may focus on selling products or services. Therefore, it is important to view content from these sites more critically. The websites listed at the end of each concept fit the general guidelines given here, but students are encouraged to consider the quality of the individual sources when evaluating information from the various sites.

HELP Health is available to **EVERYONE** for a Lifetime, and it's Personal

A recent survey indicated that the Internet is the leading source of health information for Americans. Unfortunately many health websites contain false or misleading information. We all have health problems from time to time and need good information.

If you or a family member has a health problem, what steps will you take to get information that you know to be accurate?

Strategies for Action

Being a good consumer requires time, information, and effort. With time and effort, you can gain the information you need to make good decisions about the products and services you purchase. In Lab 23A, you will evaluate an exercise device, a food supplement, a magazine article, or a Web site. In Lab 23B, you will evaluate a health/wellness or fitness club. Taking the time to investigate a product will help you save money and help you avoid making poor decisions that affect your health, fitness, and wellness. When you are making decisions about products or services, it is a good idea to begin your investigation well in advance of the day when a decision is to be made. Salespeople often suggest that "this offer is only good today." They know that people often make poor decisions when under time pressure, and they want you to make a decision today so that they will not lose a sale.

Web Resources

Additional websites with information related to Concept 23 are available at the associated Web link.

Center for Science in the Public Interest **www.cspinet.org**
Federal Trade Commission **www.ftc.gov**
Food and Drug Administration **www.fda.gov**
Healthfinder **www.healthfinder.gov**
National Council against Health Fraud **www.ncahf.org**
National Institutes of Health, Health Information **http://health.nih.gov/**
Office of Dietary Supplements **http://ods.od.nih.gov**
Quackwatch **www.quackwatch.org**
U.S. Consumer Information Center **www.pueblo.gsa.gov**

Suggested Readings

Selected readings and references are listed below. A more comprehensive list is available at the Web link.

Anderson, G. M., D. Juurlink, and A. S. Detsky. 2008. Newly approved does not always mean new and improved. *Journal of the American Medical Association* 299(13):1598–1600.
Avoid injury on or near equipment. 2010. Available at **www.consumerreports.org/health/healthy-living/fitness** /equipment/treadmills/treadmills/exercise-equipment-safety/exercise-equipment-safety.htm
Barrett, S., et al. 2007. *Consumer Health: A Guide to Intelligent Decisions.* 8th ed. New York: McGraw-Hill Higher Education.
Bausell, R. B. 2007. *Snake Oil Science: The Truth about Complementary and Alternative Medicine.* Oxford: Oxford University Press.
Brokowski, L. 2009. Evaluation of pharmacist use and perception of Wikipedia as a drug information resource. *Annals of Pharmacotherapy* 43(11):1912–1913.
Consumer Reports. 2010. Dangerous Supplements. *Consumer Reports* 75(9):16.
Corbin, C. B. 2007. Dietary supplements: Making informed decisions. *ACSM's Health & Fitness Journal* 11(5):1–6.
Fox, S., and S. Jones. 2009. *The Social Life of Health Information: America's Pursuit of Health Takes Place on a Widening Network of Both Online and Offline Sources.* Washington, DC: Pew Internet & American Life Project. Available at **www.pewinternet.org/Reports/2009/8-The-Social-Life-of-Health-Information.aspx?r=1**
Should you buy this now? Usually not, based on our tests of 15 infomercial products. 2010. *Consumer Reports* 75(2):16–20.
Swaim, D. P. 2009. Exercise equipment: Assessing the advertised claims. *ACSM's Health and Fitness Journal* 13(5):8–11.
Treadmills and ellipticals: Our latest tests find 14 top machines. 2010. *Consumer Reports* 75(2):32–38.

Lab 23A Practicing Consumer Skills: Evaluating Products

Name	Section	Date

Purpose: To evaluate an exercise device, a book, a magazine article, an advertisement, a food supplement, or a website

Procedures

1. Evaluate an exercise device, a book, an article, a newspaper or magazine advertisement, a food supplement, or a website. Place an X in the circle by the item you choose to evaluate. Attach a copy if you evaluate an advertisement.
2. Read each of the 10 evaluation factors for the item you selected. Place an X in the circle by the factors that describe the item you are evaluating.
3. Total the number of X marks to determine a score for the item being evaluated. The higher the score, the more likely it is to be safe and/or effective.
4. Answer the questions in the Conclusions and Implications section.

Results

Directions: Place an X in the circle by the product you evaluated. Place an X over the circle by each true statement. Provide information about the product in the space provided.

Exercise Device

1. The exercise device requires effort consistent with the FIT formula.

2. The exercise device is safe and the exercise done using the device is safe.

3. There are no claims that the device uses exercise that is effortless.

4. Exercise using the device is fun or is a type that you might do regularly.

5. There are no claims using gimmick words, such as *tone, cellulite, quick,* or *spot fat reduction.*

6. The seller's credentials are sound.

7. The product does something for you that cannot be done without it.

8. You can return the device if you do not like it (the seller has been in business for a long time).

9. The cost of the product is justified by the potential benefits.

10. The device is easy to store or you have a place to permanently use the equipment without storing it.

Exercise Device

Name of device: _____
_____
_____

Description and manufacturer:
_____
_____
_____

Advertisement

Source: _____
_____
_____

Book or Article

Author(s): _____
_____
_____

Journal article or book title: _____
_____
_____

Journal name or name of publisher:
_____
_____

Date of publication: _____
_____
_____

Book/Article/Advertisement

1. The credentials of the author are sound. He or she has a degree in an area related to the content of the book or magazine.*

2. The facts in the article are consistent with the facts described in this book.

3. The author does not claim "quick" or "miraculous" results.

4. There are no claims about the spot reduction of fat or other unfounded claims.

5. The author/advertisement is not selling a product.

6. Reputable experts are cited.

7. The article does not promote unsafe exercises or products.

8. New discoveries from exotic places are not cited.

9. The article/advertisement does not rely on testimonials by nonexpert, famous people.

10. The author/advertisement does not make claims that the AMA, the FDA, or another legitimate organization is trying to suppress information.

*Not applicable for advertisement.

487

Food Supplement

1. The seller is not the prime source of product information.

2. The seller has been in business for a long time and has a good reputation.

3. There is scientific evidence of product effectiveness.

4. There is clear evidence about the side effects of the active ingredients.

5. The long-term effectiveness and safety of the product are cited.

6. You are sure of the content of the product.

7. You have information that the manufacturer is reputable.

8. The known benefits are worth the cost.

9. There is evidence that you can get benefits from this product that cannot be obtained from good food.

10. There are no claims that use quack words or claims about conspiracies against the product by reputable organizations.

Food Supplement

Name: _____
_____
_____

Purported benefit: _____
_____
_____

Manufacturer/seller: _____
_____
_____

Dose and active ingredient: _____
_____
_____

Web Site

Web address: _____
_____
_____

Type of information provided: ____
_____
_____

Organization or person responsible for information: _____
_____
_____

Web Site

1. The site does not sell products associated with information provided.

2. The provider is a person, an organization (org), or a governmental agency (gov) with a sound reputation.

3. The site does not use quack words.

4. The site does not try to discredit well-established organizations or governmental agencies.

5. The site does not rely on testimonials, celebrities, or people with unknown credentials.

6. The site is well regarded by experts, and has a high rating at http://navigator.tufts.edu.

7. The site has a history of providing good information.

8. The site provides complete information that is documented by research.

9. No claims of quick cures or miracle results are made.

10. The site provides information consistent with information provided in this text.

Conclusions and Implications

Total the number of Xs for the device, book/magazine, advertisement, food supplement, or website: [ ]

In several sentences, give your assessment of the product. Did it score well? Would you use/buy the product? Explain.

Lab 23B Evaluating a Health/Wellness or Fitness Club

Name		Section	Date

Purpose: To practice evaluating a health club (various combinations of the words *health, wellness,* and *fitness* are often used for these clubs)

Procedures

1. Choose a club and make a visit.
2. Listen carefully to all that is said and ask lots of questions.
3. Look carefully all around you as you are given the tour of the facilities; ask what the exercises or the equipment does for you, or ask leading questions, such as, "Will this take inches off my hips?"
4. As soon as you leave the club, rate it, using Chart 1. Space is provided for notes in Chart 1.

Chart 1 ▶ Health Club Evaluation Questionnaire

Directions: Place an X over a "yes" or "no" answer. Make notes as necessary.

	Yes	No	Notes
1. Were claims for improvement in weight, figure/physique, or fitness realistic?	○	○	
2. Was a long-term contract (1 to 3 years) encouraged?	○	○	
3. Was the sales pitch high-pressure to make an immediate decision?	○	○	
4. Were you given a copy of the contract to read at home?	○	○	
5. Did the fine print include objectionable clauses?	○	○	
6. Did they ask you about medical readiness?	○	○	
7. Did they sell diet supplements as a sideline?	○	○	
8. Did they have passive equipment?	○	○	
9. Did they have cardiovascular training equipment or facilities (cycles, track, pool, aerobic dance)?	○	○	
10. Did they make unscientific claims for the equipment, exercise, baths, or diet supplements?	○	○	
11. Were the facilities clean?	○	○	
12. Were the facilities crowded?	○	○	
13. Were there days and hours when the facilities were open but would not be available to you?	○	○	
14. Were there limits on the number of minutes you could use a piece of equipment?	○	○	
15. Did the floor personnel closely supervise and assist clients?	○	○	
16. Were the floor personnel qualified experts?	○	○	
17. Were the managers/owners qualified experts?	○	○	
18. Has the club been in business at this location for a year or more?	○	○	

Results

1. Score the chart as follows:

    A. Give 1 point for each "no" answer for items 2, 3, 5, 7, 8, 10, 12, 13, and 14
        and place the score in the box.

        Total A [ ]

    B. Give 1 point for each "yes" answer for items 1, 4, 6, 9, 11, and 18
        and place the score in the box.

        Total B [ ]

        Total A and B above and place the score in the box.

        Total A and B [ ]

    C. Give 1 point for each "yes" answer for items 15, 16, and 17
        and place the score in the box.

        Total C [ ]

2. A total score of 12–15 points on items A and B suggests the club rates at least fair, compared with other clubs.

3. A score of 3 on item C indicates that the personnel are qualified and suggests that you could expect to get accurate technical advice from the staff.

4. Regardless of the total scores, you would have to decide the importance of each item to you personally, as well as evaluate other considerations, such as cost, location, and personalities of the clients and the personnel, to decide if this would be a good place for you or your friends to join.

Conclusions and Implications: In several sentences, discuss your conclusion about the quality of this club and whether you think it would fit your needs if you wanted to belong.

Toward Optimal Health and Wellness: Planning for Healthy Lifestyle Change

Health Objectives for the Year 2020

- Attain high-quality, longer lives free of preventable disease, injury, and premature death.
- Achieve health equity, eliminate disparities, and improve the health of all groups.
- Create social and physical environments that promote good health for all.
- Promote quality of life, healthy development, and healthy behaviors across all stages of life.
- Increase public awareness and understanding of the determinants of health, disease, and disability.
- Improve the health literacy of the population.

- Increase percentage of college students receiving information on priority risk behavior areas.
- Increase percentage of people with health-care providers who involve them in decisions about health care.
- Increase counseling by physicians.
- Increase recycling.
- Increase proportion of adults who have social support.
- Increase screening and treatment of mental health problems.

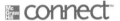

| FITNESS AND WELLNESS   http://connect.mcgraw-hill.com

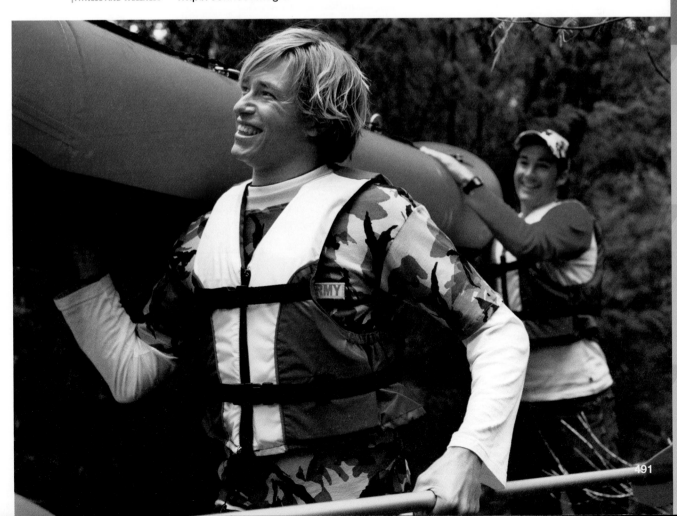

In addition to healthy lifestyles, other factors such as heredity, health care, the environment, cognitions and emotions, and personal actions and interactions contribute to good health, wellness, and fitness.

The broad vision of Healthy People 2020 is to cre-ate "a society in which all people live long, healthy lives." Two major missions of the 2020 objectives are "to identify nationwide health improvement priorities and increase public awareness and understanding of the determinants of health, disease and disability and the opportunity for progress." The first concept in this book introduced you to a model that explained the many factors influencing health, wellness, and fitness (see Figure 1).

The focus of this book has been on changing factors over which you have control. For this reason, much of the discussion has centered on changing lifestyles, because lifestyles impact health, wellness, and fitness more than any of the other factors. Still, other factors are important. In this final concept, the focus is on providing additional strategies for action related to the "changeable" factors in the model.

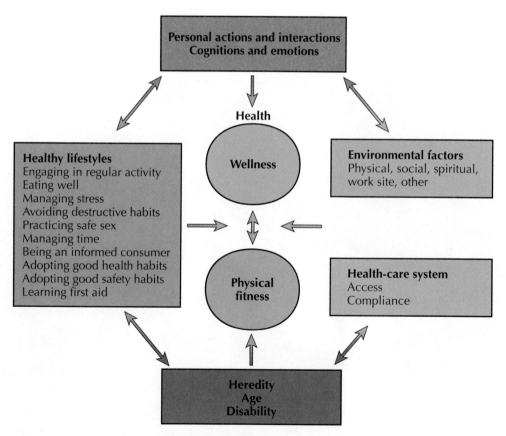

Figure 1 ▶ Determinants of health, fitness, and wellness.

Strategies for Action

Consider strategies for taking advantage of your heredity. You are aware that heredity is a factor affecting all aspects of fitness as well as your health and wellness. You can use several strategies to overcome negative predispositions and to take advantage of positive ones:

- *Learn about your family history.* If members of your family have had specific diseases or health problems, make sure you inform your physician. Investigate to see if the conditions might affect you.
- *Take action to diminish risk factors for which you have a predisposition.* For example, if you have a family history of Type II diabetes, do regular activity, eat well, and keep your body fat level in the good fitness zone.
- *Take advantage of your hereditary strengths.* Self-assessments can help you see where you have strength and account for weaknesses. Build on your strengths and find ways to compensate for your weaknesses. For example, people who have fewer fast-twitch muscle fibers will probably not be great sprinters but often have more slow-twitch fibers, which favor endurance performances, such as distance running.

Consider strategies for using the health-care system effectively. Consider the information

FEATURE 1   in Table 1 concerning health care. Evidence indicates that medical illiteracy and lack of health-care information are linked to higher than normal death rates. Do a self-assessment of your current use of health care (see Lab 24A). Develop a plan using some of the following strategies (see Lab 24B):

Table 1 ▶ Facts about Personal Physicians and Health Insurance

- More women than men have a regular physician.
- More than half of young men have no personal doctor.
- Three times more women than men have visited a doctor in the past year.
- Women are more aware of health issues than men.
- Nearly half of men wait a week or more to see a doctor when ill.
- Many men see sickness as "unmanly."
- Married men see doctors more frequently than single men because their wives prompt them.
- Lack of health insurance results in fewer doctor's visits, less frequent health screening, and less access to prescribed medicine.

- *Get periodic medical exams.* Do not wait until something is wrong before you seek medical advice. After 40 years of age, a yearly preventive physical exam is recommended. Younger people should have an exam at least every 2 years. Mammograms for women and prostate tests (PSA) for men are recommended. Breast and testicular self-exams are also important.
- *Immunize.* Public health officials estimate that many lives were saved by immunization for H1N1 (swine flu) during 2009. See web feature for more information.
- *Investigate and then identify a regular doctor or doctors.* Check with other physicians you know and trust for referrals. Check with your state medical board and national directories (e.g., Directory of Board Certified Medical Specialists, www.abms.org) for specialist certifications or fellowships.
- *Investigate and then choose an emergency care center and a hospital.* Choose an accredited emergency center near your home and a hospital that is accredited and grants privileges to your personal doctors.
- *Be there, or have others present, when those you care about are in the hospital.* Medical mistakes cause nearly 100,000 unnecessary deaths each year. According to the National Patient Safety Foundation (www.npsf.org), watching staff to ensure good hygiene, asking

Technology Update
Online Second Opinions and Wellness Feedback

Medical Second Opinions. Getting a second opinion when facing a challenging medical problem is highly recommended. The Cleveland Clinic, a well-respected medical institution, has begun offering online medical services. Among them is a system for getting online second opinions. *MyConsult*® allows you to get a second opinion online for over 600 life-threatening or life-altering diagnoses. For more information, access **www.eclevelandclinic.org**.

Worksite Wellness Online. Intel, a large computer chip maker, has partnered with Core Performance to develop a work-site wellness information tracking system that allows fitness and wellness information to be entered on exercise machines and stored as personal records. The equipment is connected to the Internet, and records of fitness (e.g., weight, body fat, blood pressure) and exercise behaviors (e.g., duration, exercise intensity) are stored in private personal files. For more information, visit the associated Web link.

In the News

Healthiest Cities and States

In recent years numerous organizations have conducted surveys to determine which cities and states are the healthiest. All use indicators such as access to health care, percentage of people insured, health-care costs, resources (e.g., parks, work-site wellness programs), environmental quality, and personal fitness and health (e.g., percent over-weight, personal fitness). Results vary depending on the organization doing the polling, but one thing is clear: in all polls, the South ranked lowest (both cities and states). The extreme Northeast, upper Midwest, and West often rank best. For women, Burlington, Vermont, and Bethesda-Gaithersburg-Frederick, Maryland, ranked first and second. Find out how your city or state ranks. For more information go to the associated Web link.

about medications and treatments, and telling a nurse or doctor if things look wrong can help eliminate mistakes. Learn the nurses' routines so you know how to find them when necessary.

- **Ask questions.** Do not be afraid to speak up. Prepare questions for doctors and other medical personnel. The American College of Surgeons suggests several questions before surgeries: What are the reasons for the surgery? Are there alternatives? What will happen if I don't have the procedure? What are the risks? What are the long-term effects and problems? How will the procedure impact my quality of life and future health?
- **If you have doubts about medical advice, get a second opinion.** As many as 30 percent of original diagnoses are incorrect or differ from second opinions. Do worry about offending your doctor by getting another opinion. Good doctors encourage this.
- **Communicate with your physician.** Prepare a list of all medications and supplements that you take and make all physicians aware of them. Share records of past medical treatments.
- **Use medications properly and be well informed about the medicines you take.** Preventable adverse reactions to medicines account for more than 1.5 million deaths each year. When medicine is prescribed, ask for details. Ask why the medicine was prescribed and the nature of side effects. Ask if the medicine interacts with other medicines or supplements. Read all inserts that come with the medicine and ask your doctor and pharmacist about correct dosage and information concerning when to take the medication. The FDA recently simplified drug inserts to help you understand the information that comes with medicine.

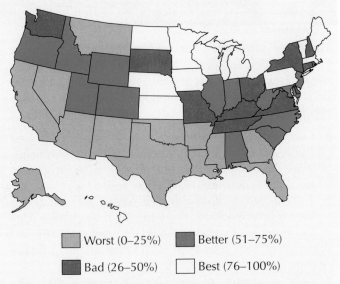

▢ Worst (0–25%)	▢ Better (51–75%)
▢ Bad (26–50%)	▢ Best (76–100%)

Figure 2 ▶ Percentage of people by state with insurance coverage.

- **Safely dispose of old medicine.** Throwing old medicine in the trash is often unsafe for the environment and can be dangerous to other people and animals. Contact a health center to determine the best way to dispose of old medicine.
- **Become familiar with the symptoms of common medical problems.** If symptoms persist, seek medical help. Many deaths can be prevented if early warning signs of medical problems are heeded.
- **If medical advice is given, comply.** People commonly stop taking medicine when symptoms stop rather than taking the full amount of medicine prescribed.
- **Be cautious when using the Internet for health information.** If you use the Internet for health information, be sure to use reliable websites (see Concept 23). Seek information from more than one source.
- **Make your wishes for health care known.** Have a medical power of attorney. This document spells out the treatments you desire in the case of severe illness. Without such a document, your loved ones may not be able to make decisions consistent with your wishes. Be sure your loved ones have a similar document so that you can help them carry out their wishes.
- **Get medical insurance.** Find a way to get health insurance. People who think they save money by avoiding the payment of insurance premiums place themselves (and their families) at risk and may not really save money. Recent statistics show that uninsured people pay 2.5 times more for hospital services than health insurance companies pay for people they insure and pay 3 times more than Medicaid-allowed costs (see Figure 2).
- **Stay home when you are sick.** Most companies (62 percent) urge employees to stay at home when they are sick to prevent spreading sickness to others. Forty percent of employees say they have gotten the flu at work. Still, 40 percent of employees say they

feel pressure to go to work when sick. Sick workers are less productive, and working when sick lengthens recovery time.

- **Take steps to avoid "superbugs" both in medical institutions and at home.** The most recent studies indicate that nearly 100,000 people a year become infected with the superbug MRSA (often pronounced "MURSA"). MRSA is a type of drug-resistant staph infection. Approximately 20,000 people die from this superbug each year. About 85 percent of MRSA infections are associated with the health-care system (visits to doctors, health-care facilities, and hospitals). To avoid MRSA and other infections, check hospitals and health-care facilities for incidence records and compare them to national

rates published by the CDC. Check to see that hand sanitizers are available and used. Watch health-care professionals to be sure they wash their hands before and after exams. Use hand sanitizers and wash your hands regularly.

(i) **Consider strategies for improving your environment.** Consider the information in FEATURE 2 Table 2 when trying to improve environments related to wellness.

- **Strategies for interacting with the physical environment.** Avoid polluted environments, such as smoke-filled establishments; choose a living location low in pollution; keep your home free of pollutants

---

Table 2 ▶ Environmental Factors Influencing Health, Wellness, and Fitness

Physical Environment

The physical environment in which you live has both direct and indirect effects on your health and wellness. Here are some examples:

- *Pollution.* Air pollution (increased ozone, hydrocarbons, and particulates) and water pollution both have negative effects on health. Smoking in public places is a source of pollution.
- *Urban sprawl and population growth.* Sprawl reduces opportunities for healthy lifestyles, such as walking and biking, and increases the need for auto travel. Population growth results in greater housing density and can result in less community and home safety. Urban growth places great demands on sanitation systems and contributes to land pollution.

Social Environment

A healthy social environment offers opportunities for friendly interactions in a supportive environment, including the following:

- *Sense of community.* Being a part of the greater community is important to social and mental health.
- *Opportunities for supportive personal relationships.* We all need friendly personal interactions. Support by others, especially family members, can help in managing stress and in adopting healthy lifestyles.
- *Time availability.* We tend to take time for what we think is important. Social interactions require that time be spent with other people.
- *Removal from abusive environments.* If relationships become abusive, you may have to remove yourself and others at risk and seek help from others.

Spiritual Environment

A positive environment provides each person with opportunities to find spiritual fulfillment, for example:

- *Opportunities for spiritual development.* Reading spiritual materials, prayer, meditation, and discussions with others (of similar and dissimilar beliefs) all provide opportunities to clarify and solidify spiritual beliefs.
- *Access to spiritual community and leadership.* Finding a community for worship and/or spiritual support has been shown to be comforting and a path to fulfillment for many. Spiritual fulfillment may benefit from consultation with those with experience and expertise.

Intellectual Environment

Environments that foster learning and sound critical thinking are important to intellectual wellness. Factors to consider include the following:

- *Access to accurate information.* Whether the source is formal education or self-learning, access to accurate information is essential. Of course, good information is beneficial only if used.
- *Stimulation for effective thinking.* Sometimes we can become lazy, failing to evaluate information effectively. Seeking environments that stimulate critical thinking is important.

Work Environment

The work environment is a combination of the physical, social, intellectual, and spiritual environments. Factors that lead to a healthy work environment include the following:

- *Healthy physical and social environment.* A healthy work environment includes an adequate, well-lit, pollution-free workspace and reasonable work hours. Good relationships with bosses and co-workers and adequate work breaks are key elements of a healthy social work environment.
- *Opportunity and support for healthy lifestyles.* Many companies have work-site wellness programs, which include opportunities for physical activity and other healthy lifestyle change. Programs that have quality professional leadership have been shown to reduce absenteeism, reduce health-care costs, and increase job satisfaction.

Environment Supporting Healthy Lifestyles

Environments that promote healthy lifestyles can enhance health and wellness. Factors to consider include the following:

- *Active environments.* If we are to promote healthy lifestyles at home, work, and school, it is important to create environments that encourage active lifestyles. Examples include providing safe, open recreational areas and work-site wellness programs.
- *People working together.* Changes designed to promote healthy lifestyles require the efforts of many people. Cooperative efforts by groups with well-defined goals are most likely to be successful. Many communities have created health coalitions to create these environments.

(regularly check filters, avoid use of toxic products); and seek out environments that are conducive to physical activity (see Concept 6) and healthy eating (see Concept 15).

- **Strategies for the social environment.** Find a social community that accommodates your personal and family needs; get involved in community affairs, including those that affect the environment; build relationships with family and friends; provide support for others so that their support will be there for you when you need it; use time-management strategies to help you allocate time for social interactions.
- **Strategies for the spiritual environment.** Pray, meditate, read spiritual materials, participate in spiritual discussions, find a place to worship, provide spiritual support for others, seek spiritual guidance from those with experience and expertise, keep a journal, experience nature, honor relationships, help others.
- **Strategies for the intellectual environment.** Make decisions based on sound information, question simple solutions to complex problems, seek environments that stimulate critical thinking.
- **Strategies for the work environment.** Choose a job that has a healthy physical environment, including adequate space, lighting, and freedom from pollution (tobacco smoke), as well as a healthy social, spiritual, and intellectual environment and one that has a worksite wellness program led by professionals.
- **Strategies for finding an environment that supports healthy lifestyles.** Choose a place to live that is near parks and playgrounds and has sidewalks, bike paths, jogging trails, and swimming facilities; join a gym or health club; avoid environments that limit choices to fast food and food with empty calories; find a social environment that reinforces healthy lifestyles.

Consider strategies for adopting healthy lifestyles. Statistics show that more than half of early deaths are caused by unhealthy lifestyles. For this reason, changing lifestyles is the focus of this book. We emphasize priority healthy lifestyles such as being regularly active, eating well, managing stress, avoiding destructive behaviors, and practicing safe sex because they are factors over which we have some control, and if adopted, they have considerable impact on health, wellness, and fitness. Other healthy lifestyles not emphasized in this book are described in Table 3.

- **Use the six steps to help you plan lifestyle programs.** In Concept 2 you learned about the six steps involved in planning for healthy lifestyle change. The labs at the end of this concept are designed to help you create plans for a variety of lifestyles using the six steps. Lab 24A helps you assess many of the factors that influence health, wellness, and fitness so that you can identify areas in which you especially need to prepare lifestyle change plans. Lab 24B is designed to help you prepare plans for making lifestyle change from the list presented in Figure 1

HELP Health is available to Everyone for a Lifetime, and it's **PERSONAL**

The American College of Sports Medicine uses the American Fitness Index to determine which a city's "healthy living" rating. They use positive personal-health indicators such as the number of people who exercise regularly, eat well, and get good health care as well negative indicators such as the number of people who smoke and who have chronic health problems. Also considered are environmental factors such as parks, public transportation, recreational facilities, fitness centers, and farmer's markets.

Use the personal-health and environmental factors (see above) to rate the area where you live (area within a 10-minute drive).

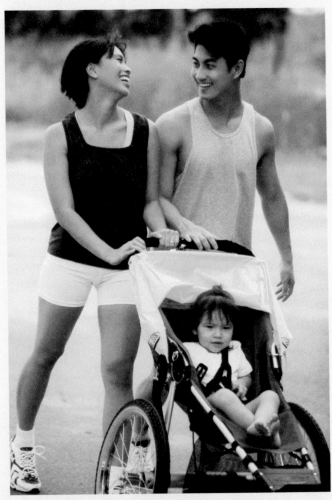

Make it a priority to find ways to remain active throughout your life.

Table 3 ▶ Other Healthy Lifestyles

Lifestyle	Examples
Adopting good personal health habits. Many of these habits, important to optimal health, are considered to be elementary because they are often taught in school or in the home at an early age. In spite of their importance, many adults regularly fail to adopt these behaviors.	• Brushing and flossing teeth • Regular bathing and hand washing • Adequate sleep • Care of ears, eyes, and skin
Protecting your ears. Researchers fear a future epidemic of hearing loss because of exposure to loud music, especially among young adults.	• *Limit exposure to loud sounds, including live and recorded music.* • *Be aware that maximum volume on an MP3 player greatly increases risk of hearing loss.* Maximum volume on one of these devices is 120 decibels, equal to a live concert or sporting event and just lower than a jet engine or sound of a gunshot.
Adopting good safety habits. Unintentional injuries cost Canadians about $8.7 billion per year, and in the United States, the cost of injury and violence is $224 billion a year. Thousands of people die each year and thousands more suffer disabilities or problems that detract from good health and wellness. Not all accidents can be prevented, but we can adopt habits to reduce risk.	• *Automobile accidents.* Wear seat belts, avoid using the phone while driving, do not drink and drive, and do not drive aggressively. • *Water accidents.* Learn to swim, learn CPR, wear life jackets while boating, do not drink while boating. • *Others.* Store guns safely, use smoke alarms, use ladders and electrical equipment safely, and maintain cars, bikes, and motorcycles properly.
Protecting your skin. Adolescents and young adults of college age are especially likely to overexpose themselves to the sun and at tanning facilities. Skin cancer is the leading form of cancer and its principal cause is exposure to the sun and UVA/UVB rays from other sources. Exposure to the sun and tanning devices are the main causes of aging skin.	• *Limit sun exposure (e.g., wear protective clothing, hats, sunglasses).* • *Use sunscreen with high SPF and that meet proposed FDA rules (see www.skincancer.org/Sunscreen).* • *Use EGO rule when applying sunscreen.* Apply it early, apply it generously, and apply it often. • *Avoid use of tanning devices.* WHO now classifies them as a carcinogen equal to smoking in risk.
Learning first aid. Many deaths could be prevented and the severity of injury could be reduced if those at the sites of emergencies were able to administer first aid.	• Learn cardiopulmonary resuscitation (CPR). New research shows that chest compression alone saves lives even without mouth-to-mouth breathing. • Learn the Heimlich maneuver to assist people who are choking. • Learn basic first aid.

(e.g., eating well, managing stress). Lab 24C is designed to help you plan a personal physical activity program.

- *Use self-management skills.* Learning and using self-management skills, discussed in Concept 2 and throughout the book, can help you adopt and maintain healthy lifestyles.
- *Formal steps can become less formal with experience.* Few of us will go through life doing formal fitness assessments every month, writing down goals weekly, or self-monitoring activity daily. However, the more a person does self-assessments, the more he or she is aware of personal fitness status. This awareness reduces the need for frequent testing. For example, a person who does regular heart rate monitoring knows when he or she is in the target zone without counting heart rate every minute. A person who has frequently used skinfold measures to self-assess fatness can develop a good sense of body fatness with less frequent measurements. The same is true of other self-management

skills. With experience, you can use the techniques less formally.

Consider your cognitions and emotions when planning strategies for action. Much of the information in this book is designed to help you make good decisions about health, wellness, and fitness. Using the guidelines presented throughout this book and using self-management skills can help you make good decisions. As noted in Concept 1, it is also important to consider your emotions when making decisions. Consider these guidelines:

- *Collect and evaluate information before you act.* Become informed before you make important decisions. Get information from reliable sources and consult with others you trust.
- *Emotions are important to making certain decisions but should not be used instead of good decision-making processes.* Fear and anger are two emotions

Table 4 ▶ Actions and Interactions That Influence Wellness	
Dimension of Wellness	**Influential Factors**
Physical wellness	Pursuing behaviors that are conducive to good physical health (being physically active and maintaining a healthy diet)
Social wellness	Being supportive of family, friends, and co-workers and practicing good communication skills
Emotional wellness	Balancing work and leisure and responding proactively to challenging or stressful situations
Intellectual wellness	Challenging yourself to continually learn and improve in your work and personal life
Spiritual wellness	Praying, meditating, or reflecting on life
Total wellness	Taking responsibility for your own health

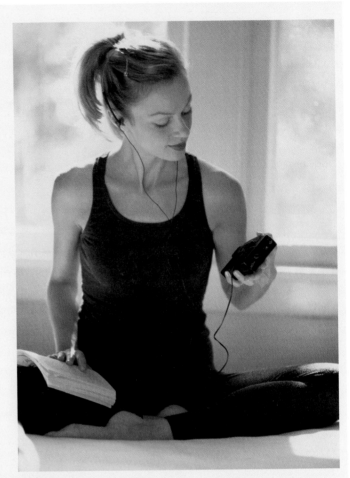

Good planning and a positive attitude can help in making lifestyle changes.

that can affect your judgment and influence your ability to make decisions. Even love for another person can influence your actions. Get control of your emotions, or seek guidance from others you trust, before making important decisions in emotionally charged situations.

- *Resist pressure to make quick decisions when there is no need to decide quickly.* Salespeople often press for a quick decision to get a sale. Take some time to think before making a quick decision that may be based on emotion rather than critical thinking. Of course, some decisions must be made when emotions are charged (e.g., medical care in an emergency), but, when possible, delaying a decision can be to your advantage.
- *Use stress-management techniques to help you gain control when you must make decisions in emotionally charged situations.* Practice stress-management techniques (see Concepts 16 and 17) so that you can use them effectively when needed.

Consider strategies for taking action and benefiting from interactions. In the end, it is what you do that counts. You can learn everything there is to know about fitness, health, and wellness, but if you do not take action and take advantage of your interactions with people and your environments, you will not benefit (see Figure 1). The following are some strategies for taking action and interacting effectively:

- *Plan your actions and interactions.* Use the information in this book to plan your actions. Seek

environments that produce positive interactions. People who plan are not only more likely to act but also more likely to act effectively.
- *Put your plans into action.* Do not put off until tomorrow what you can do today. For good plans to be effective, they must be implemented. Actions and interactions that influence various dimensions of wellness are described in Table 4. As noted in Concept 1, occupational and environmental factors are very important to personal wellness. For this reason, considerable coverage was given to these factors earlier in this concept (see Table 2); however, they are not classified as personal wellness dimensions.
- *Honor your beliefs and relationships.* Actions and interactions that are inconsistent with basic beliefs and that fail to honor important relationships can result in reduced quality of life.
- *Seek the help of others and provide support for others who need your help.* As already noted, support from friends, family, and significant others can be critical in helping you achieve health, wellness, and

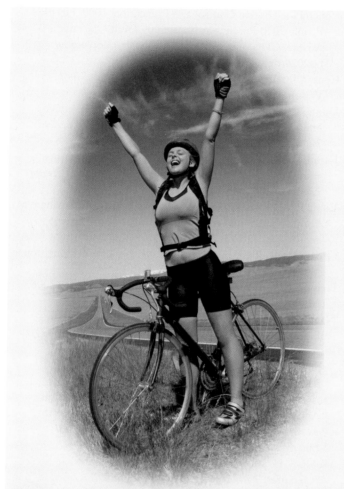

Making lifestyle changes, such as becoming more physically active, can improve your confidence and lead to other healthy lifestyle changes.

fitness. Get help. Do what you can to be there for others who need your help.

- *Consider using professional help.* Most colleges have programs through their health centers that provide free, confidential assistance or referral. Many businesses have employee assistance programs (EAP). The programs have counselors who will help you or your family members find ways to solve a particular problem. Many other programs and support groups are available to help you change your lifestyle. For example, most hospitals and many health organizations

have hotlines that provide referral services for establishing healthy lifestyles.

Consider your personal beliefs and philosophy when making decisions. Though science can help you make good decisions and solve problems, most experts tell you that there is more to it than that. Your personal philosophy and beliefs play a role. The following are factors to consider:

- *Clarify your personal philosophy and consider a new way of thinking.* The determination of whether a person is healthy, well, or fit is often subjective. Many make comparisons with other people, and such comparisons often result in setting personal standards impossible to achieve. Achieving the body fat of a model seen on television is not realistic or healthy for most people. Expecting to be able to perform as a professional athlete is not something most of us can achieve. For this reason, the standards for health, wellness, and fitness in this book are based on health criteria rather than comparative criteria. As you began your study, you were introduced to the HELP philosophy. Adhering to this philosophy can help you adopt a new way of thinking. This philosophy suggests that each person should use health (*H*) as the basis for making decisions rather than comparisons with others. This is something that everyone (*E*) can do for a lifetime (*L*). It allows each of us to set personal (*P*) goals that are realistic and possible to attain.
- *Allow for spontaneity.* The reliance on science emphasized in this book can help you make good choices. But if you are to live life fully, you sometimes must allow yourself to be spontaneous. In doing so, the key is to be consistent with your personal philosophy so that your spontaneous actions will be enriching rather than a source of future regret.
- *Believe that you can make a difference.* As noted previously, you make your own choices. Though heredity and several other factors are out of your control, the choices that you make are yours. Believing that your actions make a difference is critical to taking action and making changes when necessary, allowing you to be healthy, well, and fit for a lifetime.

Web Resources

Additional websites with information related to Concept 24 are available at the associated Web link.

American Association for Retired Persons Health Guide
 www.aarp.org/health/healthguide
American College Health Association **www.acha.org**
American Dietetics Association **www.eatright.org**
American Heart Association (search CPR)
 www.americanheart.org
Cleveland Clinic Second Opinion **www.eclevelandclinic.org**
Gallup-Healthyways Well-Being Index
 www.well-beingindex.com
Healthfinder **www.healthfinder.gov**
Healthy People 2020 **www.healthypeople.gov/hp2020**
Mayo Clinic **www.mayoclinic.com**
National Health Interview Survey
 www.cdc.gov/nchs/nhis.htm
Research America **www.researchamerica.org**
Skin Cancer Foundation **www.skincancer.org**
Superbug Information **www.cdc.gov/ncidod/dhqp/ar_mrsa**
 .html; www2a.cdc.gov/podcasts/player.asp?f=6936
U.S. Consumer Information Center **www.pueblo.gsa.gov**
World Health Organization **www.who.int**

Suggested Readings

Selected readings and references are listed below. A more comprehensive list is available at the associated Web link.

Baker, D. W. 2007. Health literacy and mortality among elderly persons. *Archives of Internal Medicine* 167(14): 1503–1509.

Bray, S. R. 2007. Self-efficacy for coping with barriers helps students stay physically active during transition to their first year at a university. *Research Quarterly for Exercise and Sport* 78(1):61–70.

Centers for Disease Control and Prevention. 2009. Healthy People 2020 Public Meetings: 2009 Draft Objectives. Atlanta: CDC. Available at **www.healthypeople.gov/ hp2020/objectives**

Central Intelligence Agency. 2009. *The World Fact Book*. Washington, DC: CIA.

Dunn, A. L. 2009. Effectiveness of lifestyle physical activity interventions to reduce cardiovascular disease. *American Journal of Lifestyle Medicine* 3:11S–18S.

Eaton, D. K., et al. 2007. Selected health status indicators and behaviors of young adults. *American Journal of Health Education* 38(2):66–75.

Eime, R. M. 2010. Does sports club participation contribute to health-related quality of life? *Medicine and Science in Sports and Exercise* 42(5):1022–1028.

Groopman, J. 2007. *How Doctors Think*. New York: Houghton Mifflin.

Heron, M. P., et al. 2008. Deaths: Preliminary data for 2006. *National Vital Statistics Reports* 56(16):1–52.

Nagao, K., et al. 2007. Cardiopulmonary resuscitation by bystanders with chest compression only (SOS-KANTO): An observational study. *Lancet* 369(9565):920–926.

Taylor, S. 2009. *Health Psychology*. 7th ed. New York: McGraw-Hill.

Trust for America's Health. 2008. Blueprint for a Healthier America. Washington, DC: Trust for America's Health. Available at **http://healthyamericans.org/report/55/ blueprint-for-healthier-america**

Woolf, S. H. 2008. The power of prevention and what it requires. *Journal of the American Medical Association* 299(20):2437–2439.

World Health Organization. 2009. Global Health Risks. Geneva: WHO. Available at **www.who.int/publications/en**

Xu, J., and R. E. Roberts. 2010. The power of positive emotions: It's a matter of life or death—Subjective well-being and longevity over 28 years in a general population. *Health Psychology* 29(1):9–19.

Lab 24A Assessing Factors That Influence Health, Wellness, and Fitness

Name		Section	Date

Purpose: To assess the factors that relate to health, wellness, and fitness

Chart 1 ▶ Assessment Questionnaire: Factors That Influence Health, Wellness, and Fitness

Factor	Very True	Somewhat True	Not True At All	Score
Heredity				
1. I have checked my family history for medical problems.	③	②	①	
2. I have taken steps to overcome hereditary predispositions.	③	②	①	
			Heredity Score =	
Health Care				
3. I have health insurance.	③	②	①	
4. I get regular medical exams and have my own doctor.	③	②	①	
5. I get treatment early, rather than waiting until problems get serious	③	②	①	
6. I carefully investigate my health problems before making decisions.	③	②	①	
			Health-Care Score =	
Environment				
7. My physical environment is healthy.	③	②	①	
8. My social environment is healthy.	③	②	①	
9. My spiritual environment is healthy.	③	②	①	
10. My intellectual environment is healthy.	③	②	①	
11. My work environment is healthy.	③	②	①	
12. My environment fosters healthy lifestyles.	③	②	①	
			Environment Score =	
Lifestyles				
13. I am physically active on a regular basis.	③	②	①	
14. I eat well.	③	②	①	
15. I use effective techniques for managing stress.	③	②	①	
16. I avoid destructive behaviors.	③	②	①	
17. I practice safe sex.	③	②	①	
18. I manage my time effectively.	③	②	①	
19. I evaluate information carefully and am an informed consumer.	③	②	①	
20. My personal health habits are good.	③	②	①	
21. My safety habits are good.	③	②	①	
22. I know first aid and can use it if needed.	③	②	①	
			Lifestyles Score =	
Personal Actions and Interactions				
23. I collect and evaluate information before I act.	③	②	①	
24. I plan before I take action.	③	②	①	
25. I am good about taking action when I know it is good for me.	③	②	①	
26. I honor my beliefs and relationships.	③	②	①	
27. I seek help when I need it.	③	②	①	
			Personal Actions/Interactions Score =	

Procedures

1. Answer each of the questions in Chart 1 on page 501. Consider the information in this concept as you answer each question. The five factors assessed in the questionnaire are from Figure 1, page 409.
2. Calculate the scores for heredity (sum items 1 and 2), health care (sum items 3–6), environment (sum items 7–12), lifestyles (sum items 13–22), and actions/interactions (sum items 23–27).
3. Determine ratings for each of the scores using the Rating Chart.
4. Record your scores and ratings in the Results chart. Record your comments in the Conclusions and Implications section.

Results

Factor	Score	Rating
Heredity		
Health care		
Environment		
Lifestyles		
Actions/interactions		

Rating Chart

Factor	Healthy	Marginal	Needs Attention
Heredity	6	4–5	Below 4
Health care	11–12	9–10	Below 9
Environment	16–18	13–15	Below 13
Lifestyles	26–30	20–25	Below 20
Actions/ interactions	13–15	10–12	Below 10

Conclusions and Implications

1. In the space below, discuss your scores for the five factors (sums of several questions) identified in Chart 1. Use several sentences to identify specific areas that need attention and changes that you could make to improve.

2. For any individual item on Chart 1, a score of 1 is considered low. You might have a high score on a set of questions and still have a low score in one area that indicates a need for attention. In several sentences, discuss actions you could take to make changes related to individual questions.

Lab 24B Planning for Improved Health, Wellness, and Fitness

Name _____

Section _____   **Date** _____

Purpose: To plan to make changes in areas that can most contribute to improved health, wellness, and fitness

Procedures

1. Experts agree that it is best not to make too many changes all at once. Focusing attention on one or two things at a time will produce better results. Based on your assessments made in Lab 24A, select two areas in which you would like to make changes. Choose one from the list related to environments and health care and one related to lifestyle change. Place a check by those areas in Chart 1 in the Results section. Because Lab 24C is devoted to physical activity, it is not included in the list. You may want to make additional copies of this lab for use in making other changes in the future.
2. Use Chart 2 to determine your Stage of Change for the changes you have identified. Since you have identified these as an area of need, it is unlikely that you would identify the stage of maintenance. If you are at maintenance, you can select a different area of changes that would be more useful.
3. In the appropriate locations, record the change you want to make related to your environment or health care. State your reasons, your specific goal(s), your written statement of the plan for change, and a statement about how you will self-monitor and evaluate the effectiveness of the changes made. In Chart 3, record similar information for the lifestyle change you identified.

Results

Chart 1 ▶

Check one in each column.

Area of Change	✔	Area of Change	✔
Health insurance		Eating well	
Medical checkups		Managing stress	
Selecting a doctor		Avoiding destructive habits	
Physical environment		Practicing safe sex	
Social environment		Managing time	
Spiritual environment		Becoming a better consumer	
Intellectual environment		Improving health habits	
Work environment		Improving safety habits	
Environment for lifestyles		Learning first aid	

Chart 2 ▶

List the two areas of change identified in Chart 1. Make a rating using the diagram at the right.

Identified Area of Change	Stage of Change Rating
1.	
2.	

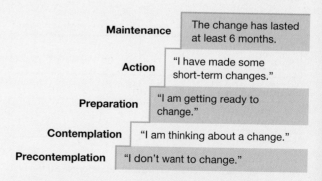

Maintenance — The change has lasted at least 6 months.

Action — "I have made some short-term changes."

Preparation — "I am getting ready to change."

Contemplation — "I am thinking about a change."

Precontemplation — "I don't want to change."

Note: Some of the areas identified in this lab relate to personal information. It is appropriate not to divulge personal information to others (including your instructor) if you choose not to. For this reason, you may choose not to address certain problems in this lab. You are encouraged to take steps to make changes independent of this assignment and to consult privately with your instructor to get assistance.

Chart 3 ▶ Making Changes for Improved Health, Wellness, and Fitness

Describe First Area of Change (from Chart 1)	Describe Second Area of Change (from Chart 1)
Step 1: State Reasons for Making Change	**Step 1: State Reasons for Making Change**

Step 2: Self-Assessment of Need for Change
List your stage from Chart 2.

Step 2: Self-Assessment of Need for Change
List your stage from Chart 2.

Step 3: State Your Specific Goals for Change
State several specific and realistic goals.

Step 3: State Your Specific Goals for Change
State several specific and realistic goals.

Step 4: Identify Activities or Actions for Change
List specific activities you will do or actions you will take to meet your goals.

Step 4: Identify Activities or Actions for Change
List specific activities you will do or actions you will take to meet your goals.

Step 5: Write a Plan; Include a Timetable
Expected start date:

Expected finish date:

Days of week and times: list times below days.

Mon.	Tue.	Wed.	Th.	Fri.	Sat.	Sun.

Location: where will you do the plan?

Step 5: Write a Plan; Include a Timetable
Expected start date:

Expected finish date:

Days of week and times: list times below days.

Mon.	Tue.	Wed.	Th.	Fri.	Sat.	Sun.

Location: where will you do the plan?

Step 6: Evaluate Your Plan
How will you self-monitor and evaluate to determine if the plan is working?

Step 6: Evaluate Your Plan
How will you self-monitor and evaluate to determine if the plan is working?

Lab 24C Planning Your Personal Physical Activity Program

Name	**Section**	**Date**

Purpose: To establish a comprehensive plan of lifestyle physical activity and to self-monitor progress in your plan (note: you may want to reread the concept on planning for physical activity before completing this lab)

Procedures

Step 1. Establishing Your Reasons

In the spaces provided below, list several of your principal reasons for doing a comprehensive activity plan.

1.	4.
2.	5.
3.	6.

Step 2. Identify Your Needs Using Fitness Self-Assessments and Ratings of Stage of Change for Various Activities

In Chart 1, rate your fitness by placing an X over the circle by the appropriate rating for each part of fitness. Use your results obtained from previous labs or perform the self-assessments again to determine your ratings. If you took more than one self-assessment for one component of physical fitness, select the rating that you think best describes your true fitness for that fitness component. If you were unable to do a self-assessment for some reason, check the "No Results" circle.

Chart 1 ▶ Rating for Self-Assessments

Health-Related Fitness Tests	Rating				
	High-Performance Zone	Good Fitness Zone	Marginal Zone	Low Zone	No Results
1. Cardiovascular: 12-minute run (Chart 6, page 133)	○	○	○	○	○
2. Cardiovascular: step test (Chart 2, page 131)	○	○	○	○	○
3. Cardiovascular: bicycle test (Chart 5, page 133)	○	○	○	○	○
4. Cardiovascular: walking test (Chart 1, page 131)	○	○	○	○	○
5. Cardiovascular: swim test (Chart 7, page 134)	○	○	○	○	○
6. Flexibility: sit-and-reach test (Chart 1, page 218)	○	○	○	○	○
7. Flexibility: shoulder flexibility (Chart 1, page 218)	○	○	○	○	○
8. Flexibility: hamstring/hip flexibility (Chart 1, page 218)	○	○	○	○	○
9. Flexibility: trunk rotation (Chart 1, page 218)	○	○	○	○	○
10. Strength: isometric grip (Chart 3, page 190)	○	○	○	○	○
11. Strength: 1 RM upper body (Chart 2, page 189)	○	○	○	○	○

Chart 1 ▶ Rating for Self-Assessments, *continued*

Health-Related Fitness Tests	Rating				
	High-Performance	Good Fitness	Marginal	Low	No Results
12. Strength: 1 RM lower body (Chart 2, page 189)	○	○	○	○	○
13. Muscular endurance: curl-up (Chart 4, page 190)	○	○	○	○	○
14. Muscular endurance: 90-degree push-up (Chart 4, page 190)	○	○	○	○	○
15. Muscular endurance: flexed arm support (Chart 5, page 190)	○	○	○	○	○
16. Fitness rating: skinfold (Chart 1, page 304)	○	○	○	○	○
17. Body mass index (Chart 7, page 309)	○	○	○	○	○

Skill-Related Fitness and Other Self-Assessments	Rating				
	Excellent	Very Good or Good	Fair	Poor	No Results
1. Agility (Chart 1, page 279)	○	○	○	○	○
2. Balance (Chart 2, page 280)	○	○	○	○	○
3. Coordination (Chart 3, page 280)	○	○	○	○	○
4. Power (Chart 4, page 281)	○	○	○	○	○
5. Reaction time (Chart 5, page 281)	○	○	○	○	○
6. Speed (Chart 6, page 282)	○	○	○	○	○
7. Fitness of the back (Chart 2, page 256)	○	○	○	○	○
8. Posture (Chart 2, page 259.)	○	○	○	○	○

Summarize Your Fitness Ratings Using the Results Above	Rating				
	High-Performance	Good Fitness	Marginal	Low	No Results
Cardiovascular	○	○	○	○	○
Muscular Endurance	○	○	○	○	○
Strength	○	○	○	○	○
Flexibility	○	○	○	○	○
Body fatness	○	○	○	○	○
	Excellent	Very Good or Good	Fair	Poor	No Results
Skill-related fitness	○	○	○	○	○
Posture and fitness of the back	○	○	○	○	○

Rate your stage of change for each of the different types of activities from the physical activity pyramid. Make an X over the circle beside the stage that best represents your behavior for each of the five types of activity in the lower three levels of the pyramid. A description of the various stages is provided below to help you make your ratings.

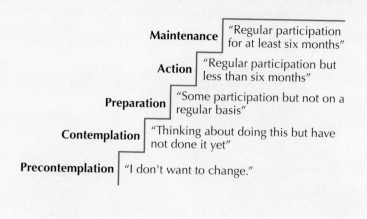

Maintenance — "Regular participation for at least six months"

Action — "Regular participation but less than six months"

Preparation — "Some participation but not on a regular basis"

Contemplation — "Thinking about doing this but have not done it yet"

Precontemplation — "I don't want to change."

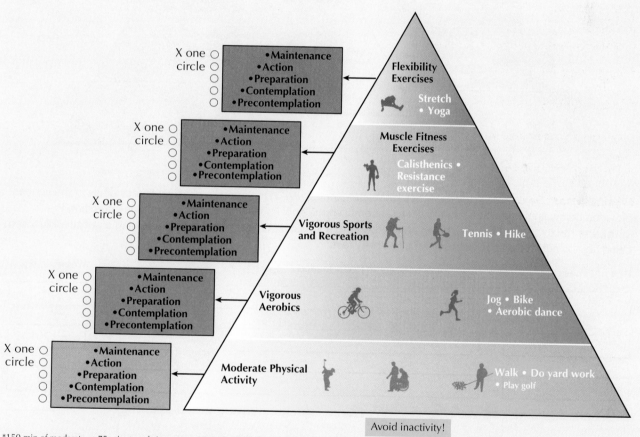

X one circle
• Maintenance
• Action
• Preparation
• Contemplation
• Precontemplation

Flexibility Exercises
Stretch • Yoga

X one circle
• Maintenance
• Action
• Preparation
• Contemplation
• Precontemplation

Muscle Fitness Exercises
Calisthenics • Resistance exercise

X one circle
• Maintenance
• Action
• Preparation
• Contemplation
• Precontemplation

Vigorous Sports and Recreation
Tennis • Hike

X one circle
• Maintenance
• Action
• Preparation
• Contemplation
• Precontemplation

Vigorous Aerobics
Jog • Bike • Aerobic dance

X one circle
• Maintenance
• Action
• Preparation
• Contemplation
• Precontemplation

Moderate Physical Activity
Walk • Do yard work • Play golf

Avoid inactivity!

*150 min of moderate or 75 minutes of vigorous activity per week is recommended; moderate and vigorous activity can be combined to meet guidelines.

In step 1, you wrote down some general reasons for developing your physical activity plan. Setting goals requires more specific statements of goals that are realistic and achievable. For people who are at the contemplation or preparation stage for a specific type of activity, it is recommended that you write only short-term physical activity goals (no more than 4 weeks). Those at the action or maintenance level may choose short-term goals to start with, or if you have a good history of adherence, choose long-term goals (longer than 4 weeks). Precontemplators are not considered because they would not be doing this activity.

Step 3. Set Specific Goals

Chart 2 ▶ Setting Goals

Physical Activity Goals. Place an X over the appropriate circle for the number of days of the week and the number of weeks for each type of activity. Write the number of exercises or activities you plan in each of the five areas.

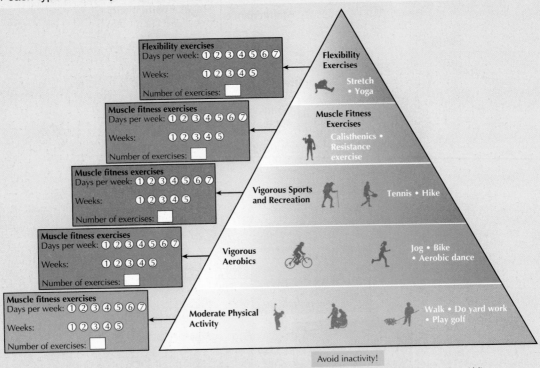

Flexibility exercises
Days per week: ① ② ③ ④ ⑤ ⑥ ⑦
Weeks: ① ② ③ ④ ⑤
Number of exercises: ☐

Muscle fitness exercises
Days per week: ① ② ③ ④ ⑤ ⑥ ⑦
Weeks: ① ② ③ ④ ⑤
Number of exercises: ☐

Muscle fitness exercises
Days per week: ① ② ③ ④ ⑤ ⑥ ⑦
Weeks: ① ② ③ ④ ⑤
Number of exercises: ☐

Muscle fitness exercises
Days per week: ① ② ③ ④ ⑤ ⑥ ⑦
Weeks: ① ② ③ ④ ⑤
Number of exercises: ☐

Muscle fitness exercises
Days per week: ① ② ③ ④ ⑤ ⑥ ⑦
Weeks: ① ② ③ ④ ⑤
Number of exercises: ☐

Flexibility Exercises — Stretch • Yoga

Muscle Fitness Exercises — Calisthenics • Resistance exercise

Vigorous Sports and Recreation — Tennis • Hike

Vigorous Aerobics — Jog • Bike • Aerobic dance

Moderate Physical Activity — Walk • Do yard work • Play golf

Avoid inactivity!

*150 min of moderate or 75 minutes of vigorous activity per week is recommended; moderate and vigorous activity can be combined to meet guidelines.

Physical Fitness Goals (for People at Action or Maintenance Only). Write specific physical fitness goals in the spaces provided below. Indicate when you expect to accomplish the goal (in weeks). Examples include improving the 12-minute run to a specific score, being able to perform a specific number of push-ups, attaining a specific BMI, and being able to achieve a specific score on a flexibility test.

Part of Fitness	Description of Specific Performance	Weeks to Goal

Step 4. Selecting Activities

In Chart 3, indicate the specific activities you plan to perform from each area of the physical activity pyramid. If the activity you expect to perform is listed, note the number of minutes or reps/sets you plan to perform. If the activity you want to perform is not listed, write the name of the activity or exercise in the space designated as "Other." For lifestyle activities, active aerobics, and active sports and recreation, indicate the length of time the activity will be performed each day. For flexibility, muscle fitness exercises, and exercises for back and neck, indicate the number of repetitions for each exercise.

Chart 3 ▶ Lifetime Physical Activity Selections

✔	Lifestyle Activities	Min./Day	✔	Active Aerobics	Min./Day	✔	Active Sports and Recreation	Min./Day
	Walking			Aerobic exercise machines			Basketball	
	Yard work			Bicycling			Bowling	
	Active housework			Circuit training or calisthenics			Golf	
	Gardening			Dance or step aerobics			Karate/judo	
	Social dancing			Hiking or backpacking			Mountain climbing	
	Occupational activity			Jogging or running (or walking)			Racquetball	
	Wheeling in wheelchair			Skating/cross-country skiing			Skating	
	Bicycling to work or store			Swimming			Softball	
	Other:			Water activity			Skiing	
	Other:			Other:			Soccer	
	Other:			Other:			Volleyball	
	Other:			Other:			Other:	
	Other:			Other:			Other:	
	Other:			Other:			Other:	
	Other:			Other:			Other:	

✔	Flexibility Exercises	Reps/Sets	✔	Muscle Fitness Exercises	Reps/Sets	✔	Exercises for Back and Neck	Reps/Sets
	Calf stretch			Bench or seated press			Back saver stretch	
	Hip and thigh stretch			Biceps curl			Single knee to chest	
	Sitting stretch			Triceps curl			Low back stretch	
	Hamstring stretch			Lat pull down			Hip/thigh stretch	
	Back stretch (leg hug)			Seated rowing			Pelvic tilt	
	Trunk twist			Wrist curl			Bridging	
	Pectoral stretch			Knee extension			Wall slide	
	Arm stretch			Heel raise			Pelvic stabilizer	
	Other:			Half-squat skiing			Neck rotation	
	Other:			Lunge			Isometric neck exercise	
	Other:			Toe press			Chin tuck	
	Other:			Crunch or reverse curl			Trapezius stretch	
	Other:			Other:			Other:	
	Other:			Other:			Other:	
	Other:			Other:			Other:	

Lab 24C

Planning Your Personal Physical Activity Program

Step 5. Preparing a Written Plan

In Chart 4, place a check in the shaded boxes for each activity you will perform for each day you will do it. Indicate the time of day you expect to perform the activity or exercise (Example: 7:30 to 8 A.M. or 6 to 6:30 P.M.). In the spaces labeled "Warm-Up Exercises" and "Cool-Down Exercises," check the warm-up and cool-down exercises you expect to perform. Indicate the number of reps you will use for each exercise.

Chart 4 ▶ My Physical Activity Plan

✔	Monday	Time	✔	Tuesday	Time	✔	Wednesday	Time
	Lifestyle activity			Lifestyle activity			Lifestyle activity	
	Active aerobics			Active aerobics			Active aerobics	
	Active sports/rec.			Active sports/rec.			Active sports/rec.	
	Flexibility exercises*			Flexibility exercises*			Flexibility exercises*	
	Muscle fitness exercises*			Muscle fitness exercises*			Muscle fitness exercises*	
	Back/neck exercises*			Back/neck exercises*			Back/neck exercises*	
	Warm-up exercises			Warm-up exercises			Warm-up exercises	
	Other:			Other:			Other:	

✔	Thursday	Time	✔	Friday	Time	✔	Saturday	Time
	Lifestyle activity			Lifestyle activity			Lifestyle activity	
	Active aerobics			Active aerobics			Active aerobics	
	Active sports/rec.			Active sports/rec.			Active sports/rec.	
	Flexibility exercises*			Flexibility exercises*			Flexibility exercises*	
	Muscle fitness exercises*			Muscle fitness exercises*			Muscle fitness exercises*	
	Back/neck exercises*			Back/neck exercises*			Back/neck exercises*	
	Warm-up exercises			Warm-up exercises			Warm-up exercises	
	Other:			Other:			Other:	

✔	Sunday	Time	✔	Warm-Up Exercises	Reps	✔	Cool-Down Exercises	Reps
	Lifestyle activity			Walk or jog 1–2 min.			Walk or jog 1–2 min.	
	Active aerobics			Calf stretch			Calf stretch	
	Active sports/rec.			Hamstring stretch			Hamstring stretch	
	Flexibility exercises*			Leg hug			Leg hug	
	Muscle fitness exercises*			Sitting side stretch			Sitting side stretch	
	Back/neck exercises*			Zipper			Zipper	
	Warm-up exercises			Other:			Other:	
	Other:			Other:			Other:	

*Perform the specific exercises you checked in Chart 3.

Step 6. Keeping Records of Progress and Evaluating Your Plan

Make copies of Chart 4 (one for each week that you plan to keep records). Each day, make a check by the activities you actually performed. Include the times when you actually did the activities in your plan. Periodically check your goals to see if they have been accomplished. At some point, it will be necessary to reestablish your goals and create a revised activity plan.

Results

After performing your plan for a specific period of time, answer the question in the space provided.

How long have you been performing the plan?

Conclusions and Implications

1. In several sentences, discuss your adherence to the plan. Have you been able to stick with the plan? If so, do you think it is a plan you can do for a lifetime? If not, why do you think you are unable to do your plan?

2. In several sentences, discuss how you might modify your plan in the future.

3. In several sentences, discuss your goals for your program. Do you think you will meet your goals? Why or why not?

Appendix A
Metric Conversion Charts

Chart 1 ▶ Traditional/Metric Measurement Conversions

	Metrics to Traditional	Traditional to Metrics
Length	centimeters to inches: cm × .39 = 1 in.	inches to centimeters: in. × 2.54 = cm
	meters to feet: m × 3.3 = ft.	feet to meters: ft. × .3048 = m
	meters to yards: m × 1.09 = yd.	yards to meters: yd. × 0.92 = m
	kilometers to miles: km × 0.6 = mi.	miles to kilometers: mi. × 1.6 = km
Weight (Mass)	grams to ounces: g × 0.0352 = oz.	ounces to grams: oz. × 28.41 = g
	kilograms to pounds: kg × 2.2 = lb.	pounds to kilograms: lb. × 0.45 = kg
Volume	milliliters to fluid ounces: ml × 0.03 = fl. oz.	fluid ounces to milliliters: fl. oz. × 29.573 = ml
	liters to quarts: l × 1.06 = qt.	quarts to liters: qt. × 0.95 = l
	liters to gallons: l × 0.264 = gal.	gallons to liters: gal. × 3.8 = l

Chart 2 ▶ 12-Minute Run Test (Scores in Meters)

Classification	Men (Age)			
	17–26	**27–39**	**40–49**	**50+**
High-performance zone	2,880+	2,560+	2,400+	2,240+
Good fitness zone	2,480–2,779	2,320–2,559	2,240–2,399	2,000–2,239
Marginal zone	2,160–2,479	2,080–2,319	2,000–2,239	1,760–1,999
Low zone	<2,160	<2,080	<2,000	<1,760

Classification	Women (Age)			
	17–26	**27–39**	**40–49**	**50+**
High-performance zone	2,320+	2,160+	2,000+	1,840+
Good fitness zone	2,000–2,319	1,920–2,159	1,840–1,999	1,680–1,839
Marginal zone	1,840–1,999	1,680–1,919	1,600–1,839	1,520–1,679
Low zone	<1,840	<1,680	<1,600	<1,520

Chart 3 ▶ 12-Minute Swim Rating Chart (Scores in Meters)

Classification	Men (Age)			
	17–26	**27–39**	**40–49**	**50+**
High-performance zone	644+	598+	552+	506+
Good fitness zone	552–643	506–597	460–551	413–505
Marginal zone	460–551	414–505	368–459	322–412
Low zone	<460	<414	<368	<322

Classification	Women (Age)			
	17–26	**27–39**	**40–49**	**50+**
High-performance zone	552+	506+	460+	414+
Good fitness zone	460–551	414–505	367–459	321–413
Marginal zone	367–459	321–413	276–366	230–320
Low zone	<367	<321	<276	<230

Chart 4 ▶ Isometric Strength Rating Scale (kg)

Classification	Men			Women		
	Left Grip	Right Grip	Total Score	Left Grip	Right Grip	Total Score
High-performance zone	57+	61+	118+	34+	39+	73+
Good fitness zone	45–56	50–60	95–117	27–33	32–38	59–72
Marginal zone	41–44	43–49	84–94	20–26	23–31	43–58
Low zone	<41	<43	<84	<20	<23	<43

Suitable for use by young adults between 18 and 30 years of age. After 30, an adjustment of 0.5 of 1 percent per year is appropriate because some loss of muscle tissue typically occurs as you grow older.

Chart 5 ▶ Power Rating Scale

Classification	Men	Women
Excellent	68 cm+	60 cm+
Very good	53–67 cm	48–59 cm
Good	42–52 cm	37–47 cm
Fair	31–41 cm	27–36 cm
Poor	<32 cm	<27 cm

Chart 6 ▶ Reaction Time Rating Scale

Classification	Score in Inches	Score in Centimeters
Excellent	>21	>52
Very good	19″–21	48–52
Good	16″–18 ¾	41–47
Fair	13″–15 ¾	33–40
Poor	<13	<33

Chart 7 ▶ Speed Rating Scale

Classification	Men		Women	
	Yards	Meters	Yards	Meters
Excellent	24+	22+	22+	20+
Very good	22–23	20–21.9	20–21	18–19.9
Good	18–21	16.5–19.9	16–19	14.5–17.9
Fair	16–17	14.5–16.4	14–15	13–14.4
Poor	<16	<14.5	<14	<13

Canada's Food Guide to Healthy Eating

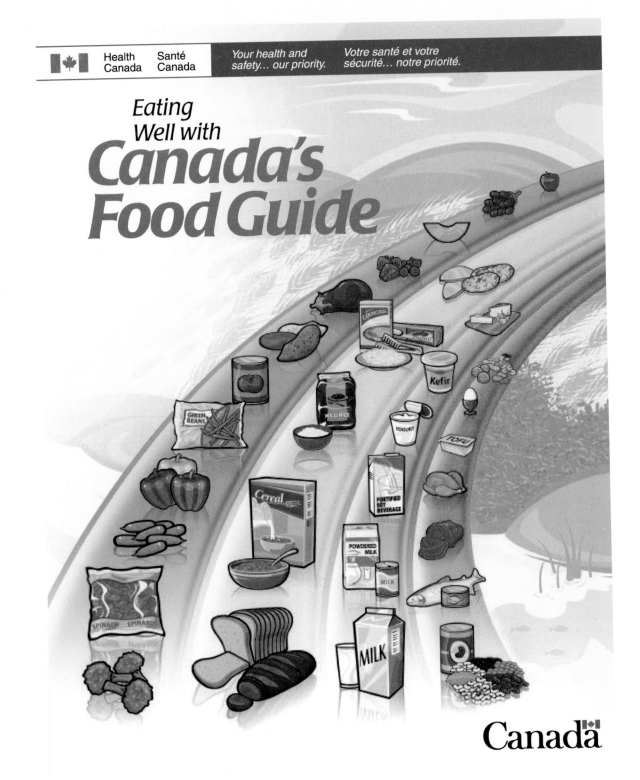

Recommended Number of Food Guide Servings per Day

Age in Years	Children			Teens			Adults				
	2-3	4-8	9-13	14-18		19-50		51+			
Sex	Girls and Boys			Females	Males	Females	Males	Females	Males		
Vegetables and Fruit	4	5	6	7	8	7-8	8-10	7	7		
Grain Products	3	4	6	6	7	6-7	8	6	7		
Milk and Alternatives	2	2	3-4	3-4	3-4	2	2	3	3		
Meat and Alternatives	1	1	1-2	2	3	2	3	2	3		

The chart above shows how many Food Guide Servings you need from each of the four food groups every day.

Having the amount and type of food recommended and following the tips in *Canada's Food Guide* will help:

- Meet your needs for vitamins, minerals and other nutrients.
- Reduce your risk of obesity, type 2 diabetes, heart disease, certain types of cancer and osteoporosis.
- Contribute to your overall health and vitality.

What is One Food Guide Serving?
Look at the examples below.

Vegetables and Fruit

Fresh, frozen or canned vegetables
125 mL (½ cup)

Leafy vegetables
Cooked: 125 mL (½ cup)
Raw: 250 mL (1 cup)

Fresh, frozen or canned fruits
1 fruit or 125 mL (½ cup)

100% Juice
125 mL (½ cup)

Grain Products

Bread
1 slice (35 g)

Bagel
½ bagel (45 g)

Flat breads
½ pita or ½ tortilla (35 g)

Cooked rice, bulgur or quinoa
125 mL (½ cup)

Cereal
Cold: 30 g
Hot: 175 mL (¾ cup)

Cooked pasta or couscous
125 mL (½ cup)

Milk and Alternatives

Milk or powdered milk (reconstituted)
250 mL (1 cup)

Canned milk (evaporated)
125 mL (½ cup)

Fortified soy beverage
250 mL (1 cup)

Yogurt
175 g
(¾ cup)

Kefir
175 g
(¾ cup)

Cheese
50 g (1 ½ oz.)

Meat and Alternatives

Cooked fish, shellfish, poultry, lean meat
75 g (2 ½ oz.)/125 mL (½ cup)

Cooked legumes
175 mL (¾ cup)

Tofu
150 g or
175 mL (¾ cup)

Eggs
2 eggs

Peanut or nut butters
30 mL (2 Tbsp)

Shelled nuts and seeds
60 mL (¼ cup)

Oils and Fats

- Include a small amount – 30 to 45 mL (2 to 3 Tbsp) – of unsaturated fat each day. This includes oil used for cooking, salad dressings, margarine and mayonnaise.
- Use vegetable oils such as canola, olive and soybean.
- Choose soft margarines that are low in saturated and trans fats.
- Limit butter, hard margarine, lard and shortening.

Make each Food Guide Serving count...
wherever you are – at home, at work or at school, at work or when eating out!

▶ **Eat at least one dark green and one orange vegetable each day.**
- Go for dark green vegetables such as broccoli, romaine lettuce and spinach.
- Go for orange vegetables such as carrots, sweet potatoes and winter squash.

▶ **Choose vegetables and fruit prepared with little or no added fat, sugar or salt.**
- Enjoy vegetables steamed, baked or stir-fried instead of deep-fried.

▶ **Have vegetables and fruit more often than juice.**

▶ **Make at least half of your grain products whole grain each day.**
- Eat a variety of whole grains such as barley, brown rice, oats, quinoa and wild rice.
- Enjoy whole grain breads, oatmeal or whole wheat pasta.

▶ **Choose grain products that are lower in fat, sugar or salt.**
- Compare the Nutrition Facts table on labels to make wise choices.
- Enjoy the true taste of grain products. When adding sauces or spreads, use small amounts.

▶ **Drink skim, 1%, or 2% milk each day.**
- Have 500 mL (2 cups) of milk every day for adequate vitamin D.
- Drink fortified soy beverages if you do not drink milk.

▶ **Select lower fat milk alternatives.**
- Compare the Nutrition Facts table on yogurts or cheeses to make wise choices.

▶ **Have meat alternatives such as beans, lentils and tofu often.**

▶ **Eat at least two Food Guide Servings of fish each week.***
- Choose fish such as char, herring, mackerel, salmon, sardines and trout.

▶ **Select lean meat and alternatives prepared with little or no added fat or salt.**
- Trim the visible fat from meats. Remove the skin on poultry.
- Use cooking methods such as roasting, baking or poaching that require little or no added fat.
- If you eat luncheon meats, sausages or prepackaged meats, choose those lower in salt (sodium) and fat.

Enjoy a variety of foods from the four food groups.

Satisfy your thirst with water!
Drink water regularly. It's a calorie-free way to quench your thirst. Drink more water in hot weather or when you are very active.

* Health Canada provides advice for limiting exposure to mercury from certain types of fish. Refer to www.healthcanada.gc.ca for the latest information.

Appendix C

Calorie, Fat, Saturated Fat, Cholesterol, and Sodium Content of Selected Fast-Food Items

Burger King	Calories	Total Fat	Sat. Fat	Chol.	Sodium
Hamburger	320	14	7	45	530
Whopper Jr.	410	23	8	50	520
Whopper	680	39	13	80	940
Chicken sandwich	660	39	11	70	1,330
Double cheeseburger	570	34	19	110	1,020
Bacon double cheeseburger	780	47	19	105	1,390
Double whopper	920	57	22	150	1,020
Double whopper with cheese	1,020	65	27	170	1,460
Fries (small—2.25 oz.)	230	11	60	0	530
Fries (medium—4 oz.)	360	18	10	0	690
Fries (large—5.5 oz.)	500	25	13	0	940
Fries (king—6 oz.)	600	30	16	0	1,140
Onion rings (medium—3.5 oz.)	320	16	8	0	460
Onion rings (king—5.5 oz.)	550	27	13	0	N/A
Coca-Cola classic (small—16 oz.)	160	0	0	0	N/A
Coca-Cola classic (med.—22 oz.)	230	0	0	0	N/A
Coca-Cola classic (large—32 oz.)	330	0	0	0	N/A
Coca-Cola classic (king—42 oz.)	430	0	0	0	N/A
Shake (medium—14 oz.)	460	8	5	30	320
Apple pie	340	14	6	0	470
Sundae pie	310	18	15	10	140

Taco Bell	Calories	Total Fat	Sat. Fat	Chol.	Sodium
Chicken fiesta burrito	370	12	4	35	1,000
Bean burrito	370	12	4	10	1,080
Chili cheese burrito	330	13	5	24	900
Chicken burrito supreme	410	16	6	45	1,120
Steak burrito supreme	420	16	6	35	1,140
7-layer burrito	520	22	7	25	1,270
Grilled stuft chicken burrito	690	29	8	70	1,900
Grilled stuft steak burrito	690	30	8	60	1,970
Chicken chalupa nacho cheese	350	19	5	25	640
Chicken chalupa baja	400	24	5	40	660
Beef chalupa nacho cheese	370	22	6	25	740
Steak chalupa baja	400	24	6	30	680
Chicken gordita supreme	300	13	5	45	530
Steak gordita supreme	300	14	5	35	550
Beef gordita supreme	300	14	5	35	550
Chicken soft taco	190	7	3	35	480
Beef soft taco	210	10	4	30	570
Steak soft taco	280	17	4	35	630
Taco supreme	260	16	6	40	350
Double decker taco supreme	420	21	8	40	760
Pintos and cheese	180	8	4	15	640
Nachos	320	18	4	5	560
Nachos supreme	440	24	7	35	800
Nachos bell grande	760	39	11	35	1,300
Chicken quesadilla	540	30	12	80	1,270
Taco salad with salsa	850	52	14	70	2,250
Shake (large—32 oz.)	1,010	29	19	115	530
Cola (small—16 oz.)	100	0	0	0	10
Cola (medium—20 oz.)	130	0	0	0	10

Jacobson, M. F. and Hurley, J.

McDonald's	Calories	Total Fat	Sat. Fat	Chol.	Sodium
Hamburger	280	10	4	30	590
Fillet o-fish	470	26	5	50	890
Crispy chicken	550	27	5	50	1,180
Cheeseburger	330	14	6	50	830
Quarter pounder	430	21	8	70	840
Big Mac	590	34	11	85	1,090
Quarter pounder with cheese	590	30	13	95	1,310
French fries (small—2.5 oz.)	210	10	3	0	140
French fries (medium—5 oz.)	450	22	8	0	290
French fries (large—6 oz.)	540	26	9	0	350
French fries (supersize—7 oz.)	610	29	10	0	390
Grilled chicken caesar salad	100	3	2	40	240
Garden salad	100	6	3	75	120
Chef salad	150	8	4	95	740
Caesar dressing	150	13	3	10	400
Thousand island dressing	130	9	2	15	350
Honey mustard	160	11	2	15	260
Coca-Cola classic (small—16 oz.)	150	0	0	0	N/A
Coca-Cola classic (med.—21 oz.)	210	0	0	0	N/A
Coca-Cola classic (large—32 oz.)	310	0	0	0	N/A
Coca-Cola classic (supersize—42 oz.)	410	0	0	0	N/A
Shake (small—14 oz.)	360	9	6	40	230
Hot fudge sundae	340	12	9	30	170
McFlurry	610	22	14	75	250
Shake (large—32 oz.)	1,010	29	19	115	530

Wendy's	Calories	Total Fat	Sat. Fat	Chol.	Sodium
Grilled chicken sandwich	300	7	2	55	740
Spicy chicken sandwich	410	14	3	65	1,280
Chicken breast fillet sandwich	430	16	3	55	750
Chicken club sandwich	470	20	5	65	940
Jr. cheeseburger	310	12	6	45	800
Jr. cheeseburger deluxe	350	16	6	45	800
Jr. bacon cheeseburger	380	19	7	55	870
Classic single with everything	410	19	7	70	920
Big bacon classic	580	30	12	100	1,460
Classic double with everything	760	45	19	175	1,730
Classic triple with everything	1,030	65	29	245	2,280
Chicken nuggets	230	16	3	30	470
French fries (small—3 oz.)	270	13	4	0	90
French fries (med.—5 oz.)	420	20	6	0	130
French fries (biggie—5.5 oz.)	470	23	7	0	150
French fries (great biggie—6.5 oz.)	570	27	8	0	180
Plain baked potato	310	0	0	0	30
Chili	210	7	3	30	800
Broccoli and cheese potato	470	14	3	5	470
Bacon and cheese potato	530	17	4	25	820
Cola (small—16 oz.)	100	0	0	0	10
Cola (med.—20 oz.)	130	0	0	0	10
Cola (biggie—32 oz.)	210	0	0	0	20
Frosty (small)	170	4	3	20	100
Frosty (large)	330	8	5	35	200

Appendix D
Calorie Guide to Common Foods

Beverages

Coffee (black)	0
Coke (12 oz.)	137
Hot chocolate, milk (1 cup)	247
Lemonade (1 cup)	100
Limeade, diluted to serve (1 cup)	110
Soda, fruit-flavored (12 oz.)	161
Tea (clear)	0

Breads and Cereals

Bagel (1 half)	76
Biscuit (2" × 2")	135
Bread, pita (1 oz.)	80
Bread, raisin ($\frac{1}{2}$" thick)	65
Bread, rye	55
Bread, white enriched ($\frac{1}{2}$" thick)	68
Bread, whole-wheat ($\frac{1}{2}$" thick)	67
Bun (hamburger)	120
Cereals, cooked ($\frac{1}{2}$ cup)	80
Corn flakes (1 cup)	96
Corn grits (1 cup)	125
Corn muffin ($2\frac{1}{2}$" diam.)	103
Crackers, graham (1 med.)	28
Crackers, soda (1 plain)	24
English muffin (1 half)	74
Macaroni, with cheese (1 cup)	464
Muffin, plain	135
Noodles (1 cup)	200
Oatmeal (1 cup)	150
Pancakes (1–4" diam.)	59
Pizza (1 section)	180
Popped corn (1 cup)	54
Potato chips (10 med.)	108
Pretzels (5 small sticks)	18
Rice (1 cup)	225
Roll, plain (1 med.)	118
Roll, sweet (1 med.)	178
Shredded wheat (1 med. biscuit)	79
Spaghetti, plain cooked (1 cup)	218
Tortilla (1 corn)	70
Waffle ($4\frac{1}{2}$" × 5")	216

Dairy Products

Butter, 1 pat ($1\frac{1}{2}$ tsp.)	50
Cheese, cheddar (1 oz.)	113
Cheese, cottage (1 cup)	270
Cheese, cream (1 oz.)	106
Cheese, Parmesan (1 tbsp.)	29
Cheese, Swiss natural (1 oz.)	105
Cream, sour (1 tbsp.)	31
Frozen custard (1 cup)	375
Frozen yogurt, vanilla (1 cup)	180
Ice cream, plain (prem.) (1 cup)	350
Ice cream soda, choc. (large glass)	455
Ice milk (1 cup)	184
Ices (1 cup)	177
Milk, chocolate (1 cup)	185
Milk, half-and-half (1 tbsp.)	20
Milk, malted (1 cup)	281
Milk, skim (1 cup)	88
Milk, skim dry (1 tbsp.)	28
Milk, whole (1 cup)	166
Sherbet (1 cup)	270
Softserve cone (med.)	335
Whipped topping (1 tbsp.)	14
Yogurt (1 cup)	150

Desserts and Sweets

Cake, angel (2" wedge)	108
Cake, chocolate (2" × 3" × 1")	150
Cake, plain (3" × $2\frac{1}{2}$")	180
Chocolate, bar	200–300
Chocolate, bitter (1 oz.)	142
Chocolate, sweet (1 oz.)	133
Chocolate, syrup (1 tbsp.)	42
Cocoa (1 tbsp.)	21
Cookies, plain (1 med.)	75
Custard, baked (1 cup)	283
Donut (1 large)	250
Gelatin, dessert (1 cup)	155
Gelatin, with fruit (1 cup)	170
Gingerbread (2" × 2" × 2")	180
Jams, jellies (1 tbsp.)	55
Pie, apple ($\frac{1}{7}$ of 9" pie)	345
Pie, cherry ($\frac{1}{7}$ of 9" pie)	355
Pie, chocolate ($\frac{1}{7}$ of 9" pie)	360
Pie, coconut ($\frac{1}{7}$ of 9" pie)	266
Pie, lemon meringue ($\frac{1}{7}$ of 9" pie)	302
Sugar, granulated (1 tsp.)	27
Syrup, table (1 tbsp.)	57

Fruit

Apple, fresh (med.)	76
Applesauce, unsweetened (1 cup)	184
Avocado, raw ($\frac{1}{2}$ peeled)	279
Banana, fresh (med.)	88
Cantaloupe, raw ($\frac{1}{2}$, 5" diam.)	60
Cherries (10 sweet)	50
Cranberry sauce, unsweetened (1 tbsp.)	25
Fruit cocktail, canned (1 cup)	170
Grapefruit, fresh ($\frac{1}{2}$)	60
Grapefruit juice, raw (1 cup)	95
Grape juice, bottled ($\frac{1}{2}$ cup)	80
Grapes (20–25)	75
Nectarine (1 med.)	88
Olives, green	72
Olives, ripe (10)	105
Orange, fresh (med.)	60
Orange juice, frozen diluted (1 cup)	110
Peach, fresh (med.)	46
Peach, canned in syrup (2 halves)	79
Pear, fresh (med.)	95
Pears, canned in syrup (2 halves)	79
Pineapple, crushed in syrup (1 cup)	204
Pineapple ($\frac{1}{2}$ cup fresh)	50
Prune juice (1 cup)	170
Raisins, dry (1 tbsp.)	26
Strawberries, fresh (1 cup)	54
Strawberries, frozen (3 oz.)	90
Tangerine ($2\frac{1}{2}$" diam.)	40
Watermelon, wedge (4" × 8")	120

Meat, Fish, Eggs

Bacon, drained (2 slices)	97
Bacon, Canadian (1 oz.)	62
Beef, hamburger chuck (3 oz.)	316
Beef pot pie	560
Beef steak, sirloin or T-bone (3 oz.)	257
Beef and vegetable stew (1 cup)	185
Chicken, fried breast (8 oz.)	210
Chicken, fried (1 leg and thigh)	305
Chicken, roasted breast (2 slices)	100
Chili, with meat (1 cup)	510
Chili, with beans (1 cup)	335
Egg, boiled	77
Egg, fried	125
Egg, scrambled	100
Fish and chips (2 pcs. fish; 4 oz. chips)	275
Fish, broiled (3" × 3" × $\frac{1}{2}$")	112
Fish stick	40
Frankfurter, boiled	124
Ham (4" × 4")	338
Lamb (3 oz. roast, lean)	158
Liver (3" × 3")	150
Luncheon meat (2 oz.)	135
Pork chop, loin (3" × 5")	284
Salmon, canned (1 cup)	145
Sausage, pork (4 oz.)	510

Shrimp, canned (3 oz.)	108
Tuna, canned (¹/₂ cup)	185
Veal, cutlet (3" × 4")	175

Nuts and Seeds

Cashews (1 cup)	770
Coconut (1 cup)	450
Peanut butter (1 tbsp.)	92
Peanuts, roasted, no skin (1 cup)	805
Pecans (1 cup)	752
Sunflower seeds (1 tbsp.)	50

Sandwiches (2 Slices of White Bread)

Bologna	214
Cheeseburger (small McDonald's)	300
Chicken salad	185
Egg salad	240
Fish fillet (McDonald's)	400
Ham	360
Ham and cheese	360
Hamburger (small McDonald's)	260
Hamburger, Burger King Whopper	600
Hamburger, Big Mac	550
Hamburger (McDonald's Quarter Pounder)	420
Peanut butter	250
Roast beef (Arby's Regular)	425

Sauces, Fats, Oils

Catsup, tomato (1 tbsp.)	17
Chili sauce (1 tbsp.)	17
French dressing (1 tbsp.)	59
Margarine (1 pat)	50
Mayonnaise (1 tbsp.)	92
Mayonnaise-type (1 tbsp.)	65
Vegetable, sunflower, safflower oils (1 tbsp.)	120

Soup, Ready-to-Serve (1 Cup)

Bean	190
Beef noodle	100
Cream	200
Tomato	90
Vegetable	80

Vegetables

Alfalfa sprouts (¹/₂ cup)	19
Asparagus (6 spears)	22
Bean sprouts (1 cup)	37
Beans, green (1 cup)	27
Beans, lima (1 cup)	152
Beans, navy (1 cup)	642
Beans, pork and molasses (1 cup)	325
Broccoli, fresh, cooked (1 cup)	60
Cabbage, cooked (1 cup)	40

Cauliflower (1 cup)	25
Carrot, raw (med.)	21
Carrots, canned (1 cup)	44
Celery, diced raw (1 cup)	20
Coleslaw (1 cup)	102
Corn, sweet, canned (1 cup)	140
Corn, sweet (med. ear)	84
Cucumber, raw (6 slices)	6
Lettuce (2 large leaves)	7
Mushrooms, canned (1 cup)	28
Onion, raw (med.)	25
Onions, French fried (10 rings)	75
Peas, field (¹/₂ cup)	90
Peas, green (1 cup)	145
Pickles, dill (med.)	15
Pickles, sweet (med.)	22
Potato, baked (med.)	97
Potato, French fried (8 sticks)	155
Potato, mashed (1 cup)	185
Radish, raw (small)	1
Sauerkraut, drained (1 cup)	32
Spinach, fresh, cooked (1 cup)	46
Squash, summer (1 cup)	30
Sweet pepper (med.)	15
Sweet potato, candied (small)	314
Tomato, cooked (1 cup)	50
Tomato, raw (med.)	30

Note: The listing of foods above is intended as only a quick reference. The MyPyramid Web site provides a way to obtain detailed reports on the calorie content of your diet. Students are encouraged to consult the MyPyramid Web site at **www.mypyramid.gov**.

Appendix E
Calories of Protein, Carbohydrates, and Fats in Foods

Food No./Food Choice	Total Calories	Protein Calories	Carbohydrate Calories	Fat Calories	Food No./Food Choice	Total Calories	Protein Calories	Carbohydrate Calories	Fat Calories
Breakfast					*Lunch*				
1. Scrambled egg (1 lg.)	111	29	7	75	1. Hamburger (reg. FF[1])	255	48	120	89
2. Fried egg (1 lg.)	99	26	1	72	2. Cheeseburger (reg. FF)	307	61	120	126
3. Pancake (1-6)	146	19	67	58	3. Doubleburger (FF)	563	101	163	299
4. Syrup (1 T[4])	60	0	60	0	4. 1/4 lb. burger (FF)	427	73	137	217
5. French toast (1 slice)	180	23	49	108	5. Doublecheese burger (FF)	670	174	134	362
6. Waffle (7-inch)	245	28	100	117	6. Doublecheese baconburger (FF)	724	138	174	340
7. Biscuit (medium)	104	8	52	44	7. Hot dog (FF)	214	36	54	124
8. Bran muffin (medium)	104	11	63	31	8. Chili dog (FF)	320	51	90	179
9. White toast (slice)	68	9	52	7	9. Pizza, cheese (slice FF)	290	116	116	58
10. Wheat toast (slice)	67	14	52	6	10. Pizza, meat (slice FF)	360	126	126	108
11. Peanut butter (1 T)	94	15	11	68	11. Pizza, everything (slice FF)	510	179	173	158
12. Yogurt (8 oz. plain)	227	39	161	27	12. Sandwich, roast beef (FF)	350	88	126	137
13. Orange juice (8 oz.)	114	8	100	6	13. Sandwich, bologna	313	44	106	163
14. Apple juice (8 oz.)	117	1	116	0	14. Sandwich, bologna-cheese	428	69	158	201
15. Soft drink (12 oz.)	144	0	144	0	15. Sandwich, ham-cheese (FF)	380	91	133	156
16. Bacon (2 slices)	86	15	2	70	16. Sandwich, peanut butter	281	39	118	124
17. Sausage (1 link)	141	11	0	130	17. Sandwich, PB and jelly	330	40	168	122
18. Sausage (1 patty)	284	23	0	261	18. Sandwich, egg salad	330	40	109	181
19. Grits (8 oz.)	125	11	110	4	19. Sandwich, tuna salad	390	101	109	180
20. Hash browns (8 oz.)	355	18	178	159	20. Sandwich, fish (FF)	432	56	147	229
21. French fries (reg.)	239	12	115	112	21. French fries (reg. FF)	239	12	115	112
22. Donut, cake	125	4	61	60	22. French fries (lg. FF)	406	20	195	191
23. Donut, glazed	164	8	87	69	23. Onion rings (reg. FF)	274	14	112	148
24. Sweet roll	317	22	136	159	24. Chili (8 oz.)	260	49	62	148
25. Cake (medium slice)	274	14	175	85	25. Bean soup (8 oz.)	355	67	181	107
26. Ice cream (8 oz.)	257	15	108	134	26. Beef noodle soup (8 oz.)	140	32	59	49
27. Cream cheese (T)	52	4	1	47	27. Tomato soup (8 oz.)	180	14	121	45
28. Jelly (T)	49	0	49	0	28. Vegetable soup (8 oz.)	160	21	107	32
29. Jam (T)	54	0	54	0	29. Small salad, plain	37	6	27	4
30. Coffee (cup)	0	0	0	0	30. Small salad, French dressing	152	8	50	94
31. Tea (cup)	0	0	0	0	31. Small salad, Italian dressing	162	8	28	126
32. Cream (T)	32	2	2	28	32. Small salad, bleu cheese	184	13	28	143
33. Sugar (t)	15	0	15	0	33. Potato salad (8 oz.)	248	27	159	62
34. Corn flakes (8 oz.)	97	8	87	2	34. Cole slaw (8 oz.)	180	0	25	155
35. Wheat flakes (8 oz.)	106	12	90	4	35. Macaroni and cheese (8 oz.)	230	37	103	90
36. Oatmeal (8 oz.)	132	19	92	21	36. Beef taco (FF)	186	59	56	71
37. Strawberries (8 oz.)	55	4	46	5	37. Bean burrito (FF)	343	45	192	106
38. Orange (medium)	64	6	57	1	38. Meat burrito (FF)	466	158	196	112
39. Apple (medium)	96	1	86	9	39. Mexican rice (FF)	213	17	160	36
40. Banana (medium)	101	4	95	2	40. Mexican beans (FF)	168	42	82	44
41. Cantaloupe (half)	82	7	73	2	41. Fried chicken breast (FF)	436	262	13	161
42. Grapefruit (half)	40	2	37	1	42. Broiled chicken breast	284	224	0	60
43. Custard pie (slice)	285	20	188	77	43. Broiled fish	228	82	32	114
44. Fruit pie (slice)	350	14	259	77	44. Fish stick (1 stick FF)	50	18	8	24
45. Fritter (medium)	132	11	54	67	45. Fried egg	99	26	1	72
46. Skim milk (8 oz.)	88	36	52	0	46. Donut	125	4	61	60
47. Whole milk (8 oz.)	159	33	48	78	47. Potato chips (small bag)	115	3	39	73
48. Butter (pat)	36	0	0	36	48. Soft drink (12 oz.)	144	0	144	0
49. Margarine (pat)	36	0	0	36					

The principal reference for the calculation of values used in this appendix was the *Nutritive Value of Foods*, published by the United States Department of Agriculture, Washington, DC, Home and Gardens Bulletin, No. 72, although other published sources were consulted, including Jacobson, M., and S. Fritschner. *The Fast-Food Guide* (an excellent source of information about fast foods). New York: Workman.

Notes:
1. FF by a food indicates that it is typical of a food served in a fast food restaurant.
2. Your portions of foods may be larger or smaller than those listed here. For this reason, you may wish to select a food more than once (e.g., two hamburgers) or select only a portion of a serving (i.e., divide the calories in half for a half portion).
3. An oz. equals 28.35 grams.
4. T = tablespoon and t = teaspoon.

Food No./Food Choice	Total Calories	Protein Calories	Carbohydrate Calories	Fat Calories	Food No./Food Choice	Total Calories	Protein Calories	Carbohydrate Calories	Fat Calories
49. Apple juice (8 oz.)	117	1	116	0	45. Broiled chicken breast	284	224	0	60
50. Skim milk (8 oz.)	88	36	52	0	46. Broiled fish	228	82	32	114
51. Whole milk (8 oz.)	159	33	48	78	47. Fish stick (1 stick FF)	50	18	8	24
52. Diet drink (12 oz.)	0	0	0	0	48. Soft drink (12 oz.)	144	0	144	0
53. Mustard (t)	4	0	4	0	49. Apple juice (8 oz.)	117	1	116	0
54. Catsup (t)	6	0	6	0	50. Skim milk (8 oz.)	88	36	52	0
55. Mayonnaise (T)	100	0	0	100	51. Whole milk (8 oz.)	159	33	48	78
56. Fruit pie	350	14	259	77	52. Diet drink (12 oz.)	0	0	0	0
57. Cheesecake (slice)	400	56	132	212	53. Mustard (t)	4	0	4	0
58. Ice cream (8 oz.)	257	15	108	134	54. Catsup (t)	6	0	6	0
59. Coffee (8 oz.)	0	0	0	0	55. Mayonnaise (T)	100	0	0	100
60. Tea (8 oz.)	0	0	0	0	56. Fruit pie (slice)	350	14	259	77
					57. Cheesecake (slice)	400	56	132	212
Dinner					58. Ice cream (8 oz.)	257	15	108	134
1. Hamburger (reg. FF)	255	48	120	89	59. Custard pie (slice)	285	20	188	77
2. Cheeseburger (reg. FF)	307	61	120	126	60. Cake (slice)	274	14	175	85
3. Doubleburger (FF)	563	101	163	299					
4. 1/4 lb. burger (FF)	427	73	137	217	*Snacks*				
5. Doublecheese burger (FF)	670	174	134	362	1. Peanut butter (1 T)	94	15	11	68
6. Doublecheese baconburger (FF)	724	138	174	412	2. Yogurt (8 oz. plain)	227	39	161	27
7. Hot dog (FF)	214	36	54	124	3. Orange juice (8 oz.)	114	8	100	6
8. Chili dog (FF)	320	51	90	179	4. Apple juice (8 oz.)	117	1	116	0
9. Pizza, cheese (slice FF)	290	116	116	58	5. Soft drink (12 oz.)	144	0	144	0
10. Pizza, meat (slice FF)	360	126	126	108	6. Donut, cake	125	4	61	60
11. Pizza, everything (slice FF)	510	179	173	158	7. Donut, glazed	164	8	87	69
12. Steak (8 oz.)	880	290	0	590	8. Sweet roll	317	22	136	159
13. French fried shrimp (6 oz.)	360	133	68	158	9. Cake (medium slice)	274	14	175	85
14. Roast beef (8 oz.)	440	268	0	172	10. Ice cream (8 oz.)	257	15	108	134
15. Liver (8 oz.)	520	250	52	218	11. Softserve cone (reg.)	240	10	89	134
16. Corned beef (8 oz.)	493	242	0	251	12. Ice cream sandwich bar	210	40	82	88
17. Meat loaf (8 oz.)	711	228	35	448	13. Strawberries (8 oz.)	55	4	46	5
18. Ham (8 oz.)	540	178	0	362	14. Orange (medium)	64	6	57	1
19. Spaghetti, no meat (13 oz.)	400	56	220	124	15. Apple (medium)	96	1	86	9
20. Spaghetti, meat (13 oz.)	500	115	230	155	16. Banana (medium)	101	4	95	2
21. Baked potato (medium)	90	12	78	0	17. Cantaloupe (half)	82	7	73	2
22. Cooked carrots (8 oz.)	71	12	59	0	18. Grapefruit (half)	40	2	37	1
23. Cooked spinach (8 oz.)	50	18	18	14	19. Celery stick	5	2	3	0
24. Corn (1 ear)	70	10	52	8	20. Carrot (medium)	20	3	17	0
25. Cooked green beans (8 oz.)	54	11	43	0	21. Raisins (4 oz.)	210	6	204	0
26. Cooked broccoli (8 oz.)	60	19	26	15	22. Watermelon (4" × 6" slice)	115	8	99	8
27. Cooked cabbage	47	12	35	0	23. Chocolate chip cookie	60	3	9	48
28. French fries (reg. FF)	239	12	115	112	24. Brownie	145	6	26	113
29. French fries (lg. FF)	406	20	195	191	25. Oatmeal cookie	65	3	13	49
30. Onion rings (reg. FF)	274	14	112	148	26. Sandwich cookie	200	8	112	80
31. Chili (8 oz.)	260	49	62	148	27. Custard pie (slice)	285	20	188	77
32. Small salad, plain	37	6	27	4	28. Fruit pie (slice)	350	14	259	77
33. Small salad, French dressing	152	8	50	94	29. Gelatin (4 oz.)	70	4	32	34
34. Small salad, Italian dressing	162	8	28	126	30. Fritter (medium)	132	11	54	67
35. Small salad, bleu cheese	184	13	28	143	31. Skim milk (8 oz.)	88	36	52	0
36. Potato salad (8 oz.)	248	27	159	62	32. Diet drink	0	0	0	0
37. Cole slaw (8 oz.)	180	0	25	155	33. Potato chips (small bag)	115	3	39	73
38. Macaroni and cheese (8 oz.)	230	37	103	90	34. Roasted peanuts (1.3 oz.)	210	34	25	151
39. Beef Taco (FF)	186	59	56	71	35. Chocolate candy bar (1 oz.)	145	7	61	77
40. Bean burrito (FF)	343	45	192	106	36. Choc. almond candy bar (1 oz.)	265	38	74	164
41. Meat burrito (FF)	466	158	196	112	37. Saltine cracker	18	1	1	16
42. Mexican rice (FF)	213	17	160	36	38. Popped corn	40	7	33	0
43. Mexican beans (FF)	168	42	82	44	39. Cheese nachos	471	63	194	214
44. Fried chicken breast (FF)	436	262	13	161					

Selected References

Web Resources and Suggested Readings are available at the end of each concept. In addition a "quick guide" to References, Web Resources, Health, Wellness and Fitness Newsletters and Journals, and Reports and Documents that contributed to the updates and changes of this edition is included below. Additional resources including Web Resources, Suggested Readings, and References used in developing the content for this book are available online at **www. mhhe.com/corbin9e**

ACSM/AHA *Guidelines for Adults*, 2007.

ACSM/AHA *Guidelines for Older Adults*, 2007.

ACSM. 2010. *Guidelines for Exercise Testing and Prescription*. 8th ed.

ACSM. 2010. *ACSM's Guidelines for Exercise Testing and Prescription*. 8th ed. Philadelphia: Lippencott, Williams & Wilkins.

ACSM. 2010. *ACSM's Resource Manual for Guidelines for Exercise Testing and Prescription*. 6th ed. Philadelphia: Lippencott, Williams & Wilkins.

Blair, S. N. 2009. Physical inactivity: The biggest public health problem of the 21st century. *British Journal of Sports Medicine* 43(1):1–2.

Cohen, D. A., et al. 2010. Not enough fruit and vegetables or too many cookies, candies, salty snacks, and soft drinks? *Public Health Reports* 125(1):88–95.

Flegal, K. M. 2010. Prevalence and trends in obesity among U.S. adults. *Journal of the American Medical Association* 303(3):235–241.

Fradkin, A., et al. 2009. Warm-up and physical performance: What is the relationship? A systematic review with meta analysis (abstract). *Medicine and Science in Sports and Exercise* 41(5 Supplement):151–152.

Haskell, W. L., et al. 2007. Physical activity and public health: Updated recommendations for adults from the ACSM and AHA. *Medicine and Science in Sports and Exercise* 39(8):1424–1434.

Lee, C. M. 2010. The social norms of alcohol-related negative consequences. *Psychology of Addictive Behaviors* 24(2): 342–348.

Lund, H. G., et al. 2010. Sleep patterns and predictors of disturbed sleep in a large population of college students. *Journal of Adolescence Health* 46:124–132.

Nelson, M. E., et al. 2007. Physical activity and public health in older adults: Recommendations from ACSM and AHA. *Medicine and Science in Sports and Exercise*. 39(8):1424–1434.

Owen, N., et al. 2010. Too much sitting: The population health science of sedentary behavior. *Exercise and Sport Sciences Reviews* 38(3): 105–113.

Pleis, J. R. and B. W. Ward. 2009. Summary health statistics for U.S. adults: National Health Interview survey. *Vital Health Statistics* 10(242): 74–75.

Rahman, S., et al. 2010. The association between obesity and low back pain: A meta-analysis. *American Journal of Epidemiology* 171(2):135–154.

Sebastiani, P., et al. 2010. Genetic signatures of exceptional longevity in humans. Science. Published online July 1, 2010, www.sciencemag.org

Sullivan, G. S. and J. P. Strode. 2010. Motivation through goal setting: A self-determined perspective. *Strategies* 23(6):19–23.

Wardlaw, G. M. 2011. *Contemporary Nutrition*. New York: McGraw-Hill Higher Education.

Web Resources

American Cancer Society   www.cancer.org

American College of Sports Medicine   www.acsm.org

American Diabetes Association   www.diabetes.org

American Heart Association   www.americanheart.org

American Medical Association   www.ama-assn.org

Centers for Disease Control and Prevention (CDC)   www.cdc.gov

FDA Food Website   www.fda.gov/Food/default.htm

Food and Drug Administration (FDA)   www.fda.gov

Health Canada   www.healthcanada.ca

Healthy People 2020   www.healthypeople.gov

Let's Move   www.letsmove.gov

National Strength and Conditioning Association   www.nsca-cc.org

President's Council on Physical Fitness, Sports and Nutrition   www.fitness.gov

Surgeon General   www.surgeongeneral.gov

World Health Organization   www.who.int

Health, Wellness, and Fitness Newsletters and Journals

ACSM's Fit Society Page   www.acsm.org/health+fitness/fit_society.ht

ACSM's Health and Fitness Journal   www.acsm.org/publications/health _fitness_journal.htm

Mayo Clinic Housecall (newsletter)   www.mayoclinic.com/health/housecall /housecall

Med Watch   www.fda.gov/medwatch

Morbidity and Mortality Weekly Reports   www.cdc.gov/mmwr

Quackwatch   www.quackwatch.org

WebMD   www.webmd.com

Reports and Documents

Centers for Disease Control and Prevention. 2009. *Healthy People 2020 Public Meetings: 2009 Draft Objectives*. Atlanta: CDC. www.healthypeople.gov/hp2020/objectives

Dietary Guidelines for Americans–2010 www.cnpp.usda.gov/dietaryguidelines.htm

International Food Information Council Foundation. 2010. 2010 Food and Health Survey. Available at www.foodinsight.org

Kovacs, M. 2009. *Dynamic Stretching: The Revolutionary New Warm-up Method to Improve Power, Performance and Range of Motion*. Berkeley, CA: Ulysses Press.

Morbidity and Mortality Weekly Reports www.cdc.gov/mmwr

National Institute of Mental Health. Accessed May 2010. *Depression*. www.nimh.nih.gov /health

National Physical Activity Plan www.physicalactivityplan.org

Surgeon General's Vision for a Healthy and Fit Nation 2010 (fact sheet) www.surgeongeneral.gov

Trust for America's Health. 2008. *Blueprint for a Healthier America*. Washington, DC: Trust for America's Health. http:// healthyamericans.org/report/55/ blueprint-for-healthier-america

United States Department of Health and Human Services, 2008. *2008 Physical Activity Guidelines for Americans*. Washington: USDHHS. www.health.gov/paguidelines.

World Health Organization. 2009. *Global Health Risks*. Geneva: WHO. www.who.int/publications/en

Selected References

Photo Credits

Index

Page numbers followed by *f* indicate figures, and page numbers followed by *t* indicate tables.

A

AA (Alcoholics Anonymous), 419
ABCD rule for self-exams, 460, 460*f*
ABC system for time management, 378, 379*t*
Abdominal hollowing, 248
Abdominal stretch, 240
Absolute endurance, 161
Absolute strength, 161
Abstinence-only education, 448
Accelerometers, 109
Acclimatization, 50–51
Acquired aging, 77
Acquired immune deficiency syndrome (AIDS), 440, 441. *See also* HIV/AIDS
ACSM. *See* American College of Sports Medicine
ACTH (adrenocorticotropic hormone), 366
Active assistance, 204
ActiveLifeMovement, 296
Active Living by Design, 110
Active workstations, 92
Activities of daily living, 102–103
Activity plans, 33
Adaptation, 362, 363
Adderall, 434
Addiction, 430, 431, 437
Adequate Intake (AI), 324*t*, 325
ADH (alcohol dehydrogenase), 411
Adherence, 22, 23
Adolescents
    alcohol use by, 415
    secondhand smoke and, 400
    sex education and, 448
    sexually explicit media and, 446
    smoking by, 401–402, 403*t*, 404
Adrenocorticotropic hormone (ACTH), 366
Aerobic capacity, 118, 267
Aerobic fitness. *See* Cardiovascular fitness
Aerobic physical activities. *See also* Physical activity
    definition of, 103
    environment and, 110–111, 115–116
    examples of, 109*f*, 110
    gaining muscle mass and, 354
    intermittent, 147–148
    moderate and vigorous, 91, 102–103, 103*t*, 141
    monitoring, 106–107, 109
    setting goals for, 111, 113–114
    tracking energy expenditure in, 107
    wearing weights during, 478
African Americans, 456, 458, 459, 463–464

Age. *See also* Older adults
    creeping obesity and, 297
    decrease in vigorous activity with, 142–143
    of drinking onset, 415
    flexibility and, 202
    muscle fitness performance and, 162
    physical activity and, 77–78, 94, 94*t*
    range of motion and, 204
    stress and, 367
    wellness and, 10
Agility, 8*f*, 279
Agonist muscles, 162, 163, 163*f*, 206, 207
AI (Adequate Intake), 324*t*, 325
AIDS (acquired immune deficiency syndrome), 440, 441. *See also* HIV/AIDS
Air pollution, exercise and, 53–54
Al-Anon, 435
Alcohol dehydrogenase (ADH), 411
Alcohol dependence, 412, 413
Alcoholic cirrhosis, 412, 413
Alcoholics Anonymous (AA), 419, 435
Alcohol use, 409–424
    alcohol abuse, 412, 413
    alcoholic beverages, 410–411, 410*f*
    alcoholism, 419
    benefits of, 411, 413
    blood alcohol concentration, 411, 413–414, 414*t*, 415*t*, 421–422
    classification of, 411–412, 411*t*
    by college students, 416–418, 416*f*, 417*t*
    detection of, 414
    driving and, 413–415, 414*t*, 415*t*
    health consequences of, 334–335, 412–413, 413*t*
    legal drinking age, 416
    in the military, 418
    perceptions about, 423–424
    physical effects of, 410–411
    risks of, 411, 412*f*
    strategies for controlling one's, 418–419
    tobacco use and, 404
    by women, 410, 412–413, 417
Alzheimer's disease, 78
Amenorrhea, 288, 289
American Cancer Society (ACS), 73–74
American College of Sports Medicine (ACSM)
    on cool-downs, 50
    "Exercise Is Medicine" program, 80
    on exercise testing and prescription, 66
    on flexibility exercise, 200, 207–208
    on pre-participation screening, 46–47, 47*t*
    on stretching, 49
    on warm-ups, 48–49

American Fitness Index, 496
American Heart Association (AHA), 327
Amino acids, 330
Anabolic steroids, 171–173, 172f
Anaerobic capacity, 265, 266
Anaerobic physical activities, 103–104
Androstenediol, 171
Androstenedione (andro), 171–172
Anemia, 119
Angina pectoris, 67
Ankle sprains, 274
Ankle weights, 478
Anorexia athletica, 294
Anorexia nervosa, 294
Antagonist muscles, 162, 163, 163f, 204
Antibodies, 441
Antioxidants, 332–333
Antiretroviral treatment (ART), 443
Anxiety, 76, 367, 376
APC gene test, 458
Appetite suppressants, 353–354
Appraisal-focused coping, 380–381, 381t, 382, 382t
Arm circles, 241
Arm lift, 253
Arm pretzel, 216
ART (antiretroviral treatment), 443
Arteries, 118, 119f, 120f
Arteriosclerosis, 67
Arthritis, 77
Artificial sweeteners, 353
Aspirin, in diabetes, 464
Assertiveness, 386
Asthma, 77
Astrand-Ryhming bicycle test, 132–133, 132f, 133f
Atherosclerosis, 67, 68–70, 68f, 69t
Avoidant coping, 380–381, 381t

B

BAC. See Blood alcohol concentration
Back. See also Back pain; Posture
    core musculature anatomy, 225, 226f
    ergonomics and, 233, 233f, 234t, 235f
    exercise guidelines for, 233–237, 235f, 237t
    healthy back and neck questionnaire, 257–258
    healthy back tests, 255–256
    planning and logging exercises for, 261–262
    posture and, 230–233, 231f, 232f, 232t, 233f
    questionable exercises and alternatives, 235, 240–246
    spine anatomy and function, 224–225, 224f
Back extension, 240
Back pain
    body mechanics and, 233, 233f
    causes and consequences of, 226–229, 228f
    core musculature and, 228
    flexibility and, 203
    medical intervention for, 229
    muscle fitness and, 162
    physical activity and, 75–76
    prevention and rehabilitation, 229–230
    strategies for action, 238
Backsaver toe touch, 100
Back scratcher, 216
Balance
    activities for, 100
    balance training, 166, 254
    definition of, 8f
    evaluating, 279, 280t
    functional training for, 271–272

Ballistic stretching, 204, 205f, 206, 208t
Bar stretch, 244
Basal cell cancers, 460–461
Basal metabolic rate (BMR), 296–297
Bass test of dynamic balance, 279
BDNG (Brain-Derived Neurotrophic Factor) gene, 377
Behavioral goals, 30–31, 32, 349
Bench press, 178
Benign tumors, 73, 454, 455
Benjamin, Regina, 66
Beta-carotene, 332, 332t
BIA (bioelectric impedance analysis), 291
Biceps curl, 178, 180
Bicycle test, 130, 132–133, 133f, 134f
Bicycling, 145
Binge drinking, 412
Bioelectric impedance analysis (BIA), 291
Biofeedback, 384
Biopsy, 454, 455
Blood
    circulation of, 118–119, 119f, 120f
    cool-downs and flow of, 49f, 50
    inflammation markers in, 70
Blood alcohol concentration (BAC)
    calculating, 421–422
    driving limits, 411, 413–414, 414t
    number of drinks and, 415t
Blood pressure, 72, 72t. See also Hypertension
Blueprint for a Healthier America, 2
BMI. See Body Mass Index
BMR (basal metabolic rate), 296–297
Bod Pod, 290–291, 290f
Body composition, 287–320. See also Obesity;
        Weight management
    assessment methods, 290–291, 290f, 303–314
    body fat location, 290, 291f, 293–294, 293f
    definition of, 6f
    energy expenditure determination, 317–320
    evaluating, 315–316
    evaluating products to change, 479–480
    gaining muscle mass, 354
    health risks from overfatness, 292–294, 292f, 293f
    losing body fat, 349–353, 349t, 352t
    maintaining, 92
    origin of fatness, 295–297, 297f
    physical activity and, 297–300, 298t, 299t
    standards for, 288–289, 289t, 304t
    strategies for action in, 300–301
    surgical sculpting, 479–480
    underweight, 293, 294–295
Body fat, 288, 291f. See also Body composition
Body Mass Index (BMI)
    calculation of, 309, 309t
    evaluating, 315–316
    health-related standards for, 289, 289t
    height-weight measurements, 308, 315
Body mechanics professionals, 235
Bodymedia FIT system, 351
Body wrapping, 477
Bone density, physical activity and, 74–75
Bone integrity, 9
"Boosts" in energy drinks, 480
Brain-Derived Neurotrophic Factor (BDNG) gene, 377
Breakfast, 335
Breast cancer, 74t, 455, 457t, 458, 469
Breast self-exams, 471–472
Built environment, 110
Bulimia, 294

C

Caffeine, 334, 433
Calcitonin, 75
Calcium, 75, 334
Calf stretches, 62, 214
Calisthenics, 167, 182–183, 197–198
Caloric balance, 298
Calories
    as energy intake, 296, 297, 297f
    expended in various activities, 299t
    in lifestyle physical activities, 108t
    public understanding of, 348
    weight control and, 347–348
Calorie sparing, 351
Calorie Tracker, 335
Cancer, 454–462
    breast, 74t, 455, 457t, 458
    cervical, 440, 445, 457t, 459–460, 469
    colon-rectal, 74t, 457t, 458
    determining risk for, 469–470
    lung, 458–459
    metastasis of, 454f, 455
    nutrition and, 322, 328
    ovarian, 459–460
    physical activity and, 73–74, 74t
    prevention of, 461, 461t, 462t
    prostate, 74t, 457t, 459
    screening guidelines for, 457t
    skin, 457t, 460–461, 460f
    statistics on, 455f
    testicular, 457t, 461–462
    tobacco use and, 399f, 401, 401t
    treatment of, 461–462
    uterine, 457t, 459–460
Cannon, Walter, 365
Capillaries, 119
Carbohydrate loading, 337
Carbohydrates, 327–329, 337, 350, 353
Carbon monoxide, 53
Carcinogens, 398, 399
Cardiovascular disease (CVD)
    alcohol use and, 412–413
    assessing risk factors for, 83–84
    atherosclerosis and, 67, 68–70, 68f, 69t
    as cause of death, 13t, 14t, 73
    heart attacks and, 67, 70–71, 70f, 71f
    marijuana and, 432
    nutrition and, 328
    physical activity and, 67–68
    Type A behavior pattern and, 369
Cardiovascular fitness, 117–138
    activities for, 100
    assessment of, 129–130, 131–138
    blood circulation and, 120f
    cardiovascular system in, 118–121, 119f, 120f, 121t
    definition of, 6f, 118
    FIT formulas for, 122–124, 123f, 124t
    health benefits and, 121–122, 122f
    heart rate and exercise monitoring, 127–129, 127f, 128f, 129f, 130
    heredity and, 126
    maximum oxygen uptake and, 121
    moderate physical activity and, 105
    muscular endurance and, 162
    obesity and, 122
    strength training and, 269
    threshold and target zones for, 124–127, 125t, 126f, 127t
    vigorous activities and, 141–142
Cardiovascular system, 118–121, 119f, 120f, 121t

CAUTION early warning signs, 462
CD4+ helper cells, 441
Cell phones, health apps for, 32
Cellulite, 479
Cervical cancer, 440, 445, 457t, 459–460, 469
Chancre sores, 446, 447
Chancroid, 447, 447t
Chantix, 405
CHD (coronary heart disease), 67–68, 71, 412–413
Chest press, 180, 186
Chewing tobacco, 398
Children
    food commercials targeting, 348
    injuries in youth athletes, 148
    moderate activities for, 106
    obesity in, 296
    physical activity pyramid and, 93
    programs to increase activity in, 348
    secondhand smoke and, 400–401
    stress in, 363–364
Chin tuck, 212, 250
Chlamydia, 444, 444t, 445
Chlamydia pneumonia heat shock protein (Cp-HSP60), 70
Cholesterol, 69, 69t, 330
Cigarettes. See Tobacco use
Circuit resistance training (CRT), 169
Clinical exercise test, 46–47, 46f
Clothing, for exercise, 47, 47t, 52, 53, 275
Club drugs, 432, 433
Cocaine, 426–427, 427t, 431, 432–433
Cognitive re-appraisal, 382, 382t
Cold weather exercise, 52–53, 52t
College students
    alcohol use by, 416–418, 416f, 417t
    creeping obesity in, 297, 301
    drug use by, 431f
    employment rates of, 378f
    with preexisting health concerns, 467
    sexually transmitted infections in, 448
    smoking by, 404
    stress in, 363t, 364, 365f
Colonoscopy, 458
Colon-rectal cancer, 74t, 457t, 458, 469
Community resource audits, 115–116
Complete proteins, 330
Complex carbohydrates, 327, 353
Compression of illness, 78
Concentric contractions, 164–165
Conduction, 50
Congestive heart failure, 67
Connective tissue, 201
Conscientiousness, 370
Continuous aerobic activities, 147–148
Continuous passive motion (CPM) tables, 476
Contract-relax-antagonist-contract (CRAC) technique, 205f, 206, 208t
Contraindicated movements, 233–234, 236f, 237t
Control, stress and, 363, 369
Convection, 50
Cool-downs, 50, 51, 61–62
Cooper, Ken, 141
Coordination, 8f, 100, 280
Coping strategies, 380–381
Core musculature anatomy, 225, 226f
Core stability, 225, 229–230
Core stabilization exercises, 248
Core strength, 163, 184–185, 197–198, 229–230
Core training, 165, 230
Coronary collateral circulation, 70–71, 71f
Coronary heart disease (CHD), 67–68, 71, 412–413

Coronary occlusion, 67, 70–71, 70*f*
Corticotropin-releasing hormone (CRH), 366
Cortisol, 367
Cotinine, 400
Cp-HSP60 (chlamydia pneumonia heat shock protein), 70
CPR training, 57, 497*t*
Crack cocaine, 433
CRAC (contract-relax-antagonist-contract) technique, 205*f*, 206, 208*t*
Cravings *vs.* hunger, 353
C-reactive protein (CRP), 70
Creatine, 173, 276
CRH (corticotropin-releasing hormone), 366
Cross-country skiing, 145–146
Cross training, 151–152
CRP (C-reactive protein), 70
Crunches (curl-ups), 182, 184, 243, 249
Crystal methamphetamine, 427–428, 427*t*, 432–433
CVD. *See* Cardiovascular disease

D

Dance aerobics, 146
Date rape drugs, 429, 429*t*, 433
Death
    actual causes of, 14, 14*t*
    alcohol use and, 412*f*
    from cancer, 455, 455*f*
    diabetes and, 463
    from injuries, 464
    major causes of, 12–13, 13*t*
    obesity and, 292–293
    from psychoactive drug use, 426, 429, 429*f*
    tobacco use as cause of, 398–399
Deep breathing, 383–384
Deep buttock stretch, 215
Definition, muscle, 160, 268, 269
Degenerated disc, 228, 228*f*
Dehydration, 50, 51
Dehydroepiandrosterone (DHEA), 171, 385
Delayed-onset muscle soreness (DOMS), 54, 55
Dementia, 78
Department of Health and Human Services (DHHS), 322
Depressant drugs, 426, 426*t*. *See also* Alcohol use
Depression
    in college students, 364
    physical activity and, 76, 376, 377
    suicide and, 466
    treatment of, 466
Designer drugs, 429, 429*t*
DHEA (dehydroepiandrosterone), 171, 385
Diabetes mellitus, 74, 462–464, 463*t*
Diaphragmatic breathing, 394
Diastolic blood pressure, 71
Diet, weight loss and, 297–298, 480. *See also* Weight management
Dietary plans, 33
Dietary Reference Intake (DRI), 324*t*, 325, 325*f*
Diet logs, 339, 341–342
Dips, 182
Disabilities, 10–11, 94, 94*t*
Disordered eating, 294–295
Distorted thinking, 382*t*
Distress, 368, 369
DOMS (delayed-onset muscle soreness), 54, 55
Dose-response relationship, 86–87, 87*f*
Double-heel click, 100
Double-leg lift, 241
Double progressive system, 170
DRI (Dietary Reference Intake), 324*t*, 325, 325*f*
Drinking games, 416–417

Driving, alcohol use and, 413–415, 414*t*, 415*t*
Drug abuse, definition of, 426, 427
Drugs, definition of, 398, 399, 410, 411
Drug use, 425–438. *See also* Psychoactive drugs
    consequences of, 429–430, 429*f*, 433
    drug classification, 426–429, 426*t*, 427*t*, 428*t*, 429*t*
    evaluating drug abuse potential, 437–438
    new drugs, 431–432
    over-the-counter drugs, 433–434
    strategies for action, 435
    trends in, 431*f*, 432
    use and abuse of, 430–434, 431*f*, 432*f*, 435
Dual-energy absorptiometry (DXA/DEXA), 290
Dual X-ray absorptiometry (DXA), 74
Dumbbell rowing, 179
Dynamic muscular endurance, 165
Dynamic strength, 165
Dynamic stretching, 204

E

Eating disorders, 294–295
Eccentric contractions, 164
Echinacea, 482
e-cigarettes, 403
Ecstasy (MDMA), 432, 433
EGO rule, 497*t*
EIM ("Exercise Is Medicine") program, 80
EKG, 47
Electrical muscle stimulators, 476
Emergency medical care, 464–465, 465*f*
Emotional storm, 71
Emotion-focused coping, 380–381, 381*t*, 382–385
Emotions
    coping strategies and, 380–381, 381*t*, 382–385
    expressing *vs.* repressing, 385
    in lifestyle changes, 497–498
Employee health promotion programs, 80, 88, 103
Empty calories, 351
Enabling factors, 24, 25–26, 25*f*, 27*t*
Endometrial cancer, 459
Endurance, muscular
    absolute, 161
    cardiovascular fitness and, 162
    dynamic, 165
    muscle fiber types and, 161
    relative, 162
    static, 165
    training for, 266–269, 268*t*
Energy balance, 298, 346
Energy bars, 276
Energy drinks, 276, 277, 480
Energy expenditure, 107, 108*t*, 317–320
Environmental factors
    in alcohol use, 415–416
    improving one's, 495–496, 495*t*
    in obesity, 346
    in wellness, 11
Ephedra, 353, 482
Epigenetics, 431
Epsom salts, 477
Ergogenic aids, 275–276
Ergonomics, 233, 234*t*, 235*f*
Error, consistent *vs.* variable, 30
Essential amino acids, 330
Essential fat, 288, 289
Ethnic groups
    cancer in, 456, 458, 459, 460
    health disparities and, 3

HIV/AIDS in, 441
  physical activity in, 94
Ethyl glucoronide (EtG), 414
Eustress, 368, 369
Evaporation, 50
Exercise, 13. *See also* Physical activity
Exercise balls, 166f
Exercise equipment, 147, 477–478
"Exercise Is Medicine (EIM)" program, 80
Exercise tests, pre-participation, 46–47, 46f
Experts, quacks *vs.*, 474–475
Extreme diets, 350–351
Extreme sports, 151

F

Facebook, 353
Fad diets, 350–351
Family history, 493
Family Smoking Prevention and Tobacco Control Act, 403
Fartlek training, 267
FAS (fetal alcohol syndrome), 413
Fast foods, 335, 359–360
Fats, dietary, 329–330, 335–336, 349
Fat substitutes, 330, 353
Fat tax, 348
Fat Translator, 335
Fatty liver, 412, 413
FDA. *See* Food and Drug Administration
Feedback, 272
Female athlete triad, 294–295
Fetal alcohol syndrome (FAS), 413
Fiber, dietary, 327–328, 329
Fibrin, 69
Fibromyalgia, 77
FICSIT study, 209
Fight-or-flight response, 365
First aid, 497t
Fitness. *See* Physical fitness
Fitness clubs, 479, 489–490
Fitnessgram method, 303, 313
Fitness zones, 95, 95t
FITT, FIT formulas, 88–89, 89f
Flat back posture, 231
Flexibility, 199–222. *See also* Stretching
  activities for, 100
  basic facts about, 200
  definition of, 6f
  endurance performance and, 268
  evaluating, 219–220
  factors influencing, 200–202, 201f
  flexibility-based activities, 209–210
  health benefits of, 202–203
  performance benefits of, 203–204
  in the physical activity pyramid, 92, 206f
  planning and logging exercises, 221–222
  safety guidelines, 210
  static *vs.* dynamic, 201–202, 202f
  strategies for action in, 211
  stretching methods, 204–206, 205f
  tests of, 217–218, 255
  thresholds and target zones, 206–209, 207f, 208t
  training for, 271–272
  worldwide trends in, 209
Fluid intake, 52, 334–335, 337
Fluid replacement beverages, 276
Folic acid, 333, 481
Food and Drug Administration (FDA)
  on dietary supplements, 480–483, 481t
  on ephedra, 353
  on food labels, 325–326, 326f
  on tobacco control, 403
Food fantasies, 355
Food labels, 325–327, 326f, 348
Forearm stretch, 216
Fortification of foods, 333
Free weights
  advantages of, 166, 166t
  exercise planning for, 195–196
  exercises for, 178–179
  on hands and wrists, 478
Freud, Sigmund, 385
Fruits, 328, 334
Functional foods, 330, 332–333, 332t

G

Gallstones, 77
Gardisil vaccine, 444–445, 459
Gender differences
  in alcohol effects, 410
  in anabolic steroid effects, 172f
  in cancer, 455f
  in flexibility, 202
  in health services use, 24
  in healthy life expectancy, 3, 3f
  in muscle fitness performance, 162
  in physical activity, 93–94, 93t, 94t
General adaptation syndrome, 366, 366t
Genetic influences
  on alcohol use, 415
  on body composition, 31, 295
  on cardiovascular fitness, 126
  on drug addiction, 430, 431
  on flexibility, 202
  on health and fitness, 9, 10f
  on high-level performance, 265
  on muscle fitness performance, 161
  physical activity *vs.*, 67
  taking advantage of heredity, 493
Genetic testing, 464
Genital herpes, 444t, 446, 447
Genital warts, 447, 447t
Gestational diabetes mellitus, 463
GHB (gamma hydroxy butyrate), 429t, 433
GI (glycemic index), 327
Global core stabilizers, 225
Glucosamine, 482
Glycemic index (GI), 327
Glycemic load, 327
Glycogen, 337
Gonorrhea, 444, 444t, 445
Google Health, 485
GPS devices, 109
Group exercise classes, 146
Growing Stronger—Strength Training for Older Adults, 162
G-Tech Backpacks, 145
Guidelines for Parents to Provide a Safe Environment for Youth Athletes, 148

H

HAART (highly active antiretroviral therapy), 443
HALE (Healthy Life Expectancy), 3, 3f
Half squat, 179, 246
Hallucinations, 428
Hallucinogens, 428–429, 428t, 433
Hamstring curl, 181
Hamstring sprains, 54

Hamstring stretches, 62, 214, 244, 247
Hands and knees balance, 185
Handwashing, 496
Hand weights, 478
Hardiness, 370, 373
HDL (high-density lipoprotein), 69, 69t, 329, 413
Head clock exercise, 242
Head nod, 248
Health. *See also* Wellness
    assessing factors in, 501–502
    definition of, 3
    determinants of, 492, 492f
    dimensions of, 4, 5t
    factors in, 9–14
    good news about, 12
    healthiest states and cities, 494
    Healthy Lifestyle Questionnaire, 15, 17–18
    HELP philosophy, 14–15
    holistic, 7
    life expectancy and, 3, 3f
    model of, 4f
    national goals for, 2
    personal actions and, 11–12
    physical activity and, 78–81, 79t, 81t
    physical fitness and, 6f, 7
    public opinion polls on, 23
    sexual activity and, 440
    wellness and, 2–7
Health-based criterion-referenced standards, 94–95
Health benefits. *See also* Physical activity benefits
    of cardiovascular fitness, 121–122, 122f
    definition of, 105
    of moderate physical activity, 105–106
    of muscle fitness, 162–163
    of stretching and flexibility, 202–203
    threshold levels for, 88, 89f
Health-care system
    effective use of, 493–495, 493t, 494t
    personal physicians, 493t
    preventive care in, 466, 467t, 493
    quality of life and, 11
    second opinions, 493–494
    unequal access in, 11
Health clubs, 479, 489–490
Health consumerism. *See* Product evaluation
Healthier Worksite Initiative, 103
Health insurance, 493t, 494, 494t
Health literacy, 485
Health on the Net (HON), 485
Health-related quality of life, 4
Health websites, 485
Healthy days, 3
Healthy Lifestyle Questionnaire, 15, 17–18
Healthy living rating, 496
Healthy People 2020 (HP2020), 2, 12, 66, 90
Heart
    anatomy of, 118–119, 119f, 120f
    physical activity and, 68, 68f
Heart attacks, 67, 70–71, 70f, 71f
Heart disease. *See* Cardiovascular disease
Heart rate
    heart rate reserve, 124, 125–127, 125t
    monitoring, 127–129, 127f, 129f, 130
    resting heart rate, 68, 118, 126f, 129, 129f
    stress and, 130
Heart rate monitors, 129
Heart rate reserve (HRR), 124, 125–127, 125t
Heat index, 51–52, 51t
Heat-related problems, 50–52, 51t, 52t

Heel sit, 213
HELP philosophy, 14–15, 26, 499
Hemoglobin, 119
Hepatitis B, 444t, 445–446
Herbals, 482
Heredity. *See* Genetic influences
Herniated disc, 228, 228f, 229
Hero exercise, 245
Herpes, 444t, 446, 447
Herpes simplex virus (HSV), 446
HGH (human growth hormone), 172–173
High altitude exercise, 53
High blood pressure. *See* Hypertension
High-density lipoprotein (HDL), 69, 69t, 329, 413
Highly active antiretroviral therapy (HAART), 443
Hip and low back stretch, 247
Hip and thigh stretch, 62, 214, 245, 247
HIV/AIDS
    high-risk sexual behavior and, 443–444
    physical activity and, 76
    prevalence of, 441
    reduction in death rates from, 13
    symptoms of, 441–442
    transmission and prevention of, 442–443, 442t
    treatment of, 443–444
    vaccine research, 443, 444
HLA B57 gene, 443
Holistic health, 7
Home exercise machines, 477–478
Homocysteine, 70
Horizontal side support, 248
Hormone replacement therapy (HRT), 75, 462
Hot tubs, 483–484
HPA (hypothalamic-pituitary-adrenal) axis, 366, 386
HPV (human papillomavirus), 440, 444–445, 444t, 446–447, 459–460
HRR (heart rate reserve), 124, 125–127, 125t
HSV (herpes simplex virus), 446
Human growth hormone (HGH), 172–173
Human immunodeficiency virus (HIV), 440, 441. *See also* HIV/AIDS
Human papillomavirus (HPV), 440, 444–445, 444t, 446–447, 459–460
Hunger, 353
Hydrogenated fats, 335–336
Hyperextension, 234, 236f
Hyperflexibility, 202–203
Hyperflexion, 234, 236f
Hyperkinetic conditions, 80, 273
Hypermobility, 202, 203
Hypertension, 67, 71–72, 72t
Hyperthermia, 50, 51
Hypertrophy, muscular, 161
Hypokinetic diseases or conditions, 7, 66–67, 81t. *See also specific diseases*
Hyponatremia, 52, 53
Hypostress, 368, 369
Hypothalamic-pituitary-adrenal (HPA) axis, 366, 386
Hypothermia, 52, 53

I

Illinois agility run, 279
Illness, definition of, 4, 5
Immune system, 76, 77f, 366, 367
Inactivity, health effects of, 90–91
Inflated garments, 477
Informed-Choice, 481t
Infrared sensors, 291–292
Inhalants, 433
Injuries
    flexibility and stretching and, 204
    joint hypermobility and, 202–203

lifestyles and, 464, 465t
microtrauma, 227
muscle fitness and, 162
overuse, 274
prevention of, 49, 237t, 271t
from resistance training, 174, 174t
RICE formula for, 54
sprains and strains, 54, 274
vigorous physical activities and, 142, 148
Inline skating, 146
Inner thigh stretch, 215
Insulin, 74, 462–463
Insulin resistance, 74
Insulin sensitivity, 74
Intellectual environment, 495t, 496
Intensity classification, 103, 103t, 109t
Interleukin-6 (IL-6), 70
Intermittent aerobic activities, 147–148
Internet
    health websites, 483, 484–485, 488
    nutrition information, 335
    second opinions, 493
    social networking, 353
    worksite wellness tracking, 493
Interval training, 266–267, 267t
Intervertebral discs, 224–225, 224f, 227–228
Intoxication, 410, 411
Iron, 333, 334
Isoflavones, 331
Isokinetic exercises, 164f, 164t, 165
Isometric abdominal test, 256
Isometric exercises, 164f, 164t, 165, 250
Isometric extensor test, 256
Isotonic exercises, 164–165, 164f, 164t

J

Jackson-Pollock method, 305, 311–312
Jacobson's progressive relaxation method, 384
Job stress, 366, 377–378
Jogging/running, 143

K

Kaposi's sarcoma, 441
Kennedy, John F., 78–80
Kettlebells, 165
Knee extension, 181
Knee pull-down, 246
Knee-to-chest exercise, 246, 247
Kyphotic curve, 230, 231f

L

Lactic acid, 265
Lacto-ovo vegetarians, 331
Last bout effect, 105
Lateral bridge tests, 256
Lateral thigh and hip stretch, 215
Lateral trunk stretch, 212
Lat pull down, 181
LDL (low-density lipoprotein), 69, 69t, 329
Lecithin, 354
Leg drop test, 255
Leg hug, 62, 213, 243
Leg kneel, 182
Leg press, 186
Leisure, 377
Leptin, 296

Let's Move!, 296
Life expectancy, 3, 3f
Lifestyle changes, 491–512
    assessing factors in wellness, 501–502
    for cancer prevention, 461, 461t, 462t
    cognitions and emotions in, 497–498
    determinants of health and wellness, 492, 492f
    for diabetes prevention, 463t
    factors promoting, 24–28, 25f
    goals in, 508
    health-care system use, 493–495, 493t, 494f
    healthy lifestyles, 497t
    improving your health environment, 495–496, 495t
    for injury prevention, 464, 465t
    interaction use in, 498
    personal beliefs and philosophy in, 499
    physical activity and, 376
    physical activity program plans, 505–512
    planning for improved health, 503–504
    relapse in, 23–24
    self-assessments in, 30, 33–35, 497
    self-management skills for, 22–23, 23f, 26t, 28–29, 40–43
    self-planning skills for, 29–35, 29t
    six steps to, 496–497
    for sleep improvement, 466
    stages of change in, 22–23, 23f, 38–39, 507
    strategies for, 497–499
    taking advantage of heredity, 493
Lifestyles
    active, 102–105, 103t, 104t, 497t
    adherence to, 22
    Healthy Lifestyle Questionnaire, 15, 17–18
    importance of, 12–14
    wellness and, 4–5, 10f, 11–12, 80
Lifting technique, 233, 234t, 235f
Ligaments, 201
Light-intensity physical activity, 106
Lipids, 69
Lipodissolve, 354
Lipoproteins, 69
Liposuction, 479–480
Local core stabilizers, 225
Locus of control, 369, 373–374
Long-slow distance (LSD) training, 266, 267
Long-term goals, 30–32
Lordotic curve, 230–232, 231f
Loud sounds, 497t
Low-density lipoprotein (LDL), 69, 69t, 329
Lower leg lift, 183
Lower trunk lift, 252
Lung cancer, 458–459, 469
Lunge, 179
Lungs, 120f

M

Machine weights, 166–167, 166t
Magnets, 476
Mainstream smoke, 400, 401
Maintenance goals, 32, 171
Malignant tumors (carcinomas), 73, 454, 455
Mammograms, 456, 458
Marching, 185, 254
Marijuana, 428–429, 428t, 432
Martial arts exercise, 146–147
Massage, 476
Mass prescription, 235
Maximum oxygen uptake (VO$_2$ max), 121
McKenzie extension exercise, 252

MDMA (ecstasy), 432, 433
Mechanical ergogenics, 276
Medical model, 11
Medwatch, 485
Melanoma, 460
Melatonin, 481t
Men. *See also* Gender differences
    breast self-exams, 471–472
    HIV/AIDS in, 442, 443–444
    muscle dysmorphia in, 295
    testicular self-exams, 471–472
Mental health, 376, 401
Mental imagery, 383–384
Menthol cigarettes, 403
Men who have sex with men (MSM), 443–444
MET (metabolic equivalents), 103, 106, 107
Metabolic fitness, 9, 288
Metabolic syndrome, 9, 72–73, 73f, 400
Metabolife, 482
Metastasis, 454, 454f, 455
Methadone, 433–434
Methamphetamine, 427–428, 427t, 432–433
MET-minutes, 142
miCoach Zone/miCoach Pacer, 145
Microtrauma, 227
Military, 364, 367, 418
Mindfulness meditation, 384–385
Mineral intake, 333–334
Moderate aerobic activity. *See* Moderate physical activity
Moderate physical activity, 101–116
    classification of, 104–105, 104t, 109t
    definition of, 102, 103
    environment and, 110–111, 115–116
    examples of, 109f, 110
    health benefits of, 105–106
    importance of, 91
    intensity of, 103–104, 103t
    monitoring, 106–107, 109
    in physical activity pyramid, 102, 102f
    recommended amount of, 106–110, 106t, 108t, 109t
    setting goals for, 111, 113–114
    tracking energy expenditure in, 107
    vigorous activity combined with, 142, 157–158
Monounsaturated fats, 329
Motor fitness, 272, 273
MRSA, 496
MTUs (muscle-tendon units), 201–202
Multiple vitamin supplements, 333
Muscle-bound, 202
Muscle cramps, 54
Muscle dysmorphia, 295
Muscle fitness. *See also* Resistance exercise
    endurance *vs.* strength in, 161
    genetics, gender, and age and, 161–162
    health benefits of, 162–163
    in the physical activity pyramid, 91–92
    planning and logging exercises, 195–198
    self-assessment of, 187–194
    technology use in, 165
Muscle implants, 480
Muscles
    agonist and antagonist, 162–163, 163f, 204, 206
    blood flow and, 49f, 50
    cardiovascular fitness and, 119, 120f
    concentric and eccentric contractions of, 164–165
    core, 225, 226f
    definition competitions, 160, 268
    gaining muscle mass, 354
    leverage in, 160–161, 161f

    location of, 176f
    skeletal muscle fiber types, 161
    stress and, 376
    tissue types, 160
Muscle-tendon units (MTUs), 201–202
Muscular endurance
    activities for, 100
    definition of, 6f
    evaluating, 188–190, 193–194
    self-assessments of, 186
    strength *vs.*, 167–169, 168f
MyFoodapedia, 335
Myofascial trigger points, 203, 227
MyPyramid, 322–323, 322f, 335, 338

N

Nanotechnology, 275
Narcotics, 426–428, 426t, 427t
National Association for Sport and Physical Education (NASPE), 90, 93
National Institute on Alcohol Abuse and Alcoholism (NIAAA), 417–418
National Institutes of Health, 485
National Physical Activity Plan, 57
Native Americans, 463–464
Natural disasters, 364–365
NEAT (non-exercise activity thermogenesis), 106, 347
Neck circling, 242
Neck pain, 226–229, 228f. *See also* Back pain
Neck rotation exercise, 250
Negative affectivity, 369
Negative self-talk, 355
Neutraceuticals (functional foods), 330, 332–333, 332t
Neutral spine, 231
Nicotine, 398, 404
Nicotine vaccine, 404
Nonessential fat, 289
Non-exercise activity thermogenesis (NEAT), 106, 347
Nutrient-dense foods, 323
Nutrition, 321–344
    analysis of, 339–342
    cancer and, 322
    carbohydrate recommendations, 327–329, 337, 350, 353
    eating management strategies, 357–358
    evaluating diets and products, 480–483
    fast foods, 335, 359–360
    fat recommendations, 329–330
    food labels, 325–327, 326f
    functional foods, 330, 332–333, 332t
    guidelines on, 322–325, 324t, 325f
    Internet information on, 335
    mineral intake, 333–334
    organic foods, 336
    performance and, 337
    protein recommendations, 330–331, 330f, 337
    selecting nutritious foods, 343–344
    sound eating practices, 335–336, 336t
    strategies for action, 338
    supplements, 480–483, 481t
    vegetarian diets, 331
    vitamin recommendations, 331–333, 333t
    water and other fluids, 334–335

O

Ober's test, 255
Obesigenic environments, 346
Obesity. *See also* Body composition
    carbohydrates and, 327
    cardiovascular fitness and, 122

costs of, 288
definition of, 289
fear of, 295
health risks from, 292–294, 292f, 293f
muscle fitness and, 162–163
origin of fatness, 295–297, 297f
physical activity and, 76, 293, 293f
prevalance of, 76, 76f, 288
social change to reverse, 296
OGTT (oral glucose tolerance test), 464
Old, definition of, 10
Older adults, activity guidelines for, 93, 106, 169. *See also* Age
Olestra, 330
Omega-3 fatty acids, 329–330
One-foot balance, 100
One-leg stretch, 62, 244
1 repetition maximum (1RM), 167–168
Online second opinions, 493
Opiate narcotics, 426–428, 427t
Opportunistic infections, 441
Optimism, 369
Oral glucose tolerance test (OGTT), 464
Oral sex, 448, 449
Organic foods, 336
Orlistat (Xenical; Alli), 353–354
Osteoporosis, 74–75, 75t, 163
Outcome goals, 31, 32, 349
Ovarian cancer, 459–460
Overhead arm stretch, 216
Overhead (military) press, 178, 180
Overlearning, 150
Overload principle, 86, 87, 169, 206–208
Overload syndrome, 273
Over-the-counter (OTC) drugs, 433–434
Overtraining, 273–275, 275f, 285–286
Overweight, 289. *See also* Body composition; Obesity
Oxycontin, 433
Oxygen debt, 265
Oxygen uptake reserve (VO₂R), 124, 125
Ozone, 53

P

Pain, 10, 77. *See also* Back pain
Panacea, 475–476
Paper ball bounce, 100
Paper ball pickup, 100
Paper drop, 100
Pap test, 459–460
Paralysis by analysis, 150, 151
Parasympathetic nervous system (PNS), 71, 365
PAR-Q (Physical Activity Readiness Questionnaire), 46–47, 59–60
Passive assistance, 204
Passive exercise, 476–477
PCDC (phosphatidylcholine deoxycholate), 353
Pectoral stretch, 212, 253
Pedometers, 107, 107f, 109, 109t
Peer influence, 417, 431, 431f
Pelvic inflammatory disease (PID), 445
Percentage of maxHR method, 126–127
Percent body fat, 288–289, 289t
% Daily Value (%DV), 326
Performance, 263–286
balance and flexibility training and, 271–272
endurance and speed training and, 266–268, 267t
ergogenic aids, 275–276
factors affecting, 264–265, 264f
flexibility and stretching and, 203–204
high-performance training guidelines, 273–274, 275f

moderate physical activity and, 105
nutrition and, 337
overtraining and, 273–275, 275f, 285–286
physical fitness and, 7, 8f
power training and, 269–271, 271t
skill-related fitness and, 272–273, 273t, 279–284
strategies for action, 277
strength and muscular endurance training and, 268–269, 268f
target and threshold levels for, 88
training characteristics, 264–265, 264f
warm-ups and, 49, 272
Periodization of training, 274, 275f
Peripheral vascular disease, 67, 72
Personal factors, in health behaviors, 24, 25, 25f
Personal goals, 30–32
Phosphorus, 333
Physical activity. *See also* Aerobic physical activities; Moderate physical activity; Physical activity benefits; Vigorous physical activity
air pollution and, 53–54
attitudes about, 54–55, 63–64
body composition and, 297–300, 298t, 299t
for body fat reduction, 298–300, 298t, 299t, 350
body weight and, 346–347, 347f
calories expended in, 299t
cardiovascular function in, 119–121, 120f, 121t
clothing for, 47, 47t, 52, 53
in cold weather, 52–53, 52t
cool-downs in, 50, 51, 61–62
depression and, 376, 377
FITT/FIT formula, 88–89, 89f
health-based criterion-referenced standards, 94–95
at high altitude, 53
in hot weather, 50–52, 51t, 52t
increase in participation in, 88
intensity classifications, 103–104, 103t, 109t
mental health and, 376
national goals for, 93–94, 93t, 94t
passive exercise, 476–477
physical activity pyramid, 89–93, 90f
pre-participation screening, 46–48, 59
principles of, 86–88, 87f
program planning, 505–512
quackery in, 475–477
reasons for avoiding, 55t
reasons for doing, 56t
shoes for, 47–48, 48f
smoking cessation and, 405
soreness and, 49, 54, 170, 203
strategies for action, 57
stress management and, 376
unsubstantiated claims in, 475–476
warm-up period before, 48–49, 61–62
workouts, 49–50
workplace, 92
Physical Activity Adherence Questionnaire, 152–153
Physical activity benefits, 65–84. *See also* Exercise
aging and, 77–78
atherosclerosis and, 67, 68–70, 68f, 69t
back pain and, 75–76
cancer and, 73–74, 74t
cholesterol and, 69
emotional/mental health and, 76
heart attacks and, 67, 70–71, 70f, 71f
heart health and, 68, 68f
hypertension and, 71–72, 72t
hypokinetic diseases and, 66–67
immune system and, 76, 77f
metabolic syndrome and, 72–73, 73f
of moderate physical activity, 105–106

Physical activity benefits (continued)
    obesity and, 76
    osteoporosis and, 74–75, 75t
    peripheral vascular disease and, 72
    during pregnancy, 77
    stroke and, 72
    Type II diabetes and, 74
Physical Activity Guidelines for Americans, 66, 93
Physical activity plans
    activity selection in, 508–509
    goals in, 508
    needs and reasons for, 505–506
    recordkeeping in, 511–512
    stages of change in, 507
    written plans, 510
Physical activity pyramid
    components of, 89–92, 90f
    considerations when using, 92–93
    moderate activities in, 102, 102f
    vigorous activities in, 140f, 141–143, 142t
Physical Activity Readiness Questionnaire (PAR-Q), 46–47, 59–60
Physical dependence, 398
Physical fitness
    definition of, 7
    determinants of, 492, 492f
    dimensions of, 6f, 7–9, 8f
    factors in, 9–14
    fitness zones, 95, 95t
    health-based criterion-referenced standards, 94–95
    health-related components, 6f, 7
    physical activity classifications and, 104–105, 104t
    self-assessment of, 97–100, 97f, 100f
    skill-related components, 7, 8f, 279–284
Physiological fatigue, 366, 367
Phytochemicals, 332, 332t
PID (pelvic inflammatory disease), 445
Pilates exercise, 210
Platelets, 69
Play, 378
PLAY 60, 348
Plyometrics, 165, 270–271, 271t
PMS (premenstrual syndrome), 77
PNF (proprioceptive neuromuscular facilitation), 205f, 206, 208t, 211
PNS (parasympathetic nervous system), 71, 365
Podcasts, 11
Pollens, 54
Polyunsaturated fats, 329
Portion sizes, 335
Positive self-talk, 355
Posttraumatic stress disorder (PTSD), 364, 367
Posture
    abdominal exercises, 249
    core stabilization exercises, 248
    correcting, 232–233, 233f
    definition of, 231
    ergonomics and, 233, 233f, 234t
    evaluating, 259–260
    factors influencing, 203, 232–233, 233f
    good standing and seated, 232, 232f
    healthy back and neck questionnaire, 257–258
    healthy back tests, 255–256
    hip and hamstring stretches, 247
    lumbar stabilization with stability balls, 254
    neck and back health and, 227, 230–233, 231f, 232f, 232t, 233f
    neck exercises, 250
    planning and logging exercises, 261–262
    questionable exercises and alternatives, 235, 240–246
    round shoulder exercises, 253
    spine anatomy and function, 224–225, 224f
    strategies for action, 238
    trunk and mobility exercises, 251–252
Power
    activities for, 7, 8f, 100
    endurance training and, 169
    evaluating, 281
    strength-related vs. speed-related, 270
    training for, 269–271, 271t
PRE. See Progressive resistance exercise
Pre-diabetes, 462–463
Predisposing factors, 25, 25f
Pregnancy
    alcohol use during, 413
    drug use in, 434
    gestational diabetes mellitus in, 463
    physical activity during, 77
Prehypertension, 71, 72t
Premenstrual syndrome (PMS), 77
Pre-participation Screening Questionnaire, 46
Press-up, 252
Prevention programs, 35
Preventive care, 466, 467t, 493
PRICE formula, 54
Principle of diminished returns, 87, 171
Principle of individuality, 88, 89
Principle of progression, 86, 87, 169–170, 207–208
Principle of rest and recovery, 87, 171
Principle of reversibility, 86, 87
Principle of specificity, 86, 87, 170–171, 270
Problem-focused coping, 380–381, 381t, 386
Prochaska, J. O., 22
Procrastination, 379, 379f
Product evaluation, 473–490
    for body composition change, 479–480
    for dietary supplements, 480–483, 481t, 488
    for diets and foods, 480
    for exercise equipment, 477–478, 487
    for health clubs and leaders, 479, 489–490
    for Internet websites, 484–485, 488
    physical activity quackery, 475–477
    practice evaluation, 487–488
    quacks and quackery, 474–475
    for saunas and baths, 483–484
    for suntans, 484
    for written materials, 484, 487
Progressive relaxation, 394
Progressive resistance exercise (PRE). See also Resistance exercise
    definition of, 160, 161
    thresholds and target zones in, 167–169, 168f, 168t
    training principles for, 169–173
    types of, 163–166, 164f, 164t
Prohormones, 171
Project MATCH, 419
Prone bridge, 256
Proprioception, 271
Proprioceptive neuromuscular facilitation (PNF), 205f, 206, 208t, 211
Prostate cancer, 74t, 457t, 459, 469
Protein recommendations, 330–331, 330f, 337
Protein supplements, 276
Provenge vaccine, 459
PSA blood test, 459
Psychedelics, 428, 428t
Psychoactive drugs. See also Alcohol use; Drug use
    club drugs, 431–432
    date rape drugs, 429, 429t, 433
    definition of, 426, 427
    depressant drugs, 426, 426t
    hallucinogens, 428–429, 428t
    marijuana, 428–429, 428t, 432

opiate narcotics, 426–428, 427t
stimulants, 426–427, 432–433
Psychological ergogenics, 276
Psychological fatigue, 366, 367
Psychology Matters, 485
PTSD (posttraumatic stress disorder), 364, 367
Pubic crab lice, 447, 447t
Pull-ups, 182
Pulse monitoring, 127–128, 127f, 128f, 130, 135–136
Purging disorder, 295
Push-ups, 100, 167, 182

Q

Quacks and quackery, 474–475. *See also* Product evaluation
Quadriceps stretch, 245
Quadruped stabilization, 256
Quality of life, 4, 5
Questionable exercises and alternatives, 235, 240–246

R

Range of motion (ROM), 200–201, 201f, 203
Range of motion (ROM) exercises, 207
Ratings of perceived exertion (RPE), 124–127, 127t, 135–136, 135t
Reaction time, 8f, 100, 281
Reciprocal inhibition, 204
Recommended Dietary Allowance (RDA), 324t, 325
Recreation, 377–378
Rectal cancer, 74t
Referred pain, 227
Reinforcing factors, 24, 25, 25f, 26–27, 28t
Relapse, 23–24, 28t
Relative muscular endurance, 162, 163
Relative strength, 162, 163
Relaxation, 56t
Relaxation techniques, 382–384, 393–394
Resilience, 367, 369–370
Resistance exercise. *See also* Progressive resistance exercise
    anabolic steroids and, 171–173, 172f
    back pain and, 230
    calisthenics, 182–183
    circuit training, 169
    core strength exercises, 184–185
    endurance performance and, 268
    equipment for, 166–167, 166t
    fallacies and facts about, 173t
    free weight exercises, 178–179
    gaining muscle mass and, 354
    health benefits of, 162–163
    muscle fiber types and, 161
    progressive, 160, 161
    resistance machine exercises, 180–181, 195–196
    safety guidelines for, 173–175, 174t
    strategies for action in, 175
    for strength training, 268–269, 268t
    thresholds and target zones in, 167–169, 168f, 168t
    training principles for, 169–173
    weight control and, 162–163, 300
    worldwide trends in, 167
Restaurant food contents, 326–327
Resting heart rate (RHR), 68, 118, 126f, 129, 129f
Reverse curl, 184, 241, 249
Reversibility, 86, 87
Rhythmical exercises, 384
RICE formula, 54, 55
Ritalin, 434
Rocker boards, 230
Rohypnol, 429t, 433

ROM (range of motion), 200–201, 201f
ROM (range of motion) exercises, 207
RPE (ratings of perceived exertion), 124–127, 127t, 135–136, 135t
Run in place, 100
Run test, 133, 133f

S

Safe sex, 448
Saturated fats, 329–330, 335–336
Saunas, 483–484
Saw Palmetto, 482
Scoliosis, 226, 227
Seafood recommendations, 330
Seated press, 186
Seated rowing, 181, 253
Seated side stretch, 62
Secondhand smoke, 400, 401, 403
Second opinions, 493–494
Sedentary death syndrome (SeDS), 66–67
Self-assessments
    of cardiovascular fitness, 129–130, 131–138
    of heart disease risk factors, 83–84
    of lifestyle change, 30, 33–35, 497
    of muscular strength, 186
    of physical fitness, 97–100, 97f, 100f
    program planning from, 505–506
    of skill-related physical fitness, 279–284
    of wellness factors, 501–502
Self-confidence, 25–27, 26t
Self-efficacy, 25–27, 369–370
Self-management skills
    for changing enabling factors, 27t
    for changing reinforcing factors, 28t
    definition of, 23
    in making lifestyle changes, 22–23, 23f, 26t, 28–29
    progress evaluation, 33–35
    Self-Management Skills Questionnaire, 40–43
    summary of labs addressing, 34t
Self-monitoring, 33
Self-planning skills
    needs identification, 30
    personal goal setting, 30–32
    program components, 32–33
    progress evaluation, 33–35
    reason clarification, 29–30, 29t
    summary of, 29t
    writing the plan, 33
Self-promoting activities, 150, 151
Self-talk, 355
Selye, Hans, 366
Sensewear Armband (SWA) monitors, 351
Serial monogamy, 448
Serostatus, 441
Set-point, 295–296
Sex education, 448
Sex enhancement supplements, 483
Sexting, 446
Sexual activity
    alcohol use and, 417
    early, 448
    lying about, 448
    oral sex, 448, 449
    sex education and, 448
Sexually transmitted infections (STIs), 439–452
    chancroid, 447, 447t
    chlamydia, 444, 444t, 445
    definition of, 440, 441
    genital herpes, 444t, 446, 447

Sexually transmitted infections (STIs) (*continued*)
genital warts, 447, 447*t*
gonorrhea, 444, 444*t*, 445
health effects of, 440–441
hepatitis B, 444*t*, 445–446
HIV/AIDS, 440, 441–444, 442*t*
human papillomavirus, 440, 444–445, 444*t*, 446–447
notification of partners, 449
prevalence of, 444, 444*t*, 445*f*
pubic crab lice, 447, 447*t*
sex education and, 448
sexually explicit media and, 447
Sexually Transmitted Infection Risk Questionnaire, 451–452
syphilis, 444, 444*t*, 446, 447
SGMA (Sporting Goods Manufacturers Association) survey, 143, 149, 149*f*
Shake sound generator, 145
Shin stretch, 214, 245
Shoes, 47–48, 48*f*
Short-term goals, 30–31
Shoulder stand bicycle, 243
Show gun meditation, 394
Sibutramine (Meridia), 353–354
Side bend exercise, 251
Side leg raises, 100, 182
Side step, 185
Sidestream smoke, 400, 401
Side stretch, 62
SIDS (sudden infant death syndrome), 400
Silicon, dietary, 413
Sitting, 90, 234*t*
Sitting stretch, 215
Sitting tucks, 184, 249
Sit-ups, 243
Skill-related fitness, 272–273, 273*t*, 279–284
Skin cancer, 457*t*, 460–461, 460*f*, 469
Skinfold measurements, 291, 291*f*, 303–307, 311–314
Sleep
deprivation and stress, 367
guidelines for good, 377*t*
lifestyle changes and, 466
physical activity and, 76
stress and, 376–377
Slimming exercises, 169
SMART goals, 30–31
Smokeless tobacco, 398, 401, 401*t*, 402
Smoking. *See* Tobacco use
Snacks, 336
SNS (sympathetic nervous system), 71, 119, 121, 365–366
Snuff, 398
Social-Ecological Model, 24
Social support
in body fat loss, 353
evaluating levels of, 395–396
improving, 495*t*, 496
in lifestyle change, 27–28, 28*t*
stress management and, 386–387
Socioeconomic status, activity and, 94, 94*t*
Sodium intake, 323, 333
Soft drinks, 348
Soldiers, PTSD among, 364, 367
Solid fats and added sugars (SoFAS), 323
Soluble fiber, 328
Somatotype, 295
Soreness, 49, 54, 170, 203
Soy foods, 331
Specificity, 86, 87, 170–171, 270
Speed, 8*f*, 100, 266–268, 267*t*, 282
Spine. *See* Back
Spine anatomy and function, 224–225, 224*f*

Spine twist, 213
Spinning, 147
Spirituality, 384–385, 495*t*, 496
Sporting Goods Manufacturers Association (SGMA) survey, 143, 149, 149*f*
Sports
extreme, 151
skill-related requirements of, 273*t*
sports fitness, 272
vigorous, 91, 141, 148–150, 149*f*
Spot-reducing, 479
Sprains, 54, 274
Squamous cell cancers, 460–461
Squatting, 185, 246
Stability balls, 254
Stage of Change Questionnaire, 38–39
Stages of change, 22–23, 23*f*, 507
Standing long jump, 100
Static endurance, 165
Static strength, 165
Static stretching, 204, 205*f*, 208*t*, 272
Steam baths, 483–484
Step aerobics, 146, 478
Step test, 131, 131*f*
Stick drop test, 281
Stick test of coordination, 280
Stiffness, 204
Stimulants, 426–427, 432–433
STIs. *See* Sexually transmitted infections
Stomach roll, 254
Straight-leg lift, 255
Strength, muscular
absolute, 161
activities for, 100
core strength, 163
definition of, 6*f*
dynamic, 165
evaluating, 188–192
muscular endurance *vs.*, 167–169, 168*f*
relative, 162
self-assessments of, 186
static, 165
training for, 268–269, 268*t*
Strength training. *See* Resistance exercise
Stress
appraisal-focused coping, 380–381, 381*t*, 382, 382*t*
biochemical markers of, 367
chronic, 366–367
coping with, 380–381, 381*t*
costs of, 366
definition of, 363
emotion-focused coping, 380–381, 381*t*, 382–385
evaluating coping strategies, 391–392
evaluating one's level of, 371–372
gene-based therapies for, 377
hardiness and locus of control, 370, 373–374
health effects of, 366–370, 368*f*
heart health and, 71
heart rate and, 130
physical activity and, 376
prevalence of, 363–364
problem-focused coping, 380–381, 381*t*, 386
reactions to, 362*f*, 365–366, 365*f*, 366*t*
relaxation techniques, 382–384, 393–394
resilience and, 367, 369–370
social support and, 386–387, 395–396
sources of, 362–365, 363*t*, 365*f*
strategies for action, 370, 387
stress reactivity and appraisals, 367–368, 376
target zone, 368, 368*f*
time management and, 378–380, 379*f*, 379*t*, 389–390

Stressors, 362–363, 363*t*
Stretching. *See also* Flexibility
  arm exercises, 216
  do and don't list for, 208*t*
  flexibility workouts *vs.*, 200
  health benefits of, 202–203
  for hip flexors and hamstrings, 247
  leg exercises, 214–215
  methods of, 204, 205*f*, 206
  muscle tension response to, 207*f*
  for performance training, 272
  in the physical activity pyramid, 206*f*
  planning and logging exercises, 221–222
  questionable exercises and alternatives, 235, 240–246
  for relaxation, 384
  safety guidelines for, 210
  stretch reflex, 207*f*
  technology in, 210, 211
  thresholds and target zones in, 206–209, 207*f*, 208*t*
  trunk exercises, 212–213
  in warm-ups, 49, 62
  warm-ups prior to, 208–209
  worldwide trends in, 209
Stretching ropes, 211
Stretch tolerance, 204
Stroke, 67, 72
Sub-threshold exercise, 90–91
Sudden infant death syndrome (SIDS), 400
Sudden sniffing death, 433
Sugars, 327
Suicide, 466
Sunscreen, 461, 497*t*
Suntans, 484
Superbugs, 496
Supine trunk twist, 251
Supplemental food labels, 326
Supplements, dietary, 480–483, 481*t*
Surgeon General's Report on Physical Activity and Health, 68
Surgeon General's Vision for a Healthy and Fit Nation, 66
Surgery, for fat reduction, 480
Susceptibility genes, 295
SWA (Sensewear Armband) monitor, 351
Swan exercise, 240
Swimming, 143–144
Swim test, 134, 134*f*
Sympathetic nervous system (SNS), 71, 119, 121, 365–366
Syndrome X, 9, 72–73, 73*t*
Synergistic effect, 426, 427
Syphilis, 444, 444*t*, 446, 447
Systolic blood pressure, 71

T

Tai chi, 209
Tans, 484
Tapering, 274, 275, 275*f*
Target zones, 88, 89*f*, 135–136, 135*f*
Technology
  active workstations, 92
  for activity monitoring, 128
  in alcohol consumption detection, 414
  biochemical markers of stress, 367
  in blood pressure measurement, 72
  epigenetic effects of cocaine, 431
  gene-based therapies for stress, 377
  genetic testing, 464
  health apps for cell phones, 32
  health websites, 485
  high-tech sneakers, 48
  HIV/AIDS vaccine research, 443, 444

  lifestyle monitoring for weight control, 351
  in muscle fitness, 165
  nicotine vaccine, 404
  online nutrition information, 335
  online second opinions, 493
  performance technology, 275
  physical activity monitoring devices, 109
  podcasts, 11
  in stretching, 210, 211
  training aids for core training, 230
  for vigorously active people, 145
  WiFi scale, 290
Television watching, health effects of, 90
Tendonitis, 54
Tendons, 201
Testicular cancer, 457*t*, 461–462
Testicular self-exams, 471–472
Tetrahydrogestrinone (THG), 172
T helper cells, 441
Thomas test, 255
3-second run, 282
Threshold of training, 88, 89*f*
"Time-dependent" aging, 77
Time management, 378–380, 379*f*, 379*t*, 389–390
TNF-a (tumor necrosis factor-a), 70
Tobacco pills, 403
Tobacco use, 397–408
  by adolescents, 401–402, 403*t*, 404
  as cause of death, 14, 14*t*, 398–399
  in cigars and pipes, 400
  as gateway, 404
  health and economic costs of, 398–401, 399*f*, 401*t*
  menthol cigarettes, 403
  nicotine, 398, 404
  public policy and, 402–403
  quitting, 22, 23–24, 404, 405
  secondhand smoke, 400, 401, 403
  smokeless, 398, 401, 401*t*, 402
  tobacco company promotion of, 403–404
  tobacco use risk questionnaire, 407–408
  trends in, 401
  in the workplace, 403
Toe touches, 242, 244
Tolerable Upper Intake Level (UL), 324*t*, 325
Tolerance, to alcohol, 412, 413
Tonus, 476, 477
Training, performance and, 264, 264*f*, 265
Trans fats, 329–330
Transtheoretical Model, 22–23, 23*f*, 24
Tricep press, 180
Triceps curl, 178
Triglycerides, 69, 69*t*
Trunk lift, 182, 251, 252
Trunk twist, 213, 251
Tumor necrosis factor-a (TNF-a), 70
12-minute run test, 133, 133*f*
12-minute swim test, 134, 134*f*
Twitter, 353
Type A behavior, 76, 368–369
Type B behavior, 368–369
Type D behavior, 369
Type I/Type II diabetes, 74, 462–463

U

UL (Tolerable Upper Intake Level), 324*t*, 325
Underfat, 288, 289
Underwater weighing, 290–291
Underweight, 293, 294–295
Unsaturated fats, 329

Upper trapezius/neck exercise, 212
Upper trapezius stretch, 250
Upper trunk lift, 251
U.S. Department of Agriculture (USDA), 322–323, 322*f*, 325, 336
USP (U.S. Pharmacopia), 481*t*
Uterine cancer, 457*t*, 459–460, 469

V

Varicose veins, 118
Vegan diets, 331
Vegetables, 328, 334
Vegetarian diets, 331
Veins, 118–119, 119*f*, 120*f*
Vending machines in schools, 348
Vertical jump test, 281
Vibrating belts, 476
Vibration boards, 165
Vicodin, 433
Video gaming, 210, 238
Vigorous aerobic activities, 91, 141
Vigorous physical activity, 139–158
    adherence assessment for, 153–154
    becoming successful in, 150–152
    benefits of, 141–142, 142*t*
    descriptions of common activities, 143–148
    injury prevention in, 142, 148
    MET-minutes and, 142
    moderate activity combined with, 142, 157–158
    participation rates in, 142–143, 144*f*, 149*f*, 151
    in the physical activity pyramid, 140*f*, 141–143, 142*t*
    planning and logging participation in, 155–156
    recreation activities, 91, 141, 151
    sports, 91, 141, 148–150, 149*f*
    strategies for action in, 151–152
    technology in, 145
    weight control and, 346
Viral load, 441
Visceral fat, 293–294, 293*f*
Vitamin B-12, 331
Vitamin C, 333, 480
Vitamin D, 75, 333, 481
Vitamins
    as antioxidants, 332
    recommended intake of, 331–333, 333*t*
    supplements, 333, 481–482, 483
VO₂ max (maximum oxygen uptake), 121
VO₂R (oxygen uptake reserve), 124, 125

W

Waist-to-hip circumference ratio, 309–310, 316
Walkability audits, 116
Walking, 103, 103*t*, 104, 110, 143
Walking test, 131, 131*f*
Wall support, 254
Wand exercise, 240, 253
Warm-up period, 48–49, 61–62
Water exercise, 147
Water intake, 52, 334–335
Water intoxication, 52
Websites, health, 483, 484–485, 488
We Can!, 296
Weighted belts, 476–477
Weight management, 345–360
    appetite suppressants, 353–354
    artificial sweeteners and fat substitutes, 353
    eating management, 347–348, 357–358
    energy balance equation and, 346
    factors influencing, 346–349, 346*f*
    fad and extreme diets, 350–351
    fast foods and, 359–360
    gaining muscle mass, 354
    goals in, 349
    guidelines for losing body fat, 349–353, 349*t*, 352*t*
    monitors for, 354
    physical activity and, 298–300, 298*t*, 299*t*, 350
    public policy and, 348
    record keeping in, 355
    regulation of body weight, 295–296
    short-term changes, 290
    smoking and, 404
    social media and, 353
    strategies for action in, 355
    supplements for, 483
    threshold and target zones for, 298, 298*t*
Wellness
    assessing factors in, 501–502
    cardiovascular fitness and, 122
    definition of, 4–5, 4*f*
    determinants of, 492, 492*f*
    dimensions of, 5, 5*f*, 5*t*, 7
    factors in, 9–14, 498*t*
    health and, 2–7
    health-care system and, 11
    lifestyles and, 4, 11–14
    muscle fitness and, 163
    physical activity and, 78–81, 79*t*, 81*t*, 105
    recreation and, 377–378
    self-perception assessment, 19–20
    sexual experience and, 440
    workplace tracking of, 493
Whirlpools, 483–484
WHO (World Health Organization), 2–3
WiFi scale, 290
Wii Fit Plus, 210, 238
Windchill factor, 52–53, 52*t*
Windmill exercise, 242
Withdrawal, 398, 399, 412, 413
Women. *See also* Gender differences
    alcohol effects on, 410, 412–413, 417
    breast self-exams, 471–472
    female athlete triad, 294–295
    HIV/AIDS in, 441, 442
    hormone replacement therapy, 75, 462
    osteoporosis in, 75
    secondhand smoke and, 400–401
    social support need by, 387
Workouts, 49–50
Workplace
    improving the work environment, 495*t*, 496
    professional help programs, 498–499
    well information tracking, 493
Workplace physical activity, 92, 103, 233, 234*t*, 236*f*
Workplace stress, 366
World Health Organization (WHO), 2–3
Wrist curl, 179
Wrist weights, 478
Writing, expressive, 385

Y

Yoga, 210, 475–476

Z

Zinc, 334
Zipper exercise, 62